Breastfeeding

A Guide for the Medical Profession

Breastfeeding

A Guide for the Medical Profession

Ruth A. Lawrence, M.D.

Associate Professor of Pediatrics and Obstetrics and Gynecology,
University of Rochester,
Rochester, New York

Second Edition

with 168 illustrations

The C. V. Mosby Company

ST. LOUIS • TORONTO • PRINCETON   1985

MOSBY

A TRADITION OF PUBLISHING EXCELLENCE

Editor: Karen Berger
Assistant editor: Sandra L. Gilfillan

The C.V. Mosby Company
11830 Westline Industrial Drive, St. Louis, Missouri 63146

Library of Congress Cataloging in Publication Data

Lawrence, Ruth A., 1924-
   Breastfeeding, a guide for the medical profession.

   Rev. ed. of: Breast-feeding, a guide for the medical
profession / Ruth A. Lawrence. St. Louis: Mosby, 1980.
   Includes bibliographies and index.
   1. Breast feeding.   2. Lactation.   3. Milk, Human.
I. Lawrence, Ruth A., 1924-   .   Breast-feeding, a guide
for the medical profession. II. Title. [DNLM: 1. Breast
Feeding. WS 125 L422b]
RJ216.L358   1985   613.2   84-11529
ISBN 0-8016-2898-9

EDP/VH/VH   9 8 7 6 5 4 3 2 1   01/A/087

Affectionately dedicated to
**Rob, Barbara, Timothy, Kathleen,
David, Mary Alice, Joan, John, and Stephen**
for their love and patient understanding
and to **Bob**
for his boundless faith, trust, and inspiration

Foreword

There would have been little need for this book had it been written at the beginning of the century, when more than 50% of the mothers in the United States breastfed infants beyond 1 year, and a wealth of experience, cultural beliefs, and information about breastfeeding was shared by young mothers, their families, and their physicians. There has, however, been so little breastfeeding in the United States for the past 4 decades that the repository of cultural information about lactation has almost disappeared. Fortunately, the feeding of human milk is once again returning to its proper position of preeminence, and the lack of practical information on breastfeeding available to parents-to-be and health-care professionals is being keenly felt.

Dr. Ruth Lawrence, a physician and mother with extensive medical and personal experience in the field, designed this manual to fill the gap for physicians, nurses, and other health-care professionals. This detailed and well-written book benefits greatly not only from the author's extensive experience running a normal and sick infant nursery but also from her special and unique personal life, rearing and breastfeeding nine healthy children of her own. Thus the author is a veteran in two areas. She beautifully documents the values of and the simple techniques and procedures for increasing, supporting, and continuing the mother's milk supply.

Health-care professionals in the United States might well ask themselves how and why we stopped the practice of breastfeeding. They might also ask themselves what factors led the educators and leaders of the medical profession to ignore (or discount) the wealth of information regarding the benefits of breastfeeding and the hazards of its discontinuation, information that has been available since early in the twentieth century. The leaders of the medical profession were extremely vocal about these benefits and hazards early in the century, and one wonders where the voices of these medical educators and leaders have been over the past 30 to 40 years. Have these voices been silent because health-care professionals believed (and convinced the general population) that modern medical science could indeed improve on nature?

Medical professionals complain that parents request too many operations, demand too many drugs, and, after medicine's best efforts, are dissatisfied with many aspects of the care provided their children. It would seem that the medical profession has over-sold the abilities of modern medical science and undersold the innate wisdom, resources, and responses of the healthy human mother.

Was another of the factors contributing to the trend away from breastfeeding that the "science of nutrition developed a reliance on measurement and analysis that encouraged the impression that prepared foods were superior because they could be measured and calculated to meet precise needs," as Dr. Lawrence suggests in Chapter 1? Working in a neonatal intensive care unit with young physicians, one gets the impression that they with their ever-ready calculators are frustrated because they do not know the precise caloric content or the total volume the breastfeeding mother gives her premature or sick infant. Are their attitudes fundamentally different from those of their paper- and pencil-pushing predecessors of a generation ago?

It does not seem possible that a reader can help but be overwhelmingly impressed by the information presented in this book. For example, Table 1-11 presents data on the difference in mortality and morbidity between artificially fed and breastfed infants and the difference in survivors to age 1 year from the end of the nineteenth century up to 1947 with *always* a marked advantage for the breastfed infant. Table 1-12 presents deaths and death rates in seven Punjab villages, which show that artificially fed infants had a mortality of 950/1000 in the first 11 months of life in contrast to 120/1000 of the breastfed infants. In this decade in rural New York state the studies of Cunningham showed again the lower incidence of respiratory and gastrointestinal illnesses in breast-fed infants compared to those fed cow's milk.

We hope this book will encourage physicians and other health-care personnel to help families realize their own strengths and resources and to adapt their child rearing to the wishes and needs of the infant or child. It will still be some time before we health-care professionals can fully readjust our expectations for growth, weight gain, development, and sleeping and feeding behavior to the standard of the breastfed infant rather than make comparisons to the bottle fed infant. We are learning that when an anxious breast-feeding mother asks why her infant does not burp often or loudly enough (or eats too frequently or has bowel movements that are too loose), we should not respond with concern or criticism of the burping technique but should say "great!" and point out that it is wise to use the behavior of the breastfed infant as our standard.

Several studies have suggested that the motor or mental development of breast fed infants may be different from bottle fed infants. There is a great opportunity for careful studies to evaluate this further at the present time. In our own research, filmed observations of mothers bottle feeding their infants have been shocking at times and have reminded us that there can be an enormous difference between the warmth, skin-to-skin contact, and multiple sensory interactions associated with breastfeeding and the situation with some bottle feedings, when the infant may be fed away from any human contact, fed when not hungry, and with an imposed rhythm and schedule that may conflict with the infant's own wishes and rhythms.

Ruth Lawrence points out that "one of the symbols of the emancipation of women that began in the 1920s was bottle feeding." Our present woman's movement is accompanied by an increased interest in breastfeeding. However, are there other features or side effects of the changing life-styles of today that will have a comparable impact on the health and well-being of a generation from now?

We will take this opportunity to comment about the association between breastfeeding and parent-infant attachment. We believe that early mother-infant contact starts a process of mother-infant interaction that gradually builds a strong affectionate tie, first of the mother to her infant and then later on of the infant to the mother. This is most likely to proceed successfully with breastfeeding, in which close contact and interaction occur repeatedly at the times the infant wishes and at a pace that fits the needs and wishes of the mother and the infant, with gratifications for both. Thus breastfeeding provides an optimal model for the development of a strong mother-infant attachment following contact immediately after birth, which in turn has been shown to be a simple maneuver to significantly increase the success of breastfeeding.

Any physician, nurse, or health-care professional who reads this book will be more convinced than ever of the importance of breastfeeding, will have solid data to support this conviction, and will be given a wealth of information about how to help mothers succeed with breastfeeding. Ruth Lawrence points out that there are many reasons why mothers may not be willing to breastfeed, and it will be necessary for us to realize that we cannot produce a change overnight in attitudes that have developed over the last 50 years.

John H. Kennell
Marshall H. Klaus

Preface
to second edition

Progress toward more universal breastfeeding continues, and with it develops a greater need to understand the science of lactation. Hundreds of research scientists are investigating the unanswered questions and reviewing old dogmas. Clinicians in all fields of medicine are coming in contact with patients with an interest in or problems surrounding lactation. Hospitals are readjusting their perinatal care to encourage and enhance breastfeeding. Community health-care programs are providing positive support and reinforcement for families.

The National Health Plan for the United States has as one of its goals that by 1990 75% of women will leave the hospital breastfeeding, and 35% will continue to breast-feed for at least 6 months. The Departments of Health and Human Services and of Agriculture as well as the Surgeon General are pursuing an active program to reach that goal.

The professional is now swamped with information, reports of research, and an avalanche of publications from many sources, some of which are conflicting. In view of this rapid transition in the past 4 years, it became apparent that a second edition of this book was needed to provide the professional with a reference of clinically applicable information synthesized from these vast resources. Once again an effort has been made to provide the scientific justification for rational management and to minimize the influence of unsubstantiated anecdotes. Further, an effort has been made to provide information about issues previously unaddressed such as employment while breastfeeding and the modality of sucking. Other topics such as drugs in breast milk and human milk for premature infants have been expanded.

I wish to thank the physicians from many parts of the world who have contacted me with information from their experiences and their questions. The response from other professionals and paraprofessionals, who found a need for further information, has also contributed to this effort.

The library searches have continued with the help of a host of University of Rochester undergraduate students who deserve credit for their perseverance and patience. The very special talent of Kathy Cook for organization and detail, however, has been a critical factor in preparing the manuscript, and I thank her.

Ruth A. Lawrence

Preface
to first edition

This book was written in an effort to provide the medical profession with an easily accessible reference for the clinical management of the mother-infant nursing couple. After many decades of championing formula for the newborn and infant, the medical profession has recognized that human milk is preferable for the human infant. The world literature reflects scientists' work on breastfeeding in the fields of nutrition, biochemistry, immunology, psychology, anthropology, and sociology. These researchers have demonstrated what most mothers have long believed: human milk is specifically designed for human infants.

Although reports in dozens of journals have contributed information valuable in the clinical management of lactation, it has remained difficult for the practitioner to gain access to it when an emergency arises. There are other topics, such as the pharmacokinetics of human milk, on which more knowledge and data are needed. This book is intended to provide the information that is available as well as identify areas of deficient information. The first part of this book is basic data on the anatomical, physiological, biochemical, nutritional, immunological, and psychological aspects of human lactation. The remainder centers on the problems of clinical management and, I hope, maximizes scientific data and minimizes anecdotal information. The goal is to provide practical information for managing individual mothers and their infants. It is also hoped that a balance has been struck between basic science, on which rational management should rest, and advice garnered by experience. Through use of the bibliographies interested readers may seek out the original works for details and supporting data.

I recognized some years ago that specific data were accumulating rapidly but remained in scattered, sometimes inaccessible, references. The increasing requests for consultation about breastfeeding sparked the idea for a more formal publication to replace the information sheets and brochures that I had been putting together. My interest in breastfeeding started during internship and residency at Yale–New Haven Hospital where Dr. Edith Jackson, Dr. Grover Powers, and Dr. Milton Senn expressed genuine concern for the declining rate of breastfeeding. Dr. Jackson provided excellent training in the art of breastfeeding for families and professionals in the rooming-in project in New Haven.

This book does not speak to world issues or the political issues of nutrition, since they have been eloquently discussed by Derrick and E.P. Patrice Jelliffe in their many works.

Throughout this book, since a nursing mother is a female, the personal pronoun *she* has been used. In referring to the infant, the choice between *he* or *she* has been made, using the male pronoun only to enhance clarity between reference to mother or child. The physician has been referred to as *he,* although I am thoroughly cognizant of the inordinate injustice perpetrated by this historical usage.

I should like to acknowledge the help and support of the many colleagues who encouraged me to investigate this subject and the hosts of nursing mothers who helped me learn what I am sharing here.

Extensive library research was done by Nancy Hess and Cathy Goodfellow, who worked as professional volunteers. Editing and tracking specific data were done by Timothy Lawrence, whom I also wish to thank. No writing is accomplished without diligent preparation of the manuscript. Loretta H. Anderson prepared many of the rough drafts. Carleen Wilenius was invaluable for her many skills with the manuscripts, not the least of which were final preparation and typing of many of the lengthy charts and bibliographies. I also wish to thank Rosemary E. Disney, who designed the cover art.

Ruth A. Lawrence

Contents

Breastfeeding

A Guide for the Medical Profession

Breastfeeding in modern medicine

There is a reason behind everything in nature.
ARISTOTLE

Until recently, breastfeeding has been a subject considered too imprecise and nonspecific to justify consideration by scientists and clinicians confronted with questions of infant nutrition. Decades have been spent in the laboratory deciphering the nutritional requirements of the growing neonate. A considerably greater investment in time, talent, and money has been put toward the development of an ideal substitute for human milk. On the other hand, artificial feeding has been described as the world's largest experiment without controls.[38] On a parallel tract in the veterinary field, a careful study of the science of lactation in other species, especially bovine, has been made because of the commercial significance of a productive herd.

While expertise has produced refinements in the analysis of food constituents, it also has become possible to learn more about human milk. The traditional lip service paid to breastfeeding conceded that human milk is for human infants. A simple chart that showed the difference between human milk and cow's milk in protein, fat, and carbohydrate content and the calcium/phosphorus ratio has been used to support the statement. It was usually quickly pointed out that simple adjustments in cow's milk would actually mitigate these seeming differences. Students of pediatrics received no formal training in the management of breastfeeding and were thus ill prepared to counsel a mother who wished to nurse. Furthermore, if the process did not go smoothly and was not easily managed by the mother alone, the pediatrician was at a loss to help. Indeed, many physicians had been warned of the dangers of undernutrition associated with breastfeeding and the deviation from the "ideal" growth curve set by overfed bottle infants. When the natural process of human lactation presented a question or a concern to the physician, the advice was frequently to wean the infant to a formula that could be clinically measured and volumetrically controlled with scientific precision.

The world scientific literature, predominantly from countries other than the United States, actually has many tributes to human milk. Early writings on infant care in the 1800s and early 1900s pointed out the hazards of serious infection in bottle fed infants.

Mortality charts were clear in the difference in risk of death between breastfed and bottle fed infants.[14,15] Only in recent years have the reasons for this phenomenon been identified in terms comparable to those used to define other anti-infectious properties. The identification of specific immunoglobulins and specific influence of the pH and flora in the intestine of the breastfed infant are examples. It became clear that the infant receives systemic protection transplacentally and local intestinal tract protection orally via the colostrum. It has been further identified that the intestinal tract environment of a breastfed infant continues to afford protection against infection by influencing the bacterial flora until the infant is weaned. It has been shown that breastfed infants also have fewer respiratory infections.

Refinement in the biochemistry of nutrition has afforded an opportunity to restudy the constituents of human milk. A closer look at the amino acids in human milk has demonstrated clearly that the array is physiologically suited for the human newborn. Forced by legislation mandating mass newborn screening for phenylalanine in all hospitals, physicians were faced with the problem of the newborn who had high phenylalanine or tyrosine levels in his blood. It became apparent that many traditional formulas provided an overload of these amino acids in the diet, which some infants were unable to handle well.

Although the modern woman may be selectively chastised for abandoning breastfeeding in the past three decades because of the ready availability of prepared formulas, paraphernalia of bottles and rubber nipples, and ease of sterilization, it should be pointed out that this is not a new problem. Meticulous combing of civilized history reveals that almost every culture has had to deal with the mother who could not or would not nurse her infant. Blame cannot be placed solely at the feet of an uninformed and unsupportive medical profession or at the feet of the formula manufacturers.

Hammurabi's code from about 1800 BC contained regulations on the practice of wet nursing, that is, nursing another woman's infant, often for hire. Throughout Europe spouted feeding cups have been found in the graves of infants dating from about 2000 BC. Paralleling the information about ancient feeding techniques is the problem of abandoned infants. Well-known biblical stories report such events, as do accounts from Rome during the time of the early popes. In fact, so many abandoned infants were discovered that foundling homes were started. French foundling homes in the 1700s were staffed by wet nurses who were carefully selected and their lives and activities controlled.

If one looks back to Spartan times,[33] it was required that a Spartan woman, even if she was the wife of a king, nurse her eldest son; plebians were to nurse all their children. Plutarch reported that a second son of King Themistes inherited the kingdom of Sparta only because he was nursed with his mother's milk. The eldest son had been nursed by a stranger and therefore was rejected. Hippocrates is said to have written on the subject of nursing, declaring, "One's own milk is beneficial, other's harmful" (Fig. 1-1).

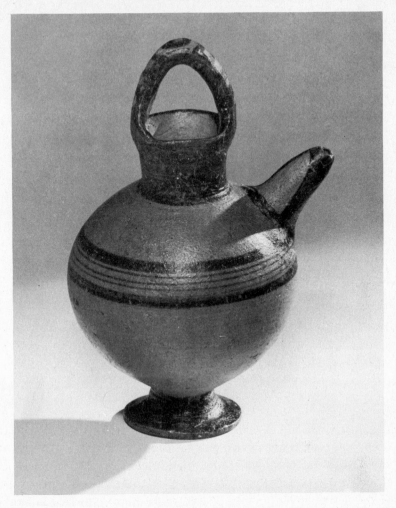

Fig. 1-1. Infant's feeding bottle from Cyprus. Circa 500 BC. Unglazed pottery. Although ancient Egyptian feeding flasks are almost unknown, specimens of Greek origin are fairly common in infant burials.

In eighteenth century France, both before and during the revolution that swept Louis XVI from the throne and brought Napoleon to power, infant feeding included maternal nursing, wet nursing, artificial feeding with the milk of animals, and feeding of pap and panada. *Panada* is from the French *panade,* bread, and means a food consisting of bread, water or other liquid, and seasoning, boiled to the consistency of pulp (Fig. 1-2). The majority of infants, especially in Paris, were placed out with wet nurses. The reason given for this widespread practice was that maternal nursing was "not the custom." Mothers wished to "guard their beauty and freshness." In 1718, Dionis wrote "today not only ladies of nobility, but yet the rich and the wives of the least of the artisans

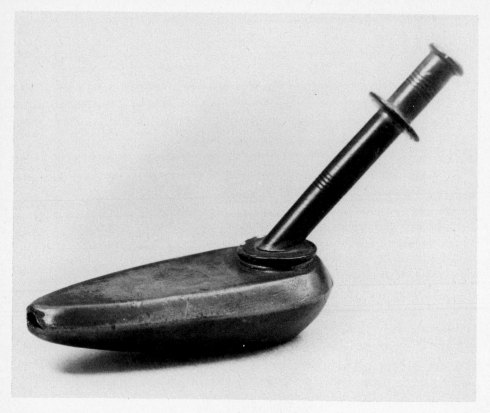

Fig. 1-2. Pewter pap spoon. Circa 1800 AD. Thin pap was placed in bowl. Tip of bowl was placed in child's mouth. Flow could be controlled by placing finger over open end of hollow handle. If contents were not taken as rapidly as desired, one could blow down handle.

have lost the custom of nursing their infants.'' As early as 1705 there were laws controlling wet nursing. The laws required wet nurses to register, forbade them to nurse more than two infants in addition to their own, and stipulated that there be a crib for each infant to prevent the nurse from taking them to bed and chancing suffocation.*

A more extensive historical review would reveal other examples of social problems in achieving adequate care of infants. Long before our modern society there were women who failed to accept the biologic role as nursing mothers, and society failed to provide adequate support for nursing mothers (Fig. 1-3).

According to Phillips,[25] breastfeeding was more common and of longer duration in stable, hard-working eras and rarer in periods of ''social dazzle'' and lowered moral

---

*It is interesting to note that at the National Convention of France of 1793 laws were passed to provide relief for infants of indigent families. The provisions are quite similar to those in our present-day welfare programs.[8]

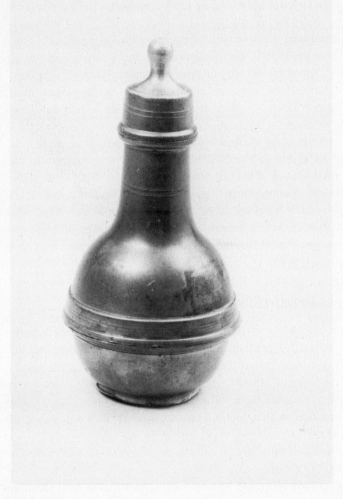

Fig. 1-3. Infant's feeding bottle. English. Circa 1780 AD. This pewter feeder is of type common to England, France, and Holland from 1600 to 1800.

standards. Urban mothers have had greater access to alternatives, and rural women have had to continue to breastfeed in greater numbers.

Reasons given for the decrease in breastfeeding in this century have been reviewed by sociologists. Urbanization and technological advances have affected social, medical, and dietary trends throughout the world. The social influences include the changing pattern of family life—smaller, isolated families that are separated from the previous generation. In medicine, the emphasis has been on disease and its treatment, especially as it relates to laboratory study and hospital care. The science of nutrition has developed a reliance on measurement and analysis, which has encouraged the impression that prepared foods are superior because they can be measured and calculated to meet precise needs.

If recent statistics are reviewed, there are encouraging trends. The acceptance or rejection of breastfeeding is being influenced in the Western world to a greater degree by the knowledge of the benefits of human lactation. Cultural rejection, negative attitudes about convenience, and lack of support from health professionals are being replaced by interest in child rearing and preparation for childbirth. This has created a system that encourages a prospective mother to consider the options for herself and her infant. The attitude in the Western world toward the female breast as a sex object to the exclusion of its ability to nurture has influenced young mothers in particular not to nurse. The emancipation of women, which began in the 1920s, was symbolized by short hair, short skirts, contraceptives, cigarettes, and bottle feeding. In the second half of this century, women have sought to be well informed, and many wish the right to choose how they feed their infant. Within the boundaries of medical prudence, the medical profession should be prepared with adequate information to support the mother's desire to breastfeed.

FREQUENCY OF BREASTFEEDING

Data collected in the 1970s[21,32] in the Ross National Mothers Survey MR 77-48, which included 10,000 mothers, revealed a general trend toward breastfeeding (Tables 1-1 and 1-2). In 1975, 33% of the mothers started out breastfeeding, and 15% were still nursing at 5 to 6 months. In 1977, the figures indicated that 43% of the mothers left the hospital nursing, and 20% were still nursing at 5 to 6 months. Other studies have shown a regional variation, with a higher percentage of mothers nursing on the West Coast than in the East.

A continuation of the study of milk-feeding patterns in 1981 in the United States by Martinez and Dodd[21] showed a sustained trend toward breastfeeding in the 55% of 51,537 new mothers contacted by mail. Although mothers who breastfeed continue to be more highly educated and have a higher income, the greatest increase in breastfeeding occurred among women with less education. From 1971 to 1981, breastfeeding in the hospital more than doubled (from 24.7% to 57.6%), with an average rate of gain of 8.8%. The incidence of breastfeeding at 1 week of age was 56.4%. For infants 2 months old breastfeeding more than tripled (from 13.9% to 44.2%) in the 10-year period.

The recent trend in infant feeding among mothers who participated in the Women, Infants, and Children (WIC) Program was analyzed separately by Martinez and Stahl[22] from the data collected by questionnaires mailed quarterly. The responses represented 4.8% of the total U.S. births in 1977 and 14.1% of the total U.S. births in 1980 (Table 1-3). WIC participants in 1977, including those who supplemented with formula or cow's milk, were breastfeeding in the hospital in 33.6% of cases. There was a steady and significant increase in the frequency of breastfeeding to 40.4% in 1980 ($p < .05$).

Table 1-1. Estimated percentages of infants receiving various types of milks and formulas*

Feeding	Age (mo)							
	0 to 1	1 to 2	2 to 3	3 to 4	4 to 5	5 to 6	6 to 9	9 to 12
Breastfed	20	15	12	10	8	5	2	<1
Milk-based formula†	64	65	59	49	41	29	3	1
Milk-free formulas†	10	10	10	10	8	6	2	1
Evaporated milk formulas	4	4	3	—	—	—	—	—
Evaporated milk and water	—	—	2	2	2	2	1	1
Fresh cow's milk	2	6	14	29	41	58	92	96

From Fomon, S.J.: What are infants fed in the United States? Pediatrics **56**:350, 1975, copyright American Academy of Pediatrics, 1975.
*Estimates based on any breastfeeding on a given day of the month in question. Estimates from 1974.
†Commercially prepared.

Table 1-2. Percentage of infants at 1 week of age receiving different milks and formulas, 1955 to 1981

	Breast milk*	Prepared infant formula	Evaporated milk	Cow's milk	Total*
1955	29.2	23.2	45.9	4.1	102.4
1960	28.4	34.9	40.0	2.8	106.1
1965	26.5	59.0	17.3	1.5	104.3
1970	24.9	74.9	3.0	0.6	103.4
1975	33.4	69.2	0.7	0.3	103.6
1978	45.1	58.6	0.5	0.1	104.3
1979	49.7	54.7	0.3	0.1	104.8
1980	54.0	50.6	0.2	0.1	104.9
1981	56.4	48.5	0.2	0.1	105.2

From Ross National Mothers Survey MR77-48, 1981.
*Includes supplemental bottle feeding, i.e., formula in addition to breastfeeding.

The demographic information indicated that WIC mothers were slightly younger (18.5% < 20 years old compared with 5.4% of those not in WIC). WIC respondents did not differ significantly from nonWIC mothers in plans for postpartum employment, although they were less well educated. Of infants born to WIC mothers, 7.9% were premature; of babies born to nonWIC mothers, only 4.3% were premature when the national average was 7.1% of births.

A study of infants from an urban clinic population in California that served 86% Hispanic, 6.3% white, 4.0% Asian, and 1.8% black clients showed that only 20.8% of babies received any breast milk and only 13.1% were exclusively breastfed in the first 3 months of life.[20] The American Indian populations of Pima and Papago tribes in Arizona were studied retrospectively in 1978 to identify the role of sociodemographic factors in the trends in breastfeeding and bottle feeding.[13] Findings included a significant decline in breastfeeding from 1949 to 1977, with a tendency for an increased rate in the

Table 1-3.   Milk fed to infants of WIC participants

	N	Breast milk (%)*	Prepared infant formula (%)	Cow's milk evaporated milk (%)
In hospital				
1977	932	33.6	71.7	0.3
1978	2,000	34.5	69.3	0.1
1979	2,465†	37.0	68.6	0.5
1980	3,424	40.0†‡	65.2†‡	0.2
% change				
1977-1980		+19.0	−9.1	−33.3
At 2 mo of age				
1977	932	22.5	79.3	2.9
1978	2,000	22.9	78.6	2.5
1979	2,463	24.4	78.6	1.9
1980	3,421	28.5†‡	75.7†‡	2.5
% change				
1977-1980		+26.7	−4.5	−13.8
At 5 and 6 mo of age				
1977	248	12.5	74.6	17.6
1978	1,265	11.2	74.5	18.0
1979	2,353	12.2	76.7	14.2†
1980	3,225	14.4*	79.4†‡	11.0†‡
% change				
1977-1980		+15.2	+6.4	−37.5

Modified from Martinez, G.A., and Stahle, D.A.: Am. J. Pub. Health **72:**68, 1982.
*Includes supplemental feeding, i.e., formula or cow's milk in addition to breastfeeding.
†Significant difference between preceding year and current year, $p < .05$.
‡Significant difference between year 1977 and year 1980, $p < .05$.

last few years among younger women. Bottle feeding was more common among higher–birth order infants and among women of pure tribal background.

In another study, families belonging to a prepaid Group Practice Health Care Plan in upstate New York were interviewed.[1] Infants were breastfed in 26% of the white, 26% of the black, and 18% of the Hispanic families. Percentages correlated with educational and income levels. The infant-feeding practices of middle-class mothers in Seattle were studied by retrospective home interview and revealed that 87% were breastfeeding during the first 5 weeks.[24]

The international trends have also received considerable attention, and data on all countries but Russia are available in *The International Breast Feeding Compendium,* 1984.[37] Because studies vary in methodology, there is no accurate way to generalize. Breastfeeding patterns in low-income countries, as extracted from world fertility surveys and secondary sources, indicate that in all but a few countries most children are breastfed for a few months at least, and in 53% of the 83 countries listed the incidence is 90% or higher. Most localized trend data in both developed and third-world countries reveal increasing frequency of breastfeeding since the 1970s.

A study by Fitzpatrick and Kevany[10] in 1975 reported only 16% of all babies to be breastfed at a few days of age in Dublin, Ireland. Sloper et al.[31] reported similar results from Oxford in the same year: 14% of the babies were breastfed at discharge from the hospital, and another 13% were receiving combined breastfeeding and bottle feeding. The national trend data for Belgium, Canada, Finland, Sweden, and the United Kingdom are beginning to show an increase in breastfeeding in the hospital.

DURATION OF BREASTFEEDING

Coupled with concerns about the decreasing number of mothers who nurse their infants when they leave the hospital is the concern about duration of breastfeeding. There is a sharp decline by age 6 months; in 1977 this decline was from 43% to 20%. Other studies that have looked at duration more closely have noted an appreciable decline shortly after discharge from the hospital.

Before evaluating the duration of breastfeeding in the industrialized world, it is wise to consider that there are two types of breastfeeding, as Newton[23] points out—unrestricted breastfeeding and token breastfeeding.

Unrestricted breastfeeding usually means that the infant is put to the breast immediately following delivery and nursed on demand thereafter. The infant is put to the breast without rules or limitations. There may be 10 or 12 feedings a day in the early weeks, with the number gradually decreasing over the first year of life. Breast milk continues to be a major source of nourishment in infancy in these infants.

Token breastfeeding, in contrast, is characterized by constant restrictions on the time and duration of nursing. Usually the feedings are scheduled. Even the amount of mother-infant contact is limited initially, such as in hospitals where newborns are kept in a central nursery and taken out only for feedings. The infant is often offered water or glucose water by rubber-nippled bottle, which confuses the infant while he is trying to establish his sucking techniques. Feeding by the clock may mean that the infant is too frantic from crying or not yet awake enough to suckle. The whole process is inhibited, and a secure milk supply may not be established.

If one examines the duration of breastfeeding, there is a difference between unrestricted and token-feeding groups. There are also cultural differences. In societies that have yet to be caught up in industrialization and continue to maintain ancient cultural patterns of child rearing, the duration is well beyond a year. A study of 46 such societies reported by Ford[12] revealed that weaning at about 2 to 3 years of age occurred in three fourths of them. One fourth of the groups began weaning at 18 months of age, and one culture started at 6 months. A similar anthropologic investigation of primitive child-rearing practices found a distinct correlation between the time of weaning and the behavior of the tribes.[12] Where weaning was delayed, there were peaceful tribes. In contrast, tribes that abruptly weaned their infants at 6 months of age and practiced other rigid disciplinary practices were warlike.

In the United States and Europe at the beginning of this century, over 50% of the infants were breastfed beyond 1 year of age. The Plunket Society of New Zealand

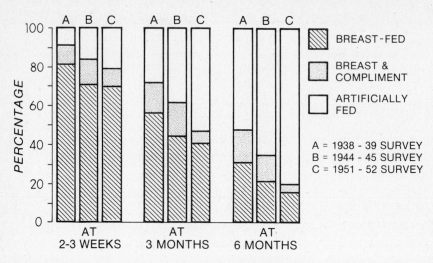

Fig. 1-4. Breastfeeding in New Zealand. A summary of the results of the Plunket Society's surveys of 1938 to 1939, 1944 to 1945, and 1951 to 1952. (From Deem, H., and McGeorge, M.: N.Z. Med. J. **57**:539, 1958.)

Table 1-4.   Duration of breastfeeding among 459 mothers

Duration of breastfeeding (wk)	Number of infants discontinuing breastfeeding (%)	Number of infants still breastfeeding (%)
1-2	84(18.3)	459(100)
3-4	67(14.6)	375(81.7)
5-8	93(20.3)	308(67.1)
9-12	28 (6.1)	215(46.8)
13-16	50(10.9)	187(40.7)
17-20	33 (7.0)	137(29.8)
21-25	31 (6.8)	104(22.8)
26+	73(16.0)	73(16.0)
TOTAL	459(100)	

*From Halpern, S.R., et al.: South. Med. J. **65**:100, 1972, reprinted by permission.

conducted three surveys to evaluate the extent and duration of breastfeeding.[7] These surveys showed a progressive decline in the number of nursing mothers and in the duration of nursing (Fig. 1-4).

In 1966, fewer than one in three mothers in the United States were breastfeeding when they left the hospital. Only 5% of the nation's infants are breastfed after 6 months of age. Fomon[11] has asserted that most breastfed infants receive solid foods or cow's milk supplements early.

A Texas study by Halpern et al.[16] in 1972 followed 2310 infants, of whom 459 were breastfed when discharged from the hospital. By 4 weeks of age 32.9% had been stopped and by 26 weeks (6 months) 84% were no longer breastfed (Table 1-4).

A study in Dublin by Fitzpatrick and Kevany[10] in 1977 looked at the duration of breastfeeding. Only six of nineteen infants (31.9%) were still wholly breastfeeding at 6

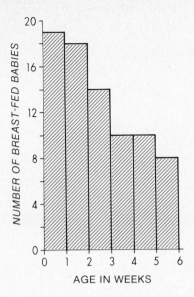

Fig. 1-5. Decline of breastfeeding in first 6 weeks of life. (From Fitzpatrick, C., and Kevany. J.: J. Irish Med. Assoc. **70:**3, 1977.)

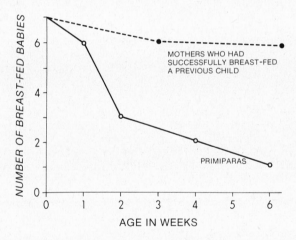

Fig. 1-6. Duration of breastfeeding in primiparas compared with mothers who have successfully breastfed a previous child. (From Fitzpatrick, C., and Kevany. J.: J. Irish Med. Assoc. **70:**3, 1977.)

weeks; two were given some bottle feedings, and eleven (57.9%) had been weaned by 6 weeks (Fig. 1-5). A higher rate of success was experienced in mothers who had nursed a previous infant (Fig. 1-6). The rapid decline was attributed to lack of appropriate advice, including the early introduction of solid foods, and lack of psychological support while in the hospital (Fig. 1-7). A similar study in Boston in 1960 had shown a mean duration of nursing to be 3½ months. Cole[2] conducted a two-part survey in a Boston

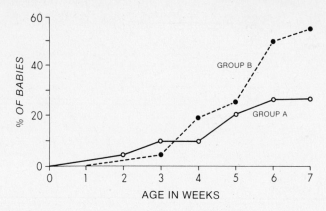

Fig. 1-7. Group A, breastfeeding; Group B, bottle feeding. (From Fitzpatrick, C., and Kevany, J.: J. Irish Med. Assoc. **70:**3, 1977.)

Table 1-5. Mother's education and projected feeding choice*†

Feeding choice	High school (%)	Some college or degree (%)	Graduate work or professional degree (%)
Breast	44 (44)	90 (62)	55 (65)
Bottle	55 (56)	55 (38)	29 (35)
TOTAL	99	145	84

From Cole, J.P.: Clin. Pediatr. **16:**352, 1977.
*Corrected chi-square = 10.33 with 2 df.
†$p = 0.01$.

suburb in 1977 that included 332 pregnant women and 140 new mothers—51% intended to breastfeed, 42% intended to bottle feed, and 1% was undecided. There was a correlation between education of the mother and incidence of breastfeeding, with 44% of high school graduates, 62% of college graduates, and 65% of those with postgraduate education desiring to breastfeed (Table 1-5). Other researchers made similar observations in the 1970s, noting that 40% of the upper- and middle-class mothers breastfeed, compared with 15% in lower classes.

The duration of breastfeeding for 140 women was studied. By the time the infant was 4 weeks of age, 80% of the women were still nursing, but only 58.6% were still breastfeeding beyond 4 months. The most frequent reasons given for stopping were (1) not enough milk, (2) felt tired, and (3) infant's physician told mother to stop. This study also pointed out the pivotal role for the pediatrician in the successful maintenance of lactation as well as the importance of the postpartum environment.

The 1981 Milk Feeding Pattern survey by Martinez and Dodd[21] reported on the duration of breastfeeding. The rate of infants breastfed at ages 3 to 4 months was 35.2%, a fourfold increase from 1971; at 5 and 6 months of age the rate was 26.8% in

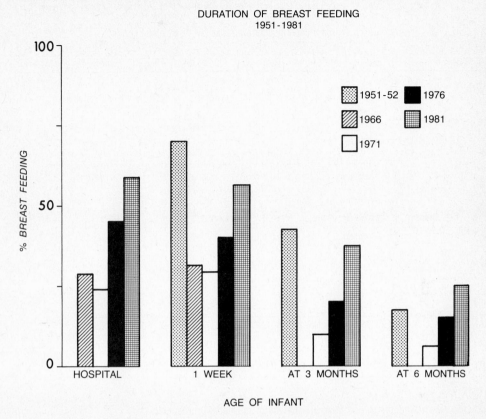

Fig. 1-8. Duration of breastfeeding (1951 to 1981). (Based on data from Woo-Lun, M., Gussler, J., and Smith, N., editors: The international breastfeeding compendium, ed. 3, Columbus, Ohio, 1984, Ross Laboratories.)

1981 and only 5.5% in 1971 (Fig. 1-8). Data collected by telephone follow-up further revealed rates of 18% at 8 months, 13% at 10 months; and 9% at 12 months (Table 1-6). The maternal demographic data on duration of breastfeeding in this study further supported the trend of higher educational level and higher income for mothers breast-feeding at 6 and 12 months (Table 1-7). More multiparas than primiparas continued to breastfeed, but duration was negatively affected by maternal employment. The influence of maternal employment in this survey was significant ($p < .01$). For every 100 mothers employed full time and breastfeeding in the hospital, 19.8% were still breastfeeding at 6 months postpartum, whereas among mothers not employed and breastfeeding in the hospital, 50.1% were still breastfeeding at 6 months postpartum. The employed mothers in most studies tend to be in better educated, higher socioeconomic groups than those who are unemployed. Thus, it is not necessarily employment alone that deters the lower socioeconomic group from breastfeeding.

Table 1-6.   Percentage of infants receiving different milks by year of survey*

	1971	1981	ARG 1971-1981
In hospital			
Breast	24.7	57.6†	8.8
CM/EM	0.9	0.1†	(19.7)
Prepared formula	77.4	48.4†	—
Total‡	103.0	106.1	
At age 2 mo			
Breast	13.9	44.2†	12.3
CM/EM	14.8	1.8†	(19.0)
Prepared formula	74.1	61.4†	(1.9)
Total‡	102.8	107.4	—
At ages 5 and 6 mo			
Breast	5.5	26.8†	17.2
CM/EM	68.1	17.0†	(13.0)
Prepared formula	28.0	63.7†	8.6
Total‡	101.6	107.5	—
At age 12 mo			
Breast	—	9.0	—
CM/EM		84.8	
Prepared formula		13.7	
TOTAL‡		107.5	

From Martinez, G.A., and Dodd, D.A.: Pediatrics 71:166, 1983, copyright American Academy of Pediatrics 1983.
*Values in parentheses indicate loss, i.e., a decrease. Abbreviations used are ARG, annual rate of gain; CM/EM, cow's milk/evaporated milk.
†Trend significant, $p < .01$.
‡Total includes supplemental bottle feeding and multiple milk usage.

Table 1-7.   Percentage of infants breastfeeding by selected maternal demographic characteristics, 1981

	1971	1981	ARG 1971-1981
Parity			
Primiparous	62.4*	24.2*	7.2
Multiparous	53.0	25.8	10.3
Education			
Grade and high school	50.8*	19.7*	7.0*
College	74.0	38.3	13.4
Employment			
Not employed	59.5*	29.8*	9.7*
Employed	50.9†	10.1†	4.0‡
Income			
<$15,000	49.4*	19.2*	7.9
$15,000-$24,999	61.0	28.0	9.1
≥$25,000	65.6	30.1	10.8
TOTAL (all infants)	57.6	25.1	9.0

From Martinez, G.A., and Dodd, D.A.: Pediatrics 71:166, 1983, copyright American Academy of Pediatrics 1983.
*Differences within category significant, $p < .01$.
†Refers to employment status at time of survey, i.e., when infants were 6 months of age, employment on a full-time basis. Data are for three quarters of 1981.
‡Refers to employment status at time of survey, i.e., when infants were 12 months of age. Employed represents mothers with full-time employment.

Table 1-8. Comparison of mother's plans for infant feeding expressed during third trimester of pregnancy with practice adopted at birth (study 1)

	Number (%) of respondents (n = 976)		
	Breastfed	Formula fed	Undecided
Plan for infant feeding	504 (52)	421 (43)	51 (5)
Feeding practice in hospital*			
Breastfed	482 (96)	13 (3)	28 (55)
Formula fed	22 (4)	408 (97)	23 (45)

From Sarett, H.P., Bain, K.R., and O'Leary, J.C.: Am. J. Dis. Child. 137:719, 1983, copyright 1983, American Medical Association.
*A total of 523 mothers (54%) breastfed their infants, and 453 mothers (46%) formula fed their infants.

Table 1-9. Time of choice of breastfeeding or formula feeding in telephone survey of recent mothers of young infants (study 2)

	% of respondents			
Time of decision	Total (n = 200)	Breastfeeding (n = 112)	Formula feeding (n = 84)	Feeding both (n = 4)
Before pregnancy	49	55	43	—
First trimester	29	31	24	75
Second trimester	7	8	7	—
Third trimester	8	5	12	—
After delivery	7	1	14	25

From Sarett, H.P., Bain, K.R., and O'Leary, J.C.: Am. J. Dis. Child. 137:719, 1983, copyright 1983, American Medical Association.

A similar study in the United States on infant-feeding trends reported by Sarett et al.[28] in 1983 indicated that 85% to 92% of mothers decide on a feeding method before the end of the second trimester, and 96% to 97% feed their infant as previously planned (Tables 1-8 and 1-9). Between 1976 and 1980 more mothers than in previous years were breastfeeding for 6 months or longer and solid food was being introduced later. West[35] reported in 1980 that of 239 breastfeeding mothers in Edinburgh only 5% were breastfeeding at 12 weeks, with the greatest decline in the first 6 weeks, and 46% were breastfeeding at 22 weeks. Duration was influenced by social class but not by the age of the mother. Reasons offered for terminating breastfeeding are noted in Table 1-10. Return to work was a reason for discontinuing in only 5 of the 116 women. One hundred, or 86%, of the mothers who stopped by 22 weeks would have liked to continue but felt they had insufficient milk or other unsurmountable problems. Unrelated to length of breastfeeding, a large percentage of all the survey mothers felt they could have benefited by more assistance from health-care professionals.

MORBIDITY AND MORTALITY STUDIES IN BREASTFED AND ARTIFICIALLY FED INFANTS

Assessing the mortality of breastfed compared with bottle fed infants is difficult to do today because many breastfed infants also receive supplements of cow's milk and

Table 1-10. Reasons for discontinuing breastfeeding

Reason	Duration of breastfeeding (wk)			Total (116)*
	<6 (49)*	6-11 (39)*	12-22 (28)*	
Inadequate milk supply	28	18	12	58
Baby unsettled after breastfeeds	18	11	2	31
Very frequent feeds required	17	8	4	29
Breastfeeding was too tiring	13	5	2	20
Painful nipples	14	2	1	17
Baby refused the breast	9	4	2	15
Unable to go out	6	4	0	10
Too time consuming	7	2	1	10
Illness of mother	3	6	0	9
Breast abscess	2	3	1	6
Return to work	0	3	2	5
Dislike of breastfeeding	5	0	0	5
Insufficient privacy at home	2	1	0	3
Illness of baby	2	1	0	3
Other factors†				
Anxiety, lack of confidence	6	2	1	9
Breast problems—mastitis, engorgement	1	5	0	6
Older children upset or jealous	3	0	0	3
Contraceptive pill reduced milk supply	0	1	1	2
Anticoagulant therapy	1	0	0	1

From West, C.P.: J. Biosoc. Sci. 12:325, 1980.
*No. of women.
†Not listed but volunteered by the mothers.

Table 1-11. Mortality rates and survivorship to age 1 year in breastfed and artificially fed infants*

Study area	Date	Mortality (per 1000)		Survivors to age 1 yr (per 1000)		
		Breastfed	Artificially fed	Breastfed	Artificially fed	Difference
Berlin, Germany	1895-1896	57	376	943	624	319
Barmen, Germany	1905	68	379	932	621	311
Hanover, Germany	1912	96	296	904	704	200
Boston, Mass.	1911	30	212	970	788	182
Eight U.S. cities†	1911-1916	76	255	924	745	179
Paris, France	1900	140	310	860	690	170
Cologne, Germany	1908-1909	73	241	927	759	168
Amsterdam, Holland	1904	144	304	856	696	160
Liverpool, England	1905	84	134	916	866	144
Eight U.S. cities‡	1911-1916	76	215	924	785	139
Derby, England	1900-1903	70	198	930	802	128
Chicago, Ill.	1924-1929	2	84	998	916	82
Liverpool, England	1936-1942	10	57	990	943	47
Great Britain	1946-1947	9	18	991	982	9

From Knodel, J.: Science 198:1111, 1977, copyright 1977 by the American Association for the Advancement of Science.
*Most of these rates do not include deaths in the first few days or weeks of life; mortality is therefore underestimated and survival overestimated. Only the rates for the eight U.S. cities in 1911-1916 represent mortality from birth; deaths that occurred before any feeding are proportionally allocated to the two feeding categories. The rates for Berlin, Barmen, Hanover, Cologne, and the eight U.S. cities were derived by applying life table techniques to mortality given by single months of age.
†Comparison of breastfed infants with infants artificially fed from birth.
‡Comparison of breastfed infants with all infants artificially fed in the period of observation.

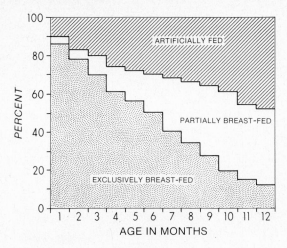

Fig. 1-9. Percentage of infants who are breastfed, partially breastfed, and artificially fed by age in months. (Modified from Woodbury, R. M.: Am. J. Hyg. **2**:668, 1922.)

solid foods. The risk of death in the first year of life has diminished in civilized countries in this century, since the advent of antibiotics and many other advances in pediatric care. Data from previous decades and other nations do show a significant difference, however.[14,15] Knodel[19] presented a complete table, including rates from cities in Germany, France, England, Holland, and the United States (Table 1-11). Mortality among breastfed infants is clearly lower than that among bottle fed infants. Knodel pointed out that early neonatal deaths, in the first week or so of life, were excluded.

In another study in 1922, Woodbury[36] reported mortality of infants by type of feeding. Mortality is lower at all ages for breastfed infants (Fig. 1-9). Overwhelming evidence of the impact of human milk on mortality is displayed in the widely publicized statistics currently available on third-world countries, where infant formulas are rapidly replacing human milk. The death rate is higher, malnutrition starts earlier and is more severe, and the incidence of infection is greater in formula fed infants (Figs. 1-10 and 1-11). Data from the work of Scrimshaw et al.[30] show mortality of 950/1000 live births in the artificially fed infants and 120/1000 in breastfed infants. The data were collected in Punjab villages from 1955 through 1959. The deaths were predominantly due to diarrheal disease (Table 1-12). The Pan American Health Organization has reported similar correlations between malnutrition, infection, and mortality. In Puffer and Serrano's[27] 1973 work in São Paulo, the death rates among breastfed infants were lower and the proportions due to diarrheal disease and malnutrition were also less.

The incidence of illness, or morbidity, among artificially fed infants in third world countries is equally as dramatic as the mortality. Kanaaneh's[18] observations in Arab villages in Israel showed hospitalization rates to vary with method of feeding. Only 0.5% of breastfed infants required hospitalization, whereas infants fed more than 3

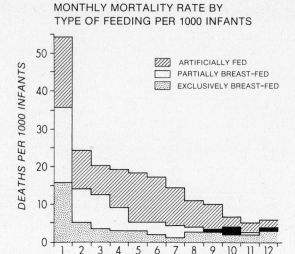

Fig. 1-10. Death rate/1000 infants by type of feeding and age in months. (Modified from Woodbury, R. M.: Am. J. Hyg. 2:668, 1922.)

Table 1-12.   Deaths and death rates by feeding regimen in seven Punjab villages, 1955-1959

Feeding regimen	Newborn infants		Neonatal deaths*		Postneonatal deaths†		Infant mortality‡	
	Number	% of total	Number	Deaths/ 1000	Number	Deaths/ 1000	Number	Deaths/ 1000
No food given	16	2.1	16	1000.0	—	—	16	1000.0
Artificial feeding from birth	20	2.6	15	750.0	4	200.0	19	950.0
Breastfed at birth	739	95.3	34	46.0	555	74.4	89	120.4
TOTAL	775	100.0	65	83.9	559	76.1	124	160.0

From Scrimshaw, N.S., Taylor, C.E., and Gordon, J.E.: WHO monograph no. 29, Geneva, 1968, World Health Organization.
*0 to 28 days inclusive.
†29 days to 11 months inclusive.
‡0 to 11 months inclusive.

months but less than 6 months at the breast had a 2.9% hospitalization rate, and infants who were bottle fed had a 24.8% rate. This is a fiftyfold difference (Table 1-13).

Demonstrating the differences in morbidity between infants fed by breast and those fed by bottle has become even more complex in industrialized countries since the resurgence of breastfeeding. Among the confounding variables are the inherent differences between the mothers who choose to breastfeed and those who choose to bottle feed.[29] Although many investigators have recognized the necessity of controlling these variables, none has succeeded totally because there is an unavoidable factor of self-selection

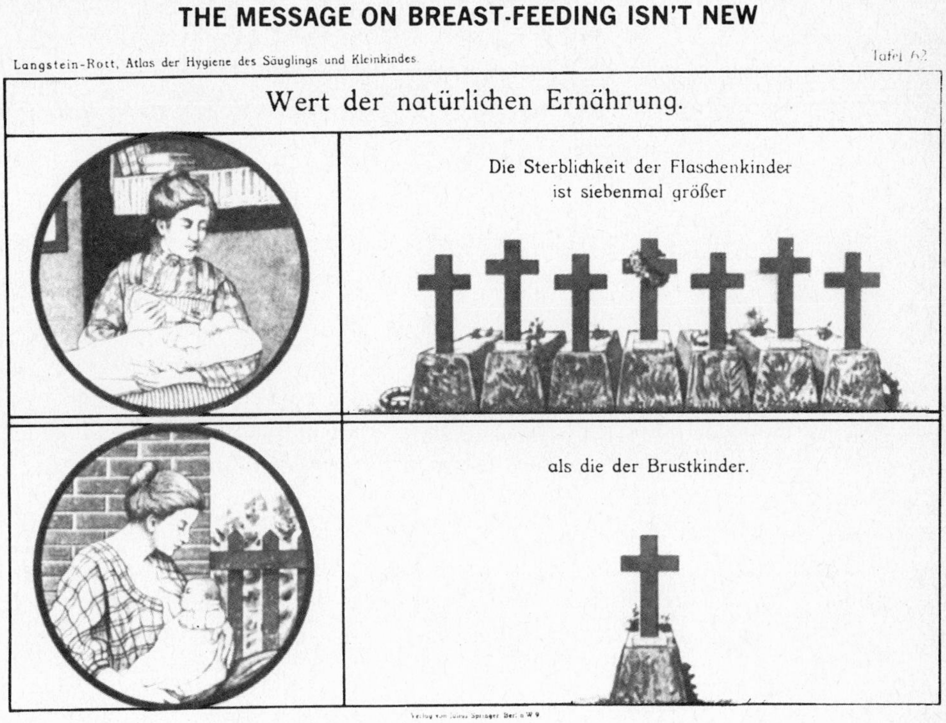

THE MESSAGE ON BREAST-FEEDING ISN'T NEW

Langstein-Rott, Atlas der Hygiene des Säuglings und Kleinkindes   Tafel 62

Wert der natürlichen Ernährung.

Die Sterblichkeit der Flaschenkinder ist siebenmal größer

als die der Brustkinder.

Verlag von Julius Springer Berlin W 9

Fig. 1-11. Poster used in 1918 to educate parents on the value of breastfeeding. Title is *Value of Natural Feeding*. Text explains that mortality of bottle fed infants (Flaschenkinder) is seven times higher than that of breastfed infants (Brustkinder). (From Langstein, R.: Atlas der Hygiene des Sauglings und Kleinkindes, Berlin, 1918, Julius Springer Verlag.)

Table 1-13. Incidence of infants hospitalized for severe diarrhea from three Arab villages in Israel, analyzed by feeding schedule

Method of feeding	Hospitalization rate (%)
Breastfed only (6 mo)	0.5
Breastfed only (3 mo, <6 mo)	2.9
Mixed >3 mo	7.0
Bottle only (3 mo)	24.8

From Kanaaneh, H.: J. Trop. Pediatr. 18:302, 1972.

that makes random assignment of infants impossible. There is a one-way flow of infants from the breastfed group to the bottle fed group, since a baby may change from breast to bottle but rarely from bottle to breast. Documenting breastfeeding practices is difficult when there is the possibility that some bottle feedings are included or that solid foods have been introduced. Investigators[9,17,18,27] have reported differences between breastfed

Table 1-14. Significant episodes of illness according to feeding mode at onset of illness (Cooperstown, 1979)

Illness	Breast	Artificial
Otitis media	3.7*	9.1
Lower respiratory infection	1.1	5.6
Diarrhea, vomiting	3.5	6.9
Hospital admissions	1.0	3.0
Total episodes of illness	8.2	21.1

From Cunningham, A.S.: Breastfeeding and morbidity in industrialized countries: an update. In Jelliffe, D.B., and Jelliffe, E.F.P., editors: Advances in international maternal and child health, vol. 1, Oxford, 1981, Oxford University Press.
*Episodes per 1000 patient-weeks.

and bottle fed infants in the incidence of morbidity associated with diarrhea, respiratory infections, otitis media, and pneumonia; they have also compared breastfed and bottle fed infants seen in clinics and emergency rooms or hospitalized in the first year of life. This extensive material has been reviewed by Cunningham.[5,6] The majority of reports demonstrate a significant advantage for the breastfed group. The relationship between breastfeeding or bottle feeding and respiratory illness in the first year of life among nearly 2000 cohort children was reported by Watkins et al.[35] in England. There was a significant advantage to breastfeeding. Mothers who smoked were less likely to breast-feed, but even when smoking was considered the breastfeeding advantage remained. Young et al.[39] reported on 1000 infants in the Yale Harvard Research Project in Tunisia who were followed from birth to 26 months and found breastfed infants to have fewer infections, illnesses, and allergies. Correlation of infections in the first postnatal year among 251 babies was made by Holmes et al.[17] with infant-feeding mode, socioeconomic status of the family, maternal educational level, maternal age, and factors including maternal smoking habit and number of siblings. The education of the mother, not the feeding mode, was the most significant variable.

Cunningham undertook a study in rural upstate New York to determine the impact of feeding on the health of the infant. Of 326 infants studied, 162 were fed proprietary formula and 164 were breastfed at birth, with only 4% still breastfed at 1 year of age. Breastfeeding was associated with significantly less illness during the first year of life. The protection was greatest during the early months, increased with the duration of breastfeeding, and appeared more striking for serious illness. (Tables 1-14 and 1-15). Breastfeeding was associated with a higher level of parental education, but controlling for that factor, the difference in morbidity is even more significant.

In the United States, diarrheal disease is uncommon in breastfed infants, and the treatment is usually to continue to breastfeed. Similarly, breastfed infants have fewer episodes of respiratory illness and otitis media. When afflicted with such febrile illnesses, the breastfed infant does not become dehydrated and rapidly toxic.

Despite the clear-cut data on mortality and morbidity from past generations and from

Table 1-15. Significant episodes of illness, regardless of feeding mode at onset of illness (Cooperstown, 1979)

Months of life	Breastfed	Limited breast	Artificially fed
1-2	0.7*	3.8	11.8
3-4	5.9	11.3	16.0
5-6	7.4	20.0	20.5
7-8	18.5	16.3	21.5
9-10	14.1	22.5	21.2
11-12	11.9	20.0	19.8
First year	58.5	93.8	110.8

From Cunningham, A.S.: Breastfeeding and morbidity in industrialized countries: an update. In Jelliffe, D.B., and Jelliffe, E.F.P., editors: Advances in international maternal and child health, vol. 1, Oxford, 1981, Oxford University Press.
*Episodes per 100 patients.

cultures seemingly remote from industrialized and medically sophisticated societies, present-day pediatricians may still discount any but the psychologic advantages of breastfeeding.

REFERENCES

1. Andrew, E.M., Clancy K.L., and Katz, M.G.: Infant feeding practices of families belonging to a prepaid group practice health care plan, Pediatrics **65**:978, 1980.
2. Cole, J.P.: Breastfeeding in Boston suburbs in relation to personal-social factors, Clin. Pediatr. **16**:352, 1977.
3. Cunningham, A.S.: Morbidity in breast-fed and artificially fed infants, J. Pediatr. **90**:726, 1977.
4. Cunningham, A.S.: Morbidity in breast-fed and artificially fed infants. II, J. Pediatr. **95**:685, 1979.
5. Cunningham, A.S.: Breastfeeding and morbidity in industrialized countries: an update. In Jelliffe, D.B., and Jelliffe, E.F.P., editors: Advances in international maternal and child health, vol. 1, Oxford, 1981, Oxford University Press.
6. Cunningham, A.S.: Breastfeeding, bottle feeding and illness, an annotated bibliography. Personal communication, 1983.
7. Deem, H., and McGeorge, M: Breastfeeding, N.Z. Med. J. **57**:539, 1958.
8. Drake, T.G.H.: Infant welfare laws in France in the 18th century, Ann. Med. Hist. **7**:49, 1935.
9. Fallot, M.E., Boyd, J.L., and Oski, F.A.: Breastfeeding reduces incidence of hospital admissions for infections in infants, Pediatrics **65**:1121, 1980.
10. Fitzpatrick, C., and Kevany, J.: The duration of breast feeding, J. Irish Med. Assoc. **70**:3, 1977.
11. Fomon, S.J.: What are infants fed in the United States? Pediatrics **56**:350, 1975.
12. Ford, C.S.: A comparative study of human reproduction, anthropology publ. no. 32, New Haven, Conn., 1945, Yale University Press.
13. Forman, M.R., et al: The PIMA infant feeding study: the role of sociodemographic factors in the trend in breast- and bottle-feeding, Am. J. Clin. Nutr. **35**:1477, 1982.
14. Grulee, C.G., Sanford, H.N., and Herron, P.H.: Breast and artificial feeding, JAMA **103**:735, 1934.
15. Grulee, C.G., Sanford, H.N., and Schwartz, H.: Breast and artificially fed infants, JAMA **104**:1986, 1935.
16. Halpern, S.R., et al.: Factors influencing breast-feeding: notes on observations in Dallas, Texas, South. Med. J. **65**:100, 1972.
17. Holmes, G.E., Hassanein, K.M., and Miller, H.C.: Factors associated with infections among breast-fed babies and babies fed proprietary milks, Pediatrics **72**:300, 1983.
18. Kanaaneh, H: The relationship of bottle feeding to malnutrition and gastroenteritis in a preindustrial setting, J. Trop. Pediatr. **18**:302, 1972.
19. Knodel, J.: Breast feeding and population growth, Science **198**:1111, 1977.

20. Magnus, P.D., and Galindo, S.: The paucity of breast-feeding in an urban clinic population, Am. J. Public Health **70:**75, 1980.

21. Martinez, G.A., and Dodd, D.A.: 1981 milk feeding patterns in the United States during the first 12 months of life, Pediatrics **71:**166, 1983.

22. Martinez, G.A., and Stahle, D.A.: The recent trend in milk feeding among WIC infants, Am. J. Public Health **72:**68, 1982.

23. Newton, N.: Psychologic differences between breast and bottle feeding. In Jelliffe, D.B., and Jeliffe, E.F.P., editors: Symposium, the uniqueness of human milk, Am. J. Clin. Nutr. **24:**993, 1971.

24. Peters, D.C., and Worthington-Roberts, B.: Infant feeding practices of middle-class breastfeeding and formula feeding mothers, Birth **9:**91, 1982.

25. Phillips, V.: Infant feeding through the ages, Keeping Abreast J. **1:**296, 1976.

26. Popkin, B.M., Bilsborrow, R.E., and Akin, J.S.: Breast-feeding patterns in low-income countries, Science **218:**1088, 1982.

27. Puffer, R.R., and Serrano, C.V.: Patterns of mortality in childhood, scientific pub. no. 262, Washington, D.C., 1973, Pan American Health Organization.

28. Sarett, H.P., Bain, K.R., and O'Leary, J.C.: Decisions on breast-feeding or formula feeding and trends in infant-feeding practices, Am. J. Dis. Child. **137:**719, 1983.

29. Sauls, H.S.: Potential effects of demographic and other variables in studies comparing morbidity of breast-fed and bottle-fed infants, Pediatrics **64:**523, 1979.

30. Scrimshaw, N.S., Taylor, C.E., and Gordon, J.E.: Interaction of nutrition and infection, WHO monograph no. 29, Geneva, 1968, World Health Organization.

31. Sloper, K., McKean, L., and Baum, J.D.: Patterns of infant feeding in Oxford, Arch. Dis. Child. **49:**749, 1974.

32. Stone, R.J.: Ross National Mothers Survey, MR 77-48, Columbus, Ohio, Ross Laboratories. Personal communication, 1978.

33. Taylor, J.: The duty of nursing children. In Ratner, H: The nursing mother: historical insights from art and theology, Child. Fam. **8(4):**19, 1949.

34. Watkins, C.J., Leeder, S.R., and Corkhill, R.T.: The relationship between breast and bottle feeding and respiratory illness in the first year of life, J. Epidemiol. Community Health **33:**180, 1979.

35. West, C.P.: Factors influencing the duration of breast-feeding, J. Biosoc. Sci. **12:**325, 1980.

36. Woodbury, R.M.: The relation between breast and artificial feeding and infant mortality, Am. J. Hyg. **2:**668, 1922.

37. Woo-lun, M., Gussler, J., and Smith, N., editors: The international breast-feeding compendium, ed. 3, Columbus, Ohio, 1984, Ross Laboratories.

38. World Health Organization: Contemporary patterns of breast-feeding, Report on the WHO collaborative study on breast-feeding, Geneva, 1981, World Health Organization.

39. Young, H.B., et al.: Milk and lactation: Some social and developmental correlates among 1,000 infants, Pediatrics **69:**169, 1982.

Anatomy of the human breast

The mammary gland, as the breast is medically termed, got its name from *mamma,* the Latin word for breast. Mammary glands begin to develop in the 6-week-old embryo, continuing their proliferation until milk ducts are developed by the time of birth. Embryologically, the mammary glands develop as ingrowths of the ectoderm into the underlying mesodermal tissue.[6] In the human embryo, a thickened raised area of the ectoderm can be recognized in the region of the future gland at the end of the fourth week of pregnancy. The thickened ectoderm becomes depressed into the underlying mesoderm, and thus the surface of the mammary area soon becomes flat and finally sinks below the level of the surrounding epidermis. The mesoderm in contact with the ingrowth of the ectoderm is compressed, and its elements become arranged in concentric layers, which at a later stage give rise to the stroma of the gland. The ingrowing mass of ectoderm cells soon becomes flask shaped and then grows out into the surrounding mesoderm as a number of solid processes that represent the future ducts of the gland. These processes, by dividing and branching, give rise to the future lobes and lobules and, much later, to the alveoli. The mammary area becomes gradually raised again in its central part to form the nipple. A lumen is formed in each part of the branching system of cellular processes after 32 weeks of gestation, and near term about 15 to 25 mammary ducts form the fetal mammary gland (Fig. 2-1). The secretion of a fluid resembling milk may take place at birth as a result of maternal hormones that have passed across the placenta into the fetal circulation. The lactiferous sinuses appear before birth as swellings of the developing ducts. In prepuberty these are epithelial-lined ducts that will bud out to form alveoli when stimulated by hormones of menarche (Fig. 2-1).

The breast is made up of glandular tissue, supporting connective tissue, and protective fatty tissue. Right after birth the newborn's breast may even be swollen and secret-

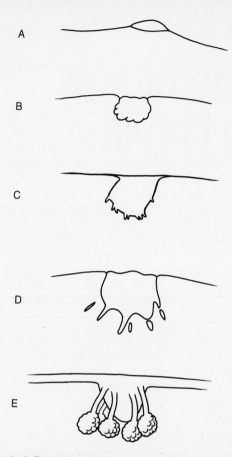

Fig. 2-1. Evolution of the nipple. **A,** Thickening of epidermis with formation of primary bud. **B,** Growth of bud into mesenchyme. **C,** Formation of solid secondary buds. **D,** Formation of mammary pit and vacuolation of buds to form epithelial-lined ducts. **E,** Lactiferous ducts proliferate. Areola is formed. Nipple is inverted initially. (Modified from Weatherly-White, R.C.A.: Plastic surgery of the female breast, Hagerstown, Md., 1980, Harper & Row, Publishers, Inc.)

ing a small amount of milk, known as witch's milk. This very common phenomenon among both male and female infants is caused by the stimulation of the infant's mammary glands by the same hormones produced by the placenta to prepare the mother's breast for lactation. This subsides quickly and from then on the mammary glands are inactive until shortly before the onset of puberty, when hormones begin to stimulate growth again.

The breast is located in the superficial fascia between the second rib and sixth intercostal cartilage and is superficial to the pectoralis major muscle. It tends to overlap this muscle inferiorly to become superficial to the external oblique and serratus anterior muscles. It measures 10 to 12 cm in diameter. It is located horizontally from the para-

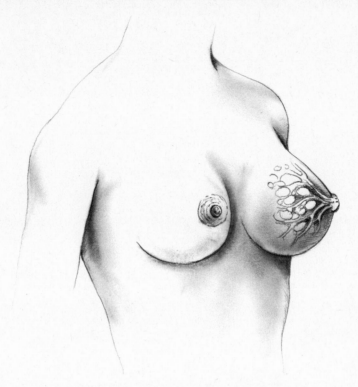

Fig. 2-2. Mammary gland in longitudinal cross section showing mature nonlactating duct system.

sternal to midaxillary line. The central thickness of the breast is 5 to 7 cm (Fig. 2-2).

At puberty the breasts in the female enlarge to their adult size, one, the left, frequently being slightly larger than the other. In a nonpregnant woman, the mature breast weighs approximately 200 g. During pregnancy there is some increased size and weight, thus near term the breast weighs between 400 and 600 g. During lactation the breast weighs between 600 and 800 g (Fig. 2-3).

The shape of the breast varies from woman to woman, just as do body build and facial characteristics. Commonly the breast is dome shaped or conic in adolescence, becoming more hemispheric and finally pendulous in the parous female. There is some projection of mammary glandular tissue into the axillary region. This is known as the tail of Spence. The presence of this mammary tissue becomes more obvious during the period of lactation. The three major structures are skin, subcutaneous tissue, and corpus mammae. The corpus mammae is the breast mass that remains after freeing the breast from the deep attachments and removing the skin, subcutaneous connective tissue, and adipose tissue.

The breast of the adult female develops from a line of glandular tissue, which is found in the fetus, known as the milk line. Hypermastia is the presence of accessory

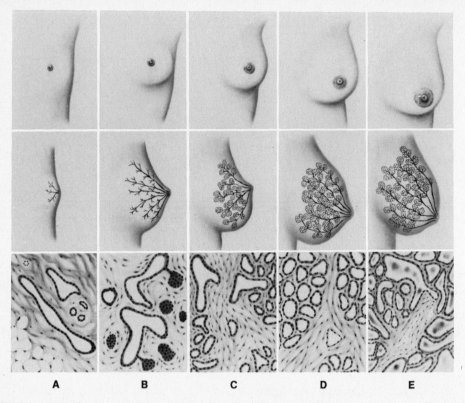

Fig. 2-3. Female breast from infancy to lactation with corresponding cross section and duct structure. A, B, and C, Gradual development of well-differentiated ductular and peripheral lobular-alevolar system. D, Ductular sprouting and intensified peripheral lobular-alveolar development in pregnancy. Glandular luminal cells begin actively synthesizing milk fat and proteins near term; only small amounts are released into lumen. E, With postpartum withdrawal of luteal and placental sex steroids and placental lactogen, prolactin is able to induce full secretory activity of alveolar cells and release of milk into alveoli and smaller ducts.

mammary glands, which are phylogenic remnants of the embryonic mammary ridge. Because of this origin, accessory nipples and glandular tissue may be found along these lines, which extend from the clavicular to the inguinal regions. Occasionally, supernumerary glands are found in the urogenital region, on the buttocks, or on the back as well. The glands are derived from the ectoderm, whereas the connective tissue stroma is mesodermal in origin (Fig. 2-4).

The accessory tissue may involve the corpus mammae, the areola, and the nipple.[8] From 2% to 6% of women have hypermastia. The response of hypermastia to pregnancy and lactation depends on the tissue present. Hyperthelia is the presence of nipple tissue without breast tissue, and hyperadenia is the presence of mammary tissue without nipples. The swelling and secretion of this tissue may produce pain during lactation. Occasionally, aberrant breast tissue can cause discomfort or embarrassment in adolescence

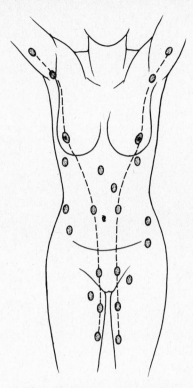

Fig. 2-4. Sites of supernumerary nipples along "milk line." Ectopic nipples, areolae, or breast tissue can develop from the groin to the axilla and upper inner arm. They can lactate or undergo malignant change. (Modified from Weatherly-White, R.C.A.: Plastic surgery of the female breast, Hagerstown, Md., 1980, Harper & Row, Publishers, Inc.)

and during menses, especially when located in the axilla.[5] In rare cases, it may be appropriate to surgically remove the tissue, a treatment well known to experienced plastic surgeons. If treatment is not initiated before pregnancy and lactation, in these cases, the symptomatology of pain and swelling will be intensified and may progress to mastitis or the necessity to terminate lactation.

Corpus mammae

The mammary gland is a conglomeration of a variable number of independent glands. Surgical dissection of many postoperative specimens has contributed more precise information about the anatomic structure.[4] The ramifications of the lactiferous ducts and stroma were carefully studied by Hicken, who reported that in 95% of women the ducts ascend into the axilla, occasionally following the brachial plexus and axillary vessels into the apex of the axilla. Ducts are found in the epigastric region in 15% of women. In rare cases, ducts cross the midline (Fig. 2-5).

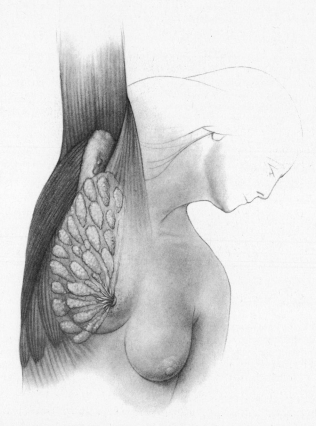

Fig. 2-5. Ramification of lactiferous ducts and mammary tissue. The ducts extend onto the upper medial aspect of the arm, to the midline, and into the epigastrium. A composite drawing from mammographic studies. (Modified from Hicken, N.F.: Arch. Surg. **40**:6, 1940.)

The morphology of the corpus mammae includes two major divisions, the parenchyma and the stroma.[1] The parenchyma includes the ductular-lobular-alveolar structures. It is composed of the alveolar gland with treelike ductular branching alveoli. The alveoli are approximately 0.12 mm in diameter. The ducts are approximately 2.0 mm in diameter. The lactiferous sinuses are 5 to 8 mm in diameter. The lobi, which are arranged like spokes converging on the central nipple, are 15 to 25 in number. Each lobus is divided again into 20 to 40 lobuli, and each lobulus is again subdivided into 10 to 100 alveoli for tubulosaccular secretory units. The stroma includes the connective tissue, fat tissue, blood vessels, nerves, and lymphatics.

The mass of tissue in the breast consists of the tubuloalveolar glands embedded in

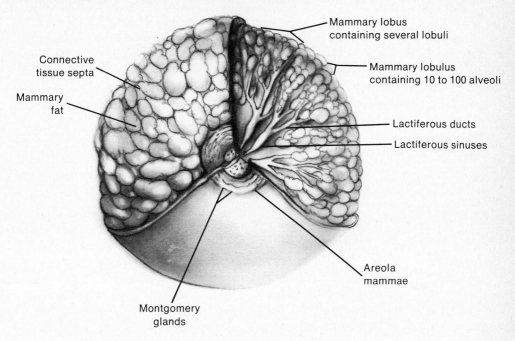

Connective
tissue septa

Mammary
fat

Mammary lobus
containing several lobuli

Mammary lobulus
containing 10 to 100 alveoli

Lactiferous ducts

Lactiferous sinuses

Areola
mammae

Montgomery
glands

Fig. 2-6. Morphology of mature breast with dissection to reveal mammary fat and duct system.

fat (the adipose tissue), giving the gland its smooth, rounded contour. The mammary fat pad is essential for the proliferation and differentiation of the mammary epithelium, providing the necessary space, support, and local control for duct elongation and, ultimately, lobuloalveolar proliferation. Each gland forms a lobe of the breast, and the lobes are separated by connective tissue septa. These septa attach to the skin. Each tubuloalveolar gland opens into a lactiferous duct, which leads into a more dilated area, the lactiferous sinus; there is a slight constriction before the sinus opens onto the surface of the nipple (Fig. 2-6). Extension of ducts within the fat pad is orderly. There is an inhibitory zone around each duct into which other ducts cannot penetrate, and development does not normally proceed beyond the duct end-bud stage before puberty.

Nipple and areola

The skin of the breast includes the nipple, the areola, and the general skin. The skin is the thin, flexible, elastic cover of the breast adherent to the fat-laden subcutaneous tissue. It contains hair, sebaceous glands, and apocrine sweat glands. The nipple, or papilla mammae, is a conic elevation located in the center of the areola at about the fourth intercostal space, slightly below the midpoint of the breast. Although very different in size, the nipples and areolae of women and men are qualitatively identical.[7] The nipple contains 15 to 25 milk ducts. Each of the tubuloalveolar glands that make up the breast opens onto the nipple by a separate opening. It also contains smooth muscle fibers and sensory nerve endings and is well supplied with sebaceous and apocrine sweat glands, but no hair. The nipple is surrounded by the areola, or areola mammae, a circular pigmented area. It is usually pink before pregnancy, turning reddish brown during pregnancy, and always maintaining some pigmentation thereafter. The areola measures 15 to 16 mm in diameter, enlarging during pregnancy and lactation. The pigmentation is due to many melanocytes distributed throughout the skin and glands. The understructure of the epidermis of the areola is not as elaborate as that of the nipple but intermediate to that of the surrounding skin.

Little or no true lobuloalveolar development occurs before the first pregnancy. A framework is laid down within which the specialized secretory cells will proliferate. The framework forms a vital part of the gland's overall developmental course, and maldevelopment or trauma during fetal or juvenile life can seriously reduce the size and secretory potential of the mature gland.

Morgagni's tubercles containing the ductular openings of the Montgomery glands are present in the areola. The Montgomery glands are large sebaceous glands with miniature ducts opening into the skin of the areola. Sweat glands and smaller free sebaceous glands are also present in the areola. The corium of the areola lacks fat, but it contains smooth muscle and collagenous and elastic connective tissue fibers in radial and circular arrangements (see Fig. 2-8). The Montgomery glands become enlarged and look like small pimples during pregnancy and lactation. They secrete a substance that lubricates and protects the nipples and areolae during nursing. After lactation, these glands recede again to their former unobtrusive state. The areola and nipple are darker than the rest of the breast, ranging from light pink in very fair-skinned women to very dark brown in others. The darker color of the areola may be some sort of visual signal to the newborn infant so that he will close his mouth on the areola, not on the nipple alone, to obtain milk. Nipple erection is induced by tactile, sensory, or autonomic sympathetic stimuli. The dermis of the nipple and the areola contains a large number of multibranched free nerve fiber endings. Local venostasis and hyperemia occur to enhance the process of erection of the nipple because the nipple and areola are rich in arterial venous anastomoses. The glabrous skin of the nipple is wrinkled, containing large papillae of the corium.

Each nipple contains 15 to 25 lactiferous ducts surrounded by fibromuscular tissue (Figs. 2-7 to 2-12). These ducts end as small orifices near the tip of the nipple. Within the nipple, the lactiferous ducts may merge. The ductular orifices, therefore, are sometimes fewer in number than the respective breast lobi. The milk ducts within the nipple dilate at the nipple base into the cone-shaped ampullae of milk sinuses. The ampullae function as temporary milk containers during lactation but contain only epithelial debris in the nonlactating state. The lining of the infundibular and ampullar parts of the lactiferous ducts consists of an eight to ten cell-layered squamous epithelium. The bulk of the nipple is composed of smooth musculature, which represents a closing mechanism for the milk ducts and sinuses of the nipple (see Fig. 2-10). The milk ducts in the nipple are embedded in stretchable and mobile connective tissue. The inner longitudinal muscular arrangements and the outer, more circular and radial, arrangements do not obstruct the milk ducts. Tangential fibers also branch off from the more circular muscular fibers of the nipple bases to the outer circular muscular range. The functions of the muscular fibroelastic system of the areola and nipple include decreasing the surface area of the

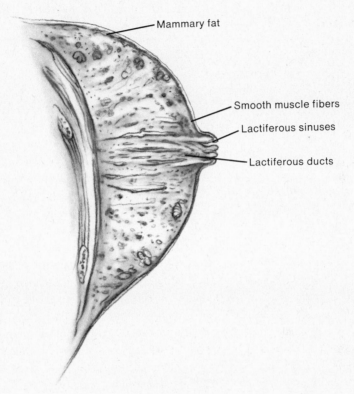

Mammary fat

Smooth muscle fibers

Lactiferous sinuses

Lactiferous ducts

Fig. 2-7. Morphology of mature breast in cross section to reveal lactiferous duct system.

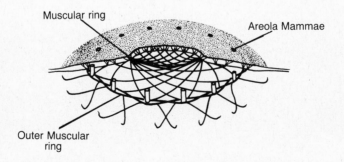

Muscular ring

Areola Mammae

Outer Muscular
ring

Fig. 2-8. The nipple and areola with smooth musculature structure.

areola, producing nipple erection, and emptying the lactiferous sinuses and ducts during nursing. When the nipple erects owing to tactile, thermal, or sexual stimulation, the system causes the nipple to become smaller, firmer, and more prominent.

The mammary tissues are enveloped by the superficial pectoral fascia, and the breast is fixed by fibrous bands to the overlying skin and the underlying pectoral fascia, which are known as Cooper's ligaments (Fig. 2-13). The glandular part of the breast is sur-

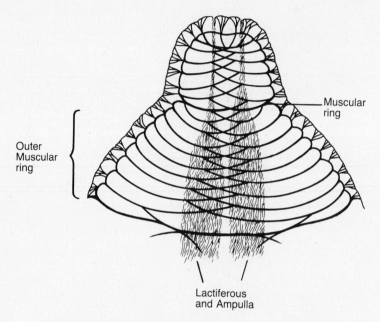

Outer Muscular ring

Muscular ring

Lactiferous and Ampulla

Fig. 2-9. Smooth musculature of areola and nipple in cross section.

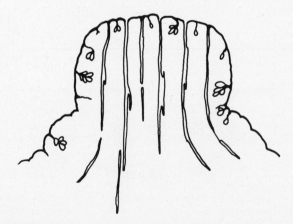

Fig. 2-10. Cross section of the nipple. The epidermis has long dermal papillae and is glabrous and heavily pigmented. Sebaceous glands are found near the tip and along the sides of the nipple.

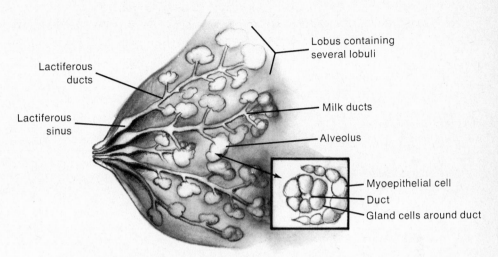

Lobus containing
several lobuli

Lactiferous
ducts

Lactiferous
sinus

Milk ducts

Alveolus

Myoepithelial cell
Duct
Gland cells around duct

Fig. 2-11. Simplified schematic drawing of duct system with cross section of myoepithelial cells around duct opening. Myoepithelial cells contract to eject milk.

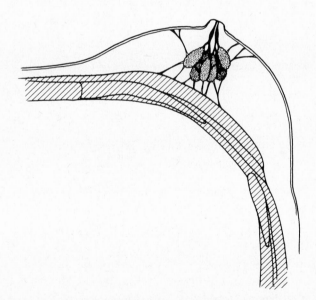

Fig. 2-12. Cross section of ligaments of breast. Ligaments of Cooper suspend the 15 to 20 lobes of the breast within a matrix of fat. They are attached to the lobes, the skin, and the deep fascia.

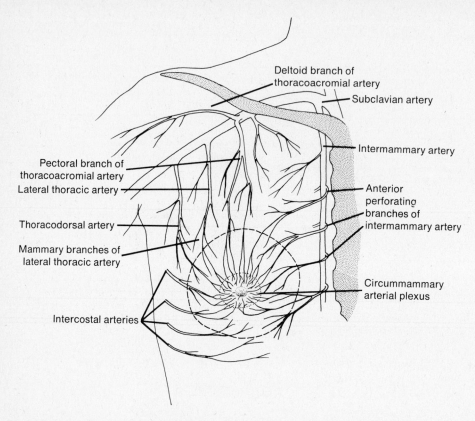

Fig. 2-13. Blood supply to mammary gland. Major blood supply from anterior perforating branches of internal mammary artery.

rounded by a fat layer that seldom extends beyond the lower border of the pectoralis major. The breast is supported by the muscles attached to the ribs, the collar bone, and the bones of the upper arm near the shoulder.

Blood supply

The blood supply to the breast is from branches of the intercostal arteries and the perforating branches of the internal thoracic artery; the third, fourth, and fifth are usually most prominent. The major blood supply to the breast is provided by the internal mammary artery and the lateral thoracic artery. There is a small supply obtained from the intercostal arteries and the arterial branches of the axillary and subclavian arteries, but this contribution is minimal, since 60% of the total breast tissue receives blood from the internal mammary artery. All the mammary branches of this artery lead transversely to the nipple and anastomoses, with branches coming from the lateral thoracic artery.[3] Anastomoses with intercostal arteries are less common, but the blood supply to the

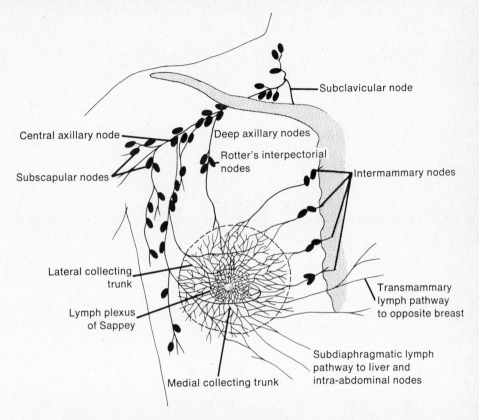

Subclavicular node

Central axillary node

Deep axillary nodes

Rotter's interpectorial nodes

Subscapular nodes

Intermammary nodes

Lateral collecting trunk

Transmammary lymph pathway to opposite breast

Lymph plexus of Sappey

Subdiaphragmatic lymph pathway to liver and intra-abdominal nodes

Medial collecting trunk

Fig. 2-14. Lymphatic drainage of mammary gland. Major drainage is toward axilla.

nipple is extensive and close to the surface, contributing to the pink color. Many areas of the breast are supplied by two or three different arterial sources. The veins end in the internal thoracic and the axillary veins. Some veins may reach the external jugular vein (Fig. 2-14).

Lymphatic drainage

The lymphatic drainage of the breast has been the subject of considerable study because of the frequency of breast cancer, but it has significance for the lactating breast as well. The lymphatic drainage can be quite extensive. The main drainage is to axillary nodes and to the parasternal nodes along the internal thoracic artery inside the thoracic cavity. The lymphatics of the breast originate in the lymph capillaries of the mammary connective tissue, which surrounds the mammary structures, and drain through the deep substance of the breast. The lymph drainage of the breast consists of the superficial, or cutaneous section, the areola, and the glandular, or deep-tissue section. Other points of

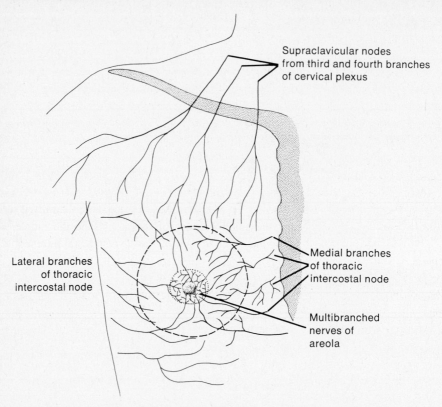

Supraclavicular nodes
from third and fourth branches
of cervical plexus

Medial branches
of thoracic
intercostal node

Lateral branches
of thoracic
intercostal node

Multibranched
nerves of
areola

Fig. 2-15. Innervation of mammary gland supraclavicular nerves and lateral and medial branches of intercostal nerves provide sensory innervation. Sympathetic and motor nerves are provided by supracervical and intercostal nerves.

drainage are to pectoral nodes between the pectoralis major and minor muscles and to the subclavicular nodes in the neck deep to the clavicle. There is some transmammary lymph drainage to the opposite breast as well as subdiaphragmatic lymphatics that lead ultimately to the liver and intra-abdominal nodes (Fig. 2-15).

Innervation of the mammary gland

The nerves of the breast are from branches of the fourth, fifth, and sixth intercostal nerves and consist of sensory fibers and sympathetic fibers innervating the smooth muscles in the nipple and blood vessels. The sensory innervation of the nipple and areola is extensive and consists of both autonomic and sensory nerves. The innervation of the corpus mammae is minimal by comparison and predominantly autonomic. There are no parasympathetic or cholinergic fibers supplying any part of the breast. There are no ganglia found in mammary tissue. Norepinephrine-containing nerve fibers are abundant among the smooth muscle cells of the nipple and at the interface between the media and adventitia of the breast arteries. Physiological observations demonstrate that the efferent nerves to these structures are sympathetic adrenergic.

The majority of the mammary nerves follow the arteries and arterioles and supply these structures. A few fibers from the perivascular networks course along the walls of the ducts. They may correspond to sensory fibers for sensing milk pressure. No innervation of mammary myoepithelial cells has been identified. It can therefore be concluded that secretory activities of the acinar epithelium depend on hormonal stimulation, such as that of prolactin, and other hormones and are not stimulated via the nervous system directly.

Stimulation of the sensory nerve fibers or sensory receptors does induce the release of adenohypophyseal prolactin and neurohypophyseal oxytocin via an afferent sensory reflex pathway whereby stimuli reach the hypothalamus. Sympathetic mammary stimulation causes the contraction of the small muscles of the areola and the nipple. The locally released norepinephrine induces stimulation of the myoepithelial adrenergic receptors, causing muscular relaxation. In the absence of parasympathetic activity, a minor physiological catamine inhibitory effect on the mammary myoepithelium may exist, which is overcome by oxytocin release during suckling, inducing myoepithelial contraction.

The supraclavicular nerves supply the sensory fibers for innervation of the upper cutaneous parts of the breast. Branches of the intercostal nerves provide the major sensory innervation of the mammary gland. The sympathetic sensory and motor fibers are derived from the supraclavicular and intercostal nerves, respectively. Sympathetic fibers only run along the mammary gland—supplying arteries to innervate the glandular body. There is relatively restricted innervation to the epidermal parts of the nipple and areola, leading to lack of superficial sensory acuity. Breast sensation was measured in a large number of women by Courtiss and Goldwyn using a device that emitted a variable current producing a burning sensation when the threshold was exceeded.[2] The areola was shown to be the most sensitive and the nipple the least sensitive, with the skin of the breast intermediate. Thus the skin in these areas responds only to major stimuli, such as sucking. The relatively large number of dermal nerve endings provides a high mammary responsiveness toward stimuli for elicitation of the sucking reflex. The neuroreflex induces adequate release of both prolactin and oxytocin. It appears that, in addition to the hormonal actions, breast nerves can also influence the mammary blood supply and milk secretion. Abnormalities of sensory or autonomic nerve distributions in the areola and nipple, therefore, could impair adequate lactation, especially in the functioning of the let-down reflex and the secretion of prolactin and oxytocin.

In summary, the somatic sensory cutaneous nerve supply of the breast includes the supraclavicular nerves and the thoracic intercostal nerves. The autonomic motor nerve supply of the breast is derived from the sympathetic fibers of the intercostal nerves, which supply the smooth musculature of the areola and the nipple. The autonomic motor nerve supply of the breast is also derived from sympathetic fibers of the accompanying

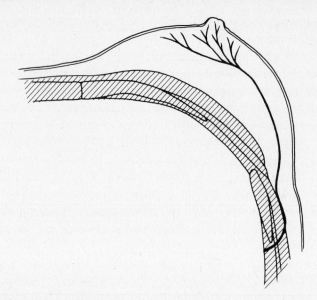

Fig. 2-16. Cross section of nerve supply of the breast and nipple. The cutaneous nerves run close to the deep fascia before turning outward toward the skin.

arteries, which innervate the smooth musculature of the inner glandular blood vessel walls to produce constriction. The nerve supply to the area of the areola and the nipple includes free sensory nerve endings, tactile corpuscles to the papillae of the corium of the nipple and areola, and the fibers around the larger lactiferous duct and in the dermis of the areola and peripheral breast. All cutaneous nerves run radially to the glandular body toward the nipple. The nerve supply to the inner gland is sparse and contains only sympathetic nerves accompanying blood vessels (Fig. 2-16).

MICROSCOPIC ANATOMY

In their structure and mode of development, the mammary glands somewhat resemble the sweat glands. During embryonic life, their differentiation is similar in the two sexes. The male experiences little additional development postnatally. The female, in contrast, experiences extensive structural change paralleling her age and the functional state of the reproductive system.

The greatest development in the female is reached by the twentieth year. Gradual changes are correlated with the menstrual cycle, and major changes accompany pregnancy and lactation.

Resting mammary gland

The mammary gland is a compound tubuloalveolar gland containing 15 to 25 irregular lobes radiating from the nipple.[1] Each lobe has a lactiferous duct (2 to 4 mm in diameter) lined by stratified squamous epithelium. The duct opens on the nipple and has an irregular angular outline. Beneath the areola each duct has a local dilation, the lactiferous sinus, and finally emerges at the end of the nipple as a 0.4 to 0.7 mm opening. Each lobe is subdivided into lobules of various orders; the smallest are elongated tubules, the alveolar ducts, covered by small saccular evaginations, the alveoli. The interlobular connective tissue is dense; however, it is more cellular, has fewer collagenous fibers, and contains almost no fat. Greater distensibility is permitted by the looser connective tissue.

The secretory portions of the gland, the alveolar ducts and the alveoli, have cuboidal or low-columnar secretory cells, resting on basal laminae and myoepithelial cells. These myoepithelial cells enclose the alveoli in a loosely meshed network with their many starlike branchings. The myoepithelial cells are stimulated by prolactin and sex steroids. The presence of myoepithelial cells has been used as evidence that the mammary gland is related to the sweat gland.

In the resting phase, epithelial structures consist of the ducts and their branches. The presence of a few alveoli budded off from the ends of ducts is still under discussion. This variance may be due to the effect of the menstrual cycle. The swelling and engorgement accompanying the menstrual cycle are associated with hyperemia and some edema of the connective tissue. Most significant is the fact that the gland does not have a single duct, but many. Each lobe is a separate compound alveolar gland whose primary ducts join into larger and larger ducts. These ducts drain into a lactiferous duct. Each lactiferous duct drains separately at the tip of the nipple.

The epidermis of the nipple and areola is invaded by unusually long dermal papillae whose capillaries richly vascularize the surface and impart the pinkish hue. Bundles of smooth muscle, placed longitudinally along the lactiferous ducts and circumferentially within the nipple and at its base, permit the erection of the nipple. In the areola are the areolar Montgomery glands, which are intermediate in their microscopic structure between sweat glands and true mammary glands. The periphery of the areola also has sweat glands and sebaceous glands (see Fig. 2-7).

Mammary gland in pregnancy

Changes in levels of circulating hormones result in profound changes in the ductular-lobular-alveolar growth during pregnancy. During the first trimester there is rapid growth and branching from the terminal portion of the duct system. As the epithelial structures proliferate, the adipose tissue seems to diminish. During this time there is increasing infiltration of the interstitial tissue with lymphocytes, plasma cells, and eosinophils. The rate of hyperplasia levels off. In the last trimester, any enlargement is the result of enlargement of the parenchymal cells and the distention of the alveoli with early colostrum, which is rich in protein and relatively low in lipid. There is a gradual accumulation of fat droplets in the secretory alveolar cells. The interlobular connective tissue is noticeably decreased and alveolar proliferation extensive. The histologic appearance of the gland is quite variable. The functional state appears to vary from dilated, thin-walled lumen to narrow-lumened, thick-walled glandular tissue. Epithelial cells vary, being flat to low columnar in shape with indistinct boundaries. Some cells protrude into the lumen of the alveoli; others are short and smooth. The lumen of the alveoli is crowded with fine granular material and lipid droplets similar to those protruding from the cells.

The former concepts of mammary gland secretion indicated that the mode of release was apocrine secretion. Apocrine secretion is the process by which the cell undergoes partial disintegration. A fat-filled portion projects into the lumen; the fat globule constricts at the base, and the cell replaces itself. Electron microscopy has shown that the cell has two distinct secretory products, formed and released by different mechanisms. The protein constituents of milk are formed and released identically to those of other protein-secreting glands, classed as merocrine glands. Secretory materials are passed out through the cell apex without appreciable loss of cytoplasm in merocrine glands. The fatty components of milk arise as lipid droplets free in the cytoplasmic matrix. The droplets increase in size and move into the apex of the cell. They project into the lumen, covered by a thin layer of cytoplasm. The droplets are ultimately cast off, enveloped by a detached portion of the cell membrane and a thin rim of subjacent cytoplasm. This process is referred to as apocrine, since it involves the loss of some cytoplasm (Fig. 2-3).

Lactating mammary gland

The lactating mammary gland is characterized by a large number of alveoli. The alveoli of the lactating gland are made up of cuboidal epithelial and myoepithelial cells. Only a small amount of connective tissue separates the neighboring alveoli. Under special preparations, lipid can be seen as small droplets within the cells. These droplets become larger and are discharged into the lumen.

The functioning of the mammary gland depends on the interplay of multiple and complex nervous and endocrine factors. Some factors are involved in the development of the mammary glands to a functional state (mammogenesis), others in the establishment of milk secretion (lactogenesis), and others in responsibility for the maintenance of lactation (galactopoiesis).

The division and differentiation of mammary epithelial cells and presecretory alveolar cells into secretory milk-releasing alveolar cells takes place in the third trimester. Stimulation of RNA synthesis promotes galactopoiesis and apocrine milk secretion into the alveoli. The DNA and RNA content of the cellular nuclei increases during pregnancy and is highest at lactation (see Fig. 2-3).

Postlactation regression of the mammary gland

If milk is not removed from the breast, the glands become greatly distended and milk production gradually ceases. Part of the decrease is due to the lack of stimulation of sucking, which initiates the neurohormonal reflex for maintenance of prolactin secretion. Perhaps a stronger effect is the engorgement of the breast with compression of blood vessels, causing diminished flow. The diminished flow results in decreased oxytocin to the myoepithelium. The alveoli are greatly distended and the epithelium flattened. The secretion remaining in the alveolar spaces and ducts is absorbed. There is a gradual collapse of the alveoli and an increase in perialveolar connective tissue. The glandular elements gradually return to the resting state. Adipose tissue increases. There are increased macrophages. The gland does not return completely to the prepregnancy state, in that the alveoli formed do not totally involute. Some appear as scattered, solid cords of epithelial cells.

Microscopically, there are increased autophagic and heterophagic processes in the first few days after weaning. Lysosomal enzymes increase, whereas nonlysosomal enzymes decrease.

Although the process of regression has been studied carefully in animals, little study has been done in the human. It is probable that slow weaning, which usually takes 3 months, has a very different timetable than abrupt weaning, in which marked involution has been intense and rapid over a matter of days or weeks.

REFERENCES

1. Bloom, W., and Fawcett, D.W.: A textbook of histology, ed. 10, Philadelphia, 1975, W.B. Saunders Co.
2. Courtiss, E.H., and Goldwyn, R.M.: Breast sensation before and after plastic surgery, Plast. Reconstr. Surg. 58:1, 1976.
3. Crafts, R.C.: A textbook of human anatomy, New York, 1966, Ronald Press Co.
4. Hicken, N.F.: Mastectomy: a clinical pathologic study demonstrating why most mastectomies result in incomplete removal of the mammary gland, Arch. Surg. 40:6, 1940.
5. Kaye, B.L.: Axillary breasts: a significant esthetic deformity, Plast. Reconstr. Surg. 53:61, 1974.
6. Knight, C.H., and Peaker, M.: Development of the mammary gland: Symposium Report No. 19, Lactation, J. Reprod. 65:521, 1982.
7. Montagna, W., and Macpherson, E.E.: Some neglected aspects of the anatomy of human breasts, J. Invest. Dermatol. 63:10, 1974.
8. Vorherr, H.: The breast: morphology, physiology, and lactation, New York, 1974, Academic Press, Inc.
9. Weatherley-White, R.C.A.: Plastic surgery of the female breast, Hagerstown, Md., 1980, Harper & Row, Publishers, Inc.

Physiology of lactation

3

Lactation is an integral part of the reproductive cycle of all mammals, including humans. The hormonal control of lactation can be described under three main headings: mammogenesis, or mammary growth; lactogenesis, or initiation of milk secretion; and galactopoiesis, or the maintenance of established milk secretion.

Under the influence of sex steroids, especially the estrogens, the mammary glandular epithelium proliferates, becoming multilayered. Buds and papillae then form. The growth of the mammary gland is a gradual process that starts during puberty. It has been shown to depend on pituitary hormones. Lobuloalveolar development and ductal proliferation also depend on an intact pituitary gland.

Mammogenesis: mammary growth

PREPUBERTAL GROWTH. The primary and secondary ducts that develop in the fetus *in utero* continue to grow in both the male and the female in proportion to growth in general. Shortly before puberty, a more rapid expansion of the duct system begins in the female. The growth of the duct system seems to depend predominantly on estrogen and does not occur in the absence of ovaries. The complete growth of the alveoli requires stimulation by progesterone as well.

Studies of hypophysectomized animals have shown failure of full mammary growth even with adequate estrogen and progesterone. It has been shown that it is the secretion of prolactin and somatotropin by the pituitary gland that effects mammary growth. Adrenocorticotropic hormone (ACTH) and thyroid-stimulating hormone (TSH) acting on the adrenal gland and the thyroid gland also play a minor role in growth of the mammary gland.

PUBERTAL GROWTH. When the hypophyseal-ovarian-uterine cycle is established, a new phase of mammary growth begins, which includes extensive branching of the system of ducts and proliferation and canalization of the lobuloalveolar units at the distal tips of the branches. Organization of the stromal connective tissue forms the interlobular septa. The ducts, ductules (terminal intralobular ducts), and alveolar structures are all formed by double layers of cells. One layer, the epithelial cells, circumscribes the lumen. The second layer, the myoepithelial cells, surrounds the inner epithelial cells and is bordered by a basement lamina.

MENSTRUAL CYCLE GROWTH.   The cyclical changes of the adult mammary gland can be associated with the menstrual cycle and the hormonal changes that control that cycle. Estrogens stimulate parenchymal proliferation, with formation of epithelial sprouts. This hyperplasia continues into the secretory phase of the cycle. Anatomically, when the corpus luteum provides increased amounts of estrogens and progesterone, there is lobular edema, thickening of the epithelial basal membrane, and secretory material in the alveolar lumen. Lymphoid and plasma cells infiltrate the stroma. Clinically, there is increased mammary blood flow in this luteal phase. This is experienced by women as fullness, heaviness, and turgescence. The breast may become nodular because of interlobular edema and ductular-acinar growth.

After the onset of menstruation and the reduction of sex steroid levels, there is limited milk-secretory prolactin action. Postmenstrual changes occur rapidly, with degeneration of glandular cells and proliferation tissue, loss of edema, and decrease in breast size. The ovulatory cycle actually enhances mammary growth in the early years of menstruation (until about age 30) because the postmenstrual regression of the glandular-alveolar growth after each cycle is not complete. These changes of ductal and lobular proliferation, which occur during the follicular phase before ovulation, continue in the luteal phase and regress after the menstrual phase, exemplifying the sensitivity of this target organ to variations in the balance of hormones.

GROWTH DURING PREGNANCY.   Hormonal influences on the breast cause profound changes during pregnancy (Fig. 3-1). Early in pregnancy a marked increase in ductular sprouting, branching, and lobular formation is evoked by luteal and placental hormones. Placental lactogen, prolactin, and chorionic gonadotropin have been identified as contributors to the accelerated growth. The dichorionic ductular sprouting has been attributed to estrogen, and lobular formation has been attributed to progesterone.

From the third month of gestation, secretory material that resembles colostrum appears in the acini. Prolactin from the anterior pituitary gland stimulates the glandular production of colostrum. By the second trimester, placental lactogen begins to stimulate the secretion of colostrum. The effectiveness of hormonal stimulation on lactation has been demonstrated by the fact that a mother who delivers after 16 weeks of gestation will secrete colostrum, even though she has had a nonviable infant.

An estrogen-mediated increase in prolactin secretion in pregnancy may produce as much as a tenfold to twentyfold increase in plasma prolactin. This effect may be partially controlled by lactogen from the placenta, which inhibits the production of prolac-

GESTATION

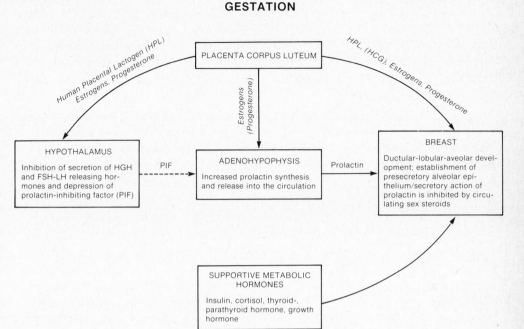

Fig. 3-1. Hormonal preparation during pregnancy of breast for lactation. (Modified from Vorherr, H.: The breast, morphology, physiology and lactation, New York, 1974, Academic Press, Inc.)

tin. Hormonal regulation of the growth and proliferation of the mammary gland cells has been carefully studied in many species.

There is a complex sequence of events, governed by hormonal action, that prepare the breast for lactation (Fig. 3-1). Estradiol 17β stimulates the ductal system of epithelial cells to elongate during pregnancy. Progesterone, in turn, induces the specific epithelial cells of the tubular invaginations to produce distinct ducts, which branch from the main tubules. The end result of the combined actions of estrogen and progesterone is a richly branched arborization of the gland. Highly differentiated secretory alveolar cells develop at the ends of these ducts, under the influence of prolactin.

Serum growth factor, which is present in normal human serum, and insulin can stimulate the stem cells of the gland to proliferate. This proliferation is enhanced by estradiol 17β. These dividing cells are further directed to the formation of alveoli by corticosteroid hormones. There are at least two types of cells identified in the epithelial layer of the gland: stem cells and secretory alveolar cells. At this point in the pregnancy, prolactin influences the production of the constituents of milk.

That the high circulating levels of prolactin are not associated with milk production is due in part to the progesterone antagonism of the stimulatory action of prolactin on casein messenger *(m)* RNA synthesis. During late pregnancy, the lactogenic receptors, which have similar affinities for both prolactin and human placental lactogen (HPL), are predominantly occupied by HPL. High doses of estradiol impair the incorporation of prolactin into milk secretory cells.

Lactogenesis: initiation of milk secretion

The breast, one of the most complex endocrine target organs, has been prepared during pregnancy and responds to the release of prolactin by producing the constituents of milk (Fig. 3-2). The lactogenic effects of prolactin are modulated by the complex interplay of pituitary, ovarian, thyroid, adrenal, and pancreatic hormones.

PROLACTIN.   Human prolactin is a significant hormone in pregnancy and lactation.[6] Prolactin also has a range of actions in various species that is greater than any other known hormone. Prolactin has been identified in many animal species whether they nurse their young or not. Because of the original association with lactation, the term describes its action, "support or stimulation of lactation." Prolactin, however, has been shown to control nonlactating responses in other species and has been identified with over 80 different physiological processes. Study of prolactin was hampered until 1970, when it became possible to separate prolactin from human growth hormone (HGH) and to isolate and characterize prolactin from human pituitary glands.[25]

Before 1971, HGH and prolactin in humans were considered to be the same hormone. Until 1971, in fact, it was thought that prolactin did not exist in humans. HGH, however, is present in the human pituitary gland in an amount 100 times that of prolactin.

In vitro, prolactin stimulates the synthesis of the *m* RNAs of specific milk proteins by binding to membrane receptors of the mammary epithelial cells. Prolactin has been demonstrated to penetrate the cytoplasm of these cells and even their nuclei. These specific actions in the gland require the presence of extracellular calcium ions. Some prolactin actually appears in the milk substrate itself, the functional significance of which is uncertain although it is thought to influence fluid and ion absorption from the neonatal jejunum.

The effect of the stimulation of protein synthesis by allowing the expression of milk protein genes is not a direct effect of the hormone, but rather the consequence of the activation of the Na/K ATPase in the plasma membrane. The intracellular concentration of potassium is kept high and sodium low compared with the concentrations in extracellular fluid. As a result, the Na/K ratio is high both in the milk and in the intracellular fluid. Further action of prolactin has been identified in the development of the immune system in the mammary gland and, possibly more directly, in the lymphoid tissue. In conjunction with estrogen and progesterone, prolactin attracts and retains IgA immunoblasts from the gut-associated lymphoid tissue for the development of the immune system for the mammary gland. A very sensitive bioassay has been developed using the in

POSTPARTUM

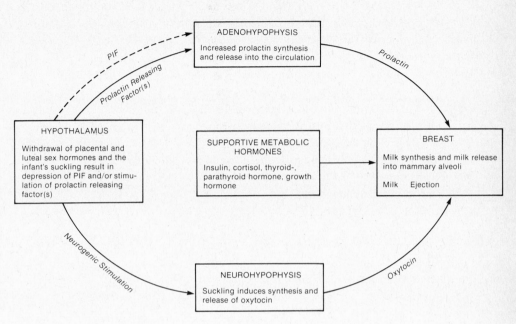

Fig. 3-2. Hormonal preparation of breast postpartum for lactation. (Modified from Vorherr, H.: The breast, morphology, physiology and lactation, New York, 1974, Academic Press, Inc.)

vitro biologic effect of prolactin to stimulate the growth of cell cultures for malignant Nb rat lymphomas.

The levels of prolactin are essentially the same in the normal human male and female. Moreover, both male and female experience a rise in prolactin levels during sleep. At puberty, the increase in estrogens causes a slight but measureable increase in prolactin. There is an increase in prolactin during the proliferative phase of the menstrual cycle but not during the secretory phase. There is also a normal diurnal variation in levels in both male and female. A number of factors, including some that are significant for the nursing mother, increase prolactin levels. Psychogenic influence and stress increase prolactin levels. Anesthesia, surgery, exercise, nipple stimulation, and sexual intercourse also produce increased amounts in both the lactating and nonlactating female. Prolactin levels increase as serum osmolality increases.

PROLACTIN-INHIBITING FACTOR. The prolactin-inhibiting factor (PIF) controls the secretion of prolactin from the hypothalamus. Prolactin thus is unusual among the pituitary hormones, since it is inhibited by a hypothalamic substance. Catecholamine levels in the hypothalamus control the inhibiting factor. The inhibiting factor is poured into the circulation as a result of dopaminergic impulses. Drugs and events that decrease catecholamines also decrease the inhibiting factor, causing a rise in prolactin. Dopamine itself can act directly on the pituitary gland to decrease prolactin secretion. Agents that increase prolactin by decreasing catecholamines and thus the PIF level include the phenothiazines and reserpine. Thyrotropin-releasing hormone (TRH) is a strong stimulator of prolactin secretion, but its physiological role is not clear, since thyrotropin levels do not rise during normal nursing. In the postpartum period, a dose of TRH will cause a marked increase in prolactin. Even the nonnursing postpartum mother will experience engorgement and milk release when stimulated with TRH. Ergot, which is frequently prescribed for the postpartum patient, inhibits prolactin secretion either by direct inhibition or by its effect on the hypothalamus.

Following are factors affecting prolactin release in normal humans[12]:

Physiologic stimuli
    Nursing in postpartum women—breast stimulation
    Sleep
    Stress
    Sexual intercourse
    Pregnancy
Pharmacologic stimuli
    Neuroleptic drugs
    TRH
    Estrogens
    Hypoglycemia
    Phenothiazines
Pharmacologic suppressors
    L-dopa
    Ergot preparations (2-Br-α-ergocryptine)
    Clomiphene citrate
    Large amounts of pyridoxine
    Monoamine oxidase inhibitors
    Prostaglandins E and $F_{2\alpha}$

In pregnancy, prolactin levels begin to rise in the first trimester and continue to rise throughout gestation. In the nonnursing mother, prolactin levels drop to normal in 2 to 3 weeks, independent of therapy to suppress lactation.

At delivery, with the expulsion of the placenta, there is an abrupt decline in estrogens and progesterone. The withdrawal of estrogen triggers the onset of lactation. Estrogens enhance the effect of prolactin on mammogenesis but antagonize prolactin in inhibiting secretion of milk. After delivery, there are low estrogen and high prolactin levels. Suckling provides a continued stimulus for prolactin release. If prolactin, essential for lactation, is diminished by hypophysectomy or medication, lactation ceases. Prolactin levels do eventually diminish to more normal levels months after parturition,

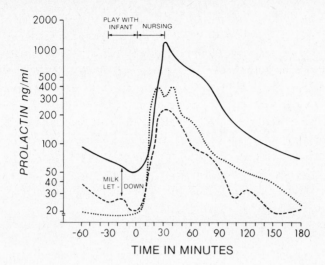

Fig. 3-3. Plasma prolactin measured by radioimmunoassay, before, during, and after period of nursing in three mothers, 22 to 26 days postpartum. Prolactin rose with suckling and not with infant contact. (Modified from Josimovich, J.B., Reynolds, M., and Cobo, E.: Lactogenic hormones, fetal nutrition, and lactation. In Josimovich, J.B., Reynolds, M., and Cobo, E.: Problems of human reproduction, vol. 2, New York, 1974, John Wiley & Sons.)

although lactation may continue. Suckling stimulates the release of adenohypophyseal prolactin and neurohypophyseal oxytocin. These hormones stimulate milk synthesis and production of milk-ejection metabolic hormones, which are also necessary in the process of milk synthesis. Thus suckling, emptying the breast, and receiving adequate precursor nutrients are essential to effective lactation (Fig. 3-3).

The most effective and specific stimulus to prolactin release is nursing. The stimulation is a result of nipple or breast manipulation, especially suckling, not a psychological effect of the presence of the infant (Fig. 3-3). The prolactin-release reflex during nipple stimulation is suppressed in some adult women, being evidenced only during pregnancy and lactation.

In the nursing mother, Tyson et al.[27] have described three types of prolactin response to nursing at the breast (Table 3-1). Stage one occurs during the first week postpartum. Prolactin levels are still elevated; thus suckling causes only small increases. The second stage is observed from the second week to the third month postpartum; baseline levels are two to three times normal and increase to ten to twenty times normal following suckling. During stage three (from the third month until weaning), prolactin levels are back to normal and suckling produces no rise in levels. It is interesting to note that milk production continues to be abundant despite only modest levels of prolactin.

Table 3-1. Prolactin levels

	Range (ng/ml)	Average (ng/ml)
Male and female (throughout menstrual life)	<25	10
Term pregnancy	200-500	200
Amniotic fluid	Up to 10,000	
Lactating women		
Stage one*	200	
Stage two†	2 times normal (resting) 10-20 times normal (during suckling)	
Stage three‡	Normal (no rise with suckling)	

Modified from Tyson, J.E.: Med. Clin. North Am. **61**:153, 1977.
*Stage one—first week postpartum.
†Stage two—second week to third month postpartum.
‡Stage three—beyond third month postpartum.

HUMAN PLACENTAL LACTOGEN AND HUMAN GROWTH HORMONE. There are three main hormones recognized in the lactogenic process: HPL, HGH, and prolactin. The progressive rise in prolactin during pregnancy parallels the rise in HPL, becoming measurable at 6 weeks gestation and increasing to 6000 ng/ml at term. This parallel action contributed to the belief that prolactin and HPL were the same. Although the principal function of HPL and prolactin in the human is a lactogenic one, no lactation appears prior to delivery.[22]

First described in 1962, HPL has been studied more than lactogens from any other species.[16] There is extensive immunologic and structural homology between HGH and HPL, which probably explains their similar biologic activities. Concentrations of HPL increase steadily during gestation and decrease abruptly with the delivery of the placenta. A large–molecular weight substance, HPL is derived from the chorion. Receptor sites that bind lactogen also bind protein and HGH.[28] HPL has been associated with mobilization of free fatty acid and inhibition of peripheral glucose utilization and lactogenic action.[24]

HGH is secreted from the anterior pituitary eosinophilic cells. These cells have been identified by staining techniques that distinguish them from those that produce prolactin. Toward the end of pregnancy, the cells that produce prolactin are noticeably more numerous, whereas those that produce HGH are "crowded out." The role of HGH in the maintenance of lactation is poorly defined and may by synergistic with prolactin and glucocorticords. It has been demonstrated that normal lactation is possible in ateliotic dwarf women in the absence of detectable quantities of HGH.[19] In order for any hormone to exert its biologic effects, however, specific receptors for the hormone must be present in the target tissue. Changes in serum concentration are without effect if receptors are not present in the mammary gland to bind the hormone.

Galactopoiesis: maintenance of established lactation

The maintenance of established milk secretion is called galactopoiesis. An intact hypothalamic-pituitary axis regulating prolactin and oxytocin levels is essential to the initiation and maintenance of lactation.[13] The process of lactation requires milk synthesis and milk release into the alveoli and the lactiferous sinuses. When the milk is not removed, effecting the diminution of capillary blood flow, the lactation process can be inhibited. Lack of sucking stimulation means lack of prolactin release from the pituitary gland. Basal prolactin levels that are enhanced by the spurts that result from sucking are necessary to maintain lactation in the first weeks postpartum. Without oxytocin, however, a pregnancy can be carried to term but the female will fail to lactate because she will fail to let-down.

Sensory nerve endings, located mainly in the areola and nipple, are stimulated by suckling. The afferent neural reflex pathway, via the spinal cord to the mesencephalon and then to the hypothalamus, produces secretion and release of prolactin and oxytocin. Hypothalamic suppression of PIF secretion causes adrenohypophyseal prolactin release. When prolactin is released into the circulation, it stimulates milk synthesis and secretion (Fig. 3-4). A conditioned milk ejection can occur in lactating women without a concomitant release of prolactin so that indeed the releases are independent, which may be significant in treating apparent lactation failure.

HORMONAL REGULATION OF PROLACTIN AND OXYTOCIN.   The release of prolactin is inhibited by PIF.[14] The PIF has not been described, but it is closely associated with dopamine. There is also evidence of either serotonin release of prolactin or catecholamine-serotonin control of prolactin release. TSH has also been shown to stimulate the release of prolactin. In addition, the release of prolactin is related to stress and sleep states. The amount of prolactin is proportional to the amount of nipple stimulation during early stages of lactation.

When suckling occurs, oxytocin is released. It enters the circulation and rapidly causes ejection of milk from alveoli and smaller milk ducts into larger lactiferous ducts and sinuses. This is the pathway of the let-down, or ejection, reflex. Oxytocin also causes contraction of the myometrium and involution of the uterus.

NEUROENDOCRINE CONTROL OF MILK EJECTION. Milk ejection involves both neural and endocrinologic stimulation and response. A neural afferent pathway and an endocrinologic efferent pathway are required.[16]

The ejection reflex depends on the existence of receptors located in the canalicular system of the breast. When the canalicules are dilated or stretched, the reflex release of oxytocin is triggered. There are tactile receptors for both oxytocin and reflex prolactin release located in the nipple. Neither the negative and positive pressures exerted by suckling nor thermal changes trigger the milk-ejection reflex. There is some minor effect of negative pressures, but tactile stimulation is the most important factor.

Studies in tactile stimulation show changes in sensitivity at puberty, during the menstrual cycle, and at parturition.[20] There is no difference in sensitivity between the sexes

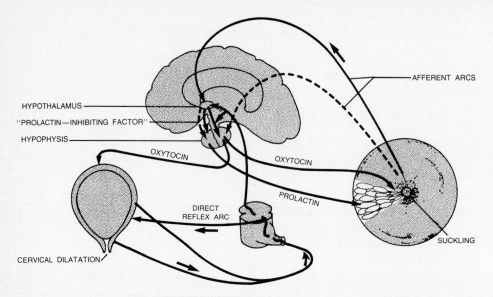

Fig. 3-4. Neuroendocrine control of milk ejection. (Modified from Vorherr, H.: The breast, morphology, physiology and lactation, New York, 1974, Academic Press, Inc.)

before puberty. In the female, tactile sensitivity increases after puberty and is increased at midcycle and during menstruation. (Midcycle peak is absent in women taking oral contraceptives). Dramatic changes occur within 24 hours of delivery after several weeks of complete insensitivity. The nipple is the more sensitive area to both touch and pain, followed by the areola; the least sensitive area is the cutaneous breast tissue. The increased sensitivity of the breast continues several days postpartum, even when the woman does not breastfeed. Estrogen treatment suppresses the induction of prolactin release on nipple stimulation, whereas on withdrawal of estrogen the prolactin response returns. Increased tactile sensitivity may be the key event activating the suckling-induced release of oxytocin and prolactin at delivery (Fig. 3-5).

The release of oxytocin by neurohypophyseal responses during lactation has been evoked both by infant's suckling and by mechanical dilation of the mammary ducts. This release of oxytocin was demonstrated to be independent of vasopressin release. Conversely, further study[13,14] demonstrated that there could be stimulation of vasopressin release independent of oxytocin release.*

Human myoepithelium, the effector tissue, is specifically stimulated by oxytocin, and this sensitivity and specificity increases throughout pregnancy. Suckling can induce milk secretion, which is under control of the adenohypophysis. In this case, oxytocin

---

*It has been shown that alcohol has an effect on the CNS in inhibiting milk ejection. This effect is dose related.

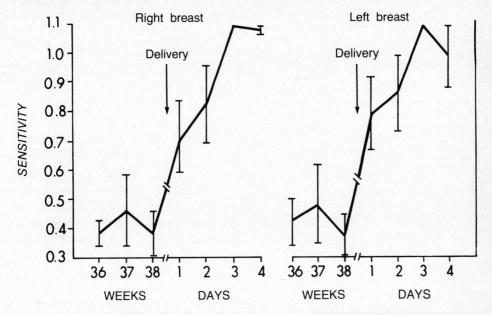

Fig. 3-5. Changes in tactile sensitivity of cutaneous breast tissue in perinatal period. Sensitivity was calculated from two-point discrimination according to the formula K-log^e. K is an arbitrary figure employed to portray low two-point discrimination values as peaks of sensitivity. (From Robinson, J.E., and Short, R.V., Br. Med. J. 1:1188, 1977.)

released by the neurohypophysis because of the suckling stimulus would cause both milk ejection and release of the anterior pituitary hormones responsible for milk secretion as well. This is probably the mechanism behind relactation and induced lactation in the woman who has never been pregnant. Mammary growth and lactogenesis may be induced by suckling, massage, and breast stimulation in many species.[5]

Suckling brings about functional changes in the offspring. When an infant sucks on an artificial nipple, he quickly decreases the amount of body movement, increases his mouth activity, and decreases crying. The suckling experience may affect infant behavior and mother-infant interaction. Nonnutritive sucking is observed in many species. In the human infant, nutritive sucking is shown to be a continuous stream of regular sucks with few, if any, pauses. Nonnutritive sucking has bursts of activity alternating with no sucking. Suckling can be altered by extraneous aural, visual, or olfactory stimuli.

Effects of suckling on the mother include the stimulation of afferent nerves for the removal of milk.[15] Reduction in sucking stimulus produces a reduction in prolactin and in milk synthesis. The lactating glands are good at adjusting the milk supply to demand, probably because of both a local and an endocrinologic mechanism. Variations in milk secretion are rapidly reflected in anatomic changes in the mammary gland. Mammary tissue shows regression after the first week or so, if unstimulated. Tissue regression proceeds at a rate parallel to the demand for secretory tissue. Thus, when suckling infant signals his needs, the breast will respond.

There are effects on maternal behavior that have been attributed to lactation. Maternal behavior is more easily defined in many other species, in which early nursing is initiated by the mother, who stimulates the neonate to suckle by grooming him. She then presents her mammary gland to the offspring so that the nipple is located with minimal effort. It has been shown that lactating females have a lessened response to stress. In the human, however, there is a strong voluntary nature to nursing behavior.

If one explores the possible spinal and brain stem pathways by which the suckling stimulus reaches the forebrain, the spinothalamic tract is the most likely. The areas of the forebrain influenced by the sucking stimulus include the hypothalamic structures that mediate oxytocin and prolactin release. The inhibition of milk ejection by visual and auditory stimuli, pinealectomy, and ventrolateral midbrain lesions in lactating rats has been studied to define further the neurohormonal pathways. In these experiments, the pineal gland appeared to mediate an inhibitory visual reflex on both oxytocin release and milk ejection.[8,18]

SYNTHESIS OF HUMAN MILK

The function of the mammary gland is unique in that it produces a material that makes tremendous demands on the maternal system without producing any physiologic advantage to the maternal organism. Because lactation is anticipated, the body prepares the breast anatomically and physiologically.[23] When lactation begins there is a marked alteration in the metabolism of the mother. There is a redistribution of the blood supply and an increased demand for nutrients, which requires an increased metabolic rate to accommodate the production. The mammary gland may have to produce milk at the metabolic expense of other organs. The supply of materials to the lactating breast for milk production and energy metabolism requires extensive cardiovascular changes in the mother. There is increased mammary blood flow, increased blood flow into the gastrointestinal tract and liver, and a high cardiac output. The mammary blood flow, cardiac output, and milk secretion are suckling dependent. Suckling induces the release of anterior pituitary hormones that act directly on breast tissue.

Milk is isosmotic with plasma in all species. Human milk differs from many other milks in that the concentration of major monovalent ions is lower and of lactose is higher. If one looks at other milks, the higher the ions, the lower the lactose, and vice versa. Many of the disparities in the intermediary metabolism among species of animals can be linked to evolutionary adaptions involving the digestive process. Nonruminants rely on glucose, derived from carbohydrate in the diet. Ruminants, because of extensive fermentation in the rumen, absorb little glucose. The microbial fermentation products, which include acetate, propionate, and butyrate, play a significant part as energy and carbon sources for tissue metabolism. Amino acids are primary substitutes for glucose in ruminants.

The biosynthesis of milk involves a cellular site where the metabolic processes occur. The epithelial cells of the gland contain stem cells and highly differentiated secretory alveolar cells at the terminal ducts. The stem cells are stimulated by HGH and insulin. Prolactin synergizes the insulin effect to stimulate the cells to secretory activity.

The cells of the acini and smaller milk ducts are active in milk synthesis and the secretion of the milk into the alveoli and smaller milk ducts. Most milk is synthesized during the process of suckling; its production is stimulated by prolactin. Cortisol plasma levels are increased during suckling as well. The secretory cells are cuboidal, changing to a cylindrical shape just before milk secretion, while cellular water uptake is increased. The cell's single nucleus is at the base in the dormant cell but migrates to the apex just prior to milk secretion.

The cytoplasm is finely granular in the resting phase, but striated as milk secretion begins. As secretion commences, the enlarged cell with its thickened apical membrane becomes clublike in shape. The tip pinches off, leaving the cell intact. The protein is thus free in the secreted solution, retaining a cap of membrane (Fig. 3-6).

Milk is therefore secreted by apocrine and merocrine mechanisms. There is minimal glandular mitosis in the lactating breast (Fig. 3-7).

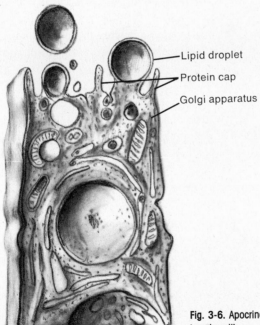

Lipid droplet
Protein cap
Golgi apparatus

Fig. 3-6. Apocrine secretory mechanism for lipids, proteins, and lactose in milk.

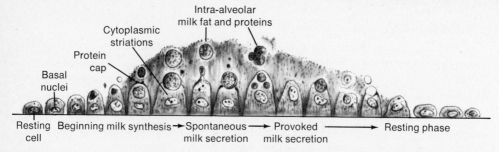

Fig. 3-7. Diagram of cycle of secretory cells from resting stage to secretion and return to resting stage. (Modified from Vorherr, H.: The breast, morphology, physiology and lactation, New York, 1974, Academic Press, Inc.)

Function of the cellular components of the lactating breast

The schematic representation of the mammary secretory cell has been described by Davis and Bowman[3] (Fig. 3-8).

NUCLEUS.   The nucleus is essential to the duplication of genetic material and the transcription of the genetic code. The nucleus is also considered a regulatory organelle in cell metabolism, transmitting the design of the enzymatic profile of the cell. The DNA and RNA content of the cellular nuclei increases during pregnancy and is highest at the time of lactation.

CYTOSOL.   The cytosol, which consists of the cytoplasm minus the mitochondrial and microsomal fractions, is also called the particle-free supernatant. The cytosol contains enzymes that involve key intermediates and cofactors essential to the process of milk synthesis.

MITOCHONDRIAL PROLIFERATION.   The alveolar cell population of the mammary gland must have a greatly expanded oxidative capacity during lactation. It is supplied by an increase in size and function of the mitochondrial population of the cell.[10] Mitochondria are increased in the epithelial cell at the onset of the lactation process. Mitochondrial proliferation has been observed in all cells with a high metabolic rate and high oxygen utilization.

During the presecretory differentiation phase in late pregnancy and early lactation, each mitochondrion undergoes a type of differentiation in which the inner membrane and matrix expand greatly. As with other cells, the mitochondria are key to the respiratory activity of the cell. Mitochondria control some cellular metabolism through differential permeability to certain anions. The citrate in the mitochondria is a major source of carbon for fatty acid biosynthesis. Mitochondria also supply the carbon for synthesis of nonessential amino acids.

MICROSOMAL FRACTION.   The microsomal fraction of the cell, which includes the Golgi apparatus, the endoplasmic reticulum, and the cell membranes, is involved in

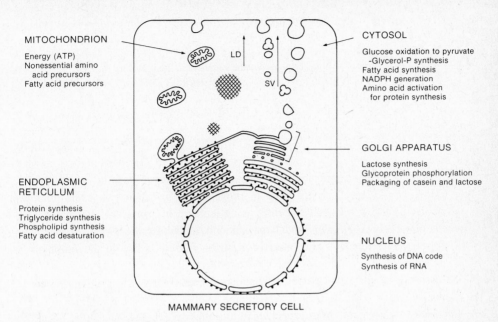

MITOCHONDRION

Energy (ATP)
Nonessential amino
   acid precursors
Fatty acid precursors

CYTOSOL

Glucose oxidation to pyruvate
   -Glycerol-P synthesis
Fatty acid synthesis
NADPH generation
Amino acid activation
   for protein synthesis

GOLGI APPARATUS

Lactose synthesis
Glycoprotein phosphorylation
Packaging of casein and lactose

ENDOPLASMIC
RETICULUM

Protein synthesis
Triglyceride synthesis
Phospholipid synthesis
Fatty acid desaturation

NUCLEUS

Synthesis of DNA code
Synthesis of RNA

MAMMARY SECRETORY CELL

Fig. 3-8. Schematic representation of cytologic and biochemical interrelationships of secretory cell of mammary gland. *LD,* Lipid droplet; *SV,* secretory vesicle.

lipid synthesis. The role of the microsomal fraction is also to assemble the constituent parts such as amino acids, glucose, and fatty acids into the final products of protein, carbohydrate, and fat for secretion.

Intermediary metabolism of the mammary gland

Following is a summary of the process of milk synthesis[29,30]

Protein—de novo synthesis → Apocrine secretion
Fat—de novo synthesis → Apocrine secretion
Lactose—synthesis from glucose → Merocrine secretion
Ions ↔ Diffusion plus active transport
Water ↔ Diffusion
Primary alveolar milk diluted → Plasma isotonicity
   by water from extracel-
   lular fluid

GLUCOSE. Glucose metabolism is a key function in milk production. Glucose serves as the main source of energy for other reactions as well as a critical source of carbon. Glucose is critical to the volume of milk produced. Glucose is also used in the production of lactose. The synthesis of lactose combines glucose and galactose, the latter originating from glucose-6-phosphate.[9]

Lactose synthesis is carried out by the following equation, as described by Turkington[26]:

$$\text{UDP-galactose} + N\text{-acetylglucosamine} \rightarrow N\text{-Acetyllactosamine} + \text{UDP} \qquad (1)$$
$$\text{UDP-galactose} + \text{Glucose} \rightarrow \text{Lactose} + \text{UDP} \qquad (2)$$

UDP is uridine diphosphogalactose. The catalyst in equation 1 is a galactosyl transferase, N-acetyllactosamine synthetase.

Most of the intracellular glucose is derived from blood sugar. A specific whey protein, α-lactalbumin, catalyzes the lactose synthesis (Fig. 3-9). It is a rate-limiting enzyme, which is inhibited by progesterone during pregnancy. In the absence of α-lactalbumin, little lactose is present. With the drop in progesterone and estrogen levels after the removal of the placenta at delivery, there is an increase in prolactin. The synthesis of α-lactalbumin becomes greater, and large amounts of lactose are produced from glucose. Progesterone regulates the onset of lactose synthesis, causing the initiation of production just as the infant is in need of nutrition.

Various aspects of lactose synthesis continue to be vigorously investigated.[9] Lactose synthesis is one of the few anabolic reactions involving glucose itself, rather than a phosphorylated derivative. Although progesterone, thyroxine, and lactogenic hormones are important in controlling synthesis, it is not known how they act in this system. The areas of ignorance about lactose synthesis remain vast.

FAT. Fat synthesis takes place in the endoplasmic reticulum. The alveolar cells are able to synthesize short-chain fatty acids, which are derived predominantly from acetate. Long-chain fatty acids, derived chiefly from blood plasma, are used in milk fat. Triglycerides are utilized from the plasma, as well as synthesized from intracellular glucose oxidized via the pentose pathway. Synthesis of fat from carbohydrate plays a predominant role in fat production in human milk.

Two enzymes, lipoprotein lipase and palmitoyl-CoA L-glycerol-3-phosphate palmitoyl transferase, increase markedly after delivery. The lipase acts at the walls of the capillaries to catalyze the lipolysis and uptake of glycerol into the epithelial cells. The transferase catalyzes the process of synthesizing glycerides to triglycerides. It is believed that the marked increase of the lipase and transferase is stimulated by prolactin. Hormonal control of the glycerol precursors and the enzymatic release of fatty acids, leading to the formation of triglycerides, has been associated not only with prolactin but also with insulin, which stimulates the uptake of glucose into the mammary cells.

Esterification of fatty acids takes place in the endoplasmic reticulum. The triglycerides subsequently accumulate into fat droplets in several cisternae. The small droplets sit on the base of the cell and coalesce to large droplets that move toward the apex of the cell. The fat droplets are engulfed in the apical membrane and project into the alveolar lumen. The droplets are discharged by apocrine secretion. Apocrine secretion involves the bulging of the cell apex to envelop the fat globules, protein, and a small amount of cytoplasm; with the pinching off, the globule becomes detached into the lumen. The membrane of the fat globule contains all the normal plasma enzymes. The fat droplets contain predominantly polar lipid and phosphatidyl choline.

Fatty acid synthesis involves a source of substrates and associated enzymes for their conversion to acetyl-CoA and NADPH in the cytoplasm of the cell and the conversion of acetyl-CoA to malonyl-CoA. The newly synthesized fatty acid is then released from the fatty acid synthetase complex.

PROTEIN.   Most proteins in milk are formed from free amino acids in the secretory

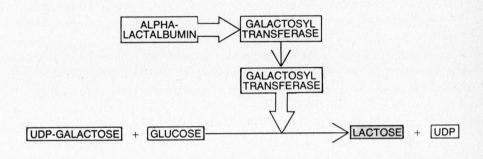

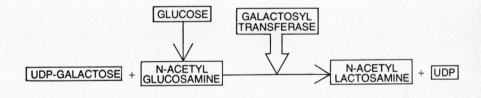

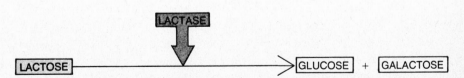

Fig. 3-9. Synthesis of lactose in mammary gland begins late in pregnancy when specific hormones and protein α-lactalbumin are present. Latter modifies enzyme galactosyl transferase, "specifying" it so that it catalyzes synthesis of lactose from glucose and galactose *(top)*. In nonlactating gland glucose and galactose *(bottom)*. (From Kretchmer, N.: Lactose and lactase, Sci. Am. **227:**71, copyright © 1972 by Scientific American, Inc. All rights reserved.)

cells of the mammary gland. The definitive data confirming the origin of milk proteins were accumulated in the past two decades. The vast majority of proteins present in normal milk are specific to mammary secretions and are not identified in any quantity elsewhere in nature.[13]

The formation of milk protein and mammary enzymes is induced by prolactin and further stimulated by insulin and cortisol. De novo synthesis of protein uses both essential and nonessential plasma amino acids. Nuclear RNAs, induced by prolactin, stimulate synthesis of messenger and transfer RNA. The *m*RNA conveys the genetic information to the protein-synthesizing centers of the cells. The transfer RNA interprets the message to assemble the amino acids in the appropriate sequence of polypeptide chains of the specific milk proteins. The newly synthesized proteins are secreted into the milk during lactation. Casein, α-lactalbumin, and β-lactoglobulin from plasma amino acids are synthesized on the ribosomes of the endoplasmic reticulum, where they are condensed and appear as visible secretory granules moving toward the cellular apex. Proteins are discharged predominantly by apocrine secretion. There is, however, some merocrine secretion, in which proteins and other cellular constituents are secreted, leaving the cell membrane intact. Protein caps or signets, protruding into alveolar lumen, have been described on the outside of the apical membrane. Protein and lactose secreted into the lumen cannot be reabsorbed (Table 3-2).

The synthesis of proteins in the mammary gland follows the general pathway of all proteins under genetic control. Induction of synthesis is under hormonal control. This process involves synthesis from amino acids via the detailed system controlled by RNA and under genetic control of DNA. There is an absolute requirement of glucocorticoid for the expression of the casein gene in the presence of prolactin. In fact, cortisol is the limiting factor for casein gene expression.[7]

IONS AND WATER.   Sodium, potassium, chloride, magnesium, calcium, phosphate, sulfate, and citrate pass the membrane of the alveolar cell in both directions. Water also passes in both directions, predominantly from the alveolar cells but also from the interstitial fluid. Plasma water passage depends on the amount of intracellular glucose available for lactose. The aqueous phase of milk is isosmotic to plasma. The major osmole of the aqueous phase of milk is lactose. The concentrations of sodium and chloride are less than those in plasma.

Human milk differs from that of many other species in that the monovalent ions are in low concentration and lactose is in high concentration.[15] The osmolarity is the same, that is, isosmotic with plasma; thus the higher the lactose, the lower the ions. It is presumed that the intracellular concentration of potassium is held high and that of sodium low by a pump on the basal membrane. The sodium and potassium ions are distributed according to the electrical potential gradient. Milk is electrically positive compared to intracellular fluid. The ratio of sodium to potassium is 1:3 in both milk and intracellular fluid. It is thought by Vorherr[30,31] that lactose secretion is responsible for the potential difference across the apical membrane, thus keeping sodium and potassium ion concentration low.

Table 3-2. Alveolar epithelial membrane permeability

Cell ↔ alveolar lumen	Cell → alveolar lumen
Glucose	Lactose
Water	Sucrose
Sodium	Citrate
Potassium	Proteins
Calcium	Fat
Chloride	
Iodine	
Phosphate	
Sulfate	

The variation among species in the concentration of lactose and ions is due to the rate of lactose synthesis, the permeability of the membrane, and the number of fixed negative charges on the membrane. The potential difference is higher in the human mammary gland than in any other species evaluated to date.

The relationship between intrastructure and function in the mammary gland changes from pregnancy to lactation. The junction between alveolar cells has attracted much interest. Cell junctions do not merely hold cells together but enable epithelia to function as permeable barriers, allowing communication between cells and coordination of activities. The three functions of cell junctions are adhesion, occlusion, and communication, which are carried out by desmosomes, tight junctions, and gap junctions respectively. Changes in tight junctions may provide the basis for a reduction in permeability between cells. For instance, at the initiation of lactation, a tight junction changing from ''leaky'' to very tight blocks the paracellular movement of lactose and ions. This requires instead transport across cells of these materials and the maintenance of control of high intracellular potassium and low intracellular sodium concentrations.[4]

Citrate is the main buffer system of milk. It is formed within the secretory cell, but how it is secreted into the milk is not clear. It is suggested that citrate and lactose are secreted by a similar route. Following the dilution of milk in the gland with isosmotic lactose, the equilibrium is restored across the apical membrane in experimental models by the entrance of sodium, potassium, and chloride into the milk. No citrate, calcium, or protein enters in excess of the normal secretion rate. Inorganic phosphate is the other major buffer system, but how it is secreted is also unknown.

Calcium, much of which is bound to casein, enters the Golgi apparatus, where it is essentially trapped, and then enters the alveolar milk by unidirectional flow.

MILK ENZYMES. Some milk enzymes enter the alveolar milk from the mammary blood capillaries via the intercellular fluid. Others come from the breakdown of the mammary secretory cells. The milk enzymes, xanthine oxidase, aldolase, and alkaline phosphatase, are contained in the fat globule, membrane, and milk serum. The most significant enzyme, lipase, splits triglycerides. Amylase, catalase, peroxidase, and alkaline and acid phosphate are not known to contribute to the infant's digestion of human milk.

CELLULAR COMPONENTS. Human milk has been called a live fluid by many and "white blood" in many ancient rites. Breast milk contains about 4000 cells/ml, which have been identified with leukocytes.[29] The cell number is particularly high in colostrum. The cells in greatest number are the macrophages, which secrete lysozyme and lactoferrin. Lymphocytes, neutrophils, and epithelial cells are also present. Lymphocytes produce IgA and interferon.

REFERENCES

1. Cowie, A.T.: Comparative physiology of lactation, Proc. R. Soc. Med. **65**:1084, 1972.
2. Cowie, A.T., Forsyth, I.A., and Hart I.C.: Hormonal control of lactation. Monographs in endocrinology, vol. 15, New York, 1980, Springer-Verlag.
3. Davis, C.L., and Bowman, D.E.: General metabolism associated with the synthesis of milk. In Larson, B.L., and Smith, V.R., editors: Lactation, vol. II, Biosynthesis and secretion of milk/diseases, New York, 1974, Academic Press, Inc.
4. Falconer, I.R., Rowe, J.M.: Effect of prolactin on sodium and potassium concentration in the mammary alveolar tissue, Endocrinology **101**:181, 1977.
5. Fournier, P.J.R., Desjardins, P.D., and Friesen, H.G.: Current understanding of human prolactin physiology and its diagnostic and therapeutic applications: a review, Am. J. Obstet. Gynecol. **118**:337, 1974.
6. Frantz, A.G.: Prolactin, Physiol. Med. **298**:201, 1978.
7. Ganguly, R., et al.: Absolute requirement of glucocorticoids for expression of the casein gene in the presence of prolactin, Proc. Natl. Acad. Sci. U.S.A. **77**:6003, 1980.
8. Hansen, S., and Gumme, B.M.: Participation of the lateral midbrain tegmentum in the neuro endocrine control of sexual behavior and lactation in the rat, Brain Res. **251**:319, 1982.
9. Healy, D.L., et al.: Prolactin in human milk: Correlation with lactose, total protein, and of lactalbumin levels, Am. J. Physiol. **238** (Endocrinol. Metab. 1):E83, 1980.
10. Jones, D.H.: The mitochondria of the mammary parenchymal cell in relation to the pregnancy-lactation cycle. In Larson, B.L., editor: Lactation, vol. IV, The mammary gland/human lactation/milk synthesis, New York, 1978, Academic Press, Inc.
11. Josimovich, J.B., and MacLaren, J.A.: Presence in the human placenta and term serum of a highly lactogenic substance immunology related to pituitary growth hormone, Endocrinology **71**:209, 1962.
12. Josimovich, J.B., Reynolds, M., and Cobo, E.: Lactogenic hormones, fetal nutrition, and lactation. In Josimovich, J.B., Reynolds, M., and Cobo, E., editors: Problems of human reproduction, vol. 2, New York, 1974, John Wiley & Sons.
13. Larson, B.L., editor: Lactation, vol. IV, The mammary gland/human lactation/milk synthesis, New York, 1978, Academic Press, Inc.
14. Larson, B.L., and Smith, V.R., editors: Lactation, vol. II, Biosynthesis and secretion of milk/diseases, New York, 1974, Academic Press, Inc.
15. Larson, B.L., and Smith, V.R., editors: Lactation, vol. III, Nutrition and biochemistry of milk/maintenance, New York, 1974, Academic Press, Inc.
16. Meites, J.: Neuroendocrinology of lactation, J. Invest. Dermatol. **63**:119, 1974.
17. Noel, G.L., Suh, H.K., and Frantz, A.G.: Prolactin release during nursing and breast stimulation in postpartum and non-postpartum subjects, J. Clin. Endocrinol. Metab. **38**:413, 1974.
18. Prilusky J., and Deis R.P.: Inhibition of milk ejection by a visual stimulus in lactating rats: implications of the pineal gland, Brain Res. **251**:313, 1982.
19. Rimoin, D.L., et al.: Lactation in the absence of human growth hormone, J. Clin. Endocrinol. Metab. **28**:1183, 1968.
20. Robinson, J.E., and Short, R.V.: Changes in breast sensitivity at puberty, during the menstrual cycle, and at parturition, Br. Med. J. **I**:1188, 1977.
21. Robyn, C., and Meuris, S.: Pituitary prolactin, lactational performance and puerperal infertility, Semin. Perinatol. **6**:254, 1982.

22. Sherwood, L.M.: Human prolactin, N. Engl. J. Med. **284:**774, 1971.
23. Smith, V.R.: Lactation, vol. I, The mammary gland/development and maintenance, New York, 1974, Academic Press, Inc.
24. Spellacy, W.N., and Buhi, W.C.: Pituitary growth hormone and placental lactogen levels measured in normal term pregnancy and at the early and late postpartum periods, Am. J. Obstet. Gynecol. **105:**888, 1969.
25. Tanaka, T., et al.: A new sensitive and specific bioassay for lactogenic hormones: measurement of prolactin and growth hormone in human serum, J. Clin. Endocrinol. Metab. **51:**1058, 1980.
26. Turkington, R.W.: Human prolactin, (editorial), Am. J. Med. **53:**389, 1972.
27. Tyson, J.E.: Mechanisms of puerperal lactation, Med. Clin. North Am. **61:**153, 1977.
28. Vigneri, R., et al.: Spontaneous fluctuations of human placental lactogen during normal pregnancy, J. Clin. Endocrinol. Metab. **40:**506, 1975.
29. Vorherr, H.: The breast, morphology, physiology and lactation, New York, 1974, Academic Press, Inc.
30. Vorherr, H.: Human lactation and breastfeeding. In Larson B.L., editor: Lactation IV. The mammary gland/human lactation/milk synthesis, New York, 1978, Academic Press, Inc.
31. Vorherr, H.: Hormonal and biochemical changes of pituitary and breast during pregnancy. In Vorherr, H., editor: Human lactation, Semin. Perinatol. **3:**193, 1979.

Biochemistry of human milk

4

The constituents of milk include a tremendous array of molecules whose descriptions continue to be refined as qualitative and quantitative laboratory techniques are perfected. Resolution of lipid chemicals has advanced dramatically in recent years, but new compounds have been identified in carbohydrate and protein as well. Some of the compounds identified may well be intermediary products in the process that occurs within the mammary cells and may be only incidental in the final product.[143]

Human and bovine milk are known in the greatest detail.[49] There is, however, much information about the milk of five other species: the water buffalo, goat, sheep, horse, and pig. There are miscellaneous data on the milk of 150 more species and no data at all on another 4000 species. Jenness and Sloan[68] have compiled a summary of 140 species from which a sampling has been extracted (Table 4-1). Jenness and Sloan have further pointed out that the constituents of milk can be divided into the following groups, according to their specificity:

Table 4-1. Constituents of milk of specific mammals

Mammalian species in taxonomic position	Total solids (g/100 g)	Fat (g/100 g)	Casein (g/100 g)	Whey protein (g/100 g)	Total protein (g/100 g)	Lactose (g/100 g)	Ash (g/100 g)
Man	12.4	3.8	0.4	0.6		7.0	0.2
Baboon	14.4	5.0			1.6	7.3	0.3
Orangutan	11.5	3.5	1.1	0.4		6.0	0.2
Black bear	44.5	24.5	8.8	5.7		0.4	1.8
California sea lion	52.7	36.5			13.8	0.0	0.6
Black rhinoceros	8.1	0.0	1.1	0.3		6.1	0.3
Spotted dolphin	31.0	18.0			9.4	0.6	—
Domestic dog	23.5	12.9	5.8	2.1		3.1	1.2
Norway rat	21.0	10.3	6.4	2.0		2.6	1.3
Whitetail jackrabbit	40.8	13.9	19.7	4.0		1.7	1.5

Modified from Jenness, R., and Sloan, R.E.: Composition of milk. In Larson, B.L., and Smith, V.R., editors: Lactation, vol. III, Nutrition and biochemistry of milk/maintenance, New York, 1974, Academic Press, Inc.

1. Constituents specific to both organ and species (example: most proteins and lipids)
2. Constituents specific to organ but not to species (example: lactose)
3. Constituents specific to species but not to organ (example: albumin and some immunoglobulins)

NORMAL VARIATIONS IN HUMAN MILK

In defining the constituents of human milk, it is important to recognize that the composition varies with the stage of lactation, the time of day, the sampling time during a given feeding, maternal nutrition, and individual variation. Many early interpretations of the content of human milk were based on spot samples or even pooled samples from multiple donors at different times and stages of lactation. Samples obtained by pumping may vary from those obtained by the suckling infant, since there is some variation in content between the various methods of pumping.

Daytime consumption of milk in a given infant has been shown by Brown et al.[8] to be 46% to 58% of the total 24-hour consumption, so that reliance on less than a 24-hour sampling may be misleading. Data from samples taken every 3 hours showed a variation in milk concentration of nitrogen, lactose, and fat, as well as in the volume of milk, by time of day (Fig. 4-1). Furthermore, there were statistically significant diurnal changes in the concentration of lactose and the volume within individual subjects, but the times of those changes were not consistent for each individual. Some individuals varied as much as twofold in volume production from day to day. These investigators also found a significant difference in the concentrations of fat and lactose and in the

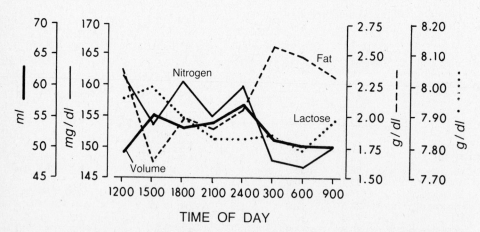

Fig. 4-1. Mean concentrations of nitrogen, lactose, and fat in human milk by time of day. (Modified from Brown, K.H., et al.: Am. J. Clin. Nutr. 35:745, 1982.)

volume of milk produced by each breast. At the extreme, the less productive breast yielded only 65% of the volume of the other breast.

The variation in the fat content has received some attention. Fat content changes during a given feeding, increasing at the end of the feeding. Fat content rises from early morning to midday; the volume increases from two to five times, according to studies by Hall.[45,46] In the later part of the first year of lactation, the fat content diminishes (Fig. 4-2). Work done by Atkinson et al.[5] and confirmed by other investigators has shown that the nitrogen content of the milk of mothers who deliver prematurely is higher than in those whose pregnancies reach full term. For a given volume of milk, the premature infant would receive 20% more nitrogen than the full-term infant if each were fed his own mother's milk. Other constituents of milk produced by mothers who deliver prematurely have also been studied and are discussed in Chapter 14.

An additional consideration in reviewing information available on the levels of various constituents of milk is the technique used to derive the data. In 1977, Hambraeus[48] reported that there was less protein in human milk than originally calculated. The present techniques of immunoassay measure the absolute amounts, whereas earlier figures were derived from calculations based on measurements of the nitrogen content. About 25% of the nitrogen in human milk is nonprotein nitrogen. Cow's milk has only 5% nonprotein nitrogen.

A major concern about variation in content of human milk is related to the mother's

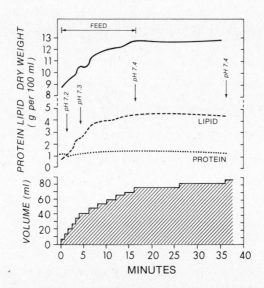

Fig. 4-2. Changes in milk composition during feeding. Continuous analysis of milk of one woman with 5-week-old infant. Infant fed at left breast while milk pumped from right breast. (Modified from Hall, B.: Lancet 1:779, April 5, 1975.)

diet. Maternal diet is of particular concern when the mother is malnourished or eats an unusually restrictive diet. Malnourished mothers have approximately the same proportions of protein, fat, and carbohydrate as well-nourished mothers, but they produce less milk. Water-soluble vitamins, ascorbic acid, thiamin, and B_{12} levels are quickly affected by deficient diets.

COLOSTRUM

The consistently identifiable stages of human milk are colostrum, transitional milk, and mature milk, and their relative contents are significant for the newborn infant and his physiological adaption to extrauterine life.

The first postpartum week's mammary secretion consists of a yellowish, thick fluid, colostrum. The residual mixture of materials present in the mammary glands and ducts at delivery and immediately after is progressively mixed with newly secreted milk, forming colostrum. Human colostrum is known to differ from mature milk in composition, both in the nature of its components and in the relative proportions of these components. Colostrum's specific gravity is 1.040 to 1.060. The mean energy value is 67 kcal/100 ml compared with the 75 kcal/100 ml of mature milk. The volume varies between 2 and 20 dl per feeding in the first 3 days. The volume also varies with the parity of the mother. Women who have had other pregnancies, particularly those who have nursed infants previously, have colostrum more readily available at delivery, and the volume increases more rapidly. The yellow color is due to β-carotene. The ash content is high, and the concentrations of sodium, potassium, and chloride are greater than in mature milk. Protein, fat-soluble vitamins, and minerals are present in greater percentages than in transitional or mature milk.

Colostrum facilitates the establishment of bifidus flora in the digestive tract. Colostrum also facilitates the passage of meconium. Meconium contains an essential growth factor for *Lactobacillus bifidus* and is the first culture medium in the sterile intestinal lumen of the newborn infant. Human colostrum is rich in antibodies, which may provide protection against the bacteria and viruses that are present in the birth canal and associated with other human contact.

The progressive changes in mammary secretion in both breastfeeding and nonbreastfeeding women between 28 and 110 days before delivery and up to 5 months after delivery were followed by Kulski and Hartman[81] to study the initiation of lactation. During late pregnancy the secretion contained higher concentrations of proteins and lower concentrations of lactose, glucose, and urea than those contained in milk secreted when lactation was well established. The concentrations of sodium, chloride, and magnesium were higher and those of potassium and calcium were lower in colostrum than in milk. The osmolarity was relatively constant throughout the study. The authors described a two-phase development of lactation with an initial phase of limited secretion in late pregnancy and a true induction of lactation in the second phase, 32 to 40 hours postpartum. Comparison with the nonlactating women revealed similar secretion during the first 3 days postpartum. This, however, was abruptly reversed during the next 6 days as mammary involution progressed. Obtaining samples in these women, however, may have served to prolong the period of production. The authors point out that although breastfeeding was not necessary for the initiation of lactation in this study, it was essential for the continuation of lactation.

The yield of milk constituents has been calculated from absolute values to demonstrate the increase in output of milk constituents during lactogenesis (Fig. 4-3). There were dramatic increases in the production of all the milk constituents. The constituents synthesized by the mammary epithelium (lactose, lactalbumin, and lactoferrin) increased at a rate greater than those for IgA or proteins derived from the serum IgG and IgM. The greatest difference in yield between day 1 and day 7 postpartum was for glucose.

A survey of the fatty acid components by Read and Sarriff[111] showed the lauric acid and myristic acid contents to be low in concentration the first few days. When the lauric and myristic acids increased, C_{18} acids decreased. Palmitoleic acid increased at the same rate as the myristic acid. From this it was concluded that the early fatty acids are derived from extramammary sources, but the breast quickly begins to synthesize fatty acids for

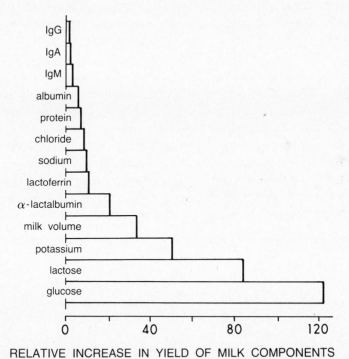

RELATIVE INCREASE IN YIELD OF MILK COMPONENTS

Fig. 4-3. Relative increase in yield of milk components from day 1 to day 7 postpartum. Values presented are for day 7 expressed as a percentage increase over day 1. (Modified from Kulski, J.K., and Hartman, P.E.: Aust. J. Exp. Biol. Med. Sci. **59:**101, 1981.)

Table 4-2. Fat distribution in milk in milligrams

Fat distribution	Colostrum (1-5 days)	Transitional (6-10 days)	Mature (after 30 days)	Cow's milk
Lipid phosphorus	2	3	4	4
Total cholesterol	27	29	20	14
Lecithin	—	—	78	57
Total fats	2900	3600	3800	3700

From Macy, I.G., and Kelly, H.J.: Human milk in infant nutrition. In Kon, S.K., and Cowie, A.T., editors: Milk the mammary gland and its secretion, vol. II, New York, 1961, Academic Press, Inc., p. 265.

the production of transitional and mature milk (Table 4-2). The total fat content may have a predictive value, since it was shown by Hytten[61] that 90% of the women whose milk contained 20 g or more of fat per feeding on the seventh day were successfully breastfeeding 3 months later. Women who only had 5 to 10 g of fat on the seventh day had an 80% dropout rate by 3 months.

Colostrum's high protein and low fat are in keeping with the needs and reserves of the newborn at birth. Although the content of total nitrogen or any amino acid in breast milk in 24 hours is grossly related to the volume produced, the concentration in milligrams per 100 ml is not so related. The relative distribution of nitrogen of the individual amino acids in each 100 ml of milk differs in each mother. The colostrum may actually reflect a transitional maternal blood picture, which is associated with nitrogen metabolism of the postpartum period. The postpartum period is one of involution of body tissue and catabolism of protein in the mother.

The mineral and vitamin reserves of the newborn infant are related to the maternal diet. A fetal supply of vitamin C, iron, and amino acids is adequate, since infant blood levels exceed those of the mother. Colostrum is rich in fat-soluble vitamin A, carotenoids, and vitamin E. The average vitamin A level on the third day can be three times that of mature milk. Similarly, carotenoids in colostrum may be ten times the level in mature milk and vitamin E may be two to three times greater than mature milk.

TRANSITIONAL MILK

The milk produced between the colostrum and mature milk stages is transitional milk; its content gradually changes. The transitional phase is considered to be approximately from 7 to 10 days postpartum to 2 weeks postpartum. The concentration of immunoglobins and total protein decreases, while the lactose, fat, and total caloric content increase. The water-soluble vitamins increase, and the fat-soluble vitamins decrease to the levels of mature milk.

In a study of transitional milks, breast milk samples were obtained from healthy mothers of term infants on the first, third, fifth, eighth, fifteenth, twenty-second, twenty-ninth, and thirty-sixth days of lactation by Hibberd et al.,[58] who defined the first day of lactation to be the third day postpartum. Twenty-four-hour samples were pooled for analysis and the remainder fed to the baby. The authors found a high degree of variability, not only between mothers but also within samples from the same mother. The maximum value in almost every case was more than twice the minimum. They were able to show, however, that the changes in composition were rapid before day 8 and then progressively less change took place until the composition was relatively stable before day 36.

MATURE MILK
Water

In almost all mammalian milks, water is the constituent in the largest quantity with the exception of the milk of some arctic and aquatic species who produce milks with high fat content (e.g., the northern fur seal produces milk with 54% fat and 65% total solids) (Table 4-1). All other constituents are dissolved, dispersed, or suspended in water. Water contributes to the temperature-regulating mechanism of the newborn because 25% of his heat loss is from evaporation of water from the lungs and skin. The lactating woman has a greatly increased obligatory water intake. If water intake is restricted during lactation, other water losses through urine and insensible loss are decreased before water for lactation is diminished. Because lactose is the regulating factor in the amount of milk produced, the secretion of water into milk is partially regulated by lactose synthesis. Investigations by Almroth[1] show that the water requirement of infants in a hot humid climate can be provided entirely by the water in human milk.

Lipids

By percentage of concentration, the second greatest constituent in milk is the lipid fraction. Milk lipids also provide the major fraction of kilocalories in human milk and are the most variable constituent.[69,70] During the course of a feeding, the fluid phase within the gland was mixed with fat droplets in increasing concentration. The fat droplets are released when the smooth muscle contracts in response to the let-down reflex. The lipid fraction is extractable by suitable solvents. Complete extraction in human milk is difficult because of the lipids bound to protein. From 30% to 55% of the kilocalories are derived from fats; this represents a concentration of 3.5 to 4.5 g/100 ml. Milk fat is dispersed in the form of droplets or globules maintained in solution by an absorbed layer or membrane. The protective membrane of the fat globules is made up of phospholipid complexes. The rest of the phospholipids found in human milk are dispersed in the skim milk fraction. The principal classes of milk lipids are readily separated by chromatography. Triglycerides, diglycerides, monoglycerides, free fatty acids, phospholipids, glycolipids, sterols, and sterol esters are found in human milk. Vitamin A esters, vitamin D, vitamin K, alkylglyceryl ethers, and glyceryl ether diesters are also in the lipid fraction but do not fall into the classes listed.

Renewed interest in defining the constituents of human milk lipid has developed in recent years as investigators look for the causes of obesity, atherosclerosis, and other degenerative diseases and their relationship to infant nutrition[37] (Table 4-3). There are a number of reports of historical value that are plagued with the technical problems of sampling.[94] Because the fat content of a feeding varies with time, spot samples give spurious results. Jensen and associates[69] have reviewed the literature exhaustively and describe the fractionated lipid constituents in detail (Table 4-4).

The average fat content of pooled 24-hour samples has been reported from various sources to vary in mature milk from 2.10% to 3.33%. Maternal diet affects the constituents of the lipids but not the total amount of fat. A minimal increase in total lipid content was observed when an extra 1000 kcal of corn oil was fed to lactating mothers.

Table 4-3. Composition of milks obtained from different mammals and the growth rate of their offspring

Species	Days required to double birth weight	Content of milk (%)			
		Fat	Protein	Lactose	Ash
Man	180	3.8	0.9	7.0	0.2
Horse	60	1.9	2.5	6.2	0.5
Cow	47	3.7	3.4	4.8	0.7
Reindeer	30	16.9	11.5	2.8	—
Goat	19	4.5	2.9	4.1	0.8
Sheep	10	7.4	5.5	4.8	1.0
Rat	6	15.0	12.0	3.0	2.0

From Hambraeus, L.: Pediatr. Clin. North Am. 24:17, 1977.

Table 4-4. Fatty acid composition of human milk lipids as of December 1976

Type	Number	Identity
Saturates		
Normal, even	10	4:0-22:0
Normal, odd	7	11:0-23:0
Monobranched	49	10:0-18:0*
Multibranched	5	12:0, 13:0, 15:0, 16:0†
Monoenes		
cis‡	59	10:1-18:1, 20:1
trans	3	16:1, 18:1, 20:1
Dienes	22	12:2-22:2 all even cis, cis, cis, trans; trans, trans; positional isomers
Polyenes		
Tri	6	18:3, 20:3, 22:3 geometric and positional isomers
Tetra	2	20:4, 22:4
Penta	2	20:5, 22:5
Hexa	1	22:6
Cyclic		
Hexane	1	11, terminal hexane
TOTAL	167	

From Jensen, R.G., Hagerty, M.M., and McMahon, K.E.: Am. J. Clin. Nutr. 31:990, 1978.
*Signifies n-acids with methyl branches.
†Signifies n-acids with three or four methyl branches.
‡Designated as cis, but not usually determined.

A diet rich in polyunsaturated fats will cause an increased percentage of polyunsaturated fats in the milk without altering the total fat content. When the mother is calorie deficient, depot fats are mobilized and milk resembles depot fat. When excessive nonfat kilocalories are fed, levels of saturated fatty acids increase as lipids are synthesized from tissue stores.[62]

Fatty acid patterns of human milk were studied by Guthrie and colleagues[40] to determine the impact of the modern diet on milk. The USDA has reported that the average American diet now includes 156 g of fat, up from 141 g in 1947. The significant change is from animal to vegetable fat, which is now 39% of total dietary fats, especially resulting from the switch from butter and lard. The original studies on human milk lipids were done from 1940 to 1950.[62] The analysis by Guthrie and co-workers[40] in 1977 shows over 56% of the fatty acids are monoenoic and polyenoic C_{18} fatty acids (i.e., 18 carbons). Oleic ($C_{18:1}$), linoleic ($C_{18:2}$), linolenic ($C_{18:3}$), and palmitic ($C_{16:0}$) acids are present in the highest amounts. The results show a change in fatty acid content to more long-chain fatty acids and a twofold to threefold increase in linoleic acid (Table 4-5). The fatty acid composition is remarkably uniform unless the maternal diet is unusually bizarre.

P/S is the ratio of polyunsaturated to saturated fats; polyunsaturated fats include $C_{18:2}$ and $C_{18:3}$, or linoleic and linolenic acid. The bovine P/S ratio is 4. The P/S ratio has shifted as a result of recent dietary changes to 1.3 from 1.35 in human milk. The P/S is significant in facilitating calcium and fat absorption. Calcium absorption is depressed by a 4:5 P/S ratio.

The breast can dehydrogenate saturated and monounsaturated fatty acids in milk synthesis. A study by Read et al.[112] of four groups of nursing mothers from different ethnic groups revealed that a high dietary intake of carbohydrate was associated with

Table 4-5. Lipid and fatty acid composition of human milk compared to literature values

		Previous studies		
Fatty acid	Guthrie et al. (1977)	Macy et al. (1953)[94]	Insull and Ahrens (1958)[62]	Glass et al. (1967)[37]
12:0 Lauric	3.8 (1.6)*	5.5	7.0	3.1
14:0 Myristic	5.2 (1.7)	8.5	8.8	5.1
16:0 Palmitic†	22.5 (2.6)	23.2	21.0	20.2
16:1 Palmitoleic†	4.1 (1.3)	3.0	2.2	5.7
18:0 Stearic	8.7 (1.4)	6.9	7.2	5.9
18:1 Oleic	39.5 (3.8)	36.5	35.8	46.4
18:2 Linoleic	14.4 (4.1)	7.8	6.4	13.0
18:3 Linolenic	2.0 (0.7)	—	—	1.4
Number of samples	110	200	11	7
TOTAL LIPID (g/100 ml)	3.1 ± 2.2	—	3.5	—

From Guthrie, H.A., Picciano, M.F., and Sheehe, D.: J. Pediatr. **90**:39, 1977.
*Percentage of total fatty acid (mean ± SD).
†n = 99; smaller number due to technical error in separating $C_{16:0}$ and $C_{16:1}$ in 11 samples.

high lauric and myristic acid levels and low linoleic and palmitic acid levels in the milk. If the diet is high in linoleic acid and the dietary carbohydrate is moderate, then there is a high level of linoleic acid in the breast milk. Other fatty acids in the diet had little effect on the milk fatty acid produced. Palmitic acid appeared to be derived from extramammary lipid.

At least 167 fatty acids have been identified in human milk (Table 4-6); possibly others are there in trace amounts. Bovine milk has been identified to have 437 fatty acids. Marked change in fatty acid composition would be the result of major dietary changes.

Essential fatty acid requirements for humans have been studied by many investigators.[113] Diets free from added fats or linoleic acid induce deficiency symptoms in infants. These symptoms include skin lesions, insufficient weight gains, and poor wound healing. Low-fat diets in newborn rats have affected cerebral function. The American Academy of Pediatrics has recommended that infant formulas contain a minimum of 3.3 g of fat/kcal (30% of total kilocalories) and 300 mg of linoleic acid (18.2)/100 kcal (about 1.7% of total kilocalories)[6] (Table 4-7). It did not set a limit on linoleic content of diet, since some human milks have 8% to 10% of the fat as linoleic acid. Studies of the milk of vegetarians (Table 4-8) have shown extremely high levels of linoleic acid,

Table 4-6. Lipids of human milk and infant formulas—composition of glyceryl ethers from neutral lipids (N) and phospholipids (P) in human milk lipids

Alkylchain	Colostrum* N	Colostrum* P	Transition milk† N	Transition milk† P	Mature milk‡ N	Mature milk‡ P	Transition milk§ N	Transition milk§ P	Mature milk§ N	Mature milk§ P
12:0			0.2	0.4						
14:0	0.5	0.7	0.5	0.7	0.9	0.8	1.5	0.7	Trace	Trace
15:0	0.5	0.4	0.5	0.4	0.5	0.6	0.9	1.1	Trace	Trace
16:0	33.8	32.5	26.0	27.7	24.8	25.3	71.6	84.9	75.8	77.4
16:1	1.5	1.7	1.1	1.6	3.2	4.6				
17:0	0.7	1.1	1.2	3.8	1.4	1.8	0.8	0.5	0.6	0.3
17:1	0.6	1.0	Trace	1.1	1.6	1.5	3.5	1.0	3.3	2.7
18:0	21.2	19.1	21.5	17.8	21.8	19.0	1.8	2.6	1.8	1.2
18:1	29.7	29.2	38.3	34.1	37.5	34.7	19.9	8.0	18.5	16.7
19:0	0.1	0.1	0.1	0.1	0.1	0.1		0.5		0.7
19:1	0.3	0.3	0.1	0.2	0.4	0.5		0.7		0.1
20:0	1.6	2.1	1.4	1.8	0.9	1.6				0.2
20:1	1.2	2.4	1.4	2.1	1.7	2.4				0.1
21:0 and 1	0.1	0.1	0.1	0.3	0.3	0.5				0.2
22:0	1.3	1.4	1.0	1.2	0.7	0.9				Trace
22:1	3.0	3.7	3.1	2.9	2.7	2.8				0.2
23.0 and 1	0.3	Trace	0.2	0.2	0.1	0.6				
24:0	0.5	0.4	0.3	0.6	Trace	0.4				
24:1	3.1	3.8	3.0	1.4	1.9					

From Jensen, R.G., Hagerty, M.M., and McMahon, K.E.: Am. J. Clin. Nutr. 31:990, 1978.
*From 1 to 2 days.
†From 3 to 7 days.
‡From 8 days to 3 months.
§2-Methoxy substituted glyceryl ethers.

Table 4-7. Fatty acid composition of some commercial infant formulas

Manufacturer	Source of fat	Fatty acid (wt %)									
		4:0-8:0	10:0	12:0	14:0	16:0	18:0	18:1	18:2	18:3	Miscellaneous
Gerber MBF*	Sesame, beef hearts				0.7	14.4	7.3	43.0	32.7	0.7	1.2
Loma Linda†											
Soyalac powder	Soy					9.8	3.3	23.2	55.7	7.4	
Soyalac, conc, liquid	Soy					9.1	3.5	21.8	57.8	7.8	
Soyalac, 87%, H₂O	Soy					8.0	3.3	22.7	59.7	6.3	
Mead Johnson*											
Enfamil 20	MCT,‡ soy, and coconut	1.9	1.1	10.0	4.1	11.1	3.8	21.1	41.1	5.9	
Pregestamil	MCT‡ and corn		20.0	(>2.9)		1.4	0.4	3.9	7.1		
Premature formula§	Corn				0.3	10.0	3.0	30.5	56.2		
Prosobee	Soy				0.3	10.6	4.7	24.4	50.3	8.5	
Ross*											
Similac powder, liquid 60/40	Coconut and corn	4.2	2.0	16.2	6.9	9.9	4.8	16.2	35.3	5.7	
Similac, concentrate, liquid RTF, Isomil	Coconut and soy	4.2	2.0	16.2	6.9	9.9	4.8	13.6	35.3	5.7	
Advance concentrate, liquid and RTF	Soy and corn	0.01	0.1	0.5	0.4	10.7	4.7	24.5	53.7	4.7	0.7
Syntex*||	Soy				0.1	8.0	4.0	28.0	54.0	5.0	
Wyeth SMA*	Oleo, coconut, safflower, and soy	2.0	1.4	14.3	5.9	13.1	7.0	39.4	13.0	1.0	0.8
Premie SMA	Oleo, coconut, safflower, and soy	10.0	4.3	14.6	5.6	10.3	5.1	34.2	14.3	1.2	0.6

Adapted from Jensen, R.G., Hagerty, M.M. and McMahon, K.E.: Am. J. Clin. Nutr. 31:990, 1978.
*Data supplied by manufacturers.
†Analyzed by Jensen et al.
‡Medium-chain TGs.
§Source of fat changed to 40% medium-chain TGs, 40% corn oil, and 20% coconut oil as of April 1977.
|| Includes Mulisoy, Neomullsoy, and carbohydrate-free formulations.

Table 4-8.   Breast milk fatty acids in vegans and omniovore controls*

Methyl esters	Vegans			Controls		
	Mean	SE	Range	Mean	SE	Range
$C_{12:0}$ Lauric	39	12.5	21-76	33	7.1	19-51
$C_{14:0}$ Myristic	68	17.0	50-118	80	5.3	68-90
$C_{16:0}$ Palmitic	166†	14.4	139-204	276	10.5	246-293
$C_{18:0}$ Stearic	52†	5.9	37-66	108	8.5	84-123
$C_{16:1}$ Palmitoleic	12†	0.9	11-15	36	5.3	25-46
$C_{18:1}$ Oleic	313	25.0	277-383	353	11.1	331-383
$C_{18:2\omega6}$ Linoleic	317†	44.5	202-397	69	8.1	56-91
$C_{18:3\omega3}$ Linolenic	15†	2.4	9-20	8	0.5	7-9

Modified from Sanders, T.A.B., et al.: Am. J. Clin. Nutr. **31**:805, 1978.
*Mean values expressed as milligrams per gram total methyl esters detected for four vegans and four omniovore controls.
†Statistical significance of difference between means shown when $p < 0.05$.

four times that of cow's milk.[120] Some researchers include other long-chain fatty acids such as $C_{20:2}$, $C_{20:3}$, $C_{24:4}$, and $C_{22:3}$ as essential nutrients because they are structural lipids in the brain and nervous tissue.[120]

One important outcome of linoleic and linolenic acids is the conversion of these compounds into longer-chain polyunsaturates. These metabolites have been shown to be important for fluidity of membrane lipids and prostaglandin synthesis. They are present in the brain and visual cells. When Gibson et al.[36] studied fatty acid composition of colostrum and mature milk at 3 to 5 days and later at 6 weeks postpartum, they reported that mature milk had a higher percentage of saturated fatty acids, including medium-chain acids, lower monounsaturates, and higher linoleic and linolenic acids and their long-chain polyunsaturated derivatives. The derivatives of these acids, often ignored by many investigators, have high biologic activity; thus, the reporting of only linoleic acid underestimates the essential fatty acid levels in human milk.

To address the issue of nutrition during brain development it is important to consider the different periods of brain development that have been described biochemically by Sinclair and Crawford.[127] First there is cell division, with the formation of neurons and glial cells, and second, myelination. Sinclair and Crawford showed in the rat brain that 50% of polyenoic acids of the gray matter lipids were laid down by the fifteenth day of life. The fatty acids characteristic of myelin lipids appeared later. Gray matter is largely composed of unmyelinated neurons, whereas white matter contains a very high proportion of myelinated conducting nerve fibers. Normal brain function depends on both.

The fatty acids characteristic of gray matter ($C_{20:4}$ and $C_{22:6}$) accumulate before the appearance of fatty acids characteristic of myelin ($C_{20:1}$ and $C_{24:1}$) in the developing brain. Arachidonic ($C_{20:4}$) and docosahexaenoic ($C_{22:6}$) acids are synthesized from linoleic and linolenic acids respectively, but the latter two must be obtained in the diet.

The essential fatty acids, linoleic and linolenic acids, may have greater significance in the quality of the myelin laid down. Dick[23] has made a very interesting observation in the geographic distribution of multiple sclerosis worldwide. He notes that the disease is rare in countries where breastfeeding is common. He postulates that the development of myelin in infancy is critical to preventing degradation later. Dick investigated the difference between human milk and cow's milk in relation to myelin production in multiple sclerosis.

Experimental allergic encephalitis is a demyelinating condition, which can be produced by shocking animals that have been sensitized to central nervous system (CNS) antigens. Newborn rats deficient in essential fatty acids are more susceptible to experimental allergic encephalitis, which has been described as resembling multiple sclerosis pathologically.

Widdowson analyzed the body fats of children from Britain and Holland. At birth, body fat was 1.3% linoleic acid for both groups of children. British infants received cow's milk formulas that contained 1.8% linoleic acid. The Dutch infants received corn-oil formulas that were 58.2% linoleic acid. The Dutch infants had body fat that was 25% linoleic acid at 1 month of age and 32% to 37% at 4 months of age. The British infants, receiving cow's milk formulas, had 3% or less linoleic acid in their body fat. The Dutch infants had lower serum cholesterol levels. The children at approximately 10 years of age appeared to be entirely normal.

CHOLESTEROL. The cholesterol content of milk is remarkably stable at 240 mg/100 g of fat when calculated by volume of fat. The range, depending on sampling techniques, is 9.0 mg to 41.0 mg/100 ml. The amount of cholesterol changed slightly over time, decreasing 1.7-fold over the first 36 days as reported by Harzer et al.,[52] stabilizing at about the fifteenth day postpartum at 20 mg/100 ml. This resulted in a change in the cholesterol/triglyceride ratio. The authors found no uniform pattern of circadian variations between mothers.

Cholesterol has been a factor of great concern because of the apparent association with risk factors for atherosclerosis and coronary heart disease. At present, commercial formulas have high P/S ratios and low cholesterol levels compared with human milk. Dietary manipulation does not change the cholesterol level in the breast milk.[109] When the dietary cholesterol level is controlled, a fall in the infant's plasma cholesterol level is, however, associated with an increase in the amount of linoleic acid in the milk.[107]

No long-range effect of serum cholesterol level has been identified, although Osborn[103] described the pathologic changes in 1500 young people (newborns to age 20). He observed the spectrum of pathologic changes from mucopolysaccharide accumulations to fully developed atherosclerotic plaques. Lesions were more frequent and severe in children who had been bottle fed. Lesions were uncommon or mild in the breastfed children. Investigations done on rats indicated that animals given high levels of cholesterol early in life were better able to cope with cholesterol in later life and maintained a lower cholesterol level.

The validity of the results of several studies done on human infants with controlled cholesterol intakes has been questioned. The mean serum cholesterol levels for the breastfed infants were significantly higher (147 mg/100 ml) than of bottle fed infants

(130 mg/100 ml). A year later, when all the infants were on regular diets, the levels were similar. There is insufficient information to determine the value or risk of cholesterol in human milk as compared with low-cholesterol milks. It appears that cholesterol absorption can be inhibited by certain substances such as orotic acid. Orotic acid is high in bovine milk and yogurt and is presumably absent in human milk. From the data available, the purpose of cholesterol in human milk has not as yet been determined, beyond the belief that the composition of human milk must be best for human infants.

LIPASES. Milk fat is almost completely digestible. The emulsion of fat in breast milk is greater than in cow's milk, resulting in smaller globules. Milk lipases play an active role in creating the emulsion, which yields a finer curd and facilitates the digestion of triacylglycerols. The newborn easily digests and completely uses the well-emulsified small fat globules of human milk. Free fatty acids are important sources of energy for the infant.

Lipase in human milk was first described in 1901. At least two different lipases (glycerol ester hydrolases) were described then. The lipases in human milk make the free fatty acids available in a large proportion even before the digestive phase of the intestine. The lipolytic milk-enzyme activity is similar to the activity of pancreatic lipase, breaking down triglycerides to free fatty acids and glycerol. One enzyme is present in the fat fraction and is inhibited by bile salts.

It appears that the function of this enzyme is to facilitate the uptake by the mammary gland of fatty acids from circulating triglycerides for incorporation with milk lipids because it is dependent in vivo on added serum for activity. Its presence in milk probably represents "leakage" from the mammary gland and it is unlikely to play a major physiologic role in the lipolysis of milk triglycerides.[56]

There are additional lipases in the skim milk fraction, and these are stimulated by bile salts. The lipase stimulated by bile salts has greater activity and splits all three ester bonds of the triglyceride. This lipase is also stable in the duodenum and contributes to the hydrolysis of the triacylglycerols in the presence of the bile salts.[56]

Investigators have continued to study the action of these lipases in the presence of bile salts.[12,43-46,56,57] The lipase remains active during passage through the stomach because it is stable above pH 3.5 and only slowly inactivated by pepsin. The optimal bile-salt concentration for activity is about 2 mmol/L which is within the physiologic range in the newborn. Bile salts protect the enzyme from tryptic activity.[56,57] It is reported that glycine rather than taurine conjugates are essential for activity. The lipid concentration and lipolytic activity increase significantly over the course of the feed, the latter remaining constant in samples collected early and late in the postpartum period.[51] The main lipolytic products are fatty acids with little specificity for different fatty acids of triglyceride. In vitro studies bile salt–stimulated lipase activity is closely controlled by components found in the milk. It is suggested by Hall and Muller[45] that human milk lipase in the small intestine complements rather than duplicates pancreatic lipase activity.

When fresh human milk is refrigerated or even placed in a deep freeze, lipolysis takes place, as demonstrated by the appearance of free fatty acids and a lowering of the pH of the milk. Apparently, even in the absence of bile salts, some lipolysis can take place. Because the fat of human milk contains a high proportion of palmitic acid in the number 2 position, it will be absorbed as a 2-monoglyceride from the intestine. Palmitic acid has been shown to have a more rapid absorption time and, in addition, does not bind calcium and interfere with calcium absorption, as does the free palmitic acid of cow's milk. The palmitic acid of cow's milk is in the number 1 and number 3 positions.

CARNITINE.   Carnitine serves as an essential carrier of acyl groups across the mitochondrial membrane to sites of oxidation, and therefore has a central role in the mitochondrial oxidation of fatty acids in the human.[102] The newborn undergoes major metabolic changes during transition from fetal to extrauterine life, including the rapid development of the capacity to oxidize fatty acids and ketone bodies as fuel alternatives to glucose. The fatty acids derived from high-fat milk and endogenous fat stores become the preferred fuel of the heart, brain, and tissues with high-energy demands. There is, in addition, a dramatic increase in serum fatty acids in the first hours of life. After the interruption of the fetoplacental circulation and in the absence of an exogenous supply of carnitine, neonatal plasma levels of free carnitines and acylcarnitines decrease very rapidly. Carnitine administration seems to act by increasing ketogenesis and lipolysis.[100] When serum carnitine and ketone body concentrations were measured in breastfed and formula-fed newborn infants, lower carnitine levels were found in infants fed formulas than in those fed breast milk.[121]

The levels of carnitine range from 70 to 95 nmol/ml in breast milk (up to 115 nmoles/ml in colostrum) and from 40 to 80 nmol/ml in commercial formula (Enfamil). Warshaw and Curry[144] suggest that the bioavailability of carnitine in human milk may be a significant factor in the higher carnitine and ketone body concentrations in breastfed babies.

The carnitine levels in human milk were followed for 50 days postpartum by Sandor et al.,[121] who found the mean level to be 62.9 nmol/ml (56.0-69.8 nmol/ml range) during the first 21 days and 35.2 $\pm$ 1.26 nmol/ml until the fortieth to fiftieth day. Levels were not related to volume of milk secreted.

Proteins

All milks have been evaluated for their protein contents, which vary from species to species. Proteins constitute 0.9% of the contents in human milk and range up to 20% in some rabbit species. Proteins of milk include casein, serum albumin, and α-lactalbumin, β-lactoglobulins, immunoglobulins, and other glycoproteins. Eight of twenty amino acids present in milk are essential and are derived from plasma. The mammary alveolar epithelium synthesizes some nonessential amino acids (Table 4-9).

Postprandial changes in plasma amino acids in breastfed infants were reported by Tikanoja[140] to be proportional to dietary intake and were highest for the branched-chain

Table 4-9. Nonprotein contents and amino acid components of human milk (compared with cow's milk, in milligrams)

Constituents	Colostrum (1-5 days)	Transitional (6-10 days)	Mature (after 30 days)	Cow's milk
Nonprotein components				
Creatine	—	—	3.3	3.1
Creatinine	—	—	2.2	0.9
Urea	—	23.3	32.2	15.1
Uric acid	—	—	4.6	1.9
Dispensable amino acids				
Alanine	—	—	35	75
Aspartic acid	—	—	116	166
Cystine	—	55	29	29
Glutamic acid	—	—	230	680
Glycine	—	—	0	11
Proline	—	—	80	250
Serine	—	—	69	160
Tyrosine	—	125	62	190
Indispensable amino acids				
Arginine	126	64	51	124
Histidine	57	38	23	80
Isoleucine	121	97	86	212
Leucine	221	151	161	356
Lysine	163	113	79	257
Methionine	33	24	23	87
Phenylalanine	105	63	64	173
Threonine	148	79	62	152
Tryptophan	52	28	22	50
Valine	169	105	90	228

From Macy, I.G., and Kelly, H.J.: Human milk and cow's milk in infant nutrition. In Kon, S.K., and Cowie, A.T., editors: Milk.: the mammary gland and its secretion, vol. II, New York, 1961, Academic Press, Inc.

amino acids. This was also found to be true for most semiessential and nonessential amino acids.[141] The blood urea levels also reflect dietary intake, with values in breastfed infants being substantially lower than levels with bottle fed infants. The sum of plasma free amino acids rose and the glycine/valine ratio fell after a feed. When breastfed and formula fed infants were compared by Järvenpää, concentrations of citrulline, threonine, phenylalanine, and tyrosine were higher in formula fed than in breastfed infants. Concentrations of taurine were lower in the formula fed infants. The peak time was different for formula-fed and breastfed infants, which points out the need to standardize sampling times.

CASEIN. It is well known that milk consists of casein, or curds, and whey proteins, or lactalbumins. The term *casein* includes a group of milk-specific proteins characterized by ester-bound phosphate, high-proline content, and low solubility at pH of 4.0 to 5.0. Caseins form complex particles or micelles, which are usually complexes of calcium caseinate and calcium phosphate. When milk clots or curdles as a result of heat, pH changes, or enzymes, the casein is transformed into an insoluble calcium caseinate–calcium phosphate complex. There are physiochemical differences between human and cow caseins. Casein has a species-specific amino acid composition.

Methionine/cysteine ratio.   The cysteine content is high in human milk, whereas it is very low in cow's milk. Instead, the methionine content is high in bovine milk, thus the methionine/cysteine ratio is two to three times greater in cow's milk than in the milk of most mammals and seven times that in human milk. Human milk is the only animal protein in which the methionine/cysteine ratio is close to 1. Otherwise, this ratio is seen only in plant proteins. Two significant characteristics of amino acid composition of human milk are the ratio between the sulfur-containing amino acids, methionine and cysteine, and the low content of the aromatic amino acids, phenylalanine and tyrosine. The newborn or premature infant is ill prepared to handle phenylalanine and tyrosine because of low levels of the specific enzymes required to metabolize them.

Taurine.   Taurine is a third sulfur-containing amino acid that has been found in high concentrations in human milk and is virtually absent in cow's milk. It is now being added to some prepared formulas. Free taurine and glutamic acid have been measured in breast milk in high concentration. Taurine has been associated in the body at all ages with bile acid conjugation; in the newborn, bile acids are almost exclusively conjugated with taurine. It has been suggested by the work of Sturman and associate[135] that taurine may also be a neurotransmitter or neuromodulator in the brain and retina. Taurine in the nutrition of the human infant was reviewed by Gaull,[35] who reports that evidence is accumulating that taurine has a more general biologic role in development and membrane stability. Taurine is found in very high concentrations in the milk of cats.[110] Kittens deprived of taurine by feeding with purified taurine-free casein diets after weaning develop retinal degeneration and blindness. The process can be reversed by feeding taurine, but not by feeding methionine, cysteine, or inorganic sulfate.[95] The structural integrity of the retina of the cat has been shown to be taurine dependent. The taurine levels were more severely depleted in the brain tissue, but its significance has not been identified yet.[134] Both humans and cats are unable to synthesize taurine to any degree. The process requires cystathionase and cysteinesulfinic acid decarboxylase, which are enzymes that convert methionine, cysteine, or cystine to taurine.

In studies of amino acid levels, only the concentrations of taurine in plasma and urine of breastfed term infants were higher than those of preterm infants fed formula. Levels in term infants were higher than those of preterm infants fed pooled human milk at a fixed volume. The effects of feeding taurine-deficient formula to the human infant are not as severe as seen in the kitten. The human infant conjugates bile acids predominantly with taurine at birth but quickly develops the capacity to conjugate with glycine. Those infants fed human milk continue to conjugate with taurine, whereas those fed formulas soon conjugate with glycine predominantly. The cat, in contrast, uses only taurine throughout life. In the human the various pools of taurine in the body cannot be predicted by measurement of plasma taurine alone. Because of the growing evidence for the role of taurine during development, the requirement for taurine for the neonate remains under investigation[134,136] although taurine has been added to some formulas.

WHEY PROTEINS.   When clotted milk stands, the clot contracts, leaving a clear fluid called "whey," which contains water, electrolytes, and proteins. The ratio of whey proteins to casein is 1.5 for breast milk and 0.2 for cow's milk, that is, 40% of human milk protein is casein and 60% lactalbumin, and cow's milk is 80% casein and 20% lactalbumin.[147]

Human milk forms a flocculent suspension with 0 curd tension. The curds are easily digested. The total amount of protein has been recently measured to be 0.9%, which is lower than the previously reported figure of 1.2%. The discrepancy is due to recalculation of the data in which the total amount of protein was determined by measuring the nitrogen content and multiplying by 6.25. Actually, it was pointed out by Macy and Kelly[93] in 1961 that 25% of the nitrogen content is nonprotein nitrogen, whereas in bovine milk 5% of the nitrogen is from nonprotein nitrogen. Hambraeus[48] has reported the composition of the nonprotein fraction to be urea, creatine, creatinine, uric acid, small peptides, and free amino acids (Table 4-10).

Closer examination of the whey proteins shows α-lactalbumin and lactoferrin to be the chief fractions, with no measurable β-lactoglobulin. β-Lactoglobulin is the chief constituent of cow's milk. The term *lactalbumin* includes a mixture of whey proteins found in bovine milk and should not be confused with α-*lactalbumin,* which is a specific protein that is part of the enzyme lactose synthetase. The α-lactalbumin content parallels lactose levels in different species. Human milk is high in both lactose and α-lactalbumin.

Table 4-10. Composition of protein nitrogen and nonprotein nitrogen in human milk and cow's milk*

		Human milk			Cow's milk
Protein nitrogen		1.43 (8.9)			5.03 (31.4)
Casein nitrogen		0.40 (2.5)		4.37 (27.3)	
Whey protein nitrogen		1.03 (6.4)		0.93 (5.8)	
α-Lactalbumin	0.42 (2.6)			0.17 (1.1)	
Lactoferrin	0.27 (1.7)			Traces	
β-Lactoglobulin	—			0.57 (3.6)	
Lysozyme	0.08 (0.5)			Traces	
Serum albumin	0.08 (0.5)			0.07 (0.4)	
IgA	0.16 (1.0)			0.005 (0.03)	
IgG	0.005 (0.03)			0.096 (0.6)	
IgM	0.003 (0.02)			0.005 (0.03)	
Nonprotein nitrogen		0.50			0.28
Urea nitrogen		0.25		0.13	
Creatine nitrogen		0.037		0.009	
Creatinine nitrogen		0.035		0.003	
Uric acid nitrogen		0.005		0.008	
Glucosamine		0.047		?	
α-Amino nitrogen		0.13		0.048	
Ammonia nitrogen		0.002		0.006	
Nitrogen from other components		?		0.074	
TOTAL NITROGEN		1.93			5.31

Courtesy Forsum, E., and Lönnerdal B.: Protein evaluation of breast milk and breast milk substitutes with special reference to the nonprotein nitrogen. Unpublished data.
*Values refer to grams of nitrogen per liter; values within parentheses to grams of protein per liter.

Lactoferrin.   Lactoferrin is an iron-binding protein that is part of the whey fraction of proteins in human milk. It is in very low amounts in bovine milk. Lactoferrin has been observed to inhibit the growth of certain iron-dependent bacteria in the gastrointestinal tract. It has been suggested that lactoferrin protects against certain gastrointestinal infections in breastfed infants. Giving iron to newborn infants appears to inactivate the lactoferrin by saturating it with iron.

IMMUNOGLOBULINS.   The immunoglobulins in breast milk are distinct from those of the serum. The main immunoglobulin in serum is IgG, which is present in the amount of 1210 mg/100 ml. IgA is found in the serum at 250 mg/100 ml, a fifth the level of IgG. The reverse is true of human colostrum and milk. Colostrum has 1740 mg of IgA/100 ml and milk has 100 mg/100 ml. Colostrum has 43 mg of IgG/100 ml and milk has 4 mg of IgG/100 ml. The IgA and IgG in human milk are derived from serum and from synthesis in the mammary gland. The IgA is secretory IgA (sIgA), the principle immunoglobulin in colostrum and milk. Secretory IgA contains an antigenic determinant associated with a secretory component. It is synthesized in the gland from two molecules of serum IgA linked by disulfide bonds. The sIgA levels are very high in colostrum the first few days and then decline rapidly, disappearing almost completely by the fourteenth day. Secretory IgA is very stable at low pH and resistant to proteolytic enzymes. It is present in the intestine of breastfed infants and provides a protective defense against infection by keeping viruses and bacteria from invading the mucosa. The protective qualities are further described in Chapter 5.

LYSOZYME.   Lysozyme is a specific protein found in high concentration in egg whites and human milk but in low concentration in bovine milk. It has been identified as a nonspecific antimicrobial factor. This enzyme is bacteriolytic against *Enterobacteriaceae* and gram-positive bacteria. It has been found in concentrations up to 0.2 mg/ml. Lysozyme is stable at 100° C and at an acid pH. Lysozyme contributes to the development and maintenance of specific intestinal flora of the breastfed infant. It will be further described under enzymes and in Chapter 5.

Carbohydrates

The predominant carbohydrate of milk is lactose, or milk sugar. It is present in high concentration (6.8 g/100 ml in human milk and 4.9 g/100 ml in bovine milk). Lactose is a disaccharide compound of two monosaccharides, galactose and glucose. Lactose is synthesized by the mammary gland. There are a number of other carbohydrates present in milk. They are classified as monosaccharides, neutral and acid oligosaccharides, and peptide- and protein-bound carbohydrates. There are small amounts of glucose (14 mg/100 ml) and galactose (12 mg/100 ml) present in breast milk also. There are other complex carbohydrates present in free form or bound to amino acids or protein, such as *N*-acetylglucosamine. The concentration of oligosaccharides is about 10 times greater than in cow's milk. This difference arises, no doubt, from biosynthetic control mechanisms yet to be described. These carbohydrates and glycoproteins possess bifidus factor activity. There is also fucose, which is not present in bovine milk and may be important to the early establishment of *L. bifidus* as gut flora. The nitrogen-containing carbohydrates are 0.7% of milk solids.

Observations have documented the fact that the enzyme for digesting lactose, lactase, is seen only in mammals, and, moreover, it gradually disappears from the intestinal tract in infancy. The tapering occurs after age 3 years and is complete by age 5 years. It is considered abnormal to maintain measurable levels of lactase in adult life. Studies[6,125] of enzyme levels in the premature and newborn intestinal tract show lactase to be one of the last to appear and thus indicate that the use of lactose by a premature under 30 weeks gestation is minimal (Table 4-11).

Lactose does appear to be specific, however, for newborn growth.[125] It has been shown to enhance calcium absorption and has been suggested as being critical to the prevention of rickets, in view of the relatively low calcium levels in human milk.[86] Lactose is a readily available source of galactose, which is essential to the production of the galactolipids, including cerebroside. These galactolipids are essential to CNS development.

Interesting correlations have been made between the amount of lactose in the milk of a species and the relative size of the brain[80] (Fig. 4-4). Excessive lactose does not make a brain bigger. It should also be noted that porpoises and dolphins have practically

Table 4-11. Amounts of disaccharides that can be hydrolyzed in vitro by the entire small intestinal mucosa at maximal velocities* in 24 hours

Gestational age (lunar months)	Number of cases	Disaccharide (g/24 hours)			Lactose	
		Maltose	Sucrose	Isomaltose	Younger than 1 day	Older than 1 day
Between 2 and 3 months	3	0.05 (0.002-0.08)	0.02 (0.0008-0.035)	0.02 (0.0005-0.03)	0.01 (0.002-0.03)	
Between 3 and 4 months	2	1 (0.5-1.5)	0.72 (0.27-1.17)	0.40 (0.19-0.62)	0.12	
4 months and 25 days	1	5.2	2.7	1.9	0.8	
6 months	1	10	6.4	3.9	0.3	
Between 7 and 8 months	6	30 (10.5-43.5)	13 (6.6-25)	8.9 (4.4-15.7)	3.8 (3-4.7)	6.4 (2.8-8.3)
Between 8 and 9 months	8	60 (43-79)	34 (28.4-45)	21.3 (16.2-28)	5.8 (4.1-8)	23.4 (13.2-33.4)
9 months and 6 days	1	68	37	26.2		14.4
10 months	3	107 (90-123)	72 (59-87)	46 (38.5-51)		62 (57-67)

From Auricchio, S., Rubino, A., and Murset, E.: Pediatrics **35**:944, 1965, copyright American Academy of Pediatrics, 1965.
*The observed velocity of the in vitro reactions was converted to apparent maximal velocities as calculated by Auricchio et al.

no lactose in their milks (0.6% and 1.3%), although they have high total solids (31.0% to 41.0%). These mammals have been considered by some to be very intelligent. The fact that lactose is found only in milk and not in other animal and plant sources enhances the significance of its high level in human milk. Lactose levels are quite constant throughout the day in a given mother's milk. Even in poorly nourished mothers, the levels of lactose do not vary. Because lactose is influential in controlling volume, the total output for the day may be diminished, but the concentration of lactose in human milk will be 6.2 to 7.2 g/100 ml (Table 4-12).[67]

Nucleotides

Nucleotides are compounds derived from nucleic acid by hydrolysis and consist of phosphoric acid combined with a sugar and a purine or pyrimidine derivative. The level

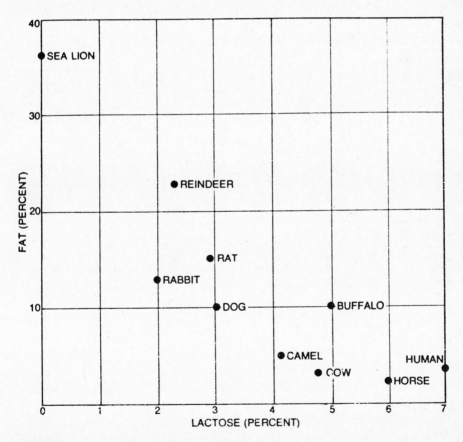

Fig. 4-4. Concentration of lactose varies with source of milk. In general, less lactose, more fat, which can also be used by newborn animal as energy source. (From Kretchmer, N.: Lactose and lactase, Sci. Am. **227**:73, copyright © 1972 by Scientific American, Inc. All rights reserved.)

Table 4-12. Fat, lactose, protein, and calcium content of mature human milk from some well-nourished and poorly nourished communities

Community	Study	Fat (g/100 ml)	Lactose (g/100 ml)	Protein (g/100) ml)	Calcium (mg/100 ml)
Well nourished					
America	Macy (1949)	4.5	6.8	1.1	34.0
Britain	Kon and Mawson (1960)	4.78	6.95	1.16	29.9
Alexandria, Egypt (healthy women)	Hanafy, et al. (1972)	4.43	6.65	1.09	—
Brazil (high economic status)	Carneiro and Dutra (1973)	3.9	6.8	1.3	20.8
Poorly nourished					
India	Belavady and Gopalan (1959)	3.42	7.51	1.06	34.2
South Africa (Bantu)	Walker, Arvidsson, and Draper (1952)	3.90	7.10	1.35	28.7
Brazil (low economic status)	Carneiro and Dutra (1973)	4.2	6.5	1.3	25.7
Ibadan, Nigeria	Naismith (1973)	4.05	7.67	1.22	—
Pakistan	Lindblad and Rahimtoola (1974)	2.73	6.20	0.8-0.9	28.4
Chimbu, New Guinea Highlands	Venkatachalam (1962)	2.36	7.34	1.01	—

Modified from Jelliffe, D.B., and Jelliffe, E.F.P.: Human milk in the modern world, Oxford, 1978, Oxford University Press.

and components of acid-soluble nucleotides of several species, including humans, have been studied, since recent work has shown a characteristic nucleotide composition in the milk that differed from that of the mammary gland. Johke[72] reviewed the existing knowledge on nucleotides in milk. The large numbers of purine and pyrimidine nucleotides present in various tissues have a number of functions in the cell. They are part of nucleic acid synthesis and metabolism and are also part of milk synthesis. It is well known that adenosine triphosphate (ATP) supplies usable energy for biosynthetic reactions.

Human milk has been recorded to have 6.1 to 9.0 μmol of free nucleotides/100 ml, according to Johke.[72] The levels in colostrum and mature milk are similar. The conspicuous difference in quality and quantity of nucleotides between the mammary gland and its secretion would indicate that nucleotides are secreted from the epithelial cells of the gland into the milk. There are distinct species differences in composition and content of nucleotides as well.[127] CMP and uracil are the nucleotides in the highest concentration in human milk, but it also contains UDP-*N*-acetyllactosamine and other oligosaccharides. Human milk contains only a trace of orotic acid and no GDP-fucose. Orotic acid is the chief nucleotide of bovine milk.[78] Nucleotide levels fall rapidly in bovine milk to minimal levels in mature bovine milk.

When the nitrogen fraction of human milk was further identified over time by Janas and Picciano,[64] a variance was noted in the pattern of nucleotides. Levels of cytidine-5'-monophosphate and adenosine-5'-monophosphate declined from 594 to 321 μg/100 ml and from 244 to 143 μg/100 ml respectively whereas levels of inosine-5'-monophosphate increased from 158 to 290 µg/100 ml. The total nucleotide nitrogen remained constant, accounting for 0.10% to 0.15% of the total nonprotein nitrogen. The average intake per day of a normal breastfed infant would be 1.4 to 2.1 mg of nucleotide nitrogen. Measurement of AMP and cyclic GMP by Skala et al.[128] showed variation in concentration within 15 minutes, which fluctuated over 24 hours. Milk concentration differed widely from maternal plasma levels collected at the same time. Whether inosine-5'-monophosphate contributes to the superior iron absorption is still unanswered (see discussion on p. 93).

Nucleotides are important in the process of protein synthesis, which is enhanced in the newborn infant by a dietary supply of nucleotides. A statistically significant increase in weight was observed by György[41] and his colleagues when weanling rats who had been fed a low-protein diet (10% casein) were given added nucleotides as compared with controls without supplements of nucleotides. A high-protein diet (20%) did not produce significant growth increase when nucleotides were added. How this applies to human infants who receive low-protein and high-nucleotide levels in breast milk needs further elaboration.

Minerals

The total ash content of milk is species specific and parallels the growth rate and body structure of the offspring. There are a number of metallic elements and organic and inorganic acids in milk. They may be present as ions, un-ionized salts, and weakly ionized salts. Some are bound to other constituents. Sodium, potassium, calcium, and magnesium are the major cations. Phosphate, chloride, and citrate are the major anions. High-lactose milks, in general, contain less total ash than low-lactose milks, which have high total salt content. This maintains osmolality close to that of serum. The high mineral content is associated with a rapid growth rate of the specific species as well.

POTASSIUM AND SODIUM.   Potassium levels are much higher than those of sodium, which are similar to the proportions in intracellular fluids (Table 4-13). Although sodium, potassium, and chloride are present as free ions, the other constituents appear as complexes and compounds. Ions can pass through the secretory cell membrane in both directions and in and out of the lumen. Intracellular sodium, chloride, and potassium are in equilibrium with the ions of the plasma and alveolar milk. An apical pumping mechanism has been calculated for chloride release, whereas sodium, potassium, and intracellular chloride pass into milk because of their electrochemical gradients. The cellular pumping mechanism maintains the ionic concentrations in the extracellular fluid and alveolar milk.

The Committee on Nutrition of the Academy of Pediatrics[16] has stated that the daily requirement for sodium for growth is 0.5 mEq/kg/day between birth and 3 months of age decreasing to 0.1 mEq/kg/day after 6 months of age (Table 4-14). To cover dermal losses, an additional 0.4 to 0.7 mEq/kg/day is needed, with little for urine and stool losses. Infants fed human milk receive enough sodium to meet their needs for growth,

Table 4-13.   Minerals in human milk and cow's milk (per 100 ml)

Minerals	Colostrum	Transitional	Mature	Cow's milk
Calcium (mg)	39.0	46.0	35.0	130.0
Chlorine (mg)	85.0	46.0	40.0	108.0
Copper (μg)	40.0	50.0	40.0	14.0
Iron (μg)	70.0	70.0	100.0	70.0
Magnesium (mg)	4.0	4.0	4.0	12.0
Phosphorus (mg)	14.0	20.0	15.0	120.0
Potassium (mg)	74.0	64.0	57.0	145.0
Sodium (mg)	48.0	29.0	15.0	58.0
Sulfur (mg)	22.0	20.0	14.0	30.0
Total ash (mg)	—	—	200.0	700.0

From Food and Nutrition Board, National Research Council, National Academy of Sciences: Recommended dietary allowances, ed. 9, Washington, D.C., 1980, U.S. Government Printing Office.

Table 4-14.   Recommended dietary intake of electrolytes for infants

Age (yr)	Sodium (mg)	Potassium (mg)	Chloride (mg)
0-0.5	115-350	350-925	275-700
0.5-1	250-750	425-1275	400-1200

From Food and Nutrition Board, National Research Council, National Academy of Sciences: Recommended dietary allowances, ed. 9, Washington, D.C., 1980, U.S. Government Printing Office.

dermal losses, and urinary losses. Studies by Keenan et al.[75,76] have demonstrated an apparent regulation of milk sodium and potassium concentrations by adrenal corticosteroids as well as a circadian rhythm in the levels.

Sodium levels in cow's milk are 3.6 times those in human milk (human, 7 mEq/L or 16 mg/dl; bovine, 22 mEq/L or 50 mg/100 ml). Hypernatremic dehydration has been associated with cow's milk feedings. Experiments with newborn rats on high salt intakes have shown that hypertension can develop.

Whether sodium levels in milk are influenced by emotional stress, as suggested by Sevy,[123] is unproven. High sodium has also been noted in the milk of infected breasts and as a result of certain maternal drugs such as reserpine. Abrupt weaning has also been reported to be associated with increased sodium levels.[50]

Potassium concentrations are 13 mEq or 51 mg/ml in human milk and 35 mEq or 137 mg/ml in bovine milk. Although the sodium and potassium contents of milk are known to depend somewhat on dietary intake, the individual and temporal variations in the milk have not been fully appreciated. The diurnal variation in milk electrolytes was found to vary between 22% and 80% by Keenan et al.,[76] and these changes varied as the lactation period progressed but were independent of mother's diet. Sodium restriction did not influence milk levels. In a longitudinal study, Hazebroek and Hofman[53] found sodium levels to fall from 20 mEq/L in the first week to 15 mEq/L. On day 8, levels were 8 mEq/L, and by the fifth week they were stabilized at 6 mEq/L.

Most attention has been paid to the role of sodium in hypertension.[15] A double-blind randomized trial was done with 245 newborns in the Netherlands assigned to a normal-sodium diet and 231 assigned to a low-sodium diet for the first 6 months of life.[59] Normal sodium intake (2.50 ± 0.95 M) was three times the low-sodium intake (0.89 ± 0.26 M). Infants in the low-sodium group had blood pressures 2.1 mm Hg lower than those in the normal sodium group. Some of the infants in each group were breastfed. The sodium/potassium ratio was 0.67 for the low-sodium group and 0.64 for the normal-sodium group. The results need confirmation. Potassium has a reciprocal relationship with sodium in many biologic functions. Potassium administration can lower elevated blood pressures in some adults.

At a constant sodium intake, decreasing the Na/K ratio in the diet by increasing potassium lowers blood pressure. The dietary Na/K ratio has an important role in determining the severity, if not the development, of salt-induced hypertension. The mechanism of potassium's antihypertensive effect is unclear, but the higher potassium and lower sodium levels of breast milk appear to be physiologically beneficial.

CHLORIDE. Little attention has been paid to the adequacy of chloride in the diet, and it has always been assumed to be sufficient until recent events focused attention on this cation.

Chloride deficiency in infants has become associated with a syndrome of failure to thrive with hypochloremia and hypokalemic metabolic alkalosis. This was first described in infants fed formula that was deficient in chloride but has also been described in a breastfed infant whose mother's milk contained less than 2 mEq/L chloride (normal >8 mEq/L).[4] This is a rare phenomenon caused by unexplained maternal production. This mother had previously successfully nourished five other infants.

TOTAL ASH. Cow's milk has three times the total salt content of human milk (Table 4-15). All the minerals that appear in cow's milk also appear in human milk. The phosphorus level is six times greater in cow's milk; the calcium level is four times higher (Table 4-16).

The renal solute load of cow's milk is considerably higher than that of breast milk. This is magnified by the metabolic breakdown products of the high protein content, which are in increased amounts, also. This is shown in the high urea levels in formula-fed infants (Table 4-17).[21] Although the mean urea levels in breast milk are 37 mg/100 ml and only 15 mg/100 ml in cow's milk, the blood urea levels in breastfed infants are about 22 mg, whereas infants fed formula are 47 mg and those fed formula plus solids are 52 mg/100 ml (Table 4-17). The plasma osmolarity of infants fed breast milk is lower and approximates the physiological level of plasma (Table 4-18).[20]

CALCIUM/PHOSPHORUS RATIO. The ratio of calcium to phosphorus is considerably lower in cow's milk (1.4) than in human milk (2.2). Many investigators have studied calcium and phosphorus values in human milk and found some variation from mother to mother and from study to study. The Ca/P ratio varied from 1.8 to 2.4, with the absolute values for calcium varying from 20 to 34 mg/100 ml and those for phosphorus varying from 14 to 18 mg/100 ml. Data compiled by Forfar[31] demonstrate the variation.

Table 4-15. Principal salt constituents in bovine and human milks

Constituent	Bovine (mg/100 ml)	Human (mg/100 ml)
Calcium	125	33
Magnesium	12	4
Sodium	58	15
Potassium	138	55
Chloride	103	43
Phosphorus	96	15
Citric acid	175	20-80
Sulfur	30	14
CO_2	20	—

From Jenness, R., and Sloan, R.E.: Composition of milk. In Larson, B.L., and Smith, V.R., editors: Lactation, vol. III., Nutrition and biochemistry of milk/maintenance, New York, 1974, Academic Press, Inc.

Table 4-16. Recommended dietary intake of minerals for infants*

Age (yr)	Calcium (mg)	Phosphorus (mg)	Magnesium (mg)	Iron (mg)	Zinc (mg)	(Iodine (μg)
0-0.5	360	240	50	10	3	40
0.5-1	540	360	70	15	5	50

From Food and Nutrition Board, National Research Council, National Academy of Sciences: Recommended dietary allowances, ed. 9, Washington, D.C., 1980, U.S. Government Printing Office.
*Because there is little information on which to base allowances, these amounts are provided in the form of ranges of recommended intakes.

Table 4-17. Statistical analysis by Student's "t" test of blood urea levels in 61 healthy infants aged 1 to 3 months

Infant group	Number	Blood urea, mean ± SE (mg/100 ml)	Individual values >40 mg/100 ml Number	Total observations (%)
A: breastfed	12	22.7 ± 1.6*	0	0‡
B: artificial milk alone	16	47.4 ± 2.0†	12	75§
C: artificial milk + solid foods	33	51.9 ± 1.8	29	88

From Davies, D.P., and Saunders, R.: Arch. Dis. Child. 48:563, 1973.
*When compared with group B and group C: $p < 0.001$ ($t = 9.7$) and $p < 0.001$ ($t = 11.5$), respectively.
†When compared with group C: $p > 0.05$ ($t = 1.6$).
‡When compared with group B and group C: $p < 0.001$ ($t = 6.9$) and $p < 0.001$ ($t = 15.5$), respectively.
§When compared with group C: $p > 0.05$ ($t = 1.1$).

Fetal and newborn plasma concentrations for calcium decline sharply from 10.4 mg/100 ml at birth to 8.5 mg/100 ml by day 4. Unlike calcium, phosphorus concentrations rise in the postnatal period. The drop in serum calcium levels in the bottle fed infants was more marked than in the breastfed infants. Infant serum phosphorus concentrations rise during the postnatal period. Those infants fed cow's milk have a greater rise than those fed human milk. When gestation is prolonged or the mother has preeclampsia, the con-

Table 4-18.   Daily protein intake (g/kg) and mean plasma osmolality

	Group A*	Group B†	Group C‡
Protein intake			
Day 7	2.1	4.6	6.8
Day 14	2.6	6.7	8.5
Day 28	ND§	ND§	ND§
Plasma osmolality			
Day 7	290.8	289.6	296.8
Day 14	287.2	291.7	298.8
Day 28	289.7	293.6	296.7

From Davies, D.P.: Arch. Dis. Child, **48:**575, 1973.
*Preterm infants fed breast milk containing 5.9% of total calories as protein.
†Preterm infants fed formula B containing 15.4% of total calories as protein.
‡Preterm infants fed formula C containing 21.1% of total calories as protein.
§ND, not determined.

Table 4-19.   Comparison of calcium and phosphorus content

	Calcium (mg/100 ml)	Phosphorus (mg/100 ml)	Ca/P
Cord blood	10.2	5.5	—
Breastfed, fourth day of life	9.5	5.3	—
Bottle fed, fourth day of life	8.0	6.0	—
Transitional breast milk	28.0	15.5	2.0
Mature breast milk	27.6	16.2	1.8

Modified from Barltrop, D., and Hillier, R.: Acta Paediatr. Scand, **63:**347, 1974.

centrations are even higher at birth. Barltrop and Hillier[7] studied the calcium and phosphorus contents of transitional and mature human milk and the corresponding infants' plasma levels (Table 4-19). No relationship between the milk composition and the plasma levels was seen on the sixth day of life.

Longitudinal studies by Greer et al.,[39] measuring calcium and phosphorus in human milk and maternal and infant sera, have shown progressive increases in infant serum calcium in association with decreasing phosphorus content of breast milk and infant serum. Maternal serum calcium also increased, although the mothers' dietary intake was below recommended levels for lactating women.

Although the Ca/P ratio has been stressed in the past, Barltrop and Hillier failed to find a statistical correlation between the calcium and phosphorus contents of plasma and corresponding breast milk Ca/P. This suggested that Ca/P ratio is not critical in the low mineral loads present in breast milk. There are extensive data to demonstrate the stress of high phosphorus and low calcium in serum of infants fed milk with a high mineral content. Lealman et al.[85] published a study of 138 infants on breast milk or cow's milk formulas. Infants fed cow's milk formulas showed changes by the sixth day of receiving the low calcium and high phosphorus levels. When human milk was fractionated and analyzed for distribution of calcium, whole milk contained 241.2 ± 61.9 μg/ml, with most of the calcium in the skim fraction. Significant amounts were also found in the fat; less than 4% was found in the casein. A low–molecular weight fraction contained 34% calcium, which may explain calcium's bioavailability. The total calcium requirements for maximum growth have been questioned by those who believe the total amount of calcium is too low in breast milk. The fact that rickets has not been seen in infants totally breastfed by well-nourished mothers is supportive circumstantial evidence. Fomon et al.[30] calculated the calcium needs for growth of premature infants to adequate stature at 1 year of age. These data clearly show breast milk to be an inadequate source of calcium for the premature infant. For each 100 g weight gain, the premature infant needs 617 mg of calcium, which would mean, assuming 65% dietary absorption, 190 mg/day of calcium, or a 600 ml intake of human milk for a 1200 g baby. A 1200 g infant would usually consume 180 ml/day of fluids.

MAGNESIUM AND OTHER SALTS.   Magnesium is present as a free ion and in complexes with casein and phosphate in caseinate micelles or citrate complexes. Cow's milk has three times as much magnesium as human milk (12 mg/100 ml compared with 4 mg/100 ml) (Table 4-15). Magnesium was measured in human milk by Fransson and Lönnerdal,[34] who found 41.4 ± 15.4 µg/ml in whole milk samples, with most of the magnesium in the skim milk fraction, but significant amounts in the fat fraction and less than 4% in the casein. The bound fraction was associated with low molecular weight proteins, thus enhancing bioavailability. Mineral intakes measured by Picciano et al.[105] were shown to increase between 1 and 3 months postpartum (1.15 to 1.36 mmol/L). Lealman and associates[85] studied the magnesium levels in the plasma of infants who received either breast milk or cow's milk formula. Breastfed infants showed an increase in magnesium levels in the first week of life, whereas the others did not, and some infants even showed a drop.

Longitudinal magnesium concentrations were measured by Greer et al.[39] in milk and maternal sera and in the infants over a 6-month period. Progressive increases in serum magnesium level were seen in the breastfed infants in association with decreasing phosphorus content of the milk. Milk magnesium levels did not change significantly between 3 and 26 weeks. The authors suggested that the rising magnesium levels in infant serum may in part be due to a decrease in dietary phosphorus in breastfed infants.

Citrate is found in the milks of many species and is three to four times higher in cow's milk than in human milk (Table 4-15). The distribution of ions and salts differs among various milks and depends on the relative concentrations of casein and citrate.

Most of the sulfur in milk is in the sulfur-containing amino acids, with only about 10% present as sulfate ion. There are some organic acids present, and they appear as anions in milk.

TRACE ELEMENTS

The recommended daily intake of trace elements for infants is given in Tables 4-16 and 4-20.

Iron.   Because of the great emphasis on iron in the modern diet, and especially in the diet of the infant in the first year of life, the iron in human milk has been closely

Table 4-20.   Recommended dietary intake of trace elements for infants*

Age (yr)	Copper (mg)	Manganese (mg)	Fluoride (mg)	Chromium (mg)	Selenium (mg)	Molybdenum (mg)
0-0.5	0.5-0.7	0.5-0.7	0.1-0.5	0.01-0.04	0.01-0.04	0.03-0.06
0.5-1	0.7-1.0	0.7-1.0	0.2-1.0	0.02-0.06	0.02-0.06	0.04-0.08

From Food and Nutrition Board, Nutritional Research Council, National Academy of Sciences: Recommended dietary allowances, ed. 9, Washington, D.C., 1980, U.S. Government Printing Office.
*Because the toxic levels for many trace elements may be only several times usual intakes, the upper levels for the trace elements given in this table should not be habitually exceeded.

scrutinized.[14] It has been determined that normal infants need 1500 mg of exogenous elemental iron in the first year of life, which can be translated into 8 to 10 mg/day (Table 4-16). Prepared infant formulas currently supply 10 to 12 mg/day. Human milk contains more iron than cow's milk, however, in that human milk has 100 μg/100 ml and cow's milk has 70 μg/100 ml. This does not meet the requirements just given. Historically, however, breastfed infants have not been anemic (Table 4-13).

Studies by Picciano and Guthrie[106] on 50 women and 350 samples of breast milk showed a variation between <0.1 and 1.6 μg of iron/ml. Age, parity, and lactation history influenced the levels in some studies.[126] The distribution of iron in various fractions of human milk of Swedish women was determined using multiple methods by Fransson and Lönnerdal,[33] who also found low levels, 0.26 and 0.73 ng/ml. The lipid fraction bound 15% to 46% of the iron; 18% to 56% of the iron was in the low molecular weight protein fraction, with only a small amount bound to lactoferrin. Feeley et al.[28] studied 102 American women by stage of lactation; 96% of the women took prenatal iron supplements. A diurnal variation was observed and a significant decrease occurred from 4 to 45 days postpartum. The authors estimated that fully breastfed infants would receive 0.10 mg/kg/day of iron, whereas Picciano and Guthrie[106] had estimated only 0.05 mg/kg/day. Siimes et al.[126] followed Finnish mothers for 9 months and noted a decline from 0.6 mg/L neonatally to a stable plateau of 0.3 mg/L at 5 months, with a large range of values for each individual. The samples were mixed from the beginning and end of each feed for a 24-hour period, thus eliminating the diurnal variation. Over 60% of the study mothers were taking iron supplements daily, and the others were taking them sporadically, so no correlation to intake was made.

The effects of maternal iron nutrition in rats during lactation was studied by Anaokar and Garry,[2] who fed three groups of dams control amounts of 250 ppm iron, high-iron diets of 2500 ppm, and no-iron diets. Milk iron concentration decreased in all diet groups during lactation. The rate of decrease was diet dependent. Furthermore, iron levels in the dams were influenced by diet and correlated with levels in their pups.

Iron absorption from human milk is more efficient and has been noted to be 49% of iron available, whereas only 10% of cow's milk iron and 4% of iron in iron-fortified formulas was absorbed.[3] Hematologic values of bottle fed infants were abnormal, whereas those of breastfed infants were not. The breastfed infants had high ferritin levels, indicating a long-term adequacy of iron assimilation (Table 4-21).[96] Studies in adults given tagged iron in human milk and in cow's milk show better absorption from the human milk solution (Table 4-22).[96] Other factors that influence iron absorption include higher amounts of vitamin C. Lactose, which promotes iron absorption, is in higher concentration in breast milk, especially as compared with prepared formulas, which may not contain lactose. Phosphorus may interfere with iron absorption, as may high protein levels. There is still considerable doubt as to whether it is physiologically sound to increase the hemoglobin of an infant with exogenous iron. All species of mammals have low iron content in their milks. All mammals investigated so far have a drop in their hemoglobin levels after birth and a gradual rise to adult levels for the species. The relationship between plasma concentration of ferritin and body iron stores has not been clearly established; the explanation of iron absorption and use in breastfed infants is still under study.

   Zinc.   Zinc has been identified as essential to the human. Its chief roles described to date are as part of the enzyme structure and as an enzyme activator. Zinc deficiency has been described as well, most recently in newborns and premature infants on hyperali-

Table 4-21.   Age, weight, and hematologic values for infants exclusively breastfed

	Patients				
Data	1	2	3	4	Normals
Age (mo)	8	9	8	18	—
Weight (kg)					
At birth	4.1	3.6	2.8	3.8	—
At time of study	11.0	10.2	9.0	12.0	—
Final weight ÷ birth weight	2.68	2.83	3.21	3.15	—
Hemoglobin (g/100 ml)	11.3	12.5	11.3	12.2	>10.5
Mean corpuscular volume (cu/μm^3)	78	82	74	80	76 ± 3
Iron (μg/100 ml)	80	77	158	73	>70
Total iron-binding capacity (μg/100 ml)	320	—	502	408	—
% Saturation	20	—	31	18	>16
Free erythrocyte porphyrins (μg/100 ml)	51	42	53	37	<70

From McMillan, J.A., Landaw, S.A., and Oski, F.A.: Pediatrics 58:686, 1976, copyright American Academy of Pediatrics, 1976.

Table 4-22.   Elemental iron and ^{59}Fe radioactivity level in milks fed to 10 adult subjects

Milk	Iron (mg/86 ml of milk)	^{59}Fe added (μg)	Total elemental iron (μg)	cpm ingested	μg/cpm ingested*
Cow's milk					
Subjects 1 to 5	74.8	0.59	75.39	2.0×10^6	3.8×10^{-5}
Subjects 6 to 10	34.4	0.60	35.00	2.5×10^6	1.4×10^{-5}
Human milk					
Subjects 1 to 5	67.1	0.45	67.55	1.5×10^6	4.5×10^{-5}
Subjects 6 to 10	51.2	0.46	51.66	2.09×10^6	2.45×10^{-5}

From McMillan, J.A., Landaw, S.A., and Oski, F.A.: Pediatrics 58:686, 1976, copyright American Academy of Pediatrics, 1976.
*Assayed at day 36. Activity was adjusted to 10 μCi on the day of ingestion of each milk solution.

mentation regimens. The chief clinical symptoms are failure to thrive and typical skin lesions. Milk has been identified as a food with bioavailable zinc. Johnson and Evans[73] studied the relative zinc availability in human breast milk, formulas, and cow's milk. Human milk had 2 μg/ml as compared with cow's milk, which had 4.1 μg/ml, and fortified formulas, which had 3 μg/ml to 5 μg/ml. The bioavailability of zinc fed to rats in various milk solutions was 59.2% for human milk, 42% for cow's milk, and 26.8% to 39% for formulas.

Zinc absorption from human milk, cow's milk, and infant formula was tested in healthy adults with labeled zinc chloride, Zn 65. The absorption was 41% from human milk, 28% from cow's milk, 31% from standard infant formula, and 14% from soy formula.[122] The dietary zinc intake of both lactating and nonlactating postpartum women was found by Moser and Reynolds[98] to be 42% recommended allowances. There was no correlation of maternal dietary zinc and maternal plasma and erythrocyte zinc with the concentrations of zinc in breast milk. Over the 6 months, breast milk zinc decreased significantly from 2.6 to 1.1 μg/ml.

Changes in hair zinc concentrations of breastfed and bottle fed infants during the first 6 months of life were measured by MacDonald et al.[92] Only the bottle fed males had a significant decline in hair zinc concentration. There was no decline of zinc in any breastfed infant, which supports the concept of the superior bioavailability of zinc in breast milk.

Picciano and Guthrie[106] studied milk from 50 mothers in 350 samples. They found zinc levels to average 3.95 μg/ml and to be consistent regardless of time of day, duration of lactation, or other variables. They estimated that breastfed infants receive 0.35 mg of zinc/kg/day.

Picciano and Guthrie[106] made additional observations on breastfed infants, comparing modern assay techniques and older data, and found zinc levels to decline slightly from the first to the third month postpartum (33.8 to 29.5 μmol/L). Human milk was fractionated and analyzed by Frannsson and Lönnerdal[34] for the distribution of zinc. Most of the zinc was found in the skim milk fraction, but significant amounts were found in the fat associated with the fat globule membrane; less than 4% was found in the casein.

Eckhert and co-workers[24] studied zinc binding in human milk and cow's milk to determine bioavailability. By gel chromatography, they showed cow's milk zinc to be associated with high–molecular weight fractions and zinc in human milk to be associated with low–molecular weight fractions. The association of zinc with low–molecular weight components of milk is related in part to protein content and composition and to the relative zinc concentration.[18] When adult females were given oral doses of zinc with human milk, cow's milk, casein hydrolysate formula, and soy-based formula, the plasma response with human milk was significantly (three times) greater than with any of the others.[11]

The low–molecular weight ligand has been proved to be readily absorbed. Breast milk has been therapeutic in the treatment of acrodermatitis enteropathica, an inherited zinc-metabolism disorder, whereas cow's milk formulas are ineffective.

Copper, selenium, aluminum, titanium, and chromium. Little is known about trace elements in human milk, but they are attracting more interest.[3] Picciano and Guthrie[106] studied copper levels in human milk and noted that the content varied considerably among women and within each woman. The range was 0.09 to 0.63 μg/ml. Copper levels were higher in the morning. Dietary supplements did not alter results. Age, parity, and lactation history showed that older mothers and multiparas had higher levels. The fully breastfed infant would receive 0.05 mg of copper/kg/day (Table 4-20).

Picciano and Guthrie[106] confirmed this work with newer bioassay techniques. Fractionated analysis by Frannsson and Lönnerdal[34] revealed whole milk concentration of copper to be 0.27 ± 0.13 μg/ml with most of the copper in the skim milk fraction, significant amounts in the fat, and little in the casein. The predominant binding was with low–molecular weight proteins, which would enhance bioavailability. Changes in hair copper concentrations were also studied among breastfed and bottle fed infants.[92] Hair copper levels rose in the first 3 months in all infants and then declined, regardless of feeding or sex of infant. The authors associated this with the redistribution of copper in early infancy (Table 4-13).

High zinc/copper ratios as they relate to dietary intakes have been associated with coronary heart disease.[77] The zinc/copper ratios of human milk are lower than those of cow's milk. Using figures from Picciano and Guthrie[106] (0.14 to 3.95:0.09 to 0.63), the ratio in human milk is 14:9. The ratio of zinc to copper in bovine milk (1000 to 6000:30 to 170) is at least 30:1.

The bioavailability of selenium depends on the sources and chemical form, and the quantitative significance is under investigation. Except for Keshan's disease, a potentially fatal cardiomyopathy seen in infants in China, there has not been a convincingly associated clinical deficiency syndrome.[47] Dietary recommendations have been based on those for adults. Dietary intakes less than the lower limits, however, should not be considered deficient, especially in breastfed infants.[148]

Selenium concentrations in human milk are consistent in samples collected from many parts of the world, according to work by Hadjimarkos and Shearer.[42] The mean value was 0.020 ppm, which was similar to the value from many parts of the United States, where the range was 0.007 to 0.033 ppm. There was a parallel between the selenium content of bovine grazing crops in the area and bovine milk levels. Alterations in bovine diet produce more marked change in the selenium in the milk produced. Bovine levels range from 0.016 to 1.27 ppm.

Selenium is considered an essential nutrient in humans. It is an integral component of glutathione peroxidase, an enzyme known to metabolize lipid peroxides, and deficiency states have been described. Questions have been raised about the detrimental effects of high selenium intake on dentition. Selenium status was assessed in infants exclusively fed human milk or infant formula for 3 months by Smith et al.[129] Foremilk samples had a mean concentration of 15.7 ng/ml, hindmilk mean concentration was 16.3 ng/ml, and mean formula concentration was 8.6 ng/ml. The breastfed infants had greater intakes and higher serum levels of selenium than the formula fed infants in the first 3 months (Table 4-20).

The concentration of chromium is highest in the organs of the newborn and declines rapidly during the first years of life. Data on chromium in human milk had been scattered and conflicting, with reports of chromium concentrations in pooled milk samples of 40 mothers to be 20 ng/ml, with a range of 5 to 40 ng/ml.[82] A longitudinal study of chromium in human milk was undertaken by Kumpulainen and Vuori.[83] Mothers collected samples at 8 to 18 days, 47 to 54 days, and 128 to 159 days postpartum, representing every feed during a 24-hour period with equal portions of fore- and hindmilk. The mean concentration was 0.39 (SD = 0.15) ng/ml and the intake 0.27 (SD = 0.11) μg/day. The values did not change over time. These values are the same as those in human serum and urine. The mothers' dietary intake averaged about 30 μg/day, which is lower than the 50 to 200 μg recommended daily allowance.

A high-density lipoprotein-cholesterol level can be increased with chromium supplementation. Chromium also is reported to have a favorable effect on serum lipid profiles. Deficiency of chromium in infancy may be an issue with low–birth weight infants or those with inadequate fetal stores.[82,83]

Fluorine. Fluorine has been widely accepted as a significant dietary factor in decreasing dental caries[104] (Table 4-20). The effect has been associated with the conversion of the enamel hydroxyapatite to fluorapatite with a reduction in acid solubility. It has been suggested that the presence of fluorine during the formation of hydroxyapatite creates less soluble, more resistant crystals. Fluorine levels in human milk are lower than in cow's milk. Ericsson et al.[27] have found lower values in human milk than previously reported. Cow's milk contains 0.03 to 0.10 mg/L and human milk contains 0.025 mg/L. Fluoridation of the water supply has shown variable results, but only a minimal effect on breast milk levels on fluorine. There was no rise in breast milk fluorine in breastfeeding mothers who had a rise in serum fluorine after an oral dose of fluoride.[25]

Fluorine excretion in milk and saliva was measured by Ericsson et al.[27] before and after ingestion of 300 ml of fluorine-enriched water (5.5 ppm). The milk levels were 0.05 ppm with little or no change measurable 2 hours following ingestion, although the concomitant saliva and blood plasma samples showed a response. More recent measurements, by newer techniques, are reported as being 0.015 μg/ml and <0.10 μg/ml of free ionic fluorine and total fluorine.[130] The authors comment on the inaccuracies at such low levels. It is interesting to note that bovine and rodent milks reflect similarly low values and lack of response to dosing. Milk products decreased the bioavailability of fluorine in adults when the fluorine was administered by oral tablet.[145]

The significant development of deciduous and permanent teeth is after birth and depends on fetal stores as well as on fluorine available in the diet. Studies comparing breastfed and bottle fed infants show a distinct difference, with fewer dental caries and better dental health in breastfed infants. The role of fluorine and other factors, such as selenium, that predispose the breastfed infant to healthier teeth have yet to be defined completely. Nursing-bottle caries add to the total dental caries of the bottle fed infant.

pH and osmolarity

The pH range in human milk is 6.7 to 7.4, with a mean of 7.1. The mean pH of cow's milk is 6.8. The caloric content of both human and cow's milk is 65 kcal/100 ml or 20 kcal/oz. The specific gravities are 1.031 and 1.032, respectively. The pH of the milk ingested has an effect on the infant and the development of metabolic acidosis, especially in episodes of dehydration.[20]

The osmolarity of human milk approximates that of human serum or 286 mosmol/ kg of water, whereas that for cow's milk is higher, 350 mosmol.[19] The renal solute load of human milk is considerably lower than that of cow's milk. Renal solute load is roughly calculated by totaling the solutes that must be excreted by the kidney. It consists primarily of nonmetabolizable dietary components, especially electrolytes, ingested in excess of body needs, and metabolic end products, mainly from the metabolism of protein. It can be estimated by adding the dietary intake of nitrogen and three minerals, sodium, potassium, and chloride. Each gram of protein is considered to yield 4 mosmol (as urea) and each milliequivalent of sodium, potassium, and chloride is 1 mosmol, according to Fomon.[29] The renal solute load of cow's milk is 221 mosmol, compared with 79 mosmol for human milk (Tables 4-18 and 4-23).

Osmoregulation in human lactation was investigated by Dearlove[22] in an effort to determine whether fluid loading was a valid clinical maneuver. It is known that an oral hypotonic fluid load results in suppression of prolactin in adults. After an intravenous hypotonic saline infusion, there was a significant correlation between serum osmolarity and prolactin. No changes in serum prolactin, milk yield, serum, or breast milk osmolarity were noted when normal lactating women were given a hypotonic fluid load in a controlled study.

Vitamins

VITAMIN A. Vitamin A content is 75 μg/100 ml or 280 international units (IU) in mature human milk and 41 μg/100 ml or 180 IU in cow's milk (Table 4-24). Thus the supply of vitamin A and its precursors, carotenoids, is considered adequate to meet the estimated daily requirement, which varies from 500 IU to 1500 IU/day if the infant consumes at least 200 ml of breast milk per day (Table 4-25). There is twice as much vitamin A in colostrum as in mature milk.

VITAMIN D. Vitamin D has always been included in the fat-soluble vitamin group because that is the form in which it had been identified in nature. The levels in human milk were 0.05 μg/100 ml, previously reported in the fat fraction. Human milk was shown by Lakdawala and Widdowson[84] in 1977 to have vitamin D in both the fat and the aqueous fractions. It was the water-soluble sulfate conjugate of vitamin D that was

Table 4-23. Dietary intake of protein, sodium chloride, and potassium and estimated renal solute load from various feedings

Feedings	Caloric density (kcal/100 ml)†	Dietary intake					Estimated renal solute load*		
		Quantity (ml)†	Protein (g)	Na (mEq)	Cl (mEq)	K (mEq)	Urea (mosmol)‡	Na + Cl + K (mosmol)	Total (mosmol)
Milks									
Whole cow milk	67	1000	33	25	29	35	132	89	221
Boiled skim milk	33	1000	46	35	40	49	184	124	308
Human milk	67	1000	12	7	11	13	48	31	79
Formulas									
SMA	100	1000	22	10	18	21	90	49	139
Similac	100	1000	24	17	24	28	97	69	166
Strained foods									
Pears	69	100	0.3	0.2	0.2	1.6	1	2	3
Applesauce	84	100	0.2	0.3	0.2	2.6	1	3	4
Beef with vegetables	104	100	6.3	1.2	1	3.1	25	5	30
Chicken with vegetables	100	100	6.3	1.1	0.9	2.1	25	4	29

From Fomon, S.J.: Infant nutrition, ed. 2, Philadelphia, 1974, W.B. Saunders Co. (Values in formulation of beef with vegetables and chicken with vegetables have been updated per personal communication with Fomon, S.J., August 6, 1984.)

*This simplified estimate of renal solute load is appropriate for use with respect to full-size but not low-birth weight infants.

†For strained foods, 100 g rather than 100 ml.

‡Assumed to account for 70% of nitrogen intake.[149]

Table 4-24. Vitamins and other constituents of human milk and cow's milk (per 100 ml)

Milk elements	Colostrum	Transitional	Mature	Cow's milk
Vitamins				
Vitamin A (μg)	151.0	88.0	75.0	41.0
Vitamin B_1 (μg)	1.9	5.9	14.0	43.0
Vitamin B_2 (μg)	30.0	37.0	40.0	145.0
Nicotinic acid (μg)	75.0	175.0	160.0	82.0
Vitamin B_6 (μg)			12.0-15.0	64.0
Pantothenic acid (μg)	183.0	288.0	246.0	340.0
Biotin (μg)	0.06	0.35	0.6	2.8
Folic acid (μg)	0.05	0.02	0.14	0.13
Vitamin B_{12} (μg)	0.05	0.04	0.1	0.6
Vitamin C (mg)	5.9	7.1	5.0	1.1
Vitamin D (μg)	—	—	0.04	0.02
Vitamin E (mg)	1.5	0.9	0.25	0.07
Vitamin K (μg)	—	—	1.5	6.0
Ash (g)	0.3	0.3	0.2	0.7
Calories (kcal)	57.0	63.0	65.0	65.0
Specific gravity	1050.0	1035.0	1031.0	1032.0
Milk (pH)	—	—	7.0	6.8

measured. Other investigators have attempted to repeat this work, but more importantly they have evaluated the biologic activity of any water-soluble metabolites. When activity is measured by an assay that measures stimulation of intestinal calcium transport, human milk is found to contain 40 to 50 IU/L of vitamin D activity. The metabolite 25-hydroxyvitamin D_3 accounts for 75% of the activity; vitamin D_2 and vitamin D_3 account for 15% activity.[60] Vitamin D sulfate, or any other as yet unidentified water-soluble metabolite of vitamin D, provides no significant biologic activity.[38]

The impact of the maternal diet content of vitamin D was measured in a double-blind study of white mothers in a temperate climate in the winter.[117] A direct relationship was seen between maternal and infant levels of 25-hydroxyvitamin D_3 and maternal diet. An additional group of infants, whose mothers' diets were unsupplemented, received 400 IU vitamin D/day had even higher serum concentrations of 25 hydroxyvitamin D_3. Clearly the levels vary and may be inadequate in human milk in some situations, especially in cold climates in the winter when there is little sunshine, especially for dark-skinned individuals. The level of 40 IU/100 ml or 1.00 μg/100 ml may provide adequate amounts in the fully breastfed infant to meet the requirements of 400 IU or 10 mg/day. See Table 4-25 for recommended daily allowances. Levels of vitamin D are also higher in colostrum than in mature milk.

VITAMIN E. Vitamin E has been a subject of much interest. Levels in colostrum are 1.5 mg/100 ml, whereas transitional milk has 0.9 mg/100 ml and mature milk has 0.25 mg/100 ml. The difference at different stages has been found to be due to α-tocopherol, because the contents of β- and γ-tocopherol are similar. Total tocopherol in mature milk correlates with total lipid and linoleic acid contents. Significantly higher tocopherol/linoleic acid ratios are found in both colostrum and transitional milk than in mature milk.[65]

Table 4-25.   Recommended daily dietary allowances for fat-soluble vitamins for infants*

Age (yr)	Weight		Height		Protein (g)	Vitamin A (μg R.E.)†	Vitamin D (μg)‡	Vitamin E (mg αT.E.)§
	(kg)	(lb)	(cm)	(in)				
0.0-0.5	6	13	60	24	kg × 2.2	420	10	3
0.5-1.0	9	20	71	28	kg × 2.0	400	10	4

From Food and Nutrition Board, National Research Council, National Academy of Sciences: Recommended dietary allowances, ed. 9, Washington, D.C., 1980, U.S. Government Printing Office.
*The allowances are intended to provide for individual variations among most normal persons as they live in the United States under usual environmental stresses. Diets should be based on a variety of common foods in order to provide other nutrients for which human requirements have been less well defined.
†Retinol equivalents. 1 retinol equivalent = 1 μg retinol or 6 μg carotene.
‡As cholecalciferol, 10 μg cholecalciferol = 400 IU vitamin D.
§α-Tocopherol equivalents 1 mg d-α-tocopherol = 1 αT.E.

Table 4-26.   Recommended daily dietary allowances for vitamins for infants*

Age (yr)	Vitamin K (μg)	Biotin (μg)	Pantothenic acid (mg)
0-0.5	12	35	2
0.5-1	10-20	50	3

From Food and Nutrition Board, National Research Council, National Academy of Sciences: Recommended dietary allowances, ed. 9, Washington, D.C., 1980, U.S. Government Printing Office.
*The allowances are intended to provide for individual variations among most normal persons as they live in the United States under usual environmental stresses. Diets should be based on a variety of common foods in order to provide other nutrients for which human requirements have been less well defined.

Cow's milk has 0.07 mg/100 ml of vitamin E (Table 4-24). Correspondingly, serum levels in breastfed infants rise quickly at birth and maintain a normal level, whereas cow's milk–fed infants have depressed levels. Vitamin E includes a group of fat-soluble compounds, α-, β-, γ-, and δ-tocopherol, and their unsaturated derivatives, α-, β-, γ-, and δ-tocotrienol. An international unit of vitamin E is equal to 1 mg of synthetic α-tocopherol or 0.74 mg of natural α-tocopherol acetate. Vitamin E is required for muscle integrity, resistance of erythrocytes to hemolysis, as well as for other biochemical and physiologic functions. The requirement for vitamin E is related to the polyunsaturated fatty acid (PUFA) content of the cellular structures and of the diet (see Table 4-25). Satisfactory plasma levels are 1 mg/100 ml, and these can be maintained by feedings with a vitamin E/PUFA ratio of 0.4 mg/g. Ordinarily, this would be supplied by 4 IU of vitamin E/day. Since human milk contains 1.8 mg/L or 40 μg of vitamin E/g of lipid, it supplies more than adequate levels of vitamin E.

VITAMIN K.   Vitamin K is in human milk at the level of 15 μg/100 ml, whereas its level in cow's milk is 60 μg/100 ml. Vitamin K is essential for the synthesis of blood clotting factors, which are normal in the serum at the time of birth. See Table 4-26 for recommended daily dietary allowances. Vitamin K is produced by the intestinal flora but takes several days in the previously sterile gut to be effective. Vitamin K–dependent clotting factors in normal breastfed infants were studied by Jimenez et al.,[71] who reported that no infant studied had clinical evidence of bleeding. The prothrombin time and partial thromboplastin time were similar in breastfed and bottle fed infants. The normotest and thrombotest were significantly prolonged in the breastfed group. The authors concluded that 5% of breastfed children have possible vitamin K deficiency. There are several case reports[89,101] of infants exclusively breastfed with no vitamin K given at birth who developed late onset hemorrhagic disease that responded to vitamin K administration. The report by O'Connor et al.[101] points out the association of vitamin K deficiency with home birth and suggests that the physician give vitamin K as recommended by the Academy of Pediatrics if it has been omitted (Table 4-26). It is recommended that all infants receive vitamin K at birth, regardless of feeding plans, to prevent hemorrhagic disease of the newborn caused by vitamin K deficiency in the first few days of life.[13]

VITAMIN C. Human milk is an outstanding source of water-soluble vitamins and reflects maternal dietary intake (Table 4-24). Increased vitamin C has been measured in the milk within 30 minutes of a bolus of vitamin C being given to the mother. Human milk contains 43 mg/100 ml (fresh cow's milk contains up to 21 mg). Levels obtained in normal lactating women 6 months postpartum were 35 mg/L in those on normal diets and 38 mg/L in those supplemented with multivitamins containing 90 mg vitamin C.[139] Levels obtained in 16 low–socioeconomic level lactating women were 53 mg/L for unsupplemented and 65 mg/L for supplemented mothers at 1 week postpartum and 61 mg/L and 72 mg/L respectively at 6 weeks postpartum. Several subjects in the unsupplemented low socioeconomic group had levels too low to provide 35 mg vitamin C/day to their infants. It is probably appropriate for pregnant women and nursing mothers to increase their intake of vitamin C. Vitamin C is part of several enzyme and hormone systems as well as of intracellular chemical reactions. It is essential to collagen synthesis (Table 4-27).

At a symposium[26] on vitamin C, it was pointed out that the body requirements for vitamin C increase during stress. Most species manufacture their own vitamin C. These include the calf; therefore, there is little vitamin C in cow's milk. The common housefly makes 10 g of vitamin C for every 70 kg of housefly weight, according to the discussion by Enloe et al.[26]

VITAMIN B COMPLEX

Vitamin B₁. Vitamin B_1, or thiamin, levels increase with the duration of lactation, but are lower in human milk (160 µg/100 ml) than in cow's milk (440 µg/100 ml). In a study by Nail et al.,[99] levels obtained by normal lactating women showed significant increases between 1 and 6 weeks postpartum, but there was no difference in levels between supplemented (1.7 mg daily) and unsupplemented women. Thiamin is essential for the use of carbohydrates in the pyruvate metabolism (cofactor in pyruvic acid decarboxylation) for fat synthesis. Insufficient thiamin produces insufficient carbohydrate oxidation with accumulation of intermediary metabolites such as lactic acid. See Table 4-27 for recommended daily allowances.

Vitamin B₂. Vitamin B_2, or riboflavin, is significant for the newborn in whom intestinal tract bacterial synthesis is minimal (see Table 4-27 for recommended daily allow-

Table 4-27. Recommended daily dietary allowances for water-soluble vitamins for infants*

Age (yr)	Vitamin C (mg)	Thiamin (mg)	Riboflavin (mg)	Niacin (mg N.E.)†	Vitamin B$_6$ (mg)	Folacin‡ (μg)	Vitamin B$_{12}$ (μg)
0-0.5	35	0.3	0.4	6	0.3	30	0.58
0.5-1	35	0.5	0.6	8	0.6	45	1.5

From Food and Nutrition Board, National Research Council, National Academy of Sciences: Recommended dietary allowances, ed. 9, Washington, D.C., 1980, U.S. Government Printing Office.
*The allowances are intended to provide for individual variations among most normal persons as they live in the United States under usual environmental stresses. Diets should be based on a variety of common foods in order to provide other nutrients for which human requirements have been less well defined.
†INF. (niacin equivalent) is equal to 1 mg of niacin or 60 mg of dietary tryptophan.
‡The folacin allowances refer to dietary sources as determined by *Lactobacillus casei* assay after treatment with enzymes ("conjugases") to make polyglutamyl forms of the vitamin.

ances). Riboflavin is involved in oxidative intracellular systems and is essential for protoplasmic growth. There are 36 μg/100 ml in human milk and 175 μg/100 ml in cow's milk (Table 4-24).

Levels obtained in normal lactating women showed significantly lower levels of riboflavin in the milk of the unsupplemented women (36.7 μg/100 ml) at 1 week as compared with the milk of the supplemented women, who received 2 mg/day in a multivitamin (80.0 μg/100 ml). There was no significant difference between 1 and 6 weeks in either group.[99]

Niacin. Niacin (nicotinamide) is an essential part of the pyridine nucleotide coenzymes and is part of the intracellular respiratory mechanisms. There is 147 μg/100 ml in human milk and 94 μg/100 ml in cow's milk (Table 4-24).

Vitamin B$_6$. Vitamin B$_6$ (pyridoxine) forms the enzyme group of certain decarboxylases and transaminases involved in metabolism of nerve tissue. The supply of vitamin B$_6$ is vital to DNA synthesis, which is needed to form the cerebrosides in the myelination of the central nervous system (see Table 4-27 for recommended daily allowances). There is 12 to 15 μg/100 ml of vitamin B$_6$ in human milk and 64 μg/100 ml in cow's milk. The principal form of B$_6$ in human milk is pyridoxal (PL), whereas pyridoxine (PN) is the principal form of vitamin B$_6$ fortification in infant formulas.[142] Levels of vitamin B$_6$ in the milk of mothers consuming more than 2.5 mg of the vitamin daily (RDA for lactating women is 2.5 mg/day) were significantly higher in the first week than were levels in the unsupplemented mother's milk. Average maternal diets in several studies were consistently below the recommended levels of vitamin B$_6$.[115] The recommended daily intake for infants under 6 months of age is 0.30 mg.

Long-term use of oral contraceptives has been shown to result in low levels of vitamin B$_6$ in maternal serum in pregnancy and at delivery and low levels in the milk of these mothers.[116] The relationship of B$_6$ supplements to suppression of prolactin and the treatment of galactorrhea is discussed under lactation failure (see Chapter 15). The doses used to suppress lactation (600 mg/day) far exceed the levels in multiple vitamins (1 to 10 mg).

Pantothenic acid.   Pantothenic acid is part of coenzyme A, a catalyst of acetylation reactions. The reaction of coenzyme A with acetic acid to form acetyl-CoA is prime to intermediary metabolism. The levels of pantothenic acid in human milk were restudied by Johnston et al.[74] because of the range of values in the literature. They found the mean to be 670 μg/100 ml in fore- and hindmilk samples. No change occurred in concentrations from 1 to 6 months postpartum. They did find a positive correlation with dietary intake. Recommended daily allowances appear in Table 4-26.

Folacin.   Folacin (folic acid) is part of the conversion of glycine to serine. It is also involved in the methylation of nicotinamide and homocystine to methionine. It is essential for erythropoiesis. There is 52 μg of folic acid/100 ml of breast milk and 55 μg/ 100 ml in cow's milk. Colostrum is relatively low in folacin, but levels increase as lactation proceeds according to newer techniques applied by Cooperman et al.,[17] who found considerable variation with a mean of 33.4 μg/100 ml. Supplementation with folic acid in deficient mothers caused prompt increase in levels in the milk. When mothers and their infants were evaluated by Tamura et al.,[137] folate levels were higher in the breastfed infants than in their mothers but there was a correlation between levels in the milk and in the infants' plasma. Folic acid has also been identified as a critical element in deficiency states during pregnancy, being associated with abruptio placentae, toxemia, and intrauterine growth failure as well as megaloblastic anemia.

Vitamin B_{12}.   Early studies reported that vitamin B_{12} is found in human milk in low concentration, 0.3 μg/100 ml, whereas cow's milk has 4.0 μg/ml. Well-nourished mothers on balanced diets appear to have adequate amounts for their infants. Microbiologic assay has demonstrated that very high concentrations of vitamin B_{12} appear in early colostrum but level off in a few days to those of serum. Colostric samples reported by Samson and McClelland[118] have a mean binding capacity of 72 ng/ml; in mature milk the capacity is one third of this value. Vitamin B_{12} levels were compared by Sandberg et al.[119] in supplemented and unsupplemented mothers and were not significantly different. Levels were 33 to 320 ng/100 ml, with a mean of 97 ng/100 ml. When nutritionally deficient low–socioeconomic group lactating women were studied by Sneed et al.,[131] supplementation with a multivitamin did indeed result in elevated vitamin B_{12} levels. This was true for folate as well.

Although cow's milk has five to ten times more vitamin B_{12} than is found in mature human milk, cow's milk has little vitamin B_{12}–binding capacity, which is substantial in human milk. Vitamin B_{12} functions in transmethylations such as synthesis of choline from methionine, serine from glycine, and methionine from homocysteine. It is involved in pyrimidine and purine metabolism. Vitamin B_{12} also affects the metabolism of folic acid. Megaloblastic anemia is a common symptom of vitamin B_{12} deficiency. Vitamin B_{12} occurs exclusively in animal tissue, is bound to protein, and is minimal or absent in vegetable protein. The minimum daily requirement for infants according to Fomon et al.[30] is 0.3 μg/day in the first year of life, when growth is rapid. (See Table 4-27.)

Enzymes

By and large, researchers have tended to dismiss the significance of enzymes in breast milk by saying that they are all destroyed by the gastric juices. Unfortunately, until recently little effort has been applied to studying the activities of enzymes in humans, although considerable data have been collected on the enzymatic activities of many milks. Jenness and Sloan[68] report 44 enzymes detected so far in bovine, human, and some other milks. Xanthine oxidase, lactoperoxidase, uridine diphosphogalactose, glucose, galactosyl transferase, ribonuclease, lipase, alkaline phosphatase, acid phosphatase, and lysozyme have been isolated, in crystalline form.

The role and significance of enzymes in human milk were reported by Shahani et al.,[124] who confirmed that there are over 20 active human-milk enzymes. More and higher levels of enzymes occur in human milk. Some enzyme levels are significantly higher in colostrum than in mature milk (Table 4-28). Most are whey proteins and contribute minimally to milk proteins. Some enzymes, like other proteins in milk, are probably produced elsewhere and are transported to the breast via the bloodstream.[63] The evidence to support the concept of local synthesis includes the demonstration of secretory tissue in the mammary gland. Amylase levels are twice as high in milk as in

Table 4-28.   Enzyme levels in human milk colostrum versus normal milk

Enzyme	Colostrum	Normal milk	Bovine milk
Adenosine triphosphatase		+	
Alanine amino transferase		2×	
Aldolase		+	
α-Amylase (diastase)*	+		
β-Amylase	1.5×		
Aspartate aminotransferase		2×	
Catalase	2×		
Cholinesterase		+	
Glucose-6-phosphate de-hydrogenase	No change		
Glucose-phosphate iso-merase	1.5×		
Inorganic pyrophosphatase	+		
Lactic dehydrogenase	+		
Lipase		+	
Lysozyme		+	3000 less
Lysozyme	No change		
Malic dehydrogenase	+		
Peroxidase	+		100×
Phosphatase, acid	3×		Same
Phosphatase, alkaline	4×		40×
Protease	2×		
Xanthine oxidase	+		10x

Modified from Shahani, K.M., Kwan, A.J., and Friend, B.A.: Am. J. Clin. Nutr. **33:**1861, 1980.
*The enzyme reported as diastase is most likely α-amylase but may also contain some β-amylase.

serum.[55,88] Casein proteins have been synthesized in vitro in cell–free mammary derived mRNA enriched systems. Mammary explants from mice, monkeys, and humans have accumulated lactose synthetase B. The enzymes of possible importance in infant digestion are those with pancreatic analogues: amylase, lipases, protease(s), and ribonuclease.[124,133,150]

AMYLASE.   Mammary amylase is present throughout lactation.[55,88] Levels are higher in colostrum than in mature milk. Milk levels are twice those of serum in the first 90 days and remain higher in serum over 6 months. When exposed to a pH of 5.3, this salivary-type amylase remains active; at a pH of 3.5, one half the original activity is present at 2 hours and one third at 6 hours. Much milk amylase activity remains in the duodenum after a meal of human milk. This is significant for the digestion of starch because pancreatic amylase is still low in infants. It has been suggested that mammary amylase may be an alternate pathway of digestion of glucose polymers as well as of starch.

DIASTASE.   Diastase catalyzes the hydrolysis of starch to maltose and may indeed be α-amylase or a mixture of α and β-amylase. There is a high level of diastase in colostrum, with an initial rapid fall and a constant level for the next 6 months. Since most infants are deficient in diastase initially, this may account for the lack of apparent digestive disturbances when starch gruels are introduced early.[122]

GLUCOSE-6-PHOSPHATE DEHYDROGENASE.   Glucose-6-phosphate dehydrogenase (G-6-PD) is rich in the milk of mothers with normal red cell dehydrogenase and absent in mothers with G-6-PD deficiency. Its levels are dependent on the increased rate of carbohydrate metabolism in the mammary gland.[122]

LACTIC AND MALIC ACID DEHYDROGENASES.   Lactic and malic acid dehydrogenase levels are high in colostrum, are lower in mature milk, and increase at the end of a feeding. The levels are higher in species with small body size, thus mice and humans have more than cows. Since there is no correlation with serum levels, it is believed to be synthesized in the mammary gland.

LACTOSE SYNTHETASE.   Lactose synthetase catalyzes the synthesis of lactose from UDP-galactose and glucose. This enzyme has two components: A-protein, a glycoprotein, and B-protein, which is a α-lactalbumin. The control mechanism for lactose biosynthesis by the A-protein and α-lactalbumin ensures that lactose is synthesized in the mammary gland only in response to specific hormones.

LIPASE.   More information has been accumulated about the activity of lipase than about other enzymes. It catalyzes the hydrolysis of glycerol esters in emulsion. A serum-stimulated lipoprotein lipase has been isolated from the "cream" and a bile salt–stimulated lipase from the skim portion.[12] The serum-stimulated lipase appears to be the result of mammary-gland leakage. The bile salt–stimulated lipase is in higher levels and resembles pancreatic lipase. It plays a significant role in the digestion of milk triacylglycerols in the intestines of infants fed human milk. It augments the low level of lipid resorption, even in low pH and high bile-salt concentrations. Human milk lipases can be activated at refrigerator temperatures.

LYSOZYME.   Lysozyme is a thermostabile nonspecific antimicrobial factor that catalyzes the hydrolysis of β-linkage between *N*-acetyl glucosamine and *N*-acetyl muramic acid in the bacterial cell wall. It is bacteriolytic toward *Enterobacteriaceae* and grampositive bacteria and is considered to play a role in the antibacterial activity of milk as well as a significant role in the development of intestinal flora. It also hydrolyzes mucopolysaccharides. Human lysozyme is antigenically and serologically different from the bovine enzyme. The content in human milk is 3000 times that in bovine milk and the activity 100 times that of bovine milk. It is considered to be a spillover product from breast epithelial cells.

PHOSPHATASES.   Acid phosphatase is similar in human and bovine milk, but alkaline phosphatase is much less active in human milk by a factor of 40. Its level increases with the increase in fat concentration and increases as the feeding progresses. Stewart et al.[132] have studied the level in 199 samples from 20 donors. There was no relationship to age, nationality, or other characteristics of the donor, except for a tendency to increase over time. They determined that alkaline phosphatase concentrations appeared to be related to the fat concentration in human milk. Levels increased as lactation progressed.

PROTEASE.   Protease catalyzes the hydrolysis of proteins. There are high levels of protease in human milk, which suggests that enzymes may provide the breastfed infant with significant digestive assistance immediately after birth.

XANTHINE OXIDASE.   Xanthine oxidase catalyzes the oxidation of purines, pyrimidines, and aldehydes. Although bovine milk contains high levels, it was only after much effort that investigators were able to identify it in human milk.[148] The activity in human milk peaks on the third day after birth and decreases with the progression of lactation. It differs from that in bovine milk in that it is not of bacterial origin and its activity is correlated with protein concentration.

Hormones

Hormones are present in human milk and in the milk of other mammals. Animal studies have shown that at least some of these hormones retain physiological activity when ingested but not when pasteurized. Although their presence was recognized in the 1930s, advances in hormone assay techniques have brought more information to light.[79] Hormones with simple structures, such as steroids and thyroxine (T_4), can pass easily into the milk from circulating blood. Peptide hormones such as hypothalamic-releasing hormones, because of their small size, would be expected to appear in milk. Of the larger–molecular weight pituitary hormones, only prolactin has been found so far. The hormones identified in human milk include gonadotropin-releasing hormone, thyroid-releasing hormone (TRH), thyroid-stimulating hormone (thyrotropin, TSH), prolactin, gonadotropins, ovarian hormones, corticosteroids, erythropoietin, cyclic adenosine monophosphate (cAMP), and cyclic guanosine monophosphate (cGMP).

The concentration of hormones changes during lactation, with prolactin decreasing over time and triiodothyronine (T_3) and T_4 increasing. There is information demonstrating that the gastrointestinal tract of suckling mammals possesses the ability to absorb various proteins with substantial preservation of their immunologic properties. The absorption of large–molecular weight hormones has been demonstrated in suckling rats and mice with measurable amounts appearing in serum and other tissues.

The thyroid hormones have received considerable attention because of the apparent protection of hypothyroid infants who are breastfed. TSH content was investigated by both direct ^{125}I-TSH radioimmunoassay and radioimmunoassay.[138] TSH was present in human milk in low concentrations comparable to those normally found in the serum of euthyroid adults. Experimentally, thyroidectomy of the lactating rat led to the disappearance of measurable T_4 and an increase in the level of TSH in the milk. In contrast, administration of T_3 decreased the TSH in the rat model.

Prolactin has been identified as a normal constituent of human milk. Levels are high in the first few days postpartum but subsequently decline rapidly. The exact mechanism by which prolactin enters the milk is unclear. Prolactin-binding sites have been identified within the alveolar cells.[54] The functional significance of prolactin also remains unclear. In rodents, milk prolactin influences fluid and ion absorption from the jejunum. It may influence gonadal and adrenal function as demonstrated in other species.

Endocrine responses in the neonate differ between breastfed and formula fed infants.[90] In a study of 34 6-day-old healthy full-term infants who were formula fed, there were significant changes in the plasma concentrations of insulin, motilin, enteroglucagon, neurotensin, and pancreatic polypeptide following a feeding. Similar levels were measured in 43 normal breastfed infants and little or no change was noted. Further, the basal levels of gastric inhibitory polypeptide, motilin, neurotensin, and vasoactive intestinal peptide were also higher in the bottle fed than in the breastfed infants. Whether pancreatic and gut hormone-release changes affect postnatal development is yet to be determined.

PROSTAGLANDINS.   In the investigation of the factors in human milk that may modify or supplement physiological functions in the neonate, the role of prostaglandins comes under review. Prostaglandins include any of a class of physiologically active substances present in many tissues and originally described in genital fluid and accessory glands. Among the many effects are those of vasodepression, stimulation of intestinal smooth muscle, uterine stimulation, aggregation of blood platelets, and antagonism to hormones influencing lipid metabolism. Prostaglandins are a group of prostanoic acids often abbreviated PGE, PGF, PGA, and PGB with numeric subscripts according to structure.

The synthesis of prostaglandins occurs when dietary linoleic acid is converted in the body by a series of steps involving chain lengthening and dehydration to arachidonic acid, the principal (but not the only) precursor of prostaglandins. Although the prostaglandins are similar in structure, the biologic effects of various prostaglandins produced from a single unsaturated fatty acid can be profoundly different and, in some cases, antagonistic.

Because of the possible beneficial effects of prostaglandins on the gastrointestinal tract of infants, several investigators[91,114] have measured levels in human milk. The measurements were made in colostrum, transitional milk, and mature milk with collections of both fore- and hindmilk. PGE and PGF have been shown to be present in breast milk in over 100 times the concentration in adult plasma (Fig. 4-5). The ratio of the principal metabolite of PGFM to PGF itself suggests a relatively long half-life (Fig. 4-6). Although prostaglandins occur in cow's milk, none was measurable in cows' milk–based formulas. Two inactive metabolites were found in milk in levels similar to those in the control adult plasma.

It is thought that prostaglandins play a role in gastrointestinal motility, possibly

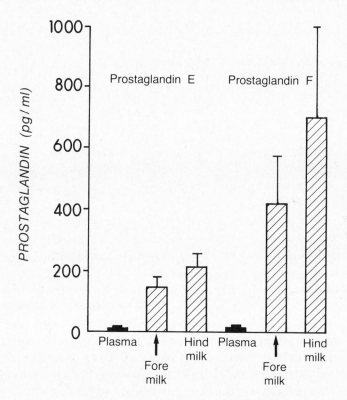

Prostaglandin E and prostaglandin F (pg/ml ± SEM) in human milk and adult plasma.

Fig. 4-5. PGE and PGF (pg/ml ± SEM) in human milk and adult plasma. (From Lucas, A., and Mitchell, M.D.: Prostaglandins in human milk, Arch. Dis. Child. 55:950, 1980.)

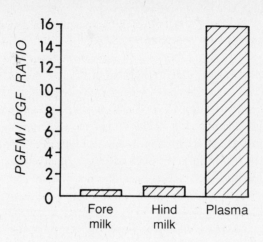

PGFM / PGF ratio in human milk and
adult plasma.

Fig. 4-6. PGFM/PGF ratio in human milk and adult plasma. (From Lucas, A., and Mitchell, M.D.: Prostaglandins in human milk, Arch. Dis. Child. **55**:950, 1980.)

assisting peristalsis physiologically. It is thought by Pickles et al.[108] that infantile diarrhea might occasionally be due to excessive prostaglandin secretion into the mother's milk during menstruation, when maternal plasma levels of PGF may be raised. The difference in stool patterns between breast and formula feeds may be partially attributable to the presence of prostaglandins in human milk and not in formulas. The role of prostaglandins in the pathogenesis of food intolerance is also under study, since prostaglandins have a cytoprotective effect on the upper bowel and reportedly are increased in patients with abnormal peristalsis and irritable bowel syndrome.[87]

BILE SALTS.   Another limiting factor in digestion in the newborn is the decreased bile-salt pool and the low concentration of bile salts in the duodenum. The presence of some biologically active substances in human milk contributes to digestion in the newborn. For this reason the role of bile salts was investigated and cholate and chenodeoxycholate were found in all samples of milk obtained from 28 lactating women in the first postpartum week.[32] In both colostrum and milk there was a predominance of cholate. Samples were randomly collected and the range of concentration was wide. The ratio of maternal serum to milk was 1:1 for cholate and 4:1 for chenodeoxycholate. The significance of these findings is under study.

EPIDERMAL GROWTH FACTOR.   Epidermal growth factor (EGF) is a small polypeptide mitogen that has been identified in many species, including humans. Of the growth factors that have been purified to date, EGF is one of the most biologically potent and best characterized as to its physical, chemical, and biologic properties. It is well established that EGF stimulates the proliferation of epidermal and epithelial tissues and has significant biologic effects in the intact mammal, particularly in the fetus and the newborn.[9,10] Effects verified in humans also include increased growth and maturation of the fetal pulmonary epithelium, stimulation of ornithine decarboxylase activity and DNA synthesis in the digestive tract, and acceleration of the healing of wounds of the corneal epithelium. Quite unrelated is the observation that EGF inhibits histamine- or pentagastrin-induced secretion of gastric acid. It has a maturational effect on duodenal mucosal cells and increased lactase activity and net calcium transport in suckling rats. EGF has been identified in plasma, saliva, urine, amniotic fluid, and milk. Human milk is known to be mitogenic for cultured cells. EGF is active when administered orally, stable in acid, and resistant to trypsin digestion.

Newborn puppies, fed their mother's milk, were found to have hyperplasia of the enteric mucosa as compared with formula fed littermates. Furthermore, the intestinal weight, length, and DNA and RNA content were greater in the puppies fed their mother's milk.

Studies of EGF in human milk first reported the fact that human milk stimulates DNA synthesis in cell cultures in which growth had been arrested.[97] The mitogenic activity of the milk was neutralized by the addition of antibody to human EGF. These findings support the concept that EGF is a major growth-promoting agent in breast milk. Actual measurements of EGF in the milk of 11 mothers who delivered at term and 20 who delivered prematurely were also done. EGF concentrations were 68 ± 19 ng/ml (mean ± SEM) in those who delivered at term and 70 ± 5 ng/ml (mean ± SEM) in the milk of those who delivered prematurely. There was no significant change over 7 weeks and no diurnal variation. The total EGF content was closely correlated with the volume of milk expressed, suggesting to the authors that EGF has a passive transport from the circulation as a function of plasma concentration.[9,10,97] Little change occurred with refrigeration or freezing. The role of EGF in promoting normal growth and functional maturation of the intestinal tract must be confirmed.

REFERENCES

1. Almroth, S.G.: Water requirements of breast-fed infants in a hot climate, Am. J. Clin. Nutr. **31:**1154, 1978.
2. Anaokar, S.G., and Garry, P.J.: Effects of maternal iron nutrition during lactation on milk iron and rat neonatal iron status, Am. J. Clin. Nutr. **34:**1505, 1981.
3. Archibald, J.G.: Trace elements in bovine milk, Dairy Sci. Abstr. **20:**212, 1958.
4. Asnes, R.S., et al.: The dietary chloride deficiency syndrome occurring in a breastfed infant, J. Pediatr. **100:**923, 1982.
5. Atkinson, S.A., Bryan, M.H., and Anderson, G.H.: Human milk: differences in nitrogen concentration in milk from mothers of term and premature infants, J. Pediatr. **93:**67, 1978.
6. Auricchio, S., Rubino, A., and Mürset, E.: Intestinal glycosidase activities in the human embryo, fetus, and newborn, Pediatrics **35:**944, 1965.
7. Barltrop, D., and Hillier, R.: Calcium and phosphorus content of transitional and mature human milk, Acta. Paediatr. Scand. **63:**347, 1974.

8. Brown, K.H., et al.: Clinical and field studies of human lactation: methodological considerations, Am. J. Clin. Nutr. **35:**745, 1982.

9. Carpenter, G.: Epidermal growth factor is a major growth-promoting agent in human milk, Science **210:**198, 1980.

10. Carpenter, G., and Cohen, S.: Epidermal growth factor, Ann. Rev. Biochem. **48:**193, 1979.

11. Casey, C.E., Walravens, P.A., and Hambidge, K.M.: Availability of zinc: loading tests with human milk, cow's milk, and infant formulas, Pediatrics **68:**394, 1981.

12. Challacombe, D.N., Edkins, S., and Brown, G.A.: Duodenal bile acids in infancy, Arch. Dis. Child. **50:**837, 1975.

13. Committee on Nutrition, American Academy of Pediatrics: Vitamin K supplementation for infants, Pediatrics **48:**483, 1971.

14. Committee on Nutrition, American Academy of Pediatrics: Commentary on breast-feeding and infant formulas, including proposed standards for formulas, Pediatrics **57:**278, 1976.

15. Committee on Nutrition, American Academy of Pediatrics: Nutrition and lactation, Pediatrics **68:**435, 1981.

16. Committee on Nutrition, American Academy of Pediatrics: Sodium intake of infants in the United States, Pediatrics **68:**445, 1981.

17. Cooperman, J.M., Dweck, H.S., and Newman, L.J.: The folate in human milk, Am. J. Clin. Nutr. **36:**576, 1982.

18. Cousins, R.J., and Smith, K.T.: Zinc-binding properties of bovine and human milk in vitro: influence of changes in zinc content, Am. J. Clin. Nutr. **33:**1083, 1980.

19. Dale, G., et al.: Plasma osmolality, sodium, and urea in healthy breast-fed and bottle-fed infants in Newcastle-upon-Tyne, Arch. Dis. Child. **50:**731, 1975.

20. Davies, D.P.: Plasma osmolality and protein intake in preterm infants, Arch. Dis. Child. **48:**575, 1973.

21. Davies, D.P., and Saunders, R.: Blood urea: normal values in early infancy related to feeding practices, Arch. Dis. Child. **48:**563, 1973.

22. Dearlove, J.C.: Prolactin, fluid balance, and lactation, Br. J. Obstet. Gynaecol. **88:**652, 1981.

23. Dick, G.: The etiology of multiple sclerosis, Proc. R. Soc. Med. **69:**611, 1976.

24. Eckhert, C.D., et al.: Zinc binding: a difference between human and bovine milk, Science **195:**789, 1977.

25. Ekstrand, J., Boreus, L.O., and de Chateau, P.: Fluoride in breast milk after oral dosing, Br. Med. J. **283:**761, 1981.

26. Enloe, C.F., and Hartley, H.L., moderators: To dose or megadose: a debate about vitamin C, Nutr. Today **13**(2):6, 1978.

27. Ericsson, Y., Hellström, I., and Hofvander, Y.: Pilot studies on the fluoride metabolism in infants on different feedings, Acta. Paediatr. Scand. **61:**459, 1972.

28. Feeley, R.M., et al.: Copper, iron, and zinc contents of human milk at early stages of lactation, Am. J. Clin. Nutr. **37:**443, 1983.

29. Fomon, S.J.: Infant nutrition, ed. 2, Philadelphia, 1974, W.B. Saunders Co.

30. Fomon, S.J., Ziegler, E.E., and Vazquez, H.D.: Human milk and the small premature infant, Am. J. Dis. Child. **131:**463, 1977.

31. Forfar, J.O.: Calcium, phosphorus, magnesium metabolism. In Forfar, J.O., editor: Aspects of neonatal metabolism, Clin. Endocrinol. Metab. **5**(1):123, 1976.

32. Forsyth, J.S., Ross, P.E., and Bouchier, I.A.D.: Bile salts in breast milk, Eur. J. Pediatr. **140:**126, 1983.

33. Fransson, G.B., and Lönnerdal, B.: Iron in human milk, J. Pediatr. **96:**380, 1980.

34. Fransson, G.B., and Lönnerdal, B.: Zinc, copper, calcium and magnesium in human milk, J. Pediatr. **101:**504, 1982.

35. Gaull, G.E.: Taurine in the nutrition of the human infant, Acta. Paediatr. Scand. (Suppl.) **269:**38, 1982.

36. Gibson, R.A., and Kneebore, G.M.: Fatty acid composition of human colostrum and mature breast milk, Am. J. Clin. Nutr. **34:**252, 1981.

37. Glass, R.L., Troolin, H.A., and Jenness, R.: Comparative biochemical studies of milks. IV. Constituent fatty acids of milk fats, Comp. Biochem. Physiol. **22:**415, 1967.

38. Greer, F.R., et al.: Water-soluble vitamin D in human milk: a myth, Pediatrics **69:**238, 1982.

39. Greer, F.R., et al.: Increasing serum calcium and magnesium concentrations in breast-fed infants: longitudinal studies of minerals in human milk and in sera of nursing mothers and their infants, J. Pediatr. **100:**59, 1982.

40. Guthrie, H.A., Picciano, M.F., and Sheehe, D.: Fatty acid patterns of human milk, J. Pediatr. **90:**39, 1977.

41. György, P.: Biochemical aspects. In Jelliffe, D.B., and Jelliffe, E.F.P., editors: The uniqueness of human milk, Am. J. Clin. Nutr. **24:**970, 1971.

42. Hadjimarkos, D.M., and Shearer, T.R.: Selenium in mature human milk, Am. J. Clin. Nutr. **26:**583, 1973.
43. Hall, B.: Activation of human milk lipase, Biochem. Soc. Trans. **3:**90, 1975.
44. Hall, B.: Changing composition of human milk and early development of appetite control, Lancet **1:**779, 1975.
45. Hall, B., and Muller, D.P.R.: Studies on the bile salt stimulated lipolytic activity of human milk using whole milk as source of both substrate and enzyme. I. Nutritional implications, Pediatr. Res. **16:**251, 1982.
46. Hall, B., and Muller, D.P.R.: Studies on bile-salt-stimulated lipolytic activity in human milk. II. Demonstration of two groups of milk with different activities, Pediatr. Res. **17:**716, 1983.
47. Hambidge, K.M.: Trace-element nutrition, Pediatr. Ann. **10:**451, 1981.
48. Hambraeus, L.: Proprietary milk versus human milk in infant feeding: a critical approach from a nutritional point of view, Pediatr. Clin. North Am. **24:**17, 1977.
49. Hambraeus, L., Forsum, E., and Lonnerdal, B.: Nutritional aspects of breast milk and cow's milk formulas. In Hambraeus, L., Hanson, L., and Macfarlane, H., editors: Symposium on food and immunology, Stockholm, 1975, Almqvist and Wiksell, p. 116.
50. Hartmann, P.E., and Kulski, J.K.: Changes in composition of mammary secretion of women after abrupt termination of breast feeding, J. Physiol. **275:**1, 1978.
51. Harzer, G., et al.: Changing patterns of human milk lipids in the course of the lactation and during the day, Am. J. Clin. Nutr. **37:**612, 1983.
52. Harzer, G., and Kauer, H.: Binding of zinc to casein, Am. J. Clin. Nutr. **35:**981, 1982.
53. Hazebroek, A., and Hofman, A.: Sodium content of breast milk in the first six months after delivery, Acta. Paediatr. Scand. **72:**459, 1983.
54. Healy, D.L., et al.: Prolactin in human milk: correlation with lactose, total protein, and α-lactalbumin levels, Am. J. Physiol. 238 (Endocrinol. Metab. 1): E83, 1980.
55. Heitlinger, L.A., et al.: Mammary amylase: a possible alternate pathway of carbohydrate digestion in infancy, Pediatr. Res. **17:**15, 1983.
56. Hernell, O., and Bläckberg, L.: Digestion of human milk lipids: physiologic significance of sn-2 monoacyl glyceral hydrolysis by bile salt-stimulated lipase, Pediatr. Res. **16:**882, 1982.
57. Hernell, O., and Olivecrona, T.: Human milk lipases. II. Bile-salt-stimulated lipase, Biochim. Biophys. Acta. **369:**234, 1974.
58. Hibberd, C.M., et al.: Variation in the composition of breast milk during the first five weeks of lactation: implications for the feeding of preterm infants, Arch. Dis. Child. **57:**658, 1982.
59. Hofman, A., Hazebroek, A., and Valkenburg, H.A.: A randomized trial of sodium intake and blood pressure in newborn infants, JAMA **250:**370, 1983.
60. Hollis, B.W., et al.: Vitamin D and its metabolites in human and bovine milk, J. Nutr. **111:**1240, 1981.
61. Hytten, F.E.: Clinical and chemical studies in human lactation. VII. The effect of differences in yield and composition of milk on the infant's weight gain and duration of breast-feeding, Br. Med. J. **1:**1410, 1954.
62. Insull, W., and Ahrens, E.H.: The fatty acids of human milk from mothers on diets taken ad libitum, Biochem. J. **72:**27, 1959.
63. Isaacs, C.E., et al.: Sulfhydryl oxidase (SHO) in human milk and induction in kidney and skin at weaning (Abstract), Pediatr. Res. **15:**112A, 1981.
64. Janas, L.M., and Picciano, M.F.: The nucleotide profile of human milk, Pediatr. Res. **16:**659, 1982.
65. Jansson, L., Åkesson, B., and Holmberg, L.: Vitamin E and fatty acid composition of human milk, Am. J. Clin. Nutr. **34:**8, 1981.
66. Järvenpää A.L., et al.: Milk protein quantity and quality in the term infant. II. Effects on acidic and neutral amino acids, Pediatrics **70:**221, 1982.
67. Jelliffe, D.B., and Jelliffe, E.F.P.: Human milk in the modern world, Oxford, 1978, Oxford University Press.
68. Jenness, R., and Sloan, R.E.: Composition of milk. In Larson, B.L., and Smith, V.R., editors: Lactation, vol. III, Nutrition and biochemistry of milk/maintenance, New York, 1974, Academic Press, Inc.
69. Jensen, R.G., Clark, R.M., and Ferris, A.M.: Composition of the lipids in human milk: a review, Lipids **15:**345, 1980.
70. Jensen, R.G., Hagerty, M.M., and McMahon, K.E.: Lipids of human milk and infant formulas: a review, Am. J. Clin. Nutr. **31:**990, 1978.
71. Jimenez, R., et al.: Vitamin K–dependent clotting factors in normal breast fed infants, J. Pediatr. **100:**424, 1982.
72. Johke, T.: Nucleotides of mammary secretions.

In Larson, B.L., editor: Lactation, vol. IV, Mammary gland/human lactation/milk synthesis, New York, 1978, Academic Press, Inc.

73. Johnson, P.E., and Evans, G.W.: Relative zinc availability in human breast milk, infant formulas, and cow's milk, Am. J. Clin. Nutr. 31:416, 1978.

74. Johnston, L., Vaughn, L., and Fox, H.M.: Pantothenic acid content of human milk, Am. J. Clin. Nutr. 34:2205, 1981.

75. Keenan, B.S., Buzek, S.W., and Garza, C.: Cortisol and its possible role in regulation of sodium and potassium in human milk, Am. J. Physiol. 244 (Endrocinol. Metab. 7): E253, 1983.

76. Keenan, B.S., et al.: Diurnal and longitudinal variations in human milk sodium and potassium: implication for nutrition and physiology, Am. J. Clin. Nutr. 35:527, 1982.

77. Klevay, L.M.: Ratio of zinc to copper in milk and mortality due to coronary artery disease: an association. In Hemphill, D.D., editor: Trace substances in environmental health, vol. VIII, Columbia, 1974, University of Missouri Press.

78. Kobata, A., Suzuoki, Z., and Kida, M.: The acid soluble nucleotides of milk. I. Quantitative and qualitative differences of nucleotide constituents in human and cow's milk, J. Biochem. 51:277, 1962.

79. Koldovsky, O.: Hormones in milk, Life Sci. 26:1833, 1980.

80. Kretchmer, N.: Lactose and lactase, Sci. Am. 227:73, 1972.

81. Kulski, J.K., and Hartmann, P.E.: Changes in human milk composition during the initiation of lactation, Aust. J. Exp. Biol. Med. Sci. 59:101, 1981.

82. Kumpulainen, J.: Determination of chromium in human milk and urine by graphite-furnace atomic absorption spectrometry, Ann. Chim. Acta. 113:355, 1980.

83. Kumpulainen, J., and Vuori, E.: Longitudinal study of chromium in human milk, Am. J. Clin. Nutr. 33:2299, 1980.

84. Lakdawala, D.R., and Widdowson, E.M.: Vitamin D in human milk, Lancet 1:167, 1977.

85. Lealman, G.T., et al.: Calcium, phosphorus, and magnesium concentrations in plasma during first week of life and their relation to type of milk feed, Arch. Dis. Child. 51:377, 1976.

86. Lengemann, F.W.: The site of action of lactose in the enhancement of calcium utilization, J. Nutr. 69:23, 1959.

87. Lessof, M.H., Anderson, J.A., and Youlten, L.J.F.: Prostaglandins in the pathogenesis of food intolerance, Ann. Allergy 51:249, 1983.

88. Lindberg, T., and Skude, G.: Amylase in human milk, Pediatrics 70:235, 1981.

89. Lorber, J., Lilleyman, J.S., and Peile, E.B.: Acute infantile thrombocytosis and vitamin K deficiency associated with intracranial haemorrhage, Arch. Dis. Child. 54:47, 1979.

90. Lucas, A., et al.: Breast vs bottle: endocrine responses are different with formula feeding, Lancet 1:1267, 1980.

91. Lucas, A., and Mitchell, M.D.: Prostaglandins in human milk, Arch. Dis. Child. 55:950, 1980.

92. MacDonald, L.D., Gibson, R.S., and Miles, J.E.: Changes in hair zinc and copper concentrations of breast fed and bottle fed infants during the first six months, Acta. Paediatr. Scand. 71:785, 1982.

93. Macy, I.G., and Kelly, H.J.: Human milk and cow's milk in infant nutrition. In Kon, S.K., and Cowie, A.T., editors: Milk: the mammary gland and its secretion, vol. II, New York, 1961, Academic Press, Inc., p. 265.

94. Macy, I.G., Kelly, H.J., and Sloan, R.E.: The composition of milks, Pub. no. 254, Washington, D.C., 1953, National Research Council.

95. Malloy, M.H., et al.: Development of taurine metabolism in Beagle pups: effects of taurine-free total parenteral nutrition, Biol. Neonate 40:1, 1981.

96. McMillan, J.A., Landaw, S.A., and Oski, F.A.: Iron sufficiency in breast fed infants and the availability of iron from human milk, Pediatrics 58:686, 1976.

97. Moran, J.R., Courtney, M.E., and Orth, D.N.: Epidermal growth factor in human milk: daily production and diurnal variation during early lactation in mothers delivering at term and at premature gestation, J. Pediatr. 103:402, 1983.

98. Moser, P.B., and Reynolds, R.D.: Dietary zinc intake and zinc concentrations of plasma, erythrocytes, and breast milk in antepartum and postpartum lactating and nonlactating women: a longitudinal study, Am. J. Clin. Nutr. 38:101, 1983.

99. Nail, P.A., Thomas, M.R., and Eakin, R.: The effect of thiamin and riboflavin supplementation on the level of those vitamins in human milk and urine, Am. J. Clin. Nutr. 33:198, 1980.

100. Novak, M., et al.: Carnitine in the perinatal

metabolism of lipids. I. Relationship between maternal and fetal plasma levels of carnitine and acylcarnitines, Pediatrics **67**:95, 1981.

101. O'Connor, M.E., et al.: Vitamin K deficiency and breast-feeding. Am. J. Dis. Child. **137**:601, 1983.

102. Orzali, A., et al.: Effect of carnitine on lipid metabolism in the newborn, Biol. Neonate **43**:186, 1983.

103. Osborn, G.R.: Relationship of hypotension and infant feeding to aetiology of coronary disease, Coll. Int. Cont. Natl. Res. Sci. **169**:193, 1968.

104. Oseid, B.J.: Breast-feeding and infant health, Clin. Obstet. Gynecol. **18**(2):149, 1975.

105. Picciano, M.F., et al.: Milk and mineral intakes of breastfed infants, Acta. Paediatr. Scand. **70**:189, 1981.

106. Picciano, M.F., and Guthrie, H.A.: Copper, iron and zinc contents of mature human milk, Am. J. Clin. Nutr. **29**:242, 1976.

107. Picciano, M.F., Guthrie, H.A., and Sheehe, D.M.: The cholesterol content of human milk, Clin. Pediatr. **17**:359, 1978.

108. Pickles, V.R., et al., Prostaglandins in endometrium and menstrual fluid from normal and dysmenorrhoeic subjects, J. Obstet. Gynaecol. Br. Commonwealth **72**:185, 1965.

109. Potter, J.M., and Nestel, P.J.: The effect of dietary fatty acids and cholesterol on the milk lipids of lactating women and the plasma cholesterol of breast-fed infants, Am. J. Clin. Nutr. **29**:54, 1976.

110. Rassin, D.K., Sturman, J.A., and Gaull, G.E.: Taurine in milk: species variation, Pediatr. Res. **11**:449, 1977.

111. Read, W.W.C., and Sarriff, A.: Human milk lipids. I. Changes in fatty acid composition of early colostrum, Am. J. Clin. Nutr. **17**:177, 1965.

112. Read, W.W.C., Lutz, P.G., and Tashjian, A.: Human milk lipids. II. The influences of dietary carbohydrates and fat on the fatty acids of mature milk: a study in four ethnic groups, Am. J. Clin. Nutr. **17**:180, 1965.

113. Read, W.W.C., Lutz, P.G., and Tashjian, A.: Human milk lipids. III. Short-term effects of dietary carbohydrate and fat, Am. J. Clin. Nutr. **17**:184, 1965.

114. Reid, B., Smith, H., and Friedman, Z.: Prostaglandins in human milk, Pediatrics **66**:870, 1980.

115. Roepke, J.L.B., and Kirksey, A.: Vitamin B_6 nutriture during pregnancy and lactation. I. Vitamin B_6 intake, levels of the vitamin in biological fluids, and condition of the infant at birth, Am. J. Clin. Nutr. **32**:2249, 1979.

116. Roepke, J.L.B., and Kirksey, A.: Vitamin B_6 nutriture during pregnancy and lactation. II. The effect of long-term use of oral contraceptives, Am. J. Clin. Nutr. **32**:2257, 1979.

117. Rothberg, A.D., et al.: Maternal-infant vitamin D relationships during breast-feeding, J. Pediatr. **101**:500, 1982.

118. Samson, R.R., and McClelland, D.B.L.: Vitamin B_{12} in human colostrum and milk, Acta. Paediatr. Scand. **69**:93, 1980.

119. Sandberg, D.P., Begley, J.A., and Hall, C.A.: The content, binding, and forms of vitamin B_{12} in milk, Am. J. Clin. Nutr. **34**:1717, 1981.

120. Sanders, T.A.B., et al.: Studies of vegans: the fatty acid composition of plasma choline phosphoglycerides, erythrocytes, adipose tissue, and breast milk, and some indicators of susceptibility to ischemic heart disease in vegans and omnivore controls, Am. J. Clin. Nutr. **31**:805, 1978.

121. Sandor, A., et al.: On carnitine content of human breast milk, Pediatr. Res. **16**:89, 1982.

122. Sandström, B., Cederblad, A., and Lönnerdal, B.: Zinc absorption from human milk, cow's milk, and infant formulas, Am. J. Dis. Child. **137**:726, 1983.

123. Sevy, S.: Acute emotional stress and sodium in breast milk, Am. J. Dis. Child. **122**:459, 1971.

124. Shahani, K.M., Kwan, A.J., and Friend, B.A.: Role and significance of enzymes in human milk, Am. J. Clin. Nutr. **33**:1861, 1980.

125. Sheehy, T.W., and Anderson, P.R.: Fetal disaccharidases, Am. J. Dis. Child. **121**:464, 1971.

126. Siimes, M.A., Vuori, E., and Kuitunen, P.: Breast-milk iron: a declining concentration during the course of lactation, Acta. Paediatr. Scand. **68**:29, 1979.

127. Sinclair, A.J., and Crawford, M.A.: The accumulation of arachidonate and docosahexaenoate in the developing rat brain, J. Neurochem. **19**:1753, 1972.

128. Skala, J.P., Koldovsky, O., and Hahn, P.: Cyclic nucleotides in breast milk, Am. J. Clin. Nutr. **34**:343, 1981.

129. Smith, A.M., Picciano, M.F., and Milner, J.A.: Selenium intakes and status of human milk and formula fed infants, Am. J. Clin. Nutr. **35**:521, 1982.

130. Smith, F.A., Hodge, H.C., and MacGregor,

J.T.: Fluoride in pregnancy. In Milunsky, A., Friedman, E.A., and Gluck, L., editors: Advances in perinatal medicine, vol. 2, New York, 1982, Plenum Publishing Co.

131. Sneed, S.M., Cane, C., and Thomas, M.R.: The effects of ascorbic acid, vitamin B_6, vitamin B_{12} and folic acid supplementation on the breast milk and maternal nutritional status of low socioeconomic lactating women, Am. J. Clin. Nutr. **34**:1338, 1981.

132. Stewart, R.A., Platou, E., and Kelly, V.J.: The alkaline phosphatase content of human milk, J. Biol. Chem. **232**:777, 1958.

133. Storrs, A.B., and Hull, M.E.: Proteolytic enzymes in human and cow milk, J. Dairy Sci. **39**:1097, 1956.

134. Sturman, J.A., Rassin, D.K., and Gaull, G.E.: Taurine in developing rat brain: transfer of ^{35}S-taurine to pups via the milk, Pediatr. Res. **11**:28, 1977.

135. Sturman, J.A., Rassin, D.K., and Gaull, G.E.: Taurine in the developing kitten: nutritional importance, Pediatr. Res. **11**:450, 1977.

136. Sturman, J.A., Rassin, D.K., and Gaull, G.E.: Taurine in development, Life Sci. **21**:1, 1977.

137. Tamura, T., Yoshimura, Y., and Arakawat, T.: Human milk folate and folate status in lactating mothers and their infants, Am. J. Clin. Nutr. **33**:193, 1980.

138. Tenore, A., et al.: Thyrotropin in human breast milk, Hormone Res. **14**:193, 1981.

139. Thomas, R.M., et al.: The effects of vitamin C, vitamin B_6, and vitamin B_{12}, folic acid, riboflavin, and thiamin on the breast milk and maternal status of well-nourished women at 6 months postpartum, Am. J. Clin. Nutr. **33**:2151, 1980.

140. Tikanoja, T.: Plasma amino acids in term neonates after a feed of human milk or formula. I. Total amino acids and glycine/valine ratios as reflectors of protein intake, Acta. Paediatr. Scand. **71**:385, 1981.

141. Tikanoja, T., et al.: Plasma amino acids in term neonates after a feed of human milk or formula. II. Characteristic changes in individual amino acids, Acta. Paediatr. Scand. **71**:391, 1982.

142. Vanderslice, J.T., et al.: Form of vitamin B_6 in human milk, Am. J. Clin. Nutr. **37**:867, 1983.

143. Vorherr, H.: The breast: morphology, physiology, and lactation, New York, 1974, Academic Press, Inc.

144. Warshaw, J.B., and Curry, E.: Comparison of serum carnitine and ketone body concentrations in breast- and in formula-fed newborn infants, J. Pediatr. **97**:122, 1980.

145. Wei, S.H.: Postnatal fluoride supplements, Curr. Ther. Dentistry **7**:390, 1980.

146. Widdowson, E.M., et al.: Body fat of British and Dutch infants, Br. Med. J. **1**:653, 1975.

147. Wing, J.P.: Human versus cow's milk in infant nutrition and health: update 1977. Curr. Probl. Pediatr. **8**(1):entire issue, 1977.

148. Young, V.R., Nahapetian, A., and Janghorbani, M.: Selenium bioavailability with reference to human nutrition, Am. J. Clin. Nutr. **35**:1076, 1982.

149. Ziegler, E.E., and Fomon, S.J.: Fluid intake, renal solute load, and water balance in infancy, J. Pediatr. **78**:561, 1971.

150. Zikakis, J.P., Dougherty, T.M., and Biasotto, N.O.: The presence and some properties of xanthine oxidase in human milk and colostrum, J. Food Sci. **41**:1408, 1976.

Host-resistance factors and immunologic significance of human milk

5

As the newborn infant prepares for existence outside the uterus, various organ systems adjust and adapt. It had been suggested that protection against infection was provided by the mother transplacentally, since it has been established that the neonate is immunologically immature at birth.

The neonate does not have sufficient innate defenses to protect himself against the highly contaminated environment he enters from the usually sterile environment of the uterus. The incidence of infection in the newborn infant is significant. It has been estimated that up to 10% of newborns are infected during delivery or in the first few months of life. It is generally believed that the newborn cannot muster the same level of defense against infection that an adult is capable of developing. The diminished phagocytic function of newborn cells is an example. This maturational defect is attributed to both cellular and extracellular factors.

Maternal antibody is transmitted to the fetus by different pathways in different species. An association has been recognized between the number of placental membranes and the relative importance of the placenta and the colostrum as sources of antibodies. By this analysis it is noted that the horse, with six placental membranes, passes little or no antibodies transplacentally and relies on colostrum for protection of the foal. Humans and monkeys, having three placental membranes, receive more of the antibodies via the placenta and less from the colostrum. The transfer of IgG in the human is accomplished, according to Bellanti and Hurtado,[5] by means of active transport mechanism of the immunoglobulin across the placenta. Bellanti and Hurtado do point out, however, that secretory IgA immunoglobulins are found in human milk and provide local protection on the mucous membranes of the gastrointestinal tract. The lowered incidence of enteric and respiratory infections seen in breastfed infants has been recognized.[35,36] It has been established by other investigations that the mammary glands and their secretion of milk are important in protecting the infant, not only through the colostrum but through mature milk from birth through the early months of life. Some information has been available for decades to support the acknowledgment of the protective role of human milk.[28] Many recent discoveries, however, have further broadened knowledge.[19]

Although the predominance of IgA in human colostrum and milk had been described, the importance of this phenomenon was not fully appreciated until the discovery that IgA is a predominant immunoglobulin present in mucosal secretions of other glands in addition to the breast. Mucosal immunity has become the subject of extensive research.[31] The data produced suggest that there may be considerable traffic of cells between secretory sites. These data support the concept of a general system of mucosa-associated lymphoid tissue (MALT), which includes the gut, lung, mammary gland, salivary and lacrimal glands, and the genital tract. This concept of MALT implies that immunization at one site may be an effective means of producing immunity at distant sites. Antibodies found in the milk have also been found in the saliva, for instance. There is evidence available to suggest that the mammary glands may act as extensions of the gut-associated lymphoid tissue (GALT) and possibly the broncho-associated (immunocompetent) lymphoid tissue (BALT). The ability of epithelial surfaces exposed to the external environment to defend against foragers has been well established for the gastrointestinal, genitourinary, and respiratory tracts. The common defense is secretory IgA. Direct contact with the antigen and the lymphoid cells of the breast is unlikely.[45]

All mysteries of the protective value of human milk, however, have not been unraveled. The protective properties of human milk can be divided into cellular factors and humoral factors for facility of discussion, although they are closely related in vivo. A wide variety of soluble and cellular components and microbial agents have been identified in human milk and colostrum (Table 5-1).

CELLULAR COMPONENTS OF HUMAN COLOSTRUM AND MILK

Cells do constitute an important postpartum component of maternal immunologic endowment. Over 100 years ago, cell bodies were described in the colostrum of animals. As with much lactation research, further study of colostral corpuscles was undertaken by the dairy industry for commercial reasons in the early 1900s. This research afforded an opportunity to make major progress in the understanding of cells in milk. Initially it was believed that these cells represented a reaction to infection in the mammary gland and were even described as ''pus cells.''

It has become clear that the cells of milk are normal constituents of that solution in all species. Cells include macrophages, lymphocytes, neutrophils, and epithelial cells, and they total 4000/mm.[3] Cell fragments and epithelial cells were examined by electron

Table 5-1.   Immunologically active components in human colostrum and milk

Soluble	Cellular	Microbial agents
Secretory component		
Immunoglobulins sigA, 7S	Monocytic phagocytes	Bacterial agents
IgA, IgG, IgM	macrophage	
Immunoregulatory mediators		
Complement	Neutrophils	Hepatitis B surface
		antigen
Chemotactic factors	B lymphocytes	Rubella
Lactoferrin	Plasma cells	Cytomegalovirus
Lysozyme	T lymphocytes	Other vaccine viruses
Lactoperoxidase	Transplantation antigens	
Interferon		
Bifidus factor		

From Ogra, S.S., and Ogra, P.L.: Components of immunology reactivity in human colostrum and milk. In Ogra, P.L., and Dayton, D., editors: Immunology of breast milk, New York, 1979, Raven Press.

microscope in fresh samples from 30 women by Brooker.[8] He found that membrane-bound cytoplasmic fragments in the sedimentation pellet outnumbered intact cells. The fragments were mostly from secretory cells that contained numerous cisternae of rough endoplasmic reticulum, lipid droplets, and Golgi vesicles containing casein micelles. Secretory epithelial cells were found in all samples and, after the second month postpartum, began to outnumber macrophages. Ductal epithelial cells were about 1% of the population of cells for the first week or so and then disappeared. All samples contained squamous epithelial cells originating from galactophores and the skin of the nipple.

Living leukocytes are normally present in human milk. The overall concentration of these leukocytes is of the same order of magnitude as that seen in peripheral blood, although the predominant cell in milk is the macrophage rather than the neutrophil. Macrophages comprise about 90% of the leukocytes, and 2000 to 3000/mm^3 are present. Lymphocytes make up about 10% of the cells (200 to 300/mm^3), which is much lower than in human blood. There are large and small lymphocytes. By indirect immunofluorescence with anti-T antibody to identify thymus-derived lymphocytes, it has been shown that 50% of human colostral lymphocytes are T cells. By immunofluorescence procedures to detect surface immunoglobulins characteristic of B-lymphocytes, 34% were identified as B-lymphocytes (Table 5-2).

Macrophages

Macrophages are large-complex phagocytes that contain lysosomes, mitochondria, pinosomes, ribosomes, and a Golgi apparatus. The monocytic phagocytes are lipid laden and were previously called the colostral bodies of Donne. They have the same functional and morphologic features as those in other human tissue sources.[50] These features include ameboid movement, phagocytosis of microorganisms (fungi and bacteria), killing of bacteria, and production of complement components C3 and C4, lysosome, and lactoferrin. Other milk macrophage activities include the following[48]:

Table 5-2.   Distinguishing characteristics of T-lymphocytes, B-lymphocytes, and macrophages

Membrane markers	T-lympho-cytes	B-lympho-cytes	Macro-phages
IgG	−	+	−
Receptor for C3 (erythrocyte-antibody-complement [EAC] rosettes)	−	+	+
Receptor for immunoglobulin or antibody-antigen complexes (Fc)	−	+	+
Thymus-specific antigens (θ, mouse thymocyte leukemia antigen, and so on)	+	−	−
Receptors for sheep red blood cells (erythrocyte [E] rosettes)	+	−	−
In vitro stimulation of DNA synthesis by mitogens			
Phytohemagglutinin (PHA)	+	−*	−
Concanavallin A (Con A)	+	−	−
Lipopolysaccharide (bacterial endotoxin)	−	+	−
Anti-immunoglobulin	−	+	−
Specific binding to antigen-coated beads	−	+	−
Mixed lymphocyte culture reactivity	+	−	−
Graft-versus-host (GVH) reaction-inducing capacity	+	−	−
Adherence to surfaces (glass, plastic)	−†	−‡	+
Phagocytic	−	−	+

From Bellanti, J.A., and Hurtado, R.C.: Immunology and resistance to infection. In Remington, J.S., and Klein, J.O., editors: Infectious diseases of the fetus and newborn infants, Philadelphia, 1976, W.B. Saunders Co.
*Some B-lymphocytes may be recruited to divide secondarily because of factors elaborated by activated T-lymphocytes. B cells may also be stimulated when the mitogen is attached to solid support.
†Except for blast cells.
‡Except for mature plasma cells or when immune complexes are attached to B cells.

Phagocytosis of latex, adherence to glass

Secretion of lysozyme, complement components

C3b-mediated erythrocyte adherence

IgG-mediated erythrocyte adherence and phagocytosis

Bacterial killing

Inhibition of lymphocyte mitogenic response

Release of intracellular IgA in tissue culture

Giant cell formation

Interaction with lymphocytes

There are data to suggest these macrophages also amplify T-cell reactivity by direct cellular cooperation or by antigen processing. The colostral macrophage has been suggested as a potential vehicle for the storage and transport of immunoglobin. A significant increase in IgA and IgG immunoglobin synthesis by colostral lymphocytes when incubated with supernatants of cultured macrophages has been reported.[51]

The macrophage may also participate in the biosynthesis and excretion of lactoperoxidase and cellular growth factors that enhance growth of intestinal epithelium and maturation of intestinal brush-border enzymes.

The mobility of macrophages is inhibited by the lymphokine migration inhibitor factor (MIF), which is produced by antigen-stimulated sensitized lymphocytes. The activities of macrophages have been demonstrated in both fresh colostrum and in colostral cell cultures.

Lymphocytes

It has been established that both T- and B-lymphocytes are present in human milk and colostrum. They synthesize IgA antibody. Human milk lymphocytes respond to mitogens by proliferation, with increased macrophage-lymphocyte interaction and the release of soluble mediators, including MIF. Cells destined to become lymphopoietic cells are derived from two separate influences, the thymus (T) and the bursa (B) or bursal equivalent tissues. The population of cells called B cells comprises the smaller part of the total. The term *B cell* is derived from its origination in a different anatomic site from the thymus; in birds it has been identified as the bursa of Fabricius. The B cells can be identified by the presence of surface immunoglobulin markers. The B cells in human milk include cells with IgA, IgM, and IgG surface immunoglobulins.

T-CELL SYSTEM.   More rapid mitotic activity occurs in the thymus gland than in any other lymphatic organ, yet 70% of the cells die within the cell substance. Thymosin has recently been identified as a hormone produced by thymic epithelial cells to expand the peripheral lymphocyte population. After emergence from the thymus gland, T cells acquire new surface antigen markers. The T cells circulate through the lymphatic and vascular systems as long-lived lymphocytes, which are called the recirculating pool. They then populate restricted regions of lymph nodes, forming thymic-dependent areas.

The significance of the leukocytes in human milk in affording immunologic benefits to the breastfed infant continues to be investigated. It is suggested that the lymphocytes can sensitize, induce immunologic tolerance, or incite graft-versus-host reactions. According to Head and Beer, lymphocytes may be incorporated into the suckling's tissues, achieving short-term adoptive immunization of the neonate.[25]

Studies of the activities of lymphocytes have been carried out by a number of investigators who collected samples of milk from lactating women at various times postpartum, examined the number of cell types present, and then studied the activities of these cells in vitro. Ogra and Ogra[44] collected samples from 200 women and measured the cell content from 1 through 180 days (Fig. 5-1). They then compared the response of T-lymphocytes in colostrum and milk with that of the T cells in the peripheral blood (Fig. 5-2).

The greatest number of cells appeared on the first day, with the counts ranging from 10,000 to 100,000/mm^3 for total cells. By the fifth day, the count had dropped to 20% of the first day's count. In addition, the number of E rosette-forming cells was determined by using sheep erythrocyte-rosetting technique. The E rosette formation (ERF) lymphocytes constituted a mean 100/mm^3 on the first day and a tenth of that by the fifth day.

At 180 days, total cells were 100,000/mm^3, lymphocytes were 10,000/mm^3, and

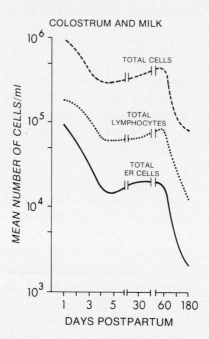

Fig. 5-1. Geometric mean concentration of total cells, lymphocytes, and E rosette-forming cells *(ER)* in the colostrum and milk of 200 lactating women. (Modified from Ogra, S.S., and Ogra, P.L.: J. Pediatr. **92:**546, 1978.)

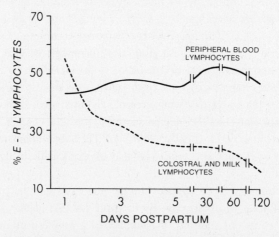

Fig. 5-2. Comparative distribution of E rosette-forming cells *(ER)* in peripheral blood and in colostrum and milk of 200 lactating women. (Modified from Ogra, S.S., and Ogra, P.L.: J. Pediatr. **92:**546, 1978.)

ERF lymphocytes were 2000/mm^3. The investigators compared the values to those in the peripheral blood of each mother (Fig. 5-2).

In a similar study, Bhaskaram and Reddy[6] sampled milk over time from 74 women and found comparable cell concentrations. They examined the bactericidal activity of the milk leukocytes and found it to be comparable to that of the circulating leukocytes in the blood, irrespective of the stage of lactation or state of nutrition of the mother.

Ogra and Ogra[44] also studied the lymphocyte proliferation responses of colostrum and milk to antigens. Their data show response to stimulation from the viral antigens of rubella, cytomegalovirus, and mumps. Analysis of cell-mediated immunity to microbial antigens shows milk lymphocytes are limited in their potential for recognizing or responding to certain infectious agents as compared with cells from the peripheral circulation. This is believed to be an intercellular action and not due to lack of external factors. On the other hand, the T cells and B cells have been shown to have unique reactivities not seen in peripheral blood. Goldblum et al.[20] were able to show a response in human colostrum to *Escherichia coli* given orally, which was not accompanied by a systemic response in the mother. This suggests that milk provides a site for local humoral or cell-mediated immunity induced at a distant site such as the gut with the reactive lymphoid cells migrating to the breast. This concept has been further refined to suggest that IgA and IgM immunoglobulin in colostrum may represent migration of specific antibody-producing cells from the gut lymphoid tissue, specifically Peyer's patches, to the mammary gland. Ogra and Ogra[43,44] suggest that the cells may be selectively accumulated in the breast during pregnancy. The responses of milk cells and their antibodies are not representative of the total immunity of the individual.[46] Head and Beer[25] have provided a scheme to describe this mechanism (Fig. 5-3). The diagram depicts the progeny of specifically sensitized lymphocytes that originated in the lymphoid tissue of the gut as they migrate to the mammary gland. As they infiltrate the mammary gland and its secretion, they supply the breast with immune cells capable of selected immune responses.

Most of these immunocompetent cells recirculate to the external mucosal surface and populate the lamina propria as antibody-producing plasma cells. A substantial number of these antigen-sensitized cells selectively home to the stroma of the mammary glands and initiate local IgA antibody synthesis against the antigens initially encountered in the respiratory or intestinal mucosa.

Parmely et al.[46] partially purified and propagated milk lymphocytes in vitro to study their immunologic function. Milk lymphocytes responded in a unique manner to stimuli known to activate T-lymphocytes from the serum. Parmely et al.[46] found milk lymphocytes to be hyporesponsive to nonspecific mitogens and histocompatible antigens on allogenic cells in their laboratory. They found them unresponsive to *Candida albicans*. Significant proliferation of lymphocytes occurred in response to K$_1$ capsular antigen of *E. coli*.[26] Lymphocytes from blood failed to respond. This supports the concept of local mammary tissue immunity at the T-lymphocyte level.

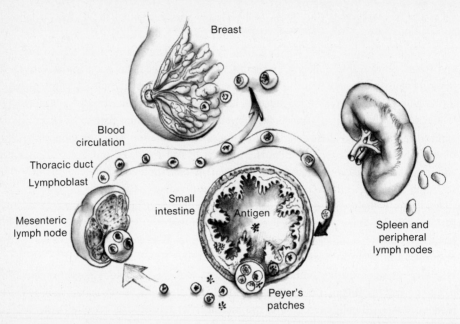

Fig. 5-3. Schematic diagram of mechanism by which progeny of specifically sensitized lymphocytes originating from gut-associated lymphoid tissue may migrate to and infiltrate mammary gland and its secretions, supplying breast with immune cells. (Modified from Head, J.R., and Beer, A.E.: The immunologic role of viable leukocytic cells in mammary exosecretions. In Larson, B.L., editor: Lactation, vol. IV. Mammary gland/human lactation/milk synthesis, New York, 1978, Academic Press, Inc.)

More recent experiments in rodents have provided evidence that T-lymphocytes reactive to transplantation alloantigens can adoptively immunize the suckling newborn. Foster nursing experiments performed in rodents have shown that newborn rats exposed to allogenic milk manifested alterations in their reactivity to skin allografts of the foster mother's strain. In animals, mothers may give their suckling newborn immunoreactive lymphocytes. The influence of maternal milk cells on the development of neonatal immunocompetence has been demonstrated in several different immunologic contexts. Congenitally, athymic nude mice nursed by their phenotypically normal mothers or normal foster mothers had increased survival. The mothers contributed their T cell–helper activity to the suckling newborn.

The accumulated research data support the concept that lymphocytes from colostrum and milk provide the human infant with immunologic benefits. Both T- and B-lymphocytes are reactive against organisms invading the intestinal tract. Investigations on allergy, necrotizing entercolitis, tuberculosis, and neonatal meningitis support the concept that milk fulfills a protective function.

Table 5-3.   Relationship of antibody type with transplacental transfer

Good passive transfer	Poor passive transfer	No passive transfer
Diphtheria antitoxin	*Haemophilus influenzae*	Enteric somatic (O) antibodies
Tetanus antitoxin	*Bordetella pertussis*	(Salmonella, Shigella, E. coli)
Antierythrogenic toxin	*Shigella flexneri*	Skin-sensitizing antibody
Antistaphylococcal antibody	Streptococcus MG	Heterophile antibody
Salmonella flagella (H) antibody		Wassermann antibody
Antistreptolysin		
All the antiviral antibodies present in maternal circulation (rubeola, rubella, mumps, poliovirus)		
VDRL antibodies		

From Bellanti, J.A., and Hurtado, R.C. Immunology and resistance to infection. In Remington, J.S., and Klein, J.O., editors: *Infectious diseases of the fetus and newborn infants*, Philadelphia, 1976, W.B. Saunders Co.

SURVIVAL OF MATERNAL MILK CELLS

Although it is clear that cells are provided in the colostrum and milk, the effectiveness and impact of these cells on the neonate depend on their ability to survive in the gastrointestinal tract. It has been demonstrated in several species, including the human, that the pH of the stomach can be as low as 0.5, but the output of HCl is minimal for the first few months, as is the peptic activity. Immediately after a feeding begins, the pH rises to 6.0 and returns to normal in 3 hours. The cells from milk tolerate this. Studies have also shown that intact nucleated lymphoid cells are found in the stomach and intestines.[27] These cells, when removed from rat stomachs, are capable of phagocytosis. Lymphoid cells in milk have been shown to traverse the mucosal wall.

When human milk is stored, however, it has been shown that the cellular components do not tolerate heating to 63° C, cooling to −23° C, or lyophilization. Although a few cells may be identified, they are not viable, according to Liebhaber et al.[34]

HUMORAL FACTORS
Immunoglobulins

All classes of immunoglobulins are found in human milk. Immunologic techniques developed in the past decade have enhanced the study of immunoglobulins through electrophoresis, chromatographics, and radioimmunoassays. More than 30 components have been identified; of these, 18 are associated with proteins in the maternal serum and the others are found exclusively in milk. Table 5-3 shows the relationship of antibody type with transplacental transfer.

The concentrations are highest in the colostrum of all species, demonstrated by the following figures developed by Michael et al.,[39] expressed in milligrams per 100 ml of colostrum:

First day	600 IgA, 80 IgG, and 125 IgM
Second day	260 IgA, 45 IgG, and 65 IgM
Third day	200 IgA, 30 IgG, and 58 IgM
Fourth day	80 IgA, 16 IgG, and 30 IgM

The main immunoglobulin in human serum is IgG; IgA is only one fifth the level of IgG. In milk, however, the reverse is true. IgA is the most important immunoglobulin in milk, not only in concentration but also in biologic activity. Of the IgA immunoglobulins, secretory IgA is the most significant and is likely synthesized in the mammary alveolar cells.

Quantitative determinations of immunoglobulins in human milk were made from milk collected at birth up to as long as 27 months postpartum by Peitersen et al.[47] The IgA content was high immediately after birth, averaging 2.7 units, dropped to 0.3 units in 2 to 3 weeks, and then remained constant (Fig. 5-4). The researchers used an arbitrary unit of expression based on the mass concentration values (g/L) developed by Behring Werke for the quantitative result. Similar observations were made on IgG levels and IgM levels, demonstrated by Figs. 5-5 and 5-6. Simultaneously, they also compared milk and serum values in 19 mothers and found the serum levels to be comparable to standard adult levels. Ogra and Ogra[42,45] have compared serum and milk levels at various times postpartum (Fig. 5-7). Samples obtained separately from the left and right breasts showed similar values. The levels remained constant during a given feeding and for a 24-hour period as a whole. In all quantitative determinations, IgA is the predominant immunoglobulin in breast milk, constituting 90% of all the immunoglobulins in colostrum and milk.

Ogra and Ogra[42,45] studied the serum of postpartum lactating mothers and nonpregnant matched controls and noted that the individual and mean concentrations of all

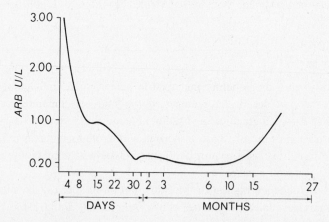

Fig. 5-4. IgA content during period of lactation. Concentration of IgA is given in arbitrary units based on mass concentration values (g/L). (Modified from Peitersen, B., et al.: Acta Paediatr. Scand. 64:709, 1975.)

classes of immunoglobulin were lower in the postpartum subjects. The levels were statistically significant in IgG, being 50 to 70 mg higher in the nonpregnant women.

It is importnat to note, in recording the fact that immunoglobulin levels, particularly IgA and IgM, are very high in colostrum and drop precipitously in the first 4 to 6 days, that the volume of mammary secretion also increases dramatically in this same period of time; thus, the absolute number is more nearly constant than it would first appear. IgG does not show this decline. Local production and concentration of IgA and probably IgM may take place in the mammary gland at the time of delivery.

IgE and IgD have also been measured in colostrum and milk. Using radioimmunoassay techniques, colostrum was found to contain concentrations of 0.5 to 0.6 IU/ml IgE in 41% of samples and less in the remainder.[1] IgD was found in all samples in concentrations of 2 to 2000 μg/100 ml. Plasma levels were poorly correlated. The findings suggest possible local mammary production rather than positive transfer. Whether IgE or IgD antibodies in breast milk have similar specificities for antigens as the IgA antibodies in milk is unanswered.[38]

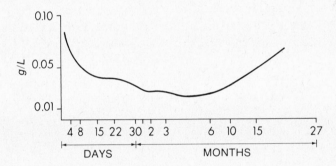

Fig. 5-5. IgG content during period of lactation recorded in arbitrary units. (Modified from Peitersen, B., et al.: Acta Paediatr. Scand. 64:709, 1975.)

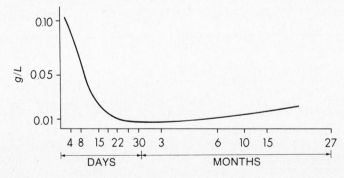

Fig. 5-6. IgM content during period of lactation. (Modified from Peitersen, B., et al.: Acta Paediatr. Scand. 64:709, 1975.)

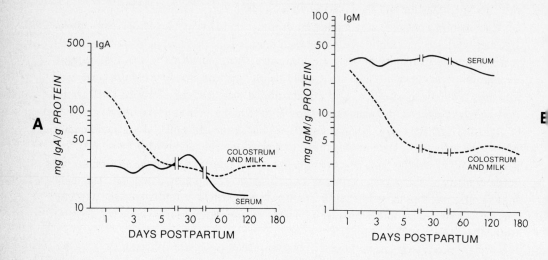

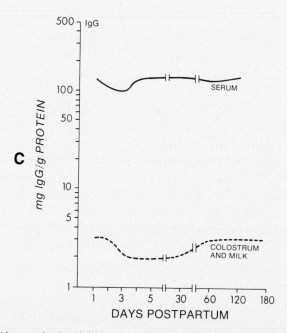

Fig. 5-7. **A,** Geometric mean levels of IgA immunoglobulin in serum and in colostrum and milk of 200 lactating women. **B,** Geometric mean levels of IgM immunoglobulin in serum and in colostrum and milk of 200 lactating women. **C,** Mean levels of IgG immunoglobulin in serum and in colostrum and milk of 200 lactating women at various times postpartum. (Modified from Ogra, S.S., and Ogra, P.L.: J. Pediatr. **92:**546, 1978.)

STABILITY OF IMMUNOGLOBULINS.   A study by Ford et al.[14] showed no change at 56° C but a 20% reduction in IgA with heating to 62.5° C for 30 minutes. IgM was totally destroyed by heat at 62.5° C. Freezing to −23° C for 4 weeks caused no alteration in IgA.

Secretory IgA differs antigenically from serum IgA. Secretory IgA can be synthesized in the nonlactating as well as in the lactating breast. It is a compact molecule and resistant to proteolytic enzymes of the intestinal tract and the low pH of the stomach. It is manufactured by the mammary gland and by the cellular lymphocytes in milk. Levels in milk are 10 to 100 times higher than in serum. Levels in cow's milk are very low, that is, a tenth the level in mature human milk (0.03 mg/100 ml). Later in life, the intestinal tract's subepithelial plasma cells secrete IgA, but this does not occur in the neonatal period.

Discussion continues as to whether antibodies are absorbed from the intestinal tract. There is, however, a wealth of evidence to demonstrate the activity of the immunoglobulins, especially secretory IgA, at the mucosal levels. These antibodies provide local intestinal protection against viruses such as poliovirus and bacteria such as *E. coli,* which may infect the mucosa or enter the body via the gut.

Bifidus factor

It has been established since the work of Tissier in 1908 on the intestinal flora of the newborn infant that the predominant bacteria of the breastfed infant are bifid bacteria. Bifid bacteria are gram-positive, nonmotile anaerobic bacilli. Many observers have shown the striking difference between the flora of the guts of breastfed and bottle fed infants. György[23] demonstrated the presence of a specific factor in colostrum and milk that supported the growth of *Lactobacillus bifidus.* Bifidus factor has been characterized as a dialyzable nitrogen-containing carbohydrate that contains no amino acid.

In vitro studies by Beerens et al.[4] showed the presence of a specific growth factor for *Bifidobacterium bifidum* in human milk, which they called BB. Other milks, including cow's milk, sheep's milk, pig's milk, and infant formulas, did not promote the growth of this species, but did show some activity supporting *B. infantis* and *B. longum.* This growth factor was found to be stable when the milk was frozen, heated, freeze-dried, and stored for 3 months (Table 5-7). There were growth-promoting factors present for the six strains studied, which varied in their resistance to physical change. Since all these factors were active in vitro, they did not require the presence of intestinal enzymes for activation. It has not been possible to show the presence of this factor in other mammalian milks; thus it is possible that it contributes to the implantation and persistence of *B. fidium* in the breastfed infant's intestine (Table 5-4).

Resistance factor

The fact that human milk protects the human infant against staphylococcal infection was well known in the preantibiotic era. The protection continued throughout the lac-

Table 5-4. Distribution of the different *Bifidobacterium* species in feces of breastfed or artificially fed infants

Feeding	Artificial	Maternal
No. of feces	39	12
No. of *Bifidobacterium* strains isolated	153	81
B. bifidum	20 = 13%	58 = 72%
B. infantis	28 = 18%	0
B. longum	91 = 60%	23 = 28%
B. adolescentis	2 = 1%	0
B. breve	12 = 8%	0

From Beerens, H., Romond, C., and Nevi, C.: Am. J. Clin. Nutr. **33:**2434, 1980.

tation period. György[23] identified the presence of an "antistaphylococcal factor" in experiments with young mice who had been stressed with staphylococci. This factor has no demonstrable direct antibiotic properties. It was termed a "resistance factor" and described as nondialyzable, thermostable, and part of the free fatty acid part of the phosphide fraction, probably $C_{18:2}$, distinct from linoleic acid.

Lysozyme

Human milk contains a nonspecific antimicrobial factor, lysozyme, which is a thermostable, acid-stable enzyme. It is found in large concentrations in the stools of breastfed infants and not in stools of formula fed infants; it thus is thought to influence the flora of the intestinal tract. Lysozyme levels show an increase over time during lactation (Fig. 5-8); this finding is more apparent in Indian women than in those of the Western world. Reddy et al.[52] studied the levels of lysozyme in well-nourished and poorly nourished women in India and found no difference between them (Table 5-5). As shown in this study, lysozyme levels increase during lactation. Levels in human milk are 14 to 39 mg/100 ml, which is 300 times the level in cow's milk (13 μg/100 ml). Lysozyme is bacteriostatic against *Enterobacteriaceae* and gram-positive bacteria.[10]

Lactoferrin

Lactoferrin is an iron-binding protein that has a strong bacteriostatic effect on staphylococci and *E. coli,* apparently by depriving the organism of iron. Lactoferrin is normally unsaturated with iron. It has been suggested that oral iron therapy can interfere with the bacteriostatic function of lactoferrin, which depends on its unsaturated state. Reddy et al.[52] showed that giving iron to the mother, however, did not interfere with the saturation of lactoferrin in the milk or, therefore, its potential microbicidal effect (Table 5-6). Lactoferrin is less than 50% saturated with iron in human milk.

The concentration of lactoferrin is high in colostrum, 600 mg/100 ml, and then progressively declines over the next 5 months of lactation, leveling off at about 180 mg/

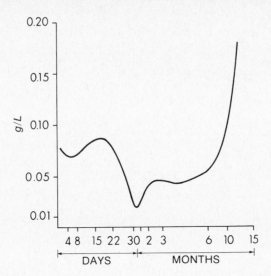

Fig. 5-8. Lysozyme content during period of lactation. In period from 15 to 27 months of lactation, lysozyme was found in only three samples, values varying considerably. (Modified from Peitersen, B., et al.: Acta Paediatr. Scand. 64:709, 1975.)

100 ml (Table 5-5). It also contains small amounts of transferrin (10 to 15 μg/ml).

Unsaturated lactoferrin has been demonstrated by Kirkpatrick et al.[30] to inhibit the growth of *C. albicans*. A combination of lactoferrin and specific antibody had a powerful bacteriostatic effect on *E. coli*. Inhibited *E. coli* appears to be markedly iron deficient. A significant factor that has been clearly demonstrated in preserving the bacteriostatic properties of human milk is that milk proteins, including lysozyme and lactoferrin, reach the duodenum without the occurrence of any digestion. They are stable in the acid pH of the stomach. Trypsin inhibitor, which has been identified in human milk, temporarily delays the hydrolysis of protein. Brock et al.[7] attempted to demonstrate a relationship between lactoferrin-mediated inhibition of *E. coli* and the presence of antibodies against the serologically important *E. coli* antigens, O, K, and H. They further investigated the role of enterobactin (enterochelin) in the ability to overcome the inhibitory effect wherein *E. coli* removes iron from lactoferrin and transferrin. The role of lactoferrin in human milk is to sequester exogenous iron reaching the gut rather than to bind or transport the endogenous iron of milk, since the iron in human milk is bound to fat and casein and not to lactoferrin.

Interferon

Colostrum cells in culture have been shown by Lawton and Shortridge[32] to be stimulated to secrete an interferon-like substance with strong antiviral activity up to 150 NIH units/ml. They did not find this property in the supernatant of colostrum or milk.

Table 5-5. Antibacterial factors in colostrum and mature milk

Group	Hemoglobin (g/100 ml)	Serum albumin (g/100 ml)	Immunoglobulins (mg/100 ml)			Lysozyme (mg/100 ml)	Lactoferrin (mg/100 ml)
			IgA	IgG	IgM		
Colostrum (1 to 5 days)							
Well-nourished women	11.5 ± 0.37	2.49 ± 0.065	335.9 ± 37.39 (17)*	5.9 ± 1.58 (17)	17.1 ± 4.29 (17)	14.2 ± 2.11 (15)	420 ± 49.0 (28)
Undernourished women	11.3 ± 0.60	2.10 ± 0.081	374.3 ± 42.13 (10)	5.3 ± 2.30 (10)	15.3 ± 2.50 (10)	16.4 ± 2.39 (21)	520 ± 69.0 (19)
Mature milk (1 to 6 months)							
Well-nourished women	12.8 ± 0.43	3.39 ± 0.120	119.6 ± 7.85 (12)	2.9 ± 0.92 (12)	2.9 ± 0.92 (12)	24.8 ± 3.41 (10)	250 ± 65.0 (17)
Undernourished women	12.6 ± 0.56	3.47 ± 0.130	118.1 ± 16.2 (10)	5.8 ± 3.41 (10)	5.8 ± 3.41 (10)	23.3 ± 3.53 (23)	270 ± 92.0 (13)

From Reddy, V., et al.: Acta Paediatr. Scand. **66:**229, 1977.
*Figures in parentheses indicate number of samples analyzed.

Table 5-6. Effect of iron therapy on lactoferrin in milk*

	Total lactoferrin (mg/100 ml)	Saturated lactoferrin (% of total)
Before iron therapy	240 ± 29.0	9.0 ± 7.15
After iron therapy	260 ± 80.0	8.6 ± 3.32

From Reddy, V., et al.: Acta Paediatr. Scand. **66**:229, 1977.
*Values are mean ± SE of eleven subjects.

Complement

The C3 and C4 components of complement, known for their ability to fuse bacteria bound to a specific antibody, are present in colostrum in low concentrations as compared with the levels in serum. IgG and IgM activate complement. C3 proactivator has been described, and IgA and IgE have been identified as stimulating the system. Activated C3 has opsonic, anaphylactic, and chemotactic properties and is important for the lysis of bacteria bound to a specific antibody.

B_{12}-binding protein

Unsaturated B_{12}-binding protein of high molecular weight has been found in very high levels in human milk and in the meconium and stools of breastfed infants as compared with infant formulas and the infants who are formula fed. The protein binding renders the B_{12} unavailable for bacterial growth of *E. coli* and bacteroides.[22]

FLORA OF THE INTESTINAL TRACT

As has been pointed out, the normal flora of the intestinal tract of the breastfed infant is *L. bifidus*. The gram-negative population in the gut is kept small.

In a prospective study of breastfed Mayan Indian infants from birth to 3 years of age,[24] bifid bacteria predominated and constituted 95% to 99% of the flora. Other culturable microorganisms were streptococci, bacteroides, clostridia, micrococci, enterococci, and *E. coli*. A change occurred when large amounts of solid foods were added at about 1 year of life. The solids were notably protein poor. *E. coli* progressively increased in numbers. *L. bifidus* metabolizes milk saccharides, producing large amounts of acetic acid, lactic acid, and some formic and succinic acids, which create the low pH of the stool of breastfed infants. The intestinal flora of bottle fed infants is gram-negative bacteria, especially coliform organisms and bacteroides.

The flora of bifid bacteria is inhibitory to certain pathogenic bacteria. Substantial clinical evidence is available to demonstrate that there is a resistance mechanism against intestinal infections from *Staphylococcus aureus, Shigella,* and *Protozoa.*

Over the past decade, newer techniques have shown that intestinal flora is *Bifidobacterium* or *Eubacterium,* which are obligatory anaerobes, and not *E. coli* as previously believed. More recently, work by Yoshioka et al.[57] in 1983, using prereduced anaerobically sterilized media, demonstrated the development of stool bacterial flora in both breastfed and bottle fed infants. In both groups, the initial colonization was the enterobacteria in concentrations of 10^9/g in specimens collected from the rectum using a sterile glass tube. Both groups of infants were also given 5% glucose water ad libitum. By day six, bifidobacteria were the predominant organisms in the breastfed infants in a ratio of 1000 to 1 with enterobacteria. In formula fed infants, the predominant organisms were enterobacteria by a ratio of 10 to 1. By 1 month of age, however, bifidobacteria were most prevalent in both groups but the number in breastfed infants was ten times that in the bottle fed infants. In the bottle fed infants, the numbers of enterobacteria, bacteroides, and staphylococci were isolated in a constant number in both groups.

Two actions are apparent. The first encourages the growth of *L. bifidus* and thus crowds out the growth of other bacteria. In the second, the number of pathogens is further kept low by the direct action of lysozyme and lactoferrin. When the number of pathogenic bacteria is kept low, the immune antibodies can keep the growth under control and prevent the absorption of bacteria through the gut wall into the bloodstream.

EVIDENCE OF EFFECTIVENESS OF HUMAN MILK IN CONTROLLING INFECTION _____

The properties of human milk do appear to control infection. There are specific disease entities that have shown a clear differential in the incidence between infants fed cow's milk and those fed human milk.[41]

Bacterial infection

Breast milk IgA has antitoxin activity against enterotoxins of *E. coli* and *Vibrio cholerae* that may be significant in preventing infantile diarrhea. Gindrat et al.[17] found antibodies against O antigen of some of the most common serotypes of *E. coli* in high titer in breast milk samples collected from healthy mothers in Sweden. The infants who had consumed reasonable amounts of breast milk with high titers of *E. coli* antibodies had antibodies in their stool.

Protection against cholera in breastfed children by antibodies in breast milk was studied by Glass et al.[19] A prospective study in Bangladesh showed cholera antibody levels to vary in the colostrum and milk. The correlation between colonization, disease, and milk antibodies led the authors to conclude that breast milk antibodies against cholera do not protect children from colonization with *V. cholera,* but they do protect against disease.

Salmonellal infection was similarly studied by France et al.[15] to evaluate the immunologic mechanisms in host colostrum and milk specific for salmonellae. Vigorous responses of colostral and milk cells against these organisms and nonspecific opsonizing capacity of the aqueous phase of colostrum and milk were demonstrated.

In studies by Gothefors et al.,[21] it was shown that *E. coli* isolated from stools of breastfed infants differed from strains found in formula fed infants in two respects: They were more sensitive to the bactericidal effect of human serum. More often, spontaneously agglutinated bacteria from other sites, such as the prepuce or periurethral area, were less sensitive in breastfed infants. These findings support the theory that breast milk favors proliferation of mutant strains, which have decreased virulence. This mutation of bacterial strains is another way breastfeeding may protect against infection.

It has been suggested that milk immunization is a dynamic process because a mother's milk has been found to contain antibody to virtually all her infant's strains of intestinal bacteria. The mother exposed to the infant's microorganisms either via the breast or the gut responds immunologically to those microorganisms and thus automatically protects her immunologically immature infant.

The orderly review of data on the presence of antibodies in human milk has produced a substantial list of affected organisms. In addition to *E. coli*, there have been identified antibodies to *Bacteroides fragilis, Clostridium tetani, Haemophilus pertussis, Diplococcus pneumoniae, Corynebacterium diphtheriae, Salmonella, Shigella, Chlamydia trachomatis, V. cholerae, S. aureus,* and several strains of *Streptococcus* (Table 5-7).

A study in Oslo by Hansen[24] of an outbreak of severe diarrhea due to *E. coli* strain 0111 showed that six severely ill children were formula fed. Two infants who were breastfed had *E. coli* strain 0111 in their stools but showed few symptoms. Their mothers had no detectable antibodies for strain 0111 in their milk, which would suggest that other factors in human milk protect the infant from serious illness when there are no antibodies in the milk. Hansen[24] also showed in another study that after colonization with a specific strain of *E. coli*, mothers had large numbers of lymphoid cells in their milk with antibodies to that *E. coli*. Their serum produced no such response. This supports the concept that antigen-triggered lymphoid cells from Peyer's patches seek out

Table 5-7. Antibacterial factors in breast milk

Factor	Shown in vitro to be active against	Effect of heat
L. bifidus growth factor	*Enterobacteriaceae,* enteric pathogens	Stable to boiling
Secretory IgA	*E. coli; E. coli* enterotoxin; *C. tetani, C. diphtheriae, D. pneumoniae, Salmonella, Shigella*	Stable at 56° C for 30 min; some loss (0-30%) at 62.5° C for 30 min; destroyed by boiling
C1-C9	Effect not known	Destroyed by heating at 56° C for 30 min
Lactoferrin	*E. coli; C. albicans*	Two-thirds destroyed at 62.5° C for 30 min
Lactoperoxidase	*Streptococcus; Pseudomonas, E. coli, S. typhimurium*	Not known; presumably destroyed by boiling
Lysozyme	*E. coli; Salmonella, M. lysodeikticus*	Stable at 62.5° C for 30 min; activity reduced 97% by boiling for 15 min
Lipid (unsaturated fatty acid)	*S. aureus*	Stable to boiling
Milk cells	By phagocytosis: *E. coli, C. albicans* By sensitized lymphocytes: *E. coli*	Destroyed by 62.5° C for 30 min

From Welsh, J.K., and May, J.T.: J. Pediatr. **94:**1, 1979.

lymphoid-rich tissue, producing IgA in the mammary gland. The mother is immunized in the gut at the same time her milk is. It has also been shown that *E. coli* enteritis can be cured by feeding human milk.

Infants with septicemia, meningitis, and urinary tract infections who were also breastfed were studied by Winberg and Wessner.[56] The infants were compared with matched controls as to the amount of breast milk consumed. The sick infants consumed significantly less breast milk. The infants who received little at the breast were given supplementary formula feeding.

A study of possible cell-mediated immunity in breastfed infants was undertaken by Schlesinger and Covelli.[53] They showed that tuberculin-positive nursing mothers had reactive T cells in their colostrum and early milk. Furthermore, eight of thirteen infants nursed by tuberculin-positive mothers had tuberculin-reactive peripheral blood T cells after 4 weeks. Cord blood had no such activity.

Viral infection

Protection against viruses has been the subject of similar studies. Breast milk contains antibodies against poliovirus, coxsackievirus, echovirus, influenza virus, reovirus, and rhinovirus.[37] It has been confirmed that human milk inhibits the growth of these viruses in tissue culture. Nonspecific substances in human milk are active against arbovirus and murine leukemia virus, according to work by Fieldsteel.[12]

A high degree of antiviral activity against Japanese B encephalitis virus as well as the two leukemia viruses has been found in human milk. The factor was found in the fat fraction and was not destroyed by extended heating, which distinguishes it from antibodies. The nonimmunoglobulin macromolecule antiviral activity in human milk is thought by Welsh et al.[55] to be due to specific fatty acids and monoglycerides (Table 5-8).

Table 5-8. Antiviral factors in breast milk

Factor	Shown in vitro to be active against	Effect of heat
Secretory IgA	Polio types 1, 2, 3, Coxsackie types A9, B3, B5; Echo types 6, 9; Semliki Forest virus, Ross River virus, rotavirus	Stable at 56° C for 30 min; some loss (0%-30%) at 62.5° C for 30 min; destroyed by boiling
Lipid (unsaturated fatty acids and monoglycerides)	Herpes simplex; Semliki Forest virus, influenza, dengue, Ross River virus, Murine leukemia virus, Japanese B encephalitis virus	Stable to boiling for 30 min
Non-immunoglobulin macromolecules	Herpes simplex; vesicular stomatitis virus	Destroyed at 60° C; stable at 56° C for 30 min; destroyed by boiling for 30 min.
	Rotavirus	Unknown
Milk cells	Induced interferon active against Sendai virus; sensitized lymphocytes? Phagocytosis?	Destroyed at 62.5° C for 30 min

From Welsh, J.K., and May, J.T.: J. Pediatr. **94**:1, 1979.

Specimens of human colostrum have been found to contain neutralizing activity against respiratory syncytial virus (RSV). RSV has become a major threat in infancy and is the most common reason for hospitalization in infancy in some developed countries. It has a high mortality. Epidemics have occurred in special-care nurseries. Statistically significant data collected by Downham[11] showed that few breastfed babies (8 of 115) were among the infants hospitalized for RSV infection, compared with uninfected controls who were breastfed (46 of 167).

The immune response to RSV was studied prospectively in 26 nursing mothers over several months by Fishaut et al.[13] Antiviral IgM and IgG were rarely found in colostrum or milk. RSV specific IgA was identified, however, in 40% to 75% of specimens. Two mothers with the disease had specific IgG, IgM, and IgA antibody in serum and nasopharyngeal secretions, but only IgA was found in their milk. This confirms that IgA antibody to specific respiratory tract pathogens is present in the products of lactation. Since RSV appears to replicate only in the respiratory tract, the authors suggest that viral-specific antibody activity in the mammary gland may be derived from the BALT.

Necrotizing enterocolitis has been a serious threat to premature infants in acute-care newborn nurseries in recent years. Animal studies have demonstrated a protective quality to breast milk. Efforts to confirm a similar relationship in human infants have been encouraging but not conclusive. Leukocytes in milk fulfill a protective function in premature infants, possibly as a consequence of their natural transplantation, according to Beer and Billingham.[3]

In a controlled prospective study of high-risk, low-birth weight infants in India using donor human milk, there were significantly fewer infections and no major infections in the group receiving human milk, although the controls experienced diarrhea, pneumonia, septicemia, and meningitis.

The relationship of sudden infant death to formula feeding is supported by circumstantial evidence and retrospective studies. The fact remains that in all series reported, sudden infant death is rare in breastfed infants. Whether this is related to protection against infection is not clear.

The apparent predisposition of bottle fed infants to purulent otitis media as compared with breastfed infants may be due to IgA-conferred immunity in human milk. It may also be due to the mechanics of bottle feeding. Of a group of infants with otitis media, 85% had had their bottles propped up, whereas only 8% of a matched bottle feeding control group who did not have otitis media had had their bottles propped. When an infant swallows fluid lying flat on the back, it is possible for him to regurgitate it into the eustachian tube.[2]

ALLERGIC PROTECTIVE PROPERTIES

In discussing the antiallergic properties of human milk, it is more difficult to identify specific protective properties.

During the neonatal period, the small intestine has increased permeability to macromolecules. Infants have more serum and secretory antibodies against dietary proteins than do children or adults. Production of secretory IgA in the intestinal tract is delayed until 6 weeks to 3 months of age. Secretory IgA in colostrum and breast milk prevents the absorption of foreign macromolecules when the infant's immune system is immature. Protein of breast milk is species specific and therefore nonallergic for the human infant. No antibody response has been demonstrated to occur with human milk in human infants. It has also been shown that macromolecules in breast milk are not absorbed.

Indirect evidence can be inferred from a demonstration of the response to cow's milk protein. Within 18 days of taking cow's milk, the infant will begin to develop antibodies. Since the advent of prepared formulas, in which the protein has been denatured by heating and drying, the incidence of cow's milk allergy has been considered to be 1%. The most reliable means of diagnosing it is by challenging with isolated cow's milk protein. Although circulating antibodies and coproantibodies have been identified, these are not reliable techniques for the clinician involved in patient care.

The allergic syndromes that have been associated with cow's milk allergy include gastroenteropathy, atopic dermatitis, rhinitis, chronic pulmonary disease, eosinophilia, failure to thrive, and sudden death, or cot death, which has been attributed to anaphylaxis to cow's milk.[29,33] The gastrointestinal symptoms have received the greatest attention and include spitting, colic, diarrhea, blood in the stools, frank vomiting, weight loss, malabsorption, colitis, and failure to thrive. Cow's milk has been associated in the gastrointestinal protein and blood loss. The diagnosis is best made by elimination from diet and, when appropriate, challenge tests. Cutaneous testing is of little help.

The association of nasal-secretion eosinophilia with infants freely fed feeding cow's milk or solid foods as compared with eosinophilia in strictly breastfed infants was shown by Murray.[40] Of free-fed infants, 32% had high eosinophilic secretions, and only 11% of breastfed infants had eosinophils in nasal secretions.

It is not surprising that many different antigenic specificities are recognized when the colostrum or milk of one species is fed to or injected into another species. Cow's milk is high on the list of food allergens, particularly in children; sensitivity to cow's milk is responsible for at least 20% of all pediatric allergic conditions, according to Gerrard.[16] Evidence exists that IgA antibodies play an important role in confining food antigens to the gut. Food antigens given to a bottle fed infant before he can make his own IgA, and when he is deprived of that in human milk and the plasma cells, may be expected to be more readily absorbed.

The association of the drop in breastfeeding and the rise in allergy was first made by Glaser.[18] He pioneered the theory of prophylactic management of allergy. The prophylactic management of the potentially allergic infant will be discussed in Chapter 16. The management of specific syndromes such as colic and colitis is discussed in Chapters 8 and 14.

REFERENCES

1. Bahna, S.I., Keller, M.A., and Heiner, D.C.: IgE and IgD in human colostrum and plasma, Pediatr. Res. **16**:604, 1982.
2. Beauregard, W.G.: Positional otitis media, J. Pediatr. **79**:294, 1971.
3. Beer, A.E., and Billingham, R.E.: Immunologic benefits and hazards of milk in maternal-paternal relationships, Ann. Intern. Med. **83**:865, 1975.
4. Beerens, H., Romond, C., and Nevi, C.: Influence of breast-feeding on bifid flora of the newborn intestine, Am. J. Clin. Nutr. **33**:2434, 1980.
5. Bellanti, J.A., and Hurtado, R.C.: Immunology and resistance to infection. In Remington, J.S., and Klein, J.O., editors: Infectious diseases of the fetus and newborn infants, Philadelphia, 1976, W.B. Saunders Co.
6. Bhaskaram, P., and Reddy, V.: Bactericidal activity of human milk leukocytes, Acta Paediatr. Scand. **70**:87, 1981.
7. Brock, J.H., et al.: Role of antibody and enterobactin in controlling growth of *Escherichia coli* in human milk and acquisition of lactoferrin- and transferrin-bound iron by *Escherichia coli,* Infect. Immun. **40**:453, 1983.
8. Brooker, B.E.: The epithelial cells and cell fragments in human milk, Cell Tissue Res. **210**:321, 1980.
9. Bullen, J.J.: Iron-binding proteins and other factors in milk responsible for resistance to *E. coli.* In Ciba Foundation Symposium no. 42, New York, 1976, Elsevier North Holland, Inc.
10. Chandon, R.C., Shahani, K.M., and Holly, R.G.: Lysozyme content of human milk, Nature **204**:76, 1964.
11. Downham, M.A.P.S., et al.: Breast feeding protects against respiratory syncytial virus infections, Br. Med. J. **2**:274, 1976.
12. Fieldsteel, A.H.: Nonspecific antiviral substance in human milk active against arbovirus and murine leukemia virus, Cancer Res. **34**:712, 1974.
13. Fishaut, M., et al.: Bronchopulmonary axis in the immune response to respiratory syncytial virus, J. Pediatr. **99**:186, 1981.
14. Ford, J.E., et al.: Influences of the heat treatment of human milk on some of its protective constituents, J. Pediatr. **90**:29, 1977.
15. France, G.L., Marmer, D.J., and Steele, R.W.: Breast feeding and *Salmonella* infection, Am. J. Dis. Child. **134**:147, 1980.
16. Gerrard, J.W.: Allergy in infancy, Allerg. Pediatr. Ann. **3**:9, October 1974.
17. Gindrat, J.J., et al.: Antibodies in human milk against *E. coli* of the serogroups most commonly found in neonatal infection, Acta Paediatr. Scand. **61**:587, 1972.
18. Glaser, J.: The dietary prophylaxis of allergic disease in infancy, J. Asthma Res. **3**:199, 1966.
19. Glass, R.I., et al.: Protection against cholera in breast-fed children by antibodies in breast milk, N. Engl. J. Med. **308**:1389, 1983.
20. Goldblum, R.M., et al.: Antibody-forming cells in human colostrum after oral immunization, Nature **257**:797, 1975.
21. Gothefors, L., Olling, S., and Winberg, J.: Breast feeding and biological properties of faecal *E. coli* strains, Acta Paediatr. Scand. **64**:807, 1975.
22. Gullberg, R.: Possible influence of vitamin B_{12} binding protein in milk on the intestinal flora in breast-fed infants. II. Contents of unsaturated B_{12} binding protein in meconium and faeces from breast-fed and bottle-fed infants, Scand. J. Gastroenterol. **9**:287, 1974.
23. György, P.: A hitherto unrecognized biochemical difference between human milk and cow's milk, Pediatrics **11**:98, 1953.
24. Hanson, L.A.: *Escherichia coli* infections in childhood: significance of bacterial virulence and immune defense, Arch. Dis. Child. **51**:737, 1976.
25. Head, J.R., and Beer, A.E.: The immunologic role of viable leukocytic cells in mammary exosecretions. In Larson, B.L., editor: Lactation, vol. IV, Mammary gland/human lactation/milk synthesis, New York, 1978, Academic Press, Inc.
26. Ho, P.C., and Lawton, J.W.M.: Human colostral cells: phagocytosis and killing of *E. coli* and *C. albicans,* J. Pediatr. **93**:910, 1978.
27. Iyengar, L., and Selvaraj, R.J.: Intestinal absorption of immunoglobulins by newborn infants, Arch. Dis. Child. **47**:411, 1972.
28. Jelliffe, D.B., and Jelliffe, E.F.P.: Human milk in the modern world, Oxford, 1978, Oxford University Press.
29. Johnstone, D.E., and Dutton, A.M.: Dietary prophylaxis of allergic disease in children, N. Engl. J. Med. **274**:715, 1966.
30. Kirkpatrick, C.H., et al.: Inhibition of growth of

Candida albicans by iron-unsaturated lactoferrin: relation to host-defense mechanisms in chronic mucocutaneous candidiasis, J. Infect. Dis. **124:**539, 1971.

31. Kleinman, R.E., and Walker, W.A.: The enteromammary immune system: an important concept in breast milk host defense, Digest. Dis. Sci. **24:**876, 1979.

32. Lawton, J.W.M., and Shortridge, K.F.: Protective factors in human breast milk and colostrum, Lancet **1:**253, 1977.

33. Lebethal, E.: Symposium on gastrointestinal and liver disease, cow's milk protein allergy, Pediatr. Clin. North Am. **22:**827, 1975.

34. Liebhaber, M., et al.: Alterations of lymphocytes and of anitbody content of human milk after processing, J. Pediatr. **91:**897, 1977.

35. Mata, L.J., and Urrutia, J.J.: Intestinal colonization of breast-fed children in a rural area of low socioeconomic level, Ann. N.Y. Acad. Sci. **176:**93, 1971.

36. Mata, L.J., and Wyatt, R.G.: Host resistance to infection. In Jelliffe, D.B., and Jelliffe, E.F.P., editors: The uniqueness of human milk, Am. J. Clin. Nutr. **24:**976, 1971.

37. Matthews, T.H.J., et al.: Antiviral activity in milk of possible clinical importance, Lancet **2:**1387, 1976.

38. McClelland, D.B.L.: Antibodies in milk, J. Reprod. Fert. **65:**537, 1982.

39. Michael, J.G., Ringenback, R., and Hottenstein, S.: The antimicrobial activity of human colostral antibody in the newborn, J. Infect. Dis. **124:**445, 1971.

40. Murray, A.B.: Infant feeding and respiratory allergy, Lancet **1:**497, 1971.

41. Narayanan, I., Prakash, K., and Gujral, V.V.: The value of human milk in the prevention of infection in the high-risk low-birth weight infants, J. Pediatr. **99:**496, 1981.

42. Ogra, P.L., Fishaut, M., and Theodore, C.: Immunology of breast milk: maternal neonatal interactions. In Freier S., and Eidelman, A.I., editors: Human milk: its biological and social value, Amsterdam, 1980, Excerpta Media International Congress, Series 518.

43. Ogra, S.S., and Ogra, P.L.: Immunologic aspects of human colostrum and milk. II. Characteristics of lymphocyte reactivity and distribution of E-rosette forming cells at different times after the onset of lactation, J. Pediatr. **92:**550, 1976.

44. Ogra, S.S., and Ogra, P.L.: Immunologic aspects of human colostrum and milk. I. Distribution characteristics and concentrations of immunoglobulins at different times after the onset of lactation, J. Pediatr. **92:**546, 1978.

45. Ogra, S.S., and Ogra, P.L.: Components of immunology reactivity in human colostrum and milk. In Ogra, P.L., and Dayton, D.H., editors: Immunology of breast milk, New York, 1979, Raven Press.

46. Parmely, M.J., Beer, A.E., and Billingham, R.E.: In vitro studies of the T-lymphocyte population of human milk, J. Exp. Med. **144:**358, 1976.

47. Peitersen, B., Bohn, L., and Andersen, H.: Quantitative determination of immunoglobulins, lysozyme, and certain electrolytes in breast milk during the entire period of lactation, during a 24-hour period, and in milk from the individual mammary gland, Acta Paediatr. Scand. **64:**709, 1975.

48. Pitt, J.: The milk mononuclear phagocyte, Pediatrics Suppl. **64:**745, 1979.

49. Pittard, W.B., III: Breast milk immunology: a frontier in infant nutrition, Am. J. Dis. Child. **133:**83, 1979.

50. Pittard, W.B., III, and Bill, K.: Immunoregulation of breast milk cells, (abstract) Pediatr. Res. **12:**485, 1978.

51. Pittard, W.B., III, Polmar, S.H., and Farnaroff, A.A.: The breast milk macrophage: a potential vehicle for immunoglobulin transport, J. Reticuloendothel. **22:**597, 1977.

52. Reddy, V., et al.: Antimicrobial factors in human milk, Acta Paediatr. Scand. **66:**229, 1977.

53. Schlesinger, J.J., and Covelli, H.D.: Evidence for transmission of lymphocyte responses to tuberculin by breast-feeding, Lancet **2:**529, 1977.

54. Stoliar, O.A., et al.: Secretory IgA against enterotoxins in breast milk, Lancet **1:**1258, 1976.

55. Welsh, J.K., Skurrie, I.J., and May, J.T.: Use of Semliki Forest virus to identify lipid-mediated antiviral activity and anti-alphavirus immunoglobulin A in human milk, Infect. Immun. **19:**395, 1978.

56. Winberg, J., and Wessner, G.: Does breast milk protect against septicaemia in the newborn? Lancet **1:**1091, 1971.

57. Yoshioka, H., Isekl, K.I., and Fujita, K.: Development and differences of intestinal flora in the neonatal period in breast-fed and bottle-fed infants, Pediatrics **72:**317, 1983.

Psychologic bonding

6

Although the previous chapters provide more than adequate information to support the urgency of breastfeeding in almost every case, the critical impact in the return to breastfeeding in modern cultures rests with the issue of the mother's role and her perception of breastfeeding as a biologic act. The maternal influences include psychophysiologic reactions during nursing, long-term psychophysiologic effects, maternal behavior, sexual behavior, and attitudes toward men. All professionals providing support care in the perinatal period need to have a clear view not only of the biologic benefits but also of their own psychologic attitudes about the breast itself. The breast has been regarded as a sex object in the Western world in this century, and its biologic benefits have been downplayed. This is clearly demonstrated by the conflicting mores that permit pornographic pictures in newspapers, movies, and nude theaters but arrest a mother, discreetly nursing her baby in public, for indecent exposure.

It has been generally accepted by proponents of breastfeeding, even before the upsurge of interest and research in bonding, that the major reason to breastfeed is to provide that special relationship and closeness that accompanies nursing. Conversely, the major contraindication to breastfeeding was lack of desire to do so. This was evidenced by the fact that it was considered more appropriate to present breastfeeding as a matter of personal choice with no compelling reasons to urge a mother to consider nursing. The concern over creating guilt in the mother who chose not to nurse has been significant to the clinician.

MOTHER-INFANT INTERACTION

The studies done in recent years to understand bonding have largely been done without reference to breastfeeding. It has been pointed out that a comprehensive book, *Attachment and Loss* by Bowlby,[7] which reviews early mother-infant interactions extensively, never mentions breastfeeding. In addition, sucking is given extensive treatment without making a distinction between bottle and breast or implying that there is an alternative to the bottle. Work by Spitz[34] and others has identified the devastating effects on the infant when he is deprived of long-term maternal contact. These investigators demonstrated major deficits in both mental and motor development, as well as general failure to thrive. What had yet to be described was the impact on the mother. Klaus and Kennell[20] have provided those data in their many writings on mother-infant interaction, which are summarized in their book, *Maternal-Infant Bonding*. There is reason to believe that the maternal-infant bond is the strongest human bond, when two major facts are considered: the infant's early growth is within the mother's body, and his survival after birth depends on her care. Although the process had not been meticulously described, it had been noted by Budin[9] that when a mother was separated from her infant and was unable to provide the early care of her sick child, she lost interest and even abandoned the infant.

The immediate emotional reactions of mothers to their newborns were studied by Robson and Kumar[30] in 193 women (two groups of primiparas $n = 112$ and $n = 41$, and one group of multiparas, $n = 40$). About 40% of the primiparas and 25% of the multiparas recalled that their predominant emotional reaction when holding their babies for the very first time had been one of indifference. Maternal affection was more likely to be lacking if the mother had had an amniotomy or painful labor or had received more than one dose of pethidine unrelated to cesarean section or forceps delivery. There was no difference between breastfeeding and bottle feeding mothers. The feelings of indifference persisted for a week or longer. This study points out that normal women may be indifferent toward their babies initially.

Klaus and Kennell[20] suggested that there is probably a critical period in which ideal bonding takes place in the human. This critical period has been described for many animal species, in which the mother rejects or even destroys her offspring if they are taken from her at a critical early postpartum time. For the goat, this time is the first 5 minutes. For the human, Kennell et al.[19] described this critical period as within the first 12 hours. Further, they noted that mothers in the United States showed different attachment behavior when permitted early contact with their premature infants compared with mothers who had first contact at 3 weeks of age. Mothers of full-term infants who were allowed contact within the first 2 hours and subsequent extra contact behaved differently at 1 month and 1 year with their babies, compared with controls. Actually, Jackson et al.[18] made similar observations in the Yale Rooming-In Unit in 1945 to 1955, but they failed to provide control observations.

The impact of early mother-infant interaction and breastfeeding on the duration of breastfeeding has been reported; no data appear to be available as to whether mothering is different between breastfeeding and bottle feeding mothers. Sosa et al.[33] reported the effect of early mother-infant contact on breastfeeding, infection, and growth. Breastfeeding mothers who were permitted early contact but not early breastfeeding were compared with mothers without early contact who also breastfed. The mothers with early contact were observed to nurse 50% longer than the controls. The early-contact infants were heavier and had fewer infections. Sosa et al.[33] conducted a similar study in Brazil, in which study each mother nursed immediately on delivery and the infant was kept beside the mother's bed until they went home. At home they had a special nurse make continual contacts to help in the breastfeeding. The control had traditional therapy, that is, contact at feeding times after an early glimpse. Infants were housed in a separate nursery. At 2 months, 77% of the early-contact mothers and only 27% of the controls were successfully nursing. It is quite possible that the early and continued contact was accompanied by increased support and assistance from the nursery staff. This added support could facilitate breastfeeding and thus be the cause of the improved outcome.

An additional study by DeChateau[14] in Sweden investigated a group of 21 mothers with early contact and 19 control mothers, all of whom were breastfeeding to begin with. The only difference in management was the first 30 minutes of early contact, since 24-hour rooming-in was provided for all mothers after 2 hours postpartum. The length of breastfeeding differed: for the early-contact group, 175 days, and for the controls, 105 days. Follow-up observations at 3 months showed different mothering behavior. The study group showed more attachment behavior, fondling, caressing, and kissing than the controls.

Unless heavy medication or difficult delivery intervenes, an infant experiences a period when his eyes are wide open, he can see, has visual preferences, turns to the spoken word, and responds to his environment. Such a period in the state of consciousness of the infant may last only seconds or minutes at a time over the next few days.

When Klaus and Kennel[20] diagramed the reciprocal interaction in the first few hours of life, they chose a nursing mother-infant couple. They included in their scheme the factors that are limited to breastfeeding, such as the transfer of lymphocytes and macrophages from mother to infant and the stimulation of oxytocin and prolactin by suckling of the infant as part of the reciprocal interaction (Fig. 6-1).

Many mothers who did not have the privilege of early contact because of hospital policy, cesarean section, or adoption of the baby, have been led to feel they have missed the single opportunity to establish model parenting. Lamb[22] and others[2,3,12] have been critical of the earlier work on the value of early contact, pointing out the weakness in study design. Lamb[22] has, however, been supportive of the trend toward humanizing childbirth to provide a rich emotional experience for parents.

BODY CONTACT AND CULTURAL TRADITION

If we look at other mammals, lactation behavior, including the duration and frequency of feedings, is species specific and predictable, because it is a generically controlled behavioral characteristic of the species. Only those animals kept in zoos or laboratories reject their young. Among higher primates, learning plays a significant role;

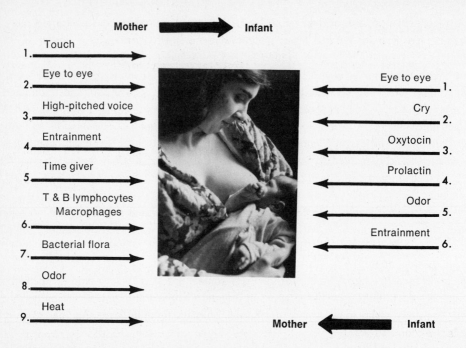

Fig. 6-1. Mother-to-infant and infant-to-mother interactions that can occur simultaneously in first days of life. (From Klaus, M.H., and Kennell, J.H.: Maternal-infant bonding: the impact of early separation or loss on family development, St. Louis, 1976, The C.V. Mosby Co.)

monkeys reared without role models have to be taught how to groom and feed their young. In the human, breastfeeding behavior is highly variable from one culture to the next. Different cultures of the world have different sets of "rules" about lactation as they do about many other aspects of life and even death. Cultural tradition dictates the initiation, frequency, and termination of breastfeeding. Learning plays a key role in the lactation process, but the learning is focused on the beliefs, attitudes, and values of the culture.

The degree of body contact permitted by the culture is a fundamental difference among these cultures. Simpson-Herbert[32] describes the degree of mother-infant body contact as the physical and social distance that mothers keep from their babies. The physical distance is viewed as a reflection of the social distance sanctioned by the culture.

Cultures prescribe how often an infant will be held or carried and how he will be carried (e.g., in the arms, a pouch, or a sling, or on a cradleboard). How the infant is clothed, where he is placed when not held, and where he spends the night are all culturally determined and also affect breastfeeding. The cultural constraints that control maternal behavior include those on the kinds and amounts of maternal clothing, acceptability of breast exposure, and beliefs on frequency and length of feedings.

Anthropologic studies of 60 societies by Whiting[37] considered mother-infant body contact. He classified these cultures as high or low in contact as follows:

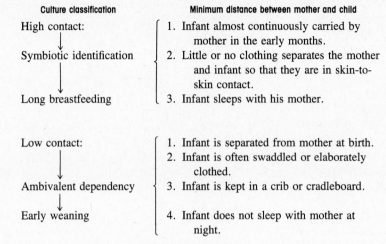

Culture classification	Minimum distance between mother and child
High contact: ↓ Symbiotic identification ↓ Long breastfeeding	1. Infant almost continuously carried by mother in the early months. 2. Little or no clothing separates the mother and infant so that they are in skin-to-skin contact. 3. Infant sleeps with his mother.
Low contact: ↓ Ambivalent dependency ↓ Early weaning	1. Infant is separated from mother at birth. 2. Infant is often swaddled or elaborately clothed. 3. Infant is kept in a crib or cradleboard. 4. Infant does not sleep with mother at night.

Other factors influence the development of cultural mores, including climate and means of food gathering. Simpson-Herbert[32] points out that when infants are heavily clothed and swaddled, as in cold climates, they are neat packages that can be put down easily. The Eskimo, however, keeps the infant inside her parka. Breastfeeding is almost continuous in warm climates where clothing is loose or absent, there is frequent holding and carrying, and the breast is readily accessible.

The diet of the hunter-gatherer society is not conducive to early weaning because meat, roots, nuts, and berries are difficult for infants to handle, whereas the softer foods of the agricultural societies can be prepared for early infant feeding.

Study of specific societies reveal that North American and European women are concerned with the beliefs that it is indecent to expose the breast, it is possible to spoil an infant with too much handling, and an early weaning is a sign of development. Western mothers keep their distance from their babies. Mothers in high–body contact societies spend at least 75% of the time in contact with their babies, while low-contact societies spend less than 25%.

PSYCHOLOGIC DIFFERENCE BETWEEN BREASTFEEDING AND BOTTLE FEEDING

Professionals have spent decades reassuring mothers that they can capture the same emotional and behavioral experience by feeding an infant a bottle as they can by feeding him at the breast and that the same warmth and love is there. Technically speaking, the same warmth is not there, because the lactating breast has been shown to be warmer than the nonlactating breast. This can be demonstrated by infrared pictures.

Newton and Newton[26] suggest that special caution should be used in evaluating statistical associative studies that purport to study the hypothesis that breastfeeding and bottle feeding are psychologic equivalents. ''Because breast-feeding involves a large measure of personal choice and because it is related to attitudinal and personality factors, no groups of breastfeeders and bottle feeders are likely to be equal in other respects. Therefore the relation of breastfeeding to any particular psychosocial measure may not be cause and effect, but simply the differences due to other uncontrolled covariables.''[26] A human mother's care of her infant is derived from a complex mixture of her genetic endowment, the response of the infant, a long history of interpersonal relationships with others, her family constellation, this and previous pregnancies, and the community and culture.

The method chosen to feed a baby is but one item in a whole style of maternal-child interaction. It is unlikely that this style is determined by the method of feeding, according to Richards.[29] Breastfeeding is a very different activity when it is carried out by a small minority from when it is commonplace.

Before reviewing specific psychologic attributes relating to breastfeeding, the distinction between styles of nursing should be considered. Newton[25] has described two distinct groups: unrestricted breastfeeding and token breastfeeding.

Unrestricted breastfeeding

Unrestricted breastfeeding means the infant is put to the breast whenever he cries or fusses. Feeding is ad lib and not by the clock, usually leading to 10 or more feedings a day. The infant receives no bottles, and solids are not introduced until the second half of the first year. Breast milk continues to be a major source of nourishment beyond the first year of life. It is interesting to note that this was routine practice in the United States in the beginning of this century as attested by writings on the subject of child rearing.

Token breastfeeding

Token breastfeeding means feeding characterized by rules and regulations. Both frequency and duration of feeding are determined by the clock. It is deemed unnecessary to permit unlimited suckling. Weaning usually occurs by the third month, if not before. Supplementary bottles and solids are not uncommon. As a result, the let-down reflex is never well established. Engorgement is not uncommon. The infant is frequently too frantic from crying or too sleepy to feed well at the appointed times.

A University of Rochester study of urban physicians revealed that many of the pediatricians prescribed solids by 3 months or earlier and suggested supplementary bottles. Most of the physicians in the family medicine program in the same community, however, provided no supplements and no solids until 6 months. Over 50% of mothers in that community who planned to breastfeed had made contact with some childbirth or breastfeeding program and chose their physician according to his practice style.

LET-DOWN REFLEX. The unrestricted breastfed infant cries and his mother has the urge to suckle him because the cry has triggered her let-down reflex. The breast is turgescent and ready for the infant. Unrestricted crying is rarely seen in these infants. With token breastfeeding such a response does not occur on schedule, and from feeding to feeding the milk supply may be little or, conversely, gushing. The infant is unable to cope with the unpredictability.

PERSONALITY DIFFERENCES BETWEEN BREASTFEEDING AND BOTTLE FEEDING MOTHERS

There are clear differences between mothers who practice unrestricted breastfeeding and those who bottle feed. There are even some distinctions between token breastfeeders and bottle feeders. It has been said that maternal personality is more important than either breastfeeding or bottle feeding per se to the development of the infant's personality. Experimenters looking at these questions have provided a wealth of somewhat conflicting information. Chamberlain[11] undertook to decipher the differences between mothers who bottle fed and those who practiced unrestricted breastfeeding with their second child. The groups were similar in age, education, parity, intelligence, and socioeconomic status. The breastfeeding mothers were less defensive about their method of feeding, were more oriented toward home life, and had higher radicalism scores. The bottle feeding mothers confirmed the hypothesis that they had problems in trying to breastfeed their first child due to inadequate lactation, possibly a psychosomatic reaction. They also had a greater incidence of sexual anomalies, as indicated from a higher surgency score. The breastfeeding mothers wanted their children to do things typical of children; the bottle feeding mothers preferred their children to be conservative and other-person oriented.

Call[10] had studied the emotional factors favoring successful breastfeeding and noted that of 104 consecutive mothers delivering at an Air Force hospital, 42.6% of the multiparas and 50% of the primiparas chose bottle feeding. Of the breastfeeding mothers, 48% of those multiparas and 40% of the primiparas were successful beyond 3 weeks. Failure was associated with engorgement, lack of let-down reflex, and psychologic conflict. The two conflicts seen in those who did not nurse and those who failed were as follows:

1. They had a conflict in accepting the biologic maternal role in relation to the infant versus other roles society holds for women. The maternal role is considered a general class attitude in middle-class American society.
2. They had a conflict regarding the functioning of the breast itself, that is, as an organ for nourishment of the young versus a sexual organ, affording the breast the same psychologic value as the penis in the male. Nursing thus became a "castration" threat.

POSTPARTUM DEPRESSION

Much has been written in the lay press about "baby blues," and many mothers will admit to a few hours or a day of incredible emotional seesawing some time in the first week after delivery. Episodes in which a mother dissolves in tears when she has "so much to be thankful for" is the usual description. This is a transient state that has been attributed to the tremendous change in hormonal levels after the delivery of the placenta. It is usually successfully treated with reassurance and rest. True postpartum depression does occur, however, and, contrary to popular fantasy, it occurs in women who are breastfeeding. The incidence of psychiatric disorders, especially depression, is known to increase postpartum.[2]

The relationship between breastfeeding and depression was studied by Kumar and Robson[21] among mothers who totally breastfed and those who totally bottle fed. No relationship was found between depression and feeding method. A prospective study following 103 women postpartum recorded a 13% incidence of marked postnatal depressive illness and an additional 16% of minor depressive illness of at least 4 weeks' duration. No correlation was made with method of feeding until the mothers were asked about their feeding methods and oral contraceptive use in an attempt to determine the influence of hormones on depression. The authors speculated that the prolactin, estrogen, and progesterone levels would vary with the amount of breastfeeding, amount of other foods consumed by the baby, and amount of hormones taken in the form of contraceptives. In this study the bottle feeders received estrogen and progesterone, but breastfeeders received only progesterone as contraceptives. Total breastfeeders who were not taking contraceptives were somewhat more likely to report depressive symptoms. Feelings of fatigue may have influenced this. The mothers least likely to be depressed were those who were likely to have normal hormonal levels, that is non–pill taking partial breastfeeders. Clearly, breastfeeding women are not immune to postpartum depression.[13]

PSYCHOPHYSIOLOGIC REACTIONS DURING NURSING

Newton and Newton[26] have equated psychophysiologic reactions during nursing to the degree of successful lactation. During unrestricted suckling the gentle stroking of the nipple occurs 3000 to 4000 times. This should result in an increase in temperature of the mammary skin and rhythmic contraction of the uterus. Failure to experience these signs is related to failure to produce adequate milk.

The long-term psychophysiologic reaction of unrestricted nursing is a more even mood cycle compared with the mood swings associated with ovulation and menstruation. Unrestricted nursing is associated with secondary amenorrhea for as long as 16 months.

From studies in animals, Thoman et al.[35] have stated, "The present experiments do indicate that there is a unique buffering system which appears to protect the lactating female from large variations in responsiveness during the process of lactating. Inasmuch as there exists considerable information that indicates that maternal factors have profound and long-lasting effects on the psychophysiologic function of offspring in adulthood, the existence of such buffering systems in the lactating females would appear to be of importance in the mother-young interaction.''

In relating the rate of success in breastfeeding to experiences at birth, Jackson et al.[18] reported that the more difficult the labor, the less successful the breastfeeding. A direct correlation has also been made with the amount of medication and anesthetic given during labor and delivery and subsequently the sleepiness of the infant and, ultimately, the inadequacy of the suckling.

Newton observed that mothers who talked to their babies on the second day nursed their babies longer, that is, beyond the second month.

IMPACT OF SOCIETY, MEDICAL PROFESSION, AND FAMILY
Society

Newton[25] has pointed out that a woman's joy in and acceptance of the female biologic role in life may be an important factor in her psychosexual behavior, which includes lactation. She found that women who wished to bottle feed also often believed that the male role was the more satisfying role. Nulliparous women who planned to breastfeed their children more often stated their satisfaction with the female role, according to Adams.[1] Breastfeeding behavior has been related to a woman's role in life as influenced by her cultural locale, education, social class, and work. Breastfeeding rates and weaning times vary in the United States by geographic area, as pointed out by Robertson.[31] The smaller the community, the longer the duration of breastfeeding. Cross-cultural studies in large cities show variation in rates of nursing. These rates are influenced by education and, in this generation, the higher the education, the higher the incidence of breastfeeding.

The attitudes of the husband, close family, and friends have an influence on the mother's attitude toward breastfeeding. More important, these attitudes influence the rate of success and the age at weaning more negatively than positively. One study showed that a grandmother's interest did not influence the mother's decision to nurse as frequently as did a friend's (peer's) decision to bottle feed.

Medical profession

The enthusiastic physician can influence the number of breastfeeding mothers in his practice; this has been demonstrated. If the physician provides knowledgeable medical and psychologic support, the success rate of the patients who intended to breastfeed will increase. Some patients who had not formed an opinion or given it any thought in their preparation for motherhood will be persuaded to try. In addition, this physician will attract patients to the practice who are already successfully breastfeeding but find their own physician unable or unwilling to support their efforts.

A study was done at the University of Rochester in a small city where over 50 pediatricians practiced. The pediatricians described their own practices according to the number of breastfeeding mothers (high, 75%; moderate, 50%; low, 25%). They were also asked when they started solid foods, general practice "regulations," and, finally, how their own children were fed. The physicians with a high incidence of breastfeeding in their practices started solids after 4 months, had few rules and regulations about the office, and usually their own children had been breastfed. The physicians with a high number of bottle feeders started solids by 6 weeks, had many rules and regulations about the practice, and their own children had been bottle fed. When asked about using lay groups to help their patients breastfeed, the female physicians were more apt than the male physicians to discredit what these mothers could do to help other mothers.

A national survey conducted among a representative sample of obstetricians, pediatricians, and family physicians by mailed questionnaire reinforced the observation that the physician's attitude and personal beliefs about breastfeeding influence the advice given.[23] It further confirmed that not all physicians were informed about current knowledge on human lactation, not all physicians discussed lactation with their pregnant patients, and not all felt it was worth counseling time when problems arose.

The family

IMPACT ON THE INFANT. For the infant, there are differences between breastfeeding and bottle feeding in the alleviation of hunger, the mother-infant interaction, oral gratification, activity, development, personality, and adaption to the environment. Often mother and baby are alone together during breastfeeding, and the mother gives her full attention to the baby with stroking and fondling. Social interaction with the baby is less frequent when he is bottle fed, and the mother is often in a distracting social situation. The breastfed infant has control of what is happening, or at least shares control, whereas the mother controls the bottle and the bouts of sucking.

Development. Early assessment of newborns in the first or second week of life shows more body activity with breastfed than bottle fed infants. They are more alert and have stronger arousal reaction. Statistics reported by Douglas[15] on age of learning to walk in Great Britain showed a distinct difference, with breastfed infants starting 2 months earlier than bottle fed. The longer the infant was nursed, the more striking the differences. Thus prolonged breastfeeding does not impede development, as has been implied by advocates of early weaning. A study in Illinois[17] in 1929 compared children exclusively breastfed for 4 months, 9 months, and over a year to bottle fed infants. The children who were exclusively breastfed for 4 and 9 months scored significantly higher on achievement tests, but the difference was reversed beyond a year. Exclusively breastfeeding beyond a year increased morbidity as well, which is in keeping with the concept that solids should be added in the second half of the first year.

Animal work has also shown a relationship of weaning time to learning skills. Since it has become evident that there are species-specific proteins and amino acids, it is possible that the brain develops more physiologically with the precise basic nutrients. Comparisons with animal species show that the more intelligent and skillful groups within a species are nursed longer.

Personality. The personality and adjustment of infants as related to their early feeding experiences have been the subject of much discussion. It must be acknowledged that the personality of the mother and the temperament of the child need to be considered. Some conflicting information is reported in studies analyzing retrospectively the effects of breastfeeding on outcome in terms of security and behavior. The emphasis has been on the duration of the breastfeeding rather than the quality of the relationship. When abrupt weaning takes place, it may be psychologically very traumatic for the infant and the mother. In animals, when the mother is stressed while lactating, the nursling's plasma cortisone levels are elevated. The psychologically depressed mother may not experience postpartum depression until the infant is weaned from the breast. It has been accepted that early experience, including feeding experience, does influence later behavior in the long run, but much more study must be done before the impact of nursing at the breast is truly understood in this complex culture today.

IMPACT ON THE FATHER. Since the birthing process moved into the hospital setting, fathers have been moved further from the nucleus of the new family. In recent years this trend has been reversed. Research on interaction with the infant had focused on the mother until Parke and associates[27] observed all three together. In the triadic situation, the father tends to hold the baby twice as much, touches the baby slightly more, but smiles significantly less than the mother. The father plays the more active role when both are present. The study was conducted with middle-class participants who had been to childbirth classes, but the same results were obtained among low-income families without preparation or the presence of the father in the labor and delivery room. The infant had to be relatively active and responsive to capture the father's attention. The investigators felt fathers were far more involved in and responsive toward their infants than our culture had acknowledged. Other studies have shown that when fathers were asked to undress their babies and establish eye contact with them in the first few days of life, they showed more caregiving behavior than did controls 3 months later.

Newton describes the early attachments of the new family as follows:

Father	interacts with baby	engrossment
Mother	interacts with baby	bonding
Baby	interacts with mother	attachment

The father has been brought back into the childbirth scene as a coach. The coach role has been described as the father's role in shared childbirth. The idea of coaching has negative connotations, since a coach is one who develops the players to work and try harder but always to win. Ideally, the father should be a partner and supporter in labor, delivery, and breastfeeding. Raphael[28] has suggested that the father may well play the role of the doula. The doula is one who provides psychologic encouragement and physical assistance to the newly delivered mother. Raphael further indicates that it is the lack of a doula to support the mother that predisposes her to failure with breastfeeding.

The stress placed on sharing responsibilities of parenthood implies an across-the-board division of labor. This implies that parenting is equal for women and men. There are complementary activities for fathers and mothers. Parents are not equally able to do all things. There is more to nurturing the infant than feeding. The father, therefore, should play a very significant role with the infant. For instance, when the infant is fussy and does not need to be fed, comforting is often best done by the father.

The father's most common negative reaction to breastfeeding according to Waletsky[36] is jealousy of the physical and emotional closeness of the nursing mother and child. The degree of jealousy may reflect how much and how happily the mother breastfeeds. Actually, fathers may express distress because they have no similar way to bring food and contentment to their baby. Male envy of female sex characteristics and reproductive capacity has been identified by Lerner[24] as "a widespread and conspicuously ignored dynamic." Improving the birth experience for husbands is a significant means of helping them feel closer to their baby and better about themselves as fathers, according to Waletsky.[36]

Fathers who object to their wives' breastfeeding may do so because they do not want to share this part of their lover with an infant. Some fathers express concern that the breasts will leak and destroy any sexual mystique. On the other hand, many men take great pride in the knowledge that their infants will be breastfed and support their wives in this effort. The decision to breastfeed should be made with the full involvement of the father in most cases.

IMPACT ON SIBLINGS. Although there is some information about siblings and breastfeeding with regard to behavior patterns, there are no known studies comparing siblings of bottle fed and breastfed infants. Just as siblings frequently wish to try the infant's bottle, they may wish to nurse at the breast. The child will reflect the mother's attitude toward the breast and nursing. If the mother nurses secretly or in private and isolates herself from the family, it may cause concern in the sibling and produce feelings of shame or guilt toward the breasts.

WHY WOMEN DO NOT BREASTFEED

Before the trend toward bottle feeding can be reversed, one has to understand why some women do not breastfeed. It cannot be blamed on society or the medical profession when a woman cannot accept this as part of the biologic role of a mother. A physician who does not understand the complexities of rejecting breastfeeding cannot hope to assist a mother to succeed in breastfeeding.

Our society has assumed that there is no valid intellectual stimulation to be had in the company of young children. Mothers are made to feel intellectually stagnant and uncreative while breastfeeding. Indeed, they are also made to feel asexual at the peak of their sexual cycle. In response, new mothers panic to maintain their social and professional ties. They feel they must produce tangible works in order to be productive. Bloom[6] points out poignantly that one of the greatest intellectual voyages of our time was undertaken when Jean Piaget sat at his son's crib and observed the child's successive attempts to grasp a rattle. A nursing mother learns about her child through many internal, subjective, and kinesthetic modes that were not open to Piaget.

Bentovim[5] has taken a systems approach, pointing out that a range of physical, psychologic, and sociologic factors are involved. A general systems-theory approach provides an explanatory model in which the elements are envisioned as interacting dynamically (Fig. 6-2). "Breast-feeding is a systemic product of many interacting factors rather than a product of individual behavior only,"[5] according to Bentovim. A good experience with breastfeeding can ensure an intense interaction and synchronous response of giving and taking. According to Brazelton,[8] this is the essence of the infant's beginning to create a secure world for himself.

Block diagram approach

Bentovim[5] has created a block diagram (Fig. 6-2) as the first step, describing quantitative and conceptual relationhips. Following the diagram, block A contains the variables relating to the mother and her characteristics that convinced her to breastfeed. Block B includes the characteristics of the family relating to breastfeeding. Block C contains variables in society that influenced the decision to breastfeed. Block D is the precipitating factors (such as pregnancy) that are acted on by A, B, and C to make the decision to breastfeed this particular infant. Block E represents the attempt to feed, which has consequences for the mother as listed in block F, for the child in block G, and for the family and society as in block H. Through neurohormonal response and sexual response, suckling can produce secondary pleasure or displeasure, shame, and anxiety. The infant responds to the mothering and attachment behavior. This interacts with the family and society, which feed back to and influence the variables in blocks A, B, and C.

This diagram (Fig. 6-2) cannot demonstrate negative and positive feedback. The same variables, however, are used to illustrate the decision-making procedure and are diagramed in Figure 6-3. Solid lines refer to positive feedback and broken lines to negative feedback. From this it is clear that beliefs and attitudes toward breastfeeding influence the choice and the success of breastfeeding. Bentovim points out that it may be possible to restore breastfeeding as the natural choice. This would depend on society's finding a system in which the breast can be accepted not only as good for the

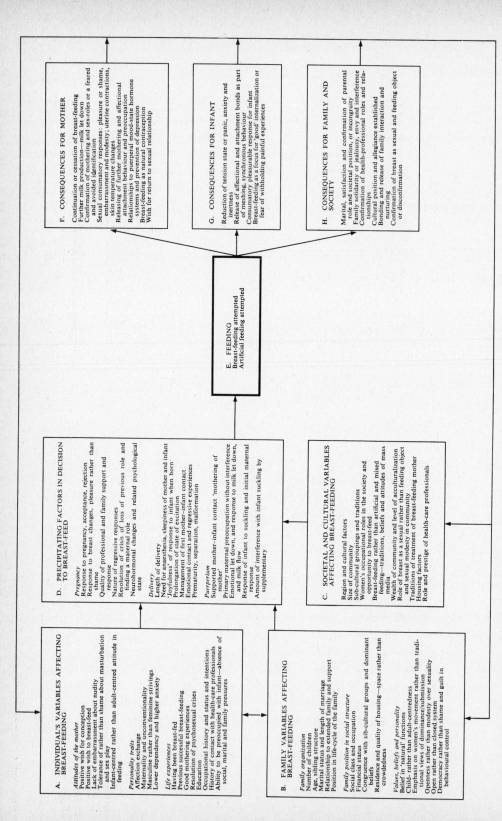

Fig. 6-2. Breastfeeding: elements of a social system. (From Bentovim, A.: Shame and other anxieties associated with breastfeeding: a systems theory and psychodynamic approach. In Ciba Foundation Symposium no. 45, breastfeeding and the mother. Amsterdam, 1976. Elsevier Scientific Publ. Co., p. 159.)

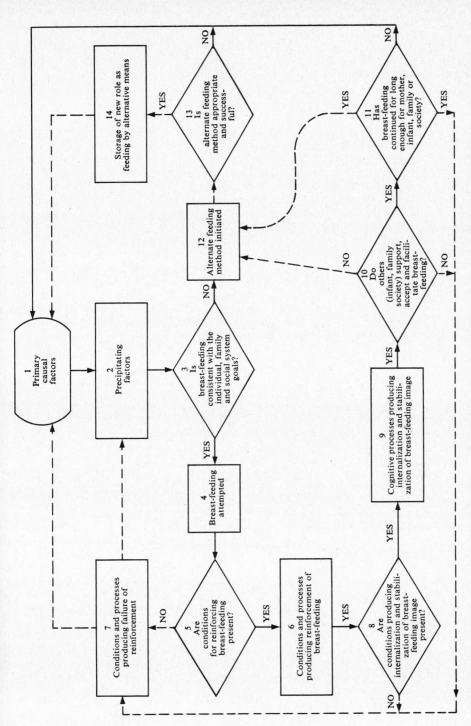

Fig. 6-3. Breastfeeding: the decision-making procedure. (From Bentovim, A.: Shame and other anxieties associated with breastfeeding: a systems theory and psychodynamic approach. In Ciba Foundation Symposium no. 45, breastfeeding and the mother, Amsterdam, 1976, Elsevier Scientific Publ. Co.)

infant and his development, but also as the object of less ambivalent and secret pleasure. Bentovim suggests, "The role of the health professionals in this area is important in that only through the right relationship with the mother will a new source of mothering be found that can act as a form of extended family for the woman to identify with and to counteract personal, family, and cultural influences."[5] Hendricks[16] confirms this view and states that the biggest block in the minds of women relates to feelings of shame associated with breastfeeding. More than half the women in the Newcastle[4] survey were prevented from breastfeeding because of a sense of shame. The shame is a result of relating the breast to concepts of sexuality.

Failure at breastfeeding

When a mother who had planned to breastfeed is unable to because of illness in herself or her baby, or when a mother begins to breastfeed and must stop, there is a grief reaction. The mother experiences a great loss. Prolonged mourning and depression are not uncommon. Some women report feeling more distant from this child than from her others if the others had been successfully breastfed. The stronger the commitment had been to breastfeed, the stronger the grief reaction. Few mothers found help, according to Richards[29] in this study, from either professionals or lay support groups. Professionals failed to understand the feeling of failure or loss. The support groups tended to magnify the guilt and sense of failure. The emotions are complex surrounding this intimate activity.

REFERENCES

1. Adams, A.B.: Choice of infant feeding technique as a function of maternal personality, J. Consult. Clin. Psychol. 23:143, 1959.
2. Alder, E.M., and Cox, J.L.: Breast feeding and post-natal depression, J. Psychosom. Res. 27:139, 1983.
3. Anisfeld, E., and Lipper, E.: Early contact, social support; and mother-infant bonding, Pediatrics 72:79, 1983.
4. Bacon, C.J., and Wylie, J.M.: Mothers' attitudes to infant feeding at Newcastle General Hospital in summer 1975, Br. Med. J. 1:308, 1976.
5. Bentovim, A.: Shame and other anxieties associated with breast feeding: a systems theory and psychodynamic approach. In Ciba Foundation Symposium no. 45, Breast feeding and the mother. Amsterdam, 1976, Elsevier Scientific Publ. Co.
6. Bloom, M.: The romance and power of breast feeding, Birth Fam. J. 8:259, 1981.
7. Bowlby, J.: Attachment and loss, London, 1969, The Hogarth Press Ltd.
8. Brazelton, T.B.: The early mother-infant adjustment, Pediatrics 32:931, 1963.
9. Budin, P.: The nursing, London, 1907, The Caxton Publishing Co.
10. Call, J.D.: Emotional factors favoring successful breast feeding of infants, J. Pediatr. 55:485, 1959.
11. Chamberlain, R.E.: Some personality differences between breast and bottle feeding mothers. Birth Fam. J. 3:31, 1976.
12. Chess, S., and Alexander, T.: Infant bonding: mystique and reality, Am. J. Orthopsychiatr. 52:213, 1982.
13. Cox, J.L., Connor, Y., and Kendall, R.E.: Prospective study of the psychiatric disorders of childbirth, Br. J. Psychiatr. 140:111, 1982.
14. deChâteau, P., et al.: A study of factors promoting and inhibiting lactation, Dev. Med. Child. Neurol. 19:575, 1977.
15. Douglas, J.W.B.: Extent of breast feeding in Great Britain in 1946 with special reference to health and survival of children, J. Obstet. Gynaecol. Br. Empire 57:335, 1950.

16. Hendrickse, R.G.: Discussion from Ciba Foundation Symposium no. 45, Breast feeding and the mother, Amsterdam, 1976, Elsevier Scientific Publ. Co.

17. Hoeffer, C., and Hardy, M.C.: Later development of breast fed and artificially fed infants, JAMA 92:615, 1929.

18. Jackson, E.B., Wilkin, L.C., and Auerbach, H.: Statistical report on incidence and duration of breast feeding in relation to personal, social and hospital maternity factors, Pediatrics 17:700, 1956.

19. Kennell, J.H., Trause, M.A., and Klaus, M.H.: Evidence for a sensitive period in the human mother. In Ciba Foundation Symposium no. 33, Parent-infant interaction, Princeton, N.J., 1975, Excerpta Medica, Associated Scientific Publishers.

20. Klaus, M.H., and Kennell, J.H.: Maternal-infant bonding: the impact of early separation or loss on family development, St. Louis, 1976, The C.V. Mosby Co.

21. Kumar, R., and Robson, K.: Neurotic disorders during pregnancy and the puerperium: preliminary report of a prospective study of 119 primigravidae. In Sandler, M.J., editor: Mental illness in pregnancy and the puerperium, London, 1978, Oxford University Press.

22. Lamb, M.: Early contact and maternal-infant bonding: one decade later, Pediatrics 70:763, 1982.

23. Lawrence, R.A.: Practices and attitudes toward breast feeding among medical professionals, Pediatrics 70:912, 1982.

24. Lerner, H.: Early origins of envy and devaluation of women: implications for sex role stereotypes, Bull. Meninger Clin. 38:538, 1974.

25. Newton, N.: Psychologic differences between breast and bottle feeding. In Jelliffe, D.B., and Jelliffe, E.F.R., editors: Symposium, the uniqueness of human milk, Am. J. Clin. Nutr. 24:993, 1971.

26. Newton, N., and Newton, M.: Psychologic aspects of lactation, N. Engl. J. Med. 277:1179, 1967.

27. Parke, R.D., O'Leary, S., and West, S.: Mother-father-newborn interaction: effects of maternal medication, labor and sex of infant, J. Perspect. Soc. Psychol. 23:243, 1972.

28. Raphael, D.: The tender gift: breastfeeding, New York, 1976, Schocken Books, Inc.

29. Richards, M.P.M.: Breast feeding and the mother-infant relationship, Acta Paedeatr. Scand. Suppl. 299:33, 1982.

30. Robson, K.M., and Kumar, R.: Delayed onset of maternal affection after childbirth, Br. J. Psychiatr. 136:347, 1980.

31. Robertson, W.O.: Breast feeding practices: Some implications of regional variations, Am. J. Public Health. 51:1035, 1961.

32. Simpson-Herbert, M.: Breast feeding and body contact, Populi 7:17, 1980.

33. Sosa, R., et al.: The effect of early mother-infant contact on breast feeding, infection and growth. In Ciba Foundation Symposium no. 45, Breast feeding and the mother, Amsterdam, 1976, Elsevier Scientific Publ. Co.

34. Spitz, R.A.: An inquiry into the psychiatric conditions in early childhood, Psychoanal. Study Child. 1:53, 1945.

35. Thoman, E.B., Wetzel, A., and Levine, S.: Lactation prevents disruption of temperature regulation and suppresses adrenocortical activity in rats, part A, Community Behav. Biol. 2:165, 1968.

36. Waletsky, L.R.: Husbands' problems with breast feeding, Am. J. Orthopsychiatr. 49:349, 1979.

37. Whiting, J.W.M.: Causes and consequences of the amount of body contact between mother and infant. In Munroe, R.L., Munroe, R.D., and Whiting, B.B., editors: Handbook of cross-culture human development, New York, 1980, Garland Publishing Co.

Contraindications to and disadvantages of breastfeeding

7

In reviewing the contraindications to breastfeeding, it is important to look at the entities that put the mother or infant at significant risk and are not remedial. Contraindications are medical; the disadvantages of breastfeeding are a second group of factors to be considered. The disadvantages tend to be social.

CONTRAINDICATIONS
Breast cancer

A mother with a diagnosis of breast cancer should not nurse her infant in the interest of having definitive treatment immediately, since prolactin levels remain very high during lactation, and the role of prolactin in the advancement of mammary cancer is still in dispute. Although endogenous prolactin by itself may not be a risk factor, it could, along with sex steroids, contribute to the acceleration of malignant growth.[19] All lumps in the lactating breast are not cancer and are not even benign tumors. The lactating breast is lumpy and the "lumps" shift day by day. If a mass is located, and the physician thinks it should be biopsied, this can be done under local anesthesia without weaning the infant. Rochester surgeons have performed many such procedures following referrals in the past 20 years without postoperative complications. The diagnosis of benign masses was made in all cases. The performance of immediate surgery relieved tremendous anxiety without unnecessarily sacrificing breastfeeding.

Is cancer more or less common in women who breastfeed? The answer is not easy to find, but in countries where breastfeeding is common, breast cancer is uncommon. In the United States, the incidence of breast cancer has steadily risen while the frequency of breastfeeding has declined. At one time it had been suggested that nursing protected a woman against breast cancer. This concept was investigated in an international study and shown to be invalid.[15] Breastfeeding, however, does not predispose a woman to cancer.[10]

The statistics associating pregnancy and breast cancer influence the picture. In an epidemiologic study, the risk of breast cancer had a linear relationship to the time interval between puberty and childbirth.[12] The risk was reduced by one third for women who bear their first child before 18 years of age compared with those women who have their first baby when they are older. The risk of breast cancer for women who become pregnant before age 20 was about half that of those who first become pregnant after 25 years of age. Births after the first full-term pregnancy did not influence the statistics. Women whose first pregnancy appeared after 30 to 35 years of age had a risk of breast cancer four times that of nulliparous women in the same age group.[29]

The critical question remains—does breastfeeding increase any child's risk of breast cancer, especially in female offspring? This haunting question, first posed by an experimental scientist, created tremendous publicity and genuine concern among physicians asked this question by patients. One needs to explore the available data.

VIRUS IN BREAST MILK.   In the laboratory, it has been reported that particles physically identical to mouse mammary tumor virus have been found in human milk. Other investigators have attempted to duplicate this work. Chopra et al.[5] reported that the particles they located in human milk resembled virus from monkey breast tumor, which had been shown to possess biophysical, biochemical, and in vitro transforming properties of known oncogenic RNA viruses. They reserved judgment on the exact identity of the particles until they could be cultured or shown to produce tumor, since they may well not be viruses. Roy-Burman et al.[22] reported their efforts to detect RNA tumor virus in human milk using milks taken from women with varied histories of viruses. They found no correlation between RNA-directed DNA polymerase activity and family history of breast cancer. They suggest, as have others, that the RNA-directed DNA polymerase activity, a reverse transcriptase, is a normal feature of lactating breast tissue. In fact, breast milk has been found to exert antiviral activity against Japanese B encephalitis virus, Friend leukemia virus, and Rauscher leukemia virus.[8]

EPIDEMIOLOGIC STUDY.   Epidemiologic data conflict with the suggestion that the tumor agent is transmitted via the breast milk. The incidence of breast cancer is low among groups that had nursed their infants, including lower economic groups, foreign-born groups, and those in sparsely populated areas.[15] The frequency of breast cancer in mothers and sisters of a woman with breast cancer is two to three times that expected by chance. This could be genetic or environmental. Cancer actually is equally common on both sides of the family of an affected woman. If breast milk were the cause, it should be transmitted from mother to daughter. When mother-daughter incidence of cancer was studied, there was no relationship found to breastfeeding.

Sarkar et al.[24] reported that human milk, when incubated with mouse mammary tumor virus, caused degradation of the particle morphology and decreasd infectivity and reverse transcriptase activity of the virions. They suggest that the significance of this destructive effect of human milk on mouse mammary tumor virus may account for the difficulty in isolating the putative human mammary tumor agent. Sanner[23] has provided data to show that the inhibitory enzymes in milk can be removed by special sedimentation technique. He ascribes the discrepancies in isolating virus particles in human milk to these factors, which inhibit RNA-directed DNA polymerase.

CURRENT POSITION. Miller and Fraumeni[17] from the Epidemiology Branch of the National Cancer Institute reviewed the information and concluded that it did not support the belief that breast cancer is related to breastfeeding and further suggested that the fear of cancer in the breastfed female offspring does not justify avoiding breastfeeding.

Morgan et al.[18] did a retrospective study by interviewing women over 60 years of age about their history of cancer and the feeding history of their daughters, as well as the incidence of cancer in their daughters. This study showed that the younger the interviewed woman was, the younger were her daughters, and the less breast cancer occurred in the daughters. However, this could be attributable to their young age. Since the incidence of breastfeeding has declined, fewer daughters have been breastfed. This factor could have skewed the results. They found breastfed women have the same breast cancer experience as nonbreastfed women. There was no increase in benign tumors, either. Daughters of breast cancer patients have an increased risk of developing benign and malignant tumors by merit of their heredity, not their breastfeeding history.

Unilateral breastfeeding (limited to the right breast) is a custom of Tanka women of the fishing villages in Hong Kong. Ing et al.[13] investigated the question, "Does the unsuckled breast have an altered risk of cancer?" They studied breast cancer data from 1958 to 1975. Breast cancer occurred equally on the left and the right breast. Comparison of patients who had nursed unilaterally with nulliparous patients and with patients who had borne children but not breastfed indicated a highly significantly increased risk of cancer in the unsuckled breast. The authors conclude that in postmenopausal women who have breastfed unilaterally, the risk of cancer is significantly higher in the unsuckled breast. They believed that breastfeeding may help protect the suckled breast against cancer.

Other authors[16] have suggested that Tanka women are ethnically a separate people and that it is possible that left-sided breast cancer is related to their genetic pool and not to their breastfeeding habits. No mention has been made of other possible influences, for instance the impact of their role as "fishermen" or any inherent trauma to the left breast.

Papaioannou,[20] in a collective review of the etiologic factors in cancer of the breast in humans, concludes, "Genetic factors, viruses, hormones, psychogenic stress, diet and other possible factors, probably in that order of importance, contribute to some extent to the development of cancer of the breast."

Wing[31] concludes in her update on human milk and health that "in view of the complete absence of any studies showing a relationship between breastfeeding and increased risk of breast cancer, the presence of virus-like particles in breast milk should not be a contraindication to breastfeeding."

Henderson et al.[12] make a similar statement and Vorherr[29] concludes that the roles of pregnancy and lactation in the development and prognosis of breast cancer are not determined.

Hepatitis B virus

The transmission of hepatitis B from mothers whose blood contains hepatitis B antigen to their infants has been described in several parts of the world.[14] Such transmission of an infectious agent from mother to infant is termed *vertical transmission*. The mode of transmission is transplacentally in utero, at delivery, or shortly after delivery. Horizontal transmission occurs between two individuals in close contact. Taiwan and Japan report a high incidence of transmission from carrier mothers to their infants, in contrast to reports from the rest of the world.[27] Follow-up from 4 to 12 months of age indicated the infants of carrier mothers in most studies remained serum negative. In the United States, the rate of transmission to infants from carrier mothers is very low.

Transmission from mothers with acute hepatitis B in pregnancy is very different. It was shown that in mothers with active disease just before, during, or after pregnancy, the infants had up to a 50% chance of being hepatitis B antigen positive. Hepatitis was acquired transplacentally or at birth, but not by breast milk because the infants were not breastfed. There is a 50% risk of hepatitis if a mother has the disease at the end of pregnancy.[7]

In addition to transplacental infection there is the risk of fecal-oral transmission at delivery and transcolostrally. Hepatitis B antigen has been found in saliva, stool, urine, prostatic fluid, and seminal fluid. Some infants do pick up the virus at birth. Hepatitis B antigen is found in breast milk.[26] Transmission by this route has not been well documented. The mothers of some infants who did become infected did not have the virus in the colostrum.[1]

Beasley et al.[2] write that although breast milk transmission is possible, their work showed no difference in frequency of antigenemia among breastfed and nonbreastfed babies in a long-term follow-up study of 147 mothers who were carriers of hepatitis B antigen. The time of transfer of the antigen from mother to infant may be during labor and delivery, when microscopic blood leaks may occur across the placenta, rather than via the breast milk.

The Redbook of the Committee on Infection of the Academy of Pediatrics[6] has stated in the 1982 edition that the benefits of breastfeeding outweigh the risks. A minority report points out that in industrialized countries, the risk of developing hepatitis B is very low, so breastfeeding would double or triple the risk of hepatitis and exceed the benefit for a child who is at low risk for any other problems.

Cytomegalovirus infection

Cytomegalovirus (CMV) has been identified in human milk of women with CMV-CF (complement fixation) antibody. Hayes and associates[11] showed 10.8% incidence at

1 to 6 days and 50% incidence at 1 to 13 weeks. There is no correlation between the presence of viruria and the finding of CMV in the milk. Breast milk ranks with cervical secretions as a potential source of CMV infection in infants according to these researchers.

β-streptococcal disease

A case of recurrent β-streptococcal disease in an infant who was breastfed has been reported. The infant was infected at birth and treated with antibiotics. Six weeks later the mother developed bilateral mastitis, and the infant became moribund 2 days later. The infant and the milk grew out β-streptococcus. In the same journal, two other cases of β-streptococcal infection in breastfed infants are reported. The same type of β-streptococcus was found in mother and infant. It is highly likely that the mother was infected by the infant. It is rare to see bilateral mastitis in humans, but in all three cases of streptococcal mastitis, it was bilateral. Any time there is streptococcal disease in the newborn, there is potential for recurrence. Bilateral mastitis should be considered a suspicious sign.

Life-threatening illnesses

Life-threatening or debilitating illness in the mother may necessitate avoiding lactation.[3] This is a clinical judgment that should be made with the mother and father, with all the facts presented. Although some woman with the same diagnosis may be able to overcome all obstacles and prove she can nurse her baby, it does not necessarily mean that this patient's situation is identical.[4] If the mother wishes some lay reading on the subject, the clinician should be familiar with the text of the material so that any apparent inconsistencies of opinion can be discussed.

DISADVANTAGES

Disadvantages to breastfeeding are those factors perceived by the mother as being an inconvenience to her, since there are no known disadvantages for the normal infant. (In the rare circumstance of galactosemia in the neonate, which involves an inability to tolerate lactose, breastfeeding is contraindicated [see Chapter 14].) In cultures in which nursing in public is commonplace, nursing is not considered inconvenient, since the infant and the feeding are always available.

The fact that the mother is committed to the infant for six to twelve feedings a day for months is overwhelming to a woman who has been free and independent. Motherhood itself, however, changes one's life-style.

Guilt from failure, shame, and other anxieties are of considerable concern. Surveys evaluating the decline of breastfeeding have revealed that feelings of shame, modesty, embarrassment, and distaste have been described. These feelings are more common in lower social groups. Research on wider sociologic and psychologic factors regarding the feelings and attitudes toward breastfeeding can have a considerable influence on the choice to breastfeed and will be helpful in dealing with these issues.

As the incidence and duration of breastfeeding increase and professionals and lay people alike are caught up in the rush to convert all parents and change all hospital routines and recommendations, a sense of balance must be maintained. It is necessary to appreciate that there are normal women who can not or will not nurse their babies. Their babies will survive and grow normally. The sharp letter by Fisher[9] brings this to focus when she describes the frustrations and disappointments of others as well as dispels what she calls the myths about breastfeeding.

The popular press[28] has drawn attention to parenting trends that divide responsibility for the infant equally between mother and father after the birth. This, of course, necessitates bottle feeding. The justification is division of labor and equal opportunity for both parents to do good things for the baby. This is probably another way of expressing breast envy and jealousy. Some husbands are jealous because they have no similar way to bring food and contentment to their infant, according to Waletzky.[30] "A certain manliness was required to foster breastfeeding in one's family when society as a whole was hostile to it," according to Pittenger and Pittenger.[21] They point out that the perinatal period is a breeding ground for marital and parental maladjustment. Many writers, on the other hand, have described participation in childbirth as a potentially beneficial experience for men. The father's feelings are useful during labor and delivery. These experiences contribute to heightened self-concepts and better adjustments to roles as husband and father. The quality of the birth experience has been cited as the major determinant of paternal attachment. Paternal attachment has led to a greater pride in breastfeeding and a more secure self-confident support person for the mother who is breastfeeding their infant. Perinatal counseling of prospective new parents may anticipate these reactions, and in turn the professional will have an opportunity to facilitate the best experience possible.

REFERENCES

1. Beasley, R.P.: Transmission of hepatitis by breast feeding (letter to the editor), N. Engl. J. Med. **292:**1354, 1975.
2. Beasley, R.P., et al.: Evidence against breast feeding as a mechanism for vertical transmission of hepatitis B, Lancet **2:**740, 1975.
3. Berger, L.R., When should one discourage breastfeeding, Pediatrics **67:**300, 1981.
4. Brewster, D.P.: You can breast feed your baby . . . even in special situations, Emmaus, Pa., 1979, Rodale Press.
5. Chopra, H., et al.: Electron microscopic detection of Simian-type virus particles in human milk, Nature N. Biol. **243:**159, 1973.
6. Committee on Infectious Disease: Report of the Committee on Infectious Disease, American Academy of Pediatrics Redbook, 19th ed., Evanston, Ill., 1982, American Academy of Pediatrics.
7. Crumpacker, C.S.: Hepatitis. In Remington, J.S., and Klein, J.O., editors: Infectious diseases of the fetus and newborn infant, Philadelphia, 1971, W.B. Saunders Co.
8. Fieldsteel, A.H.: Nonspecific antiviral substances in human milk active against arbovirus and murine leukemia virus, Cancer Res. **34:**712, 1974.
9. Fisher, P.J.: Breast or bottle: a personal choice,

(letter to the editor), Pediatrics **72:**435, 1983.

. Fraumeni, J.F., and Miller, R.W.: Breast cancer from breast feeding, Lancet **2:**1196, 1971.

. Hayes, K., et al.: Cytomegalovirus in human milk, N. Engl. J. Med. **287:**177, 1972.

. Henderson, B.E., et al.: An epidemiologic study of breast cancer, J. Nat. Cancer Inst. **53:**609, 1974.

. Ing, R., Ho, J.H.C., and Petrakis, N.L.: Unilateral breast feeding and breast cancer, Lancet **2:**124, 1977.

. Linnemann, C.C., and Goldberg, S.: HBAg in breast milk, Lancet **2:**155, 1974.

. MacMahon, B., et al.: Lactation and cancer of the breast: a summary of an international study, Bull. W.H.O. **42:**185, 1970.

. McManus, I.C.: Predominance of left-sided breast tumours, Lancet **2:**297, 1977.

. Miller, R.W., and Fraumeni, J.F.: Does breast feeding increase the child's risk of breast cancer? Pediatrics **49:**645, 1972.

. Morgan, R.W., Vakil, D.V., and Chipman, M.L.: Breast feeding, family history, and breast disease, Am. J. Epidemiol. **99:**117, 1974.

. Ory, H., et al.: Oral contraceptives and reduced risk of benign breast disease, N. Engl. J. Med. **294:**419, 1976.

. Papaioannou, A.N.: Etiologic factors in cancer of the breast in humans: collective review, Surg. Gynecol. Obstet. **138:**257, 1974.

1. Pittenger, J.E., and Pittenger, J.G.: The perinatal period: Breeding ground for marital and pa-

rental maladjustment, Keeping Abreast J. **2:**18, 1977.

22. Roy-Burman, P., et al.: Attempts to detect RNA tumour virus in human milk, Nature N. Biol. **244:**146, 1973.

23. Sanner, T.: Removal of inhibitors against RNA-directed DNA polymerase activity in human milk, Cancer Res. **36:**405, 1976.

24. Sarkar, N.H., et al.: Effect of human milk on mouse mammary tumor virus, Cancer Res. **33:**626, 1973.

25. Schreiner, R.L., Coates, T., and Shackelford, P.G.: Possible breast milk transmission of group B streptococcal infection (letter to the editor), J. Pediatr. **91:**159, 1977.

26. Smith, J.L., and Hindman, S.H.: Transmission of hepatitis by breast-feeding (letter to the editor), N. Engl. J. Med. **292:**1354, 1975.

27. Stevens, C.E., et al.: Vertical transmission of hepatitis B antigen in Taiwan, N. Engl. J. Med. **292:**771, 1975.

28. Stone, E.: A feminist fad? Ms. **11**(8):68, 1983.

29. Vorherr, H.: Pregnancy and lactation in relation to breast cancer risk, Semin. Perinatol. **3:**299, 1979.

30. Waletzky, L.R.: Husbands' problems with breastfeeding, Am. J. Orthopsychiatr. **49:**349, 1979.

31. Wing, J.P.: Human versus cow's milk in infant nutrition and health: update 1977, Curr. Prob. Pediatr. **8**(1):entire issue, November, 1977.

Management of the mother-infant nursing couple

8

Successful nursing depends on the successful association of mother and infant with appropriate support from the father and available medical resources. Since both mothers and infants vary, a simple set of rules cannot be outlined to guarantee success for everyone. In fact, one of the difficulties has been that a rigid system was established in hospitals for initiating lactation that did not fit all mother-infant couples. Furthermore, physicians do not receive formal education on breastfeeding; thus they resort to gaining information from nonmedical sources and assume that this is the only way to approach the situation.

Nowhere in medicine does one's personal interests or prejudices become more evident than in the area of counseling about childbirth and breastfeeding. Having a child does not make one an expert on the subject. As pointed out previously, the University of Rochester study of physicians revealed that there is direct correlation with the way a physician's child was fed and how the physician counsels patients. Nowhere else does personal experience influence medical management so greatly. There is a distinct difference in hospital care among nurses who have breastfed and those who have not. In addition, having had this personal experience, it is common for the professional to then assume her experience is the model to recommend for everyone. One must be especially careful in one's enthusiasm for the process not to overlook the view of a patient less inspired or actually repelled by the thought of nursing.

The field of human lactation has also attracted many paraprofessionals and lay people who make themselves available for lactation consultation. The physician must coordinate this team effort because he is ultimately responsible for the health of the mother and growth and development of the infant. He will continue in that role long after lactation has been discontinued. Lactation consultations should be asked for and responded to just as any other consultation in the health care system, with the physician selecting and contracting with the most appropriately qualified consultant available and receiving direct recommendations from the consultant.

The key to the management of the nursing couple is establishing a sense of confidence in the mother and supporting her with simple answers to questions when they arise. Good counseling also depends on understanding the science of suckling.

Management is best discussed in terms of the three stages: (1) the prenatal period, (2) the immediate postpartum, or hospital, management, and (3) the postnatal, or post-hospital, period.

THE SCIENCE OF SUCKLING

The ability to lactate is characteristic of all mammals from the most primitive to the most advanced. The divergence of suckling patterns, however, makes it urgent that the human be studied specifically to understand human patterns.[11] Some aquatic mammals such as whales nurse under water; others such as the seal and sea lion nurse on land. A variety of erect or recumbent postures are assumed by different terrestrial mammals.[23] Nursing may be continuous, as in the joey attached to a marsupial teat, or at widely different intervals characteristic of the species. The interval may be ½ hour in the dolphin, an hour in the pig, a day in the rabbit, 2 days in the tree-shrew, or a week in the northern fur seal. There are many anatomic distinctions as well. The principal mechanism of milk removal common to all mammals is the contractile response of the mammary myoepithelium under the hormonal influence of oxytocin released from the neurohypophysis.

The functional implications in all species is the effective control of milk delivery to the young in the right amount and at the appropriate intervals, which requires a storage system, exit channels, a prehensile appendage, an expulsion mechanism, and a retention mechanism. The primary, secondary, and tertiary ducts form an uninterrupted channel for the passage of milk from the alveoli to the mammary sinuses. A process of erection of the areolar region facilitates prehension by the young during suckling. The principal object of the suction produced by the facial musculature of the young is to draw the nipple into the mouth and retain it there. Positive pressure is used to expel milk from the gland by constricting action of the tongue against the hard palate and by the contractile changes in the mammary gland provided by the myoepithelial cells. Milk secretion is a continuous process, and loss of milk by leakage would be an obvious problem in any species were exit channels not capable of obstructing flow. The most universal mammalian anatomic provision to avoid milk loss is a nipple sphincter composed of smooth muscle under sympathetic nervous control (see Fig. 2-10). The sympathetic nervous stimuli also oppose milk ejection by increasing vasoconstrictor tone, thereby reducing access of circulating oxytocin to the mammary myoepithelium. Sympathetic activity also can occur during conditions of apprehension or muscular exertion. The milk-ejection reflex can be blocked by emotional disturbance or reflex excitation of the neurohypophysis. The central nervous control of milk ejection indeed suggests that restraining mechanisms exist to ensure that milk ejection can only occur under circumstances wholly conducive to the effective removal of milk by the suckling young.

In all species that have been studied, a rise in intramammary pressure and flow of milk occur as a reflex event in suckling. The excitation of the neurohypophysis results in the release of oxytocin, which is conveyed in the bloodstream to mammary capillaries, where it evokes contraction of the myoepithelium.[20] The successive ejection pressure peaks demonstrated in lactating women can be duplicated more accurately by a series of separate oxytocin injections than by the same total dose as a single injection or by a continuous infusion of the hormone. This strongly suggests that oxytocin is released from the neurohypophysis in spurts. The study of suckling patterns in all species shows a high degree of ritualization, which in turn suggests a close neural connection between cognitive or behavioral and hormonal responses.

Attention has focused on the mechanisms that control suckling behavior, on its incidence, on the events that precipitate and terminate it, on the affects of stress, and on how development modifies it. Suckling is characteristic of each species and vital for survival. Although suckling has been studied in other species with the young and the mother, much of human data has been collected using a rubber nipple and bottle. Other mammals sucked only in the nutritive mode, whether receiving milk from the nipple or not. Human infants were noted to have two distinct patterns with rubber nipples: a nutritive mode and a nonnutritive mode.[74,75] When this work was repeated using the breastfeeding model, there was no difference between nutritive and nonnutritive suckling rates but rather a continuous variation of suckling rate in response to milk-flow rate.[12] Suckling rates in other species correlate with milk composition and species-specific feeding schedules (one suck per second in great apes and four to five sucks per second in sheep and goats). In further experiments, there was a linear relationship between milk flow and suckling rate. Thus, the higher the milk flow the lower the suckling rate. In human infants younger than 12 weeks of age, suckling will terminate with sleep and be reinstated on awakening, a pattern that is well described in other species.[11] In infants older than 12 weeks, suckling is not terminated by sleep. At 12 to 24 weeks, infants will play with the nipple and explore the mother and not always elicit nipple attachment. During a given feeding from one breast during continuous measurement of milk intake, a progressive reduction in intake volume per suck and an increase in the proportion of time spent pausing between bursts of sucking was seen to occur. Using the miniature Doppler ultrasound flow transducer, Woolridge et al.[76] have studied 32 normal mother-baby pairs from 5 to 9 days postpartum. Intakes during trials averaged 34.2 g ($\pm$ 3.7 g) on the first breast and 26.2 g ($\pm$ 3.5 g) on the second breast. At the start of feeds the average suck volume was about 0.14 ml/suck, which decreases to about 0.01 ml/suck or less. The mean latency for release of milk was 2.2 minutes after the infant began to suckle. The researchers also noted that on the first breast the flow increased and stabilized after 2 minutes, with concomitant slowing and stabilizing of sucking pattern over remainder of the feed. On the second breast, the suck volume fell off dramatically toward the end of the feed (50% reduction from peak to end of feed). These observations support the theory that infants become satiated at the breast and milk remains unconsumed in the breast.[76] Over the first month of life, infants consume a given amount of fluid with decreasing investment of time. The amount of fluid per suck increases over time. The control of intake appears to come under intrinsic control during the first month of life.[61]

When sucking was studied using a multisensor nipple for recording oral variables such as lip and tongue movements and fluid flow, it was observed that fluid flow begins as the intranipple pressure decreases and tapers off as the intranipple pressure increases.[14] One flow pattern is seen in each sucking movement.

The development of the sucking response in the normal newborn with a rubber nipple transducer in a nonnutritive mode has been reported to occur immediately after birth.[2] Pressure exerted immediately was 5 torr at birth, peaking at 103 at 90 minutes. There are no data on optimal pressures nor on pressures developed with immediate breastfeeding.

The movement of the lips and tongue have been more difficult to study. A cineradiographic study of breastfeeding was done by Ardran and colleagues in 1957 and compared with a similar study of bottle feeding.[6,7] The nipples and areolas of 41 breastfeeding mothers were coated with a paste of barium sulfate in lanolin and cineradiographic films were taken with the infant at breast. These were then reviewed meticulously. The authors* concluded the following:

1. The nipple is sucked to the back of the baby's mouth and a teat is formed from the mother's breast.
2. When the jaw is raised this teat is compressed between the upper gum and the tip of the tongue resting on the lower gum. The tongue is applied to the lower surface of the teat from before backwards, pressing it against the hard palate: the teat is reduced to approximately half its former width. As the tongue moves towards the posterior edge of the hard palate the teat shortens and becomes thicker.
3. When the jaw is lowered the teat is again sucked to the back of the mouth and restored to its previous size.
4. Each cycle of jaw and tongue movement takes place in approximately 1.5 seconds. The pharyngeal cavity becomes airless and the larynx closed every time the upward movement of the tongue against the teat and hard palate is completed.
5. These movements are analogous to those seen in bottle feeding: they suggest that the contents of the ducts or cisterns of the teat are expressed into the mouth.
6. The influence of suction upon the flow of milk from the teat has not been established. It is considered that suction may be exerted during the phase of compression of the teat as the tongue is simultaneously lowered behind the teat.
7. It is suggested that the teat is formed from the nipple and the adjacent areola and underlying tissues.

---

*From Ardran, G.M., Kemp, F.H., and Lind, J.: Br. J. Radiol. **31:**156, 1958.

In a study of bottle feeding, cineradiographic films were taken of infants, lambs, and kid goats, taking a mixture of milk and barium from a bottle. The authors* concluded the following:

1. The influence of gravity is important in bottle feeding. It ensures that the bulb of the teat fills. If the hole in the teat is large enough milk drips into the mouth; when rigid teats are used this may be the only way the child can obtain an adequate supply of milk.
2. The lambs and kid goats take one teat full of milk with each jaw and tongue movement; the neck of the teat is completely occluded by approximation of the jaws and the contents of the bulb are expressed into the mouth by elevation of the tongue towards the soft palate, the tongue indenting the bulb from before backwards. Babies usually attempt this movement but in most instances are only partly successful; the teats normally supplied are too rigid and the hole is too small.
3. Following compression of the bulb of the teat by the squeezing action of the tongue, the lowering of the jaw and tongue must cause some degree of suction which may aid in the refilling of the bulb and it may also draw milk into the mouth; the amount of milk obtained in this manner may in favourable circumstances equal the amount obtained by expression.
4. During the phase of compression of the bulb of the teat by elevation of the tongue in the forepart of the mouth there is also taking place simultaneously a lowering of the tongue behind the teat which must cause some suction.
5. Factors relating to the design of different teats have been considered.
6. When milk is swallowed, naso-pharyngeal closure is made by elevation of the soft palate against the adenoidal pad on the roof of the epipharynx, the mode of closure differing from that seen in adults. The relevant variations in anatomy between infants and adults are discussed.
7. The bolus passes through the pharynx on both sides of the superior laryngeal aperture. The larynx is closed as each bolus is expressed from the pharynx and reopened just before the next bolus enters. The theory that young babies and members of the herbivora are able to continue feeding by passing food down into the oesophagus on either side of the laryngeal aperture without closing the airway is disproved.

Coordination of suck and swallow

The ability to swallow is developed in utero during the second trimester and has been well demonstrated by fetal ultrasound. Fetal swallowing of amniotic fluid is an important part of the complex regulation of amniotic fluid. The suck is actually part of the oral phase of the swallow. Little was done to examine the role of swallowing on the suckling rate until Burke[17] studied the role of swallowing in the organization of suckling behavior, albeit with a bottle and solutions of 5% and 10% sucrose solution. The author reports two major observations. "First, the frequency of swallowing in newborns increased significantly as a function of increasing concentration and amount of sucrose solution given per criterion suck. Second, there was a significant difference in the duration of the sucking interresponse times which immediately followed the onset of swallowing and the duration of interresponse times not associated with swallowing." These

---

*From Ardran, G.M., Kemp, F.H., and Lind, J.: Br. J. Radiol. **31:**11, 1958.

observations explain those of previous investigators regarding nutritive and nonnutritive sucking. It would also suggest that clinicians need to investigate the infant's swallowing reflex when dealing with a serious sucking disorder associated with failure to thrive.

Factors influencing sucking

As one manages infants with difficulty feeding, a number of rituals are often initiated to enhance infant behavior. Only a few of these have been evaluated for their effect. The effect of position of the infant, that is, flat, supine, and supported upright to 90-degree angle, was found to have no influence on the sucking pattern or pressure.[29] There was found, however, an effect of temperature. Sucking pressure decreases as environmental temperature increased from 80° F to 90° F, which may have application in encouraging an infant to nurse. This effect was shown to increase from the third to the fifth day of life. Higher sucking pressures have been recorded in the morning than in the afternoon.

When the nipple size was studied, it was observed that the large nipple elicits fewer sucks and a slower sucking rate than smaller nipples, although the volume of milk delivered is the same with all nipple sizes.[19] Although it is not possible to alter human nipple size, this knowledge may help in assessing the response of a newborn in specific situations.

The volume of each swallow was calculated during breastfeeding in 1905 by Süsswein,[67] who counted swallows and made test weighings. His observations have now been confirmed with elaborate electronic equipment.[78] The average swallow of a new newborn is 0.6 ml, which is also the exact amount drawn from a bottle equipped with a electromagnetic flowmeter transducer and a valve that responded to negative pressure at each suck in modern studies, even though the sucking mechanism between breast and bottle is different.[65] When a conventional bottle without a valve is used, the volume is reduced to ⅓ and to 0.19 ml/suck. The valve removed the need for the infant to suck against the negative pressure created in the bottle. This supports the fact that a bottle fed infant with a poor suck does better with a boat-shaped bottle, in which the distal end is kept open, or with a collapsible bag as a source of milk. The size of the hole in the nipple influenced the volume of the suck only in the valved bottle. When breastfed infants were compared with a group fed by cup from birth and a group fed by bottle, the breastfed infants had a stronger suck than either of the other two groups, who did not differ from each other in sucking skill.[23,24]

Fat content and infant sucking

The high concentration of fat in breast milk toward the end of a feed was hypothesized as a satiety signal to terminate the feeding.[39] When this was studied using high- and low-fat formulas, it was found that high-fat milk did not act to cue babies to slow or stop feeding.[28,59,60] In fact, babies appeared to feed more actively on high-fat milk, sucking in longer bursts with less resting. When human milk of low and high fat content was fed from bottles, switching the baby from low-fat breast milk to high-fat breast milk, the babies did not alter either milk intake rate or sucking patterns. To fully test the hypothesis, a study carefully observed infants switching from the first to the second breast and back to the first breast.[59,60] Infants were 2 months old and well established at exclusive breastfeeding. There was no significant difference in the time taken to attach to the new breast and the time taken to reattach to the previously sucked breast. Mean milk intake from the first breast was 91.7 g (range 58-208 g), higher than that from the second breast (mean 52.5 g, range 8-75 g). The mean fat contents before and after nursing on the first breast were 23 g/L and 52 g/L, whereas on the second breast they were 24 g/L and 48 g/L. This shows that infants will nurse when fat content is higher, contrary to the theory that increasing fat causes satiation.[59]

Studies of 3-day-old bottle fed infants fed sucrose and glucose solutions show that they manifest tongue movements of greater amplitude when fed stronger concentrations.[47,74] Sensory apparatus responsible for assessing sweetness is apparently competent in the newborn.

Breathing and sucking during feeding

Breathing and sucking during feeding were addressed by Johnson and Salisbury,[47] who studied normal full-term infants from 1 to 10 days of age, measuring breathing, sucking, and flow of fluid from a feeding bottle with a flowmeter. No infant aspirated water, but 8 of 18 infants inhaled saline. Even from a bottle, breast milk was associated with more regular breathing than was formula feeding. It has been demonstrated in other species that the newborn will become apneic when fed milk from species other than his own.

Sucking patterns are an indicator of pathologic conditions

Newborn infants whose mothers received a single dose of 200 mg secobarbital as obstetric sedation during labor sucked at significantly lower rates and pressures and consumed less nutrient than did infants whose mothers received no medication.[47] The effect persisted for 4 days. Similar effects have been seen in Brazelton's examination.[13]

The sucking rhythms of infants with a normal perinatal course were compared to those of infants with perinatal distress. The analysis showed that rhythms of nonnutritive sucking were significantly different from rhythms of normal controls even when there were no gross neurologic signs.[48,75]

Perioral stimulation facilitated nutritive sucking abilities in high-risk newborns when analyzed with 29- to 30-week gestation sick newborns with each subject serving as his own control.[49] The stimulation was applied manually with quick touch-pressure stimulus for 1 second over the buccal fat pad. Similar stimulation has been used in children with CNS dysfunction in an effort to facilitate better sucking and swallowing. Such studies have not been reported during breastfeeding.[31]

Sucking stimulus and prolactin

When lactating postpartum women nurse their infants, the prolactin level increases from a high baseline level to levels 8.5 times mean baseline at the end of the feed in the first 6 weeks postpartum. These women had normal prolactin levels before nursing 7 to 28 weeks postpartum, with an increase of six times baseline at the end of the feed. When nursing women played with but did not feed their infants, prolactin did not rise in spite of the initiation of a let-down. Substitution of a breast pump at regular intervals caused prolactin elevations similar in timing and magnitude to those induced by suckling.[58] When normal, menstruating, nonlactating adult women were stimulated with the breast pump for 30 minutes, there were significant prolactin increases in 7 of the 18 women. No response was obtained in normal men.

Stimulation of the breast with the breast pump in normal women for 2 to 14 days on a regular basis produced no increase in baseline prolactin or in prolactin response to breast stimulation. Chronic chloropromazine treatment raised basal prolactin but did not increase the response to breast stimulation in four subjects.

When the prolactin response was used as a measure of "success" in establishing lactation in the first week postpartum, there was no difference in prolactin levels between women who had been considered good producers (over 60 g per feed) by test weighings and those who were considered poor feeders (less than 60 g per feed).[44] Mothers whose infants were in the special care unit and who were using a breast pump to establish lactation had minimal prolactin response to pumping but produced a mean of 86 g of milk per pumping. A similar study had been carried out previously, in which different responses to suckling were found in prolactin levels in good, fair, and poor producers.[43] When prolactin levels were measured following use of the breast pump at uniform settings, all three groups were similar.[4] This suggests that infant suckling plays a significant role in adequate milk production.

Conclusions

Knowledge about infant suckling has been accumulating rapidly but little of it involves study of suckling at the breast. It has been established that the patterns are different mechanically. At the breast, nutritive and nonnutritive suckling vary only in rate, not in pattern. Infants can suck immediately at birth and tolerate mother's milk (colostrum) best as the pattern of respirations remains physiologic. Inadequate sucking can influence maternal production, but inadequate suckling can be improved.

PRENATAL PERIOD

It is most effective to prepare for breastfeeding well in advance of delivery. Prospective parents should consider feeding plans for the infant during the prenatal period, after the pregnancy is well established. Once quickening has occurred, the infant becomes more of a reality for the mother and she can relate to planning. Except in sophisticated cultures, the parents will not initiate this decision-making discussion, and it is appropriately introduced by the obstetrician in the second trimester. This then gives the patients plenty of time to begin planning more realistically for the infant. Particularly with first children, it is appropriate to suggest to the parents that they select a pediatrician early. They should request a prenatal conference with the pediatrician to discuss not only feeding but also other points of management and child rearing about which they might have questions. If the mother is receiving prenatal care from a family practice physician, this step is an automatic one because the parents are being groomed psychologically as well as medically for the birth.

In a University of Rochester study of feeding practices in the Rochester community, mothers were asked who and what had influenced them to feed their infants in the manner they had chosen. None of 104 consecutive mothers from two local hospitals refused to respond to questions on how they fed their infants. Fifty-four were breastfeeding and fifty were bottle feeding. The same questionnaire was given to all mothers in the study. Mothers who had elected to bottle feed had discussed feeding with their husbands before deciding in 32% of the cases and with their obstetricians in 10% of the cases; 37% had discussed feeding with neither. Only one mother had consulted her pediatrician. She was told there was no medical evidence that breastfeeding was advantageous. Mothers who had chosen to breastfeed had discussed their choice with their husbands in 80% of the cases, with their obstetricians in 38% of the cases, and with their pediatricians in 20% of the cases. Only two multiparas did not discuss feeding with any of these persons. Because some breastfeeding mothers had consulted more than one person, the figures total more than 100% (Table 8-1). This clearly demonstrates the role of the obstetrician or provider of prenatal care in a mother's decision making and also points out the need to involve both husband and wife in the discussion. These results indicate that it is necessary for the physician to initiate a discussion of feeding plans, since in most cases in which no discussion was held with the physician the mother chose bottle feeding.

Studies have suggested that some mothers make up their minds about infant feeding before they become pregnant. Usually, these mothers breastfeed. Mothers who are undecided usually have practical apprehensions about how they will manage lactation because they know nothing about it. Even in these situations, experience has shown that it is appropriate to initiate the discussion with every prepartum patient.

The mothers in the Rochester study were also asked why they had made the choice

Table 8-1. Prenatal decision making

Persons mothers consulted	Bottle feeding (%)	Breastfeeding (%)
Husband	32	80
Obstetrician	10	38
Pediatrician	2	20

they did. The reasons available to them on the questionnaire were simple, leaving opportunity for the mother to add her own (Table 8-2). Bottle feeding mothers were influenced by their mothers and friends, and fewer had attended childbirth classes. Breastfeeding mothers were less influenced by their mothers and friends, and 80% had attended childbirth classes. The significant difference was in the ''other'' reasons for the choice of feeding (Table 8-3). Bottle feeding mothers gave more negative reasons, and not one included the infant's welfare as the reason. Breastfeeding mothers all had positive reasons for nursing, and all did it because it was better for the infant in some way. A few had a second reason that involved their personal gain from nursing.

The medical profession as a group has been hesitant to take anything but a neutral position in such discussions for fear of pressuring the mother. Today the evidence is strong that there are distinct advantages to the infant as well as to the mother to breastfeed. Parents do have the right to hear the data. They can make their own choice and need not be pressured. Newton and Newton[57] have shown that parents who had negative feelings about breastfeeding were successful at breastfeeding 26% of the time. Those who were ambivalent were 35% successful. Those patients who were positive about breastfeeding had a 74% success rate under the management in the hospital. Currently,

Table 8-2.   Factors that influenced decision to breastfeed or bottle feed

Factors	Bottle feeding	Breastfeeding
Childbirth classes	44%	80%
"That's how my mother fed her babies"	40%	16%
"That's how my friends fed their babies"	30%	16%
"That's how I fed my other baby"	96% of all bottle feeding multiparas*	94% of all breastfeeding multiparas†
Other reasons	34%	68%

*60% of bottle feeding mothers were multiparas.
†53% of breastfeeding mothers were multiparas.

Table 8-3.   Reasons volunteered for the choice made

Bottle feeding		Breastfeeding	
Breastfeeding:		Best for baby	8
Did not appeal to me	3	More natural	8
Too annoying	1	More nutritional	2
Makes breasts big	1	More beneficial	2
Ties me down	2	Special immunities	2
More convenient for me	3	More satisfying	2
No medical proof for breast milk	2	Prevent allergies	3
Infant won't sleep through night if breastfed	2	Health reasons for infant	4
Best for me	3	Wanted to	2
Want to take birth control pills	1	Satisfying	3
Want to go to work	1	More convenient	2
Too nervous to breastfeed	2		
TOTAL	21		38

hospital policies and postpartum and nursery support staff are more supportive of breast-feeding, so that success rates are rising.

The prenatal discussion should also include any questions the parents may have about the lactation process and mother's ability to provide adequately for the infant. An examination of the breasts is part of good prenatal care, but the emphasis has been on ruling out cancer and not on the functional capacity of the gland. The breast tissue should be checked for lumps and cysts that might need treatment, of course. The size of the mass of mammary tissue is not correlated with the ability to produce milk. The more generous gland is usually due to a more generous fat pad. During pregnancy the fat is replaced by proliferating acini. A mother should not be discouraged from nursing because of small breasts. This may be the mother who needs most to prove herself.

Breast texture should be assessed by palpation.[26] The inelastic breast gives the impression it is firmly knit together and the overlying skin is taut and firm so it cannot be picked up. The elastic breast is looser and the overlying skin free, and the tissue is more easily picked up. Inelastic breasts are more prone to engorgement and seem improved by prepartum massaging and close attention to prevention of engorgement (Fig. 8-1).

Examination of the areola and nipple is equally important to identify any anatomic problems that may need some preparation before delivery. Gross malformations and inversion of the nipple will be easily detected, but lesser problems may go unnoticed. One must test for freedom of protrusion. When the areola is squeezed and it retracts, it indicates a "tied nipple" or inverted nipple caused by the persistence of the original invagination of the mammary dimple (Fig. 8-2).

The physician may provide literature on breastfeeding or suggest reading sources for

A   **B**

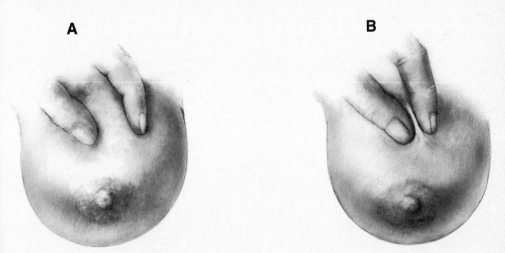

Fig. 8-1. Texture of breast tissue can be assessed by picking up skin of breast. **A,** Inelastic breast tissue; **B,** elastic breast tissue.

A   B

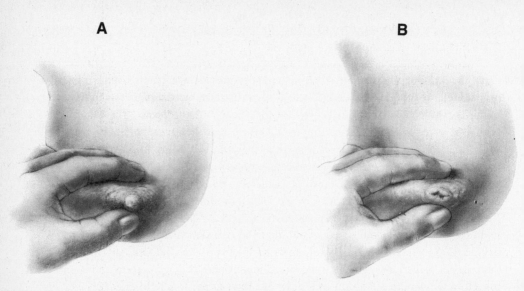

Fig 8-2. A, Normal nipple everts with gentle pressure. **B,** Inverted or tied nipple inverts with gentle pressure.

the patient. One should avoid dismissing the parents' questions by merely suggesting appropriate readings, since their personal decision making will be enhanced by open discussion with a knowledgeable professional. Although parents may have access to childbirth preparation programs in the community, the parents should not be put off to seek all their information from such sources. It often causes tremendous disappointment and misunderstanding when the parents have no opportunity to discuss with their care provider such issues as early infant contact, nursing of the infant in the delivery room, and family-centered maternity care. Although the most vocal groups on the subject of childbirth and the family in our society today lump all these options, including breastfeeding, together as a package, there are many mothers who want to breastfeed but do not wish to have rooming-in, for instance. Therefore, all patients should be provided with adequate information to make a choice in each matter separately.

The concerns most frequently expressed by mothers considering breastfeeding are related to the mother, not the infant. Mothers who are more concerned about their own well-being have more trouble adjusting to motherhood and should be provided with more support in adapting to the role. They may be helped by selecting a doula to support them, since our modern culture tends to isolate the young couple. Raphael[62] describes a doula as one of "those individuals who surround, interact with, and aid the mother at any time within the perinatal period, which includes pregnancy, birth and lactation."

Concerns most frequently expressed prenatally include the following:
1. What is the effect on the figure? Data indicate that the breast is affected by heredity, age, and pregnancy in that order and only minimally by lactation.

Women who have never borne children may "lose their figures" long before a grand multipara who nurses her infants. Pregnancy enlarges breasts temporarily, as does early lactation, but the effect is temporary. Poor diet and lack of exercise will destroy a figure in both male and female long before any other influence.

2. What is the effect on the mother's freedom? Obviously, only a mother can breastfeed the infant; however, there are ample data to support the fact that it is possible to maintain a career, keep a job, or just get away from the house and still nurse one's infant in today's world. Actually, mothers in primitive cultures have returned to the fields or some form of productivity outside the home out of sheer necessity for generations. Mothers concerned about this often are best re-assured by their peers, that is, mothers who are nursing. In communities with nursing mother groups, it is a simple referral. Employment statistics have re-vealed that women do successfully return to the work force and continue breast-feeding. Employment is rarely a reason for not breastfeeding. In most commu-nities the blue-collar mother is unemployed and bottle feeding.

3. Many women are concerned with exposing the breasts. Despite the constant bar-rage of publicity about the breast in the modern press, many women are embar-rassed to consider baring their breasts. As pointed out in Chapter 5, shame is an important consideration when helping a mother accept breastfeeding. Bentovim[10] suggests that shame and anxieties arise from the influence of one's life history and current events; thus intervention is necessary at many levels. Bacon and Wylie[8] found in their study that the most common reason for giving up breast-feeding was embarrassment. They suggest that, since their study showed a higher percentage of the high social class are breastfeeding, ". . . the higher social classes will lead the swing back to breastfeeding, just as they led the fashion to the bottle 40 years ago." The lower social classes expressed more modesty and shame toward nudity. Clothes that make discreet breastfeeding possible are read-ily available and fashionable. Considerable body exposure is not necessary for breastfeeding.

Preparation of the breasts

In addition to affording the couple an opportunity to discuss options and learn about breastfeeding and the mechanisms of lactation, the prenatal period is a time to prepare the breast for its new role as a source of nourishment for the newborn infant.[5] Many mothers do no special preparation and are very successful. Carefully controlled studies do not support the contention that fair-skinned women, especially redheads, are more prone to developing cracked, sore nipples than are others. Mothers who have had trou-ble with tender, cracked nipples when nursing a previous infant would do well to do some preparation.[22] The activity may have a good psychologic effect as well as getting the process off on a positive note for some patients.

Bathing should be as usual, with minimal or no soap directly on the nipples and thorough rinsing. Buffing the nipple with a soft towel is recommended by some but this should not be done except following a shower or bath. Persistent removal of natural oils of the nipple and areola actually predispose the skin to irritation. Montgomery glands in the areola secrete a sebaceous material for the cleansing and lubrication of the areola and nipple. This should not be removed by soaps or chemicals. Tincture of benzoin, alcohol, and other drying agents are contraindicated because they predispose the nipples to cracking during early lactation. Wearing protective brassieres, modern women do not get the friction to the nipples that looser clothing provides, which may be why cracked nipples are such a common problem. In Scandinavia, it is suggested that the pregnant woman get as much air and sunshine as possible directly on the breasts before delivery. In countries where this is not possible, a cautiously used sunlamp or hair dryer can provide the same effect. Wearing a nursing brassiere with the flaps down to expose the nipples under loose clothing will serve the same purpose.[37] In any case, aggressive and abrasive treatment of the nipples does not prevent nipple pain postpartum and may actually enhance it.[35]

The use of hydrous lanolin, which is miscible with water and thus allows normal evaporation from the skin, does no apparent harm and in controlled studies also made no difference. Use of A and D ointment prophylactically made no difference, having an effect only in the treatment of fissures later. Mothers disliked the odor of this ointment as well. Petrolatum and other ointments made the skin more macerated and susceptible to irritation. Ointment should not be applied over the end of the nipple and the ducts.[37]

Soap, alcohol, and tincture of benzoin have been shown to cause damage to tissue of areola and nipple.[56]

Gentle traction to the point of discomfort, but not pain, has been shown by some to improve perception of pain in the first week of lactation.[15] When a study was done that was carefully controlled to eliminate the subjective discrepancies of interpretation, it revealed that there was no significant difference in nipple sensitivity or trauma in those who practiced prenatal nipple rolling, application of breast cream, or expression of colostrum, as compared with those who had untreated breasts.[73] There was no increased pain or trauma among the fair-skinned participants in this study, treated or untreated. Since many women are not inclined to manipulate their breasts before delivery and might be discouraged from breastfeeding if it is implied that this must be done, physicians should prescribe treatment only when there is an indication for it. It may be appropriate to discuss this with the patient prenatally, since so many lay breastfeeding publications advise special rituals for everyone.

Preparation of the nipples

Flat nipples or inverted nipples do not preclude breastfeeding, but it is important to prescribe some form of treatment before delivery rather than wait until the infant is frustrated and the breast engorged. Flat nipples may need a consistent program of stretching, done at least twice daily during the last 6 weeks of pregnancy (Fig. 8-3). It may be more acceptable and clinically more effective for the mother to use the shield for inverted nipples as described on pages 182 and 183 (Figs. 8-4 and 8-5).

Inverted nipples (Fig. 8-2) can be diagnosed by pressing the areola between the thumb and the forefinger. A flat or normal nipple will protrude; a truly inverted nipple will retract. True inverted nipples are actually rare. Inverted nipples can be treated with

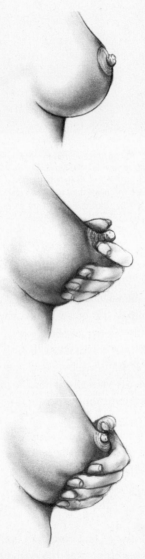

Fig. 8-3. To prepare nipple for breastfeeding during pregnancy, support breast gently with fingers while grasping nipple with thumb and index finger. Draw nipple out to point of discomfort, then release. Repeat exercise five or six times, several times a day.

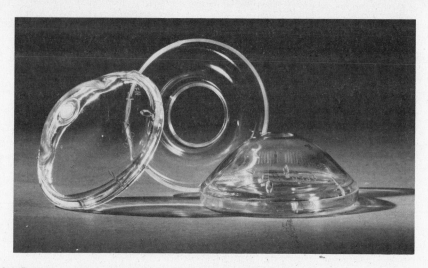

Fig. 8-4. Eschmann shields are designed for use in pregnancy and early lactation to correct flat or inverted nipples. They may also be used to correct retraction during engorgement. Shield is slipped into cup of well-fitting bra. When in position, nipple is at center of opening in bottom piece. Outer convex piece fits over it and provides protection for nipple. It should not be used to collect milk or while nursing infant. Shields should be worn during pregnancy, at first for a few hours at a time, increasing the time as pregnancy progresses. (Manufactured by Eschmann Brothers & Walsh Limited, West Sussex, England; courtesy Eschmann-Canada Ltd., Toronto, Ontario.)

massage as just described, but will respond more effectively if a nipple shield is also used when a brassiere is worn. The physician can recommend a pair of nipple shields available in any drugstore and intended for use in shielding the human nipple when the infant is nursing. The rubber nipple tip of the shield should be removed and only the plastic base with the hole in the center applied over the areola inside a well-fitting brassiere. The constant, even pressure will cause the nipple to evert through the hole. Shields can be worn daily for the last weeks or months of pregnancy. Only the plastic or glass ones should be used because the all-rubber shields pull on the skin, holding the moisture in. A special shield, which forms a plastic tent over the areola, is very effective in everting nipples. Several brands are available, with distribution in most major countries. They are available through medical supply stores and lactation centers. Because they hold the moisture in over the nipple and areola, they should only be worn a few hours at a time (Figs. 8-4 and 8-5). Many women who find nipple manipulation unappealing find the shields work very well.

Many lay publications also describe the Hoffman exercises for the inverted nipple and actually recommend exercising normal nipples. The originator of the routine reported informally after 2 years that it had been successful in his practice for flat and inverted nipples.[42] Subsequent, carefully controlled studies have not found that the exercises make a difference. The technique involves placing the thumbs or forefingers

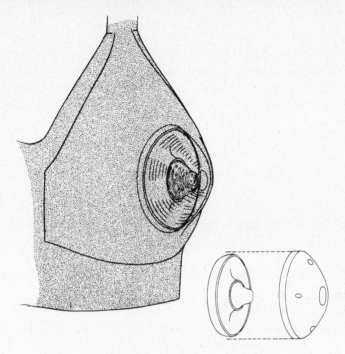

Fig. 8-5. Nipple shield is in place inside brassiere to evert nipple.

opposite each other close to the nipple and gradually pushing away from the areola. This is done in a vertical line and then a horizontal line in the form of an imaginary cross. Nipple stimulation may cause uterine contractions and is used with fetal monitoring or an "oxytocin challenge" test.

Surgical correction of permanently inverted nipples

Inverted nipples have been known to medicine for centuries and treatment has long been described to include various exercises or the use of older vigorous infants to suckle and the use of adults who hired out for this purpose in difficult cases. The first surgical procedure was described in 1873. Other techniques have since been advanced.[40,63,66] A primary indication of the inverted nipple has been the chronic occurrence of central pockets of inflammation of the nipple, leading to spread of infection and suppurative mastitis. A simple method for correction without division of the lactiferous ducts involves using a purse-string suture and traction of holding sutures. The procedure can be done in the office under local anesthesia, according to Hauben.[40] A truly inverted nipple may have fewer ducts. The microscopic pathology of severely inverted nipples indicates the ducts are abnormal.[40,63,66]

Hand expression

Some breastfeeding instructions suggest hand expressing the breast to produce a few drops of colostrum every day for the last few weeks of pregnancy. Fortunately, the instructions usually suggest the patient consult her physician first. Manual or any kind of pumping of the breasts may, indeed, stimulate the uterus to contract.

After breast stimulation at the third to fourth month of pregnancy, prolactin levels are noted to rise above the slightly elevated levels of pregnancy. At the seventh month or later, not only can lactation be induced but there is a substantial increase in prolactin levels.[58] Breast stimulation has been used to ripen the cervix and induce labor by some obstetricians. It has been the cause of premature labor. It has no particular benefit and means that the early sequestered cells are expressed away in the drops of colostrum before delivery and are lost to the infant. Occasionally, prepartum mastitis has developed from this treatment. Any seeming benefit is far outweighed by the risks.

Summary

Following is a summary of prenatal preparation:
1. During the first trimester, make the initial breast examination. Suggestions to consider how the infant is to be fed can be initiated.
2. Once the mother has experienced quickening in the second trimester, suggest that definite plans be made about feeding.
3. During the third trimester, discuss any preparations that may be appropriate, such as nipple care. Also discuss nursing immediately after delivery.

IMMEDIATE POSTPARTUM, OR HOSPITAL, PERIOD

Immediately after the placenta has separated, the establishment of lactation begins. This is a critical period because many mothers who do not receive the proper support in the hospital are driven to failure by inept management.

Nursing in the delivery room

The mother will probably want to nurse her infant immediately after birth, if she has read the current literature. If she does not ask, the obstetrician should suggest it and the delivery room staff facilitate it.

Disease-oriented physicians who have been trained to give trials of water first, hours after delivery, are always concerned that the infant may aspirate. Clinical signs of potential for aspiration include low Apgar score, increased secretions, and polyhydramnios. Actually, all infants born elsewhere in the world go straight to the breast on delivery. It has a physiologic effect on the uterus as well, causing it to contract. Because sugar water and cow's milk formulas are very irritating if aspirated, delay in feeding has been the rule in the United States, where most infants are bottle fed. Colostrum is not irritating, however, and is readily absorbed. There are a few contraindications to immediate nursing: (1) a heavily medicated mother, (2) an infant with a 5-minute Apgar score under 6, or (3) a premature infant under 36 weeks of gestation. The concern for the infant with a tracheoesophageal (TE) fistula is important, but a few precautions should suffice. If there is hydramnios or excess secretions at birth, a tube should be passed to the stomach to make sure the esophagus is patent. If all is well, the infant may nurse. If there is a TE fistula, it is a surgical emergency. Choanal atresia is another anomaly that would be of concern, but an infant cannot suck on the breast or anything if he cannot breathe through his nose. Usually an infant with choanal atresia has a low Apgar score or needs some assistance in establishing respirations.

For this first breastfeeding, it may be best to have the mother on a stretcher or a bed wide enough to have the infant lie beside her (not the delivery table). The infant should not be dangled in midair over the breast. The mother should be assisted to turn onto her side and the infant presented to the breast, with his ventral surface to the ventral surface of mother. The infant should not have to turn his head toward the breast. The mother may need assistance in holding her breast so as to present the nipple squarely into the infant's mouth, which has been stimulated to open by stroking the lips with the nipple.

Both mother and infant will do better if there is an atmosphere of tranquility in the room. The only other risk to the infant is thermal stress. If the room is air-conditioned, it may be necessary to provide a radiant warmer over the infant, especially if the infant is naked for skin-to-skin contact. Some mothers have shaking chills following the strenuous event of labor and cannot provide adequate warmth for the infant without some external source of heat.

Chilling an infant may set off a chain of events from hypothermia to hypoglycemia to tachypnea to mild acidosis to the extent of requiring a septic workup. Hypothermia, therefore, is more easily prevented than treated.

If possible, mother, father, and infant should remain together for the next hour or so. The first hour for the infant is usually one of quiet alertness, a state that will usually recur only briefly for the next few days. It is important to delay the instillation of silver nitrate drops until after this time spent with the mother. If the drops are put into the eyes, blepharospasm will prevent the infant from opening his eyes and mar the eye-to-eye contact. Only if there is a known risk of gonorrhea should the drops be put in immediately. If the mother has delivered in a birthing center, early contact and nursing should be part of the routine.

Days in the hospital

The physician should see that his patients are permitted to have their infants with them as much as they wish, within the guidelines of reasonable medical care. Only the few patients with difficult deliveries, cesarean sections with medication, postpartum complications, or eclampsia need be excluded, but the physician should make that judgment. An experienced nursing staff is critical to the management of the nursing mother at this point.[55] Advice should be reasonable and consistent, and nurses should be cautioned against interjecting their own personal opinion or experience. Key points in management should include the following:

1. Help the mother find a comfortable position. There should be no rules about sitting up or lying down.
2. Help the infant to the breast. The infant should be held so that the ventral surface of the infant faces the mother.
3. Help the mother hold her breast for her baby. The scissor hold, with index finger and thumb above and other fingers below, works well for many mothers. Fingers should be back far enough so infant can grasp the compressed areola (Fig. 8-6). If the breast is large or the hand is small, try placing the thumb on top and all the fingers under the breast supporting from the rib cage forward.[32]
4. Help the mother reposition the infant on the second breast, since moving may be hard at first.
5. If the infant falls asleep after the first breast, the mother should be shown how to break the suction with her fingers. Nonnutritive suckling while asleep is especially irritating to the nipple in the first few days. Wait a little, wake the baby, and then move him to the second side.
6. When waking an infant, unwrapping the blanket and using gentle stimulus are appropriate. Jackknifing is never appropriate and may cause regurgitation, aspiration, or trauma to vital organs.
7. Allow the infant to nurse about 5 minutes per side at first. This will usually

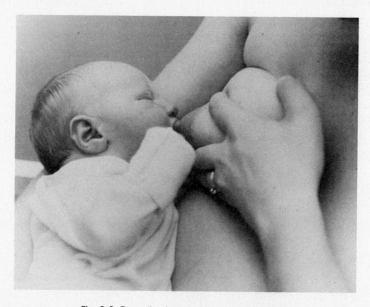

Fig. 8-6. Presenting breast while supporting infant.

assure that the infant takes both sides and will help the breasts adapt gradually. Timing should be casual and not with stopwatch rigidity. It takes 2 to 3 minutes for the let-down reflex to be effective. Frequent small feedings will provide good stimulation to the breast without stressing the mother. The milk supply is best stimulated by suckling. The policy of the nursery should be to have all breastfed infants taken to their mothers when they awaken during the night.[50]

If the physician believes that until the milk is in, the 2 AM feeding can be replaced by water in the nursery if the infant wakes up, so that the mother gets a full night's sleep, there should be a written order. A mother should be given the infant if she requests to have him. On the other hand, modern hospitals are a hubbub of activity, and with liberalized visiting hours there is no time for the mother to rest unless naps are scheduled. In the early days of the Rooming-In Unit at the Yale–New Haven Hospital, Jackson insisted that all postpartum mothers have a nap after lunch. Every day the shades were drawn and traffic decreased on the unit for an hour. This is part of mothering the mother. In primitive cultures, mothers are groomed, fed, and protected after delivery, often for weeks. Furthermore, adequate rest is essential to successful lactation. In 1953, Jackson, with her colleagues Barnes et al.,[9] prepared a classic description of the management of breastfeeding, which still remains the single most valuable source of information.

Diagnosing problems with nursing

To solve the problem of unsuccessful nursing, observe the mother feeding the infant. Often the problem is a simple one such as a mother so uncomfortable and tense that the let-down reflex will not trigger or, perhaps, an infant with a poor suck. In these cases and others the diagnosis will be made most easily by direct observation.

Understanding the mechanism of suckling in the neonate, however, is essential to recognize ineffective sucking on the part of the infant (Fig. 8-7). As the breast is offered to the infant, the lips gently clamp the areola to hold it in place as the tongue thrusts forward to grasp the nipple and areola. In a rhythmic motion, the tongue moves up against the hard palate, drawing the nipple and areola into the mouth. The cheeks fill the mouth because of the sucking fat pads and provide further negative pressure. The tongue returns to the gum and lips and draws back along the areola, compressing the collecting ductules in the areola and "milking" them as the tongue moves along the nipple, which is compressed against the hard palate, sustaining the relative negative pressure. Milk flows from the nipple and is swallowed as a response of the swallowing reflex. If the infant has a fluttering tongue, it may not be as productive in stimulating ejection. If the infant cannot coordinate suck and swallow, choking occurs. Sometimes if ejection is strong, the first rush of milk will cause choking. Stopping and starting again should solve the problem. If the infant's jaw is slightly receding, the nipple may not stay in place. Gentle support at the angle of the jaw will help.

An infant who is given a bottle or rubber nipple to suck becomes confused because

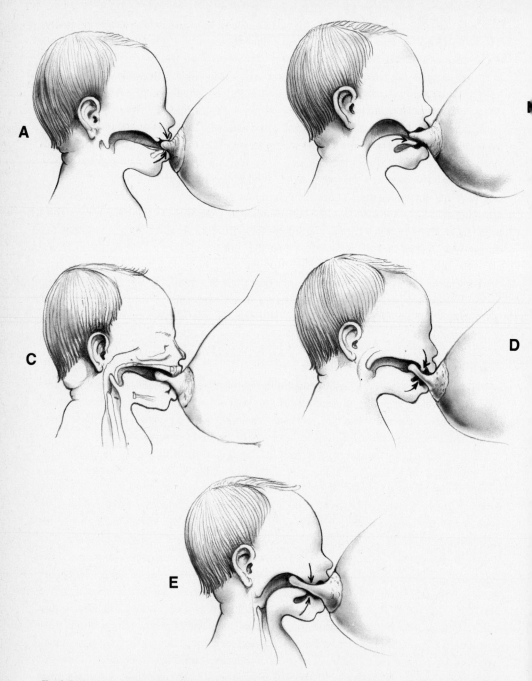

Fig. 8-7. A, Infant grasps breast (note *arrows* showing jaw action). **B,** Tongue moves forward to draw nipple in. **C,** Nipple and areola move toward palate as glottis still permits breathing. **D,** Tongue moves along nipple, pressing it against hard palate and creating pressure. **E,** Ductules under areola are milked and flow begins. Glottis closes.

the sucking action is different (Fig. 8-8). The relatively inflexible rubber nipple may keep the tongue from its usual rhythmic action. In addition, the flow may be so rapid, even without sucking, that the infant learns to put the tongue against the rubber nipple holes to slow down the flow. Some infants who have been breastfed gag when the relatively large rubber nipple is put in their mouths. When an infant uses the same tongue action he has needed for a rubber nipple at the breast, he may even push the human nipple out of the mouth. Sometimes, when he cannot grasp an engorged areola properly, he will clamp down on the nipple with his jaws, causing pain in the nipple and disrupting the ejection reflex.

When observing an infant being breastfed, take note of the following:

1. Position of mother, her body language and tension.
2. Position of infant: his ventral surface should be to mother's ventral surface, lower arm, if not swaddled, around mother's thorax; infant cannot swallow if head has to turn to breast and grasp of areola will be poor.
3. Position of mother's hand on breast.
4. Position of infant's lips on areola (cannot get all of large areola in mouth).
5. Lower lip should not be folded in so infant sucks lip.

ENGORGEMENT.   The best management of engorgement is prevention. The degree of engorgement lessens with each infant because the time at which the milk comes in seems to shorten in multiparas. The primipara suffers most from engorgement. Engorgement involves two elements: one is congestion and increased vascularity; the second is accumulation of milk. Engorgement may involve only the areola, only the body of the breast (so-called peripheral engorgement), or both.

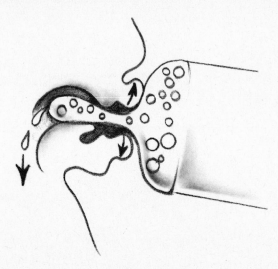

Fig. 8-8. Infant sucking on rubber nipple, which fills mouth and thus prevents tongue action and provides flow without stroking. Flow occurs even if lips not tight around rubber hub.

Areolar engorgement. When the areola is engorged, it obliterates the nipple and makes properly grasping the areola impossible for the infant. If he sucks only the nipple, it is exquisitely painful, since that is the only area of the breast where there are pain fibers. In addition, the collecting ductules are not "milked" and therefore do not empty, and the infant is frustrated by lack of milk.

The treatment is directed toward reducing the engorgement so that the infant can nurse effectively, which will further reduce the overdistended ducts. Gentle manual expression by the mother herself will usually produce a small amount of flow and soften the areola. The presence of milk on the nipple will further encourage the infant's sucking. A mother should be taught how to manually express (Fig. 8-9). By placing the thumb and forefinger at the margins of the areola and pressing back in toward the chest, and then bringing the fingers together, rhythmically stimulating the action of the infant's jaw, the flow will start and the tense tissue soften (see Appendix J). When the infant is put to the breast, the mother should compress the areola between two fingers to make it easier for the infant to grasp. Offering the breast this way makes it easier for any infant to grasp, especially when he needs encouragement to nurse (Fig. 8-10).

Peripheral engorgement. Initially, the breasts increase in vascularity and begin to swell. This usually starts in the second 24-hour period after delivery. Initially, engorgement is vascular; thus pumping mechanically is not productive and may be traumatic. The mother should be advised to wear a well-fitting but adjustable nursing brassiere that does not have thin straps or permanent plastic lining. She should wear it 24 hours a day. With moderately severe engorgement, the breasts become full, hard, and tender. The swelling starts at the clavicle and goes to the lower rib cage and from the midaxillary line to the midsternum. The breasts may even become hard, tense, and warm. The

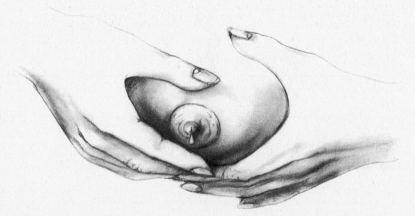

Fig. 8-9. Position for manual expression of breast. Thumbs are brought toward areola, compressing areola between thumb and supporting fingers. With areola grasped, pressure is applied toward chest wall, and then pressure is released. This compression and pressure stimulates milking action (also see Appendix J).

mother complains of throbbing and aching pain and can find no comfortable position except to lie flat on her back and very still.

Management is centered on making the mother comfortable so that she can continue to nurse and stimulate milk production as well as nourish the infant. Proper support to elevate the breasts is important. The axilla are particularly painful, probably as a result of the tension on Cooper's ligament. Cold packs may help initially to reduce vascularity. Warm packs may help some patients. Having the mother stand in a warm shower and manually express some milk at the same time may be the best preparation to feed the infant. Some find comfort in alternating hot and cold water. Aspirin may give the mother some relief and should not bother the infant. An aspirin-codeine preparation has been recommended as well. It may be necessary to provide the mother with some sleep medication. Medications should be timed so that the least amount possible reaches mother's milk and the baby. If medication is taken immediately before nursing, the pain will be relieved but the drug will not reach the milk for more than ½ hour in the case of aspirin, acetaminophen, codeine, or short-acting barbiturates.

It is important to maintain drainage during this period of engorgement to prevent back pressure from developing and eventually depressing milk production. Intraductal pressure can lead eventually to atrophy of both the secreting and myoepithelial cells and a diminishing milk supply. The best treatment is frequent breastfeeding around the clock because suckling by the infant is the most effective mechanism for removal of milk. Relief is based on establishment of flow. The infant may have trouble grasping or not be interested in nurs-

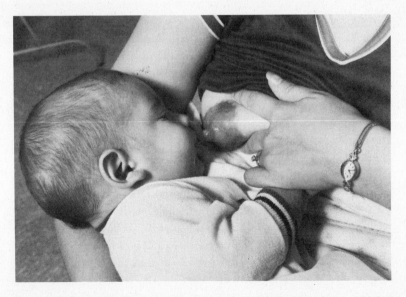

Fig. 8-10. When breast is offered to infant, areola is gently compressed between two fingers and breast supported to assure that infant is able to grasp areola adequately.

ing frequently in the first few days, so manual expression may also be necessary. Every mother should be taught this technique by the perinatal nursing staff.[64]

The mother should support the breast with her fingers and place her thumbs distally and massage gently toward the areola, rotating gradually around the breast to include all quadrants. Then, once the peripheral lobules have been softened, areolar expression as previously described should be used to encourage complete emptying of the collecting ducts in the areola. This is a procedure best done by the mother, but it may take a skilled and experienced nurse to teach this technique. The Marmet technique of manual expression of milk is illustrated in Appendix J. It may be helpful to use the Egnell pump in cases of engorgement. It is very effective because of its gentle milking action. The traditional electric pump is an instrument of unphysiologic torture because it serves merely as negative pressure suction (see Chapter 19).

Hand pumps can be used but only exert negative pressure on the areola. Unless accompanied by manual expression of the distal segments they are only temporizing. The Egnell pump does simulate the infant's stroking tongue.

Currently maternity patients are going home in 2 to 3 days or sooner, which is certainly before lactation is well established, but it may also be before engorgement is full blown. At the time when maternity floors were run so rigidly that ad lib breastfeeding was an impossible feat, it was often suggested that a mother go home and get away from the negative hospital atmosphere to a place where she could relax and concentrate on feeding the infant and resting. This is a point at which the doula, so well described by Raphael,[62] could make the difference between success and failure. It may be appropriate for the obstetrician to order the mother to have some assistance at home, whether it is her husband, her mother, or a friend. "The common denominator for success in breastfeeding is the assurance of some degree of help from some specific person for a definite period of time after childbirth," according to Raphael.[62] She studied mothers in the cycle of anxiety while she became the doula for the individuals she studied at about 6 to 10 days postpartum. The calm that can be experienced in the presence of a confident, caring person will relax the mother. The infant senses the calm and confidence and sleeps. When he feeds again, he nurses well. Breaking the cycle of panic that seizes a new mother when she finds herself home alone with a new infant who needs frequent feeding requires an ability to instill confidence.

Although the physician cannot provide the doula role, he can be sure that the family understands the need and can suggest community resources if no personal ones are available. Successful breastfeeding is not automatic, as is demonstrated by the failure rate. Some of the problems have been generated by the disturbance of the synchronization of interaction between mother and infant by rigid hospital protocol. This is continued at home when feeding is by the clock rather than by instinct. A program developed in the Rochester community for early discharge called Perinatal Homecare, where nursing, laboratory, and homemaker services are provided under insurance coverage, has proved especially conducive to successful breastfeeding.[1]

NIPPLES

Painful nipples. Presumably the nipples will adapt to the nursing experience naturally; however, often there are discomforts. It is common for the initial grasp of the nipple and sucks to cause discomfort in the first few days of lactation. It is not cause for alarm, but it requires reassurance. The sensation is created by the negative pressure on the ductules, which are not yet filled with milk. Later, when lactation is well established and the let-down reflex is experienced, mothers will describe a turgescence, which is the increased fluid pressure being relieved by suckling. Occasionally, the pain persists throughout the nursing.

Nipple pain was studied in 102 women in the first 96 hours postpartum and engorgement was most closely associated with nipple discomfort, which may be enhanced by the general discomfort of the breast. Prenatal breast preparation was unrelated to soreness. Length of time spent suckling was also unrelated. No record was kept on nonnutritive suckling, although others have found suckling without swallowing to be more stressful early in lactation. How the breast is presented to the infant is the most critical factor[32] (maternal hand position and infant squarely facing breast). This is the time to observe the feeding, looking for malpositioning or other abnormalities.

If no abnormality is found, the pain may be due to a "barracuda baby" with a vigorous suck. The breast will gradually adapt to it, and it will not last indefinitely. Sometimes the maternal tissues are unusually tender and delicate. Dry heat may help between feedings. The mother should remove the waterproofing from her brassiere and expose her breasts to air or an electric lamp with a 60-watt bulb for 20 minutes four times per day. A lamp similar to the perineal lamp can be used in the hospital.

Even more effective is the use of an electric hair dryer, set on warm and fanned across the breast about 6 to 8 inches away. This brings remarkable comfort and can be done sitting, standing, or lying down. Many patients bring hair dryers to the hospital with them. The breast will be moist with milk right after a feeding. This should not be wiped away but allowed to dry. Many cultures treat irritation of the skin with human milk. The drying effect of the treatment will help counteract the increase in moisture experienced in the first days of lactation.

Nipple shields. Nipple shields should not be used unless all else has failed, since it often becomes hard to wean the infant back. The infant becomes confused in learning his sucking routine. Glass or plastic with a rubber nursing nipple works well and has the advantage that the mother can see the milk through the glass or plastic. The effect of a traditional red rubber nipple shield referred to as "Mexican Hat" was compared to a new thin latex nipple shield. Normal mothers with no problems lactating nursed their infants using the shields.[77] The Mexican Hat shield reduced the milk transfer by 58% and increased the infants' sucking rate and time spent resting. The thin latex shield reduced milk by 22% and had no effect on sucking patterns. These findings would suggest that new thin latex nipple shields could be used effectively when shields are necessary.

Small or flat nipples.   When the nipples are small or flat, care to flatten the breast and areola between two fingers to provide as much nipple as possible to the infant will assist him in getting a hold. Sometimes a shield is necessary to draw the nipple out, but the shield should be removed and the infant placed directly on the breast for the rest of the feeding. Once engorgement is diminished and nursing is well established, small or flat nipples are usually no longer a problem.

Large nipples.   Large nipples are occasionally a problem with a small infant or an infant with an indecisive suck. A shield may help the infant cope at first, but it is best just to work patiently with the infant. Manual expression, which softens the areola to make it more pliable, before putting the infant to the breast, often helps.

Cracked nipples.   Whenever the mother complains of nipple pain on nursing, the nipple should be examined in good light to look for cracks or subepithelial petechiae, which may be the precursor to cracking. Taking a thorough history about care of the breast is important to identify the use of soaps, oils, ointments, or other self-prescribed treatments. Watching the nursing process may identify abnormal positioning at the breast. If there are true cracks, however, therapy is indicated. In the precracked stage, dry heat between nursings will be most effective. When true fissures have developed, Barnes et al.[9] recommend that the infant be taken off the affected breast for 24 to 48 hours, nursing only on the other side. That is drastic treatment and, in our experience, opening both sides of the nursing brassiere at feedings and beginning to nurse on the opposite side first will permit the initial let-down to occur "atraumatically"; then the infant can be put carefully to the affected breast. The heat treatments will assist in the therapy. When nursing has to be stopped on a given breast, it sets up a chain reaction of engorgement, reduced flow, and plugging of the ducts. A nipple shield should be tried before the nursing on a breast is stopped.

A very successful treatment described by Young,[79] which has now been adopted as a hospital routine in New Zealand, is the use of the mother's milk on the cracked nipple. A small amount is expressed and applied gently to the nipple and areola and allowed to dry on. Healing is rapid, and the success rate is excellent.*

The application of any ointment that must be removed before nursing has disadvantages, since the removal is traumatic. A and D ointment and hydrous lanolin, which do not have to be removed, are the most effective of the ointments. The indiscriminate use of ointment, however, can be the cause of nipple pain and, as with many dermatologic problems, the initial treatment of the physician may be to discontinue previous treatments. Some ointments suggested as breast creams contain antibiotics, astringents, bismuth subnitrate, or petrolatum, all of which are contraindicated. These creams are available over the counter.

Following is a summary of management of sore, painful, or cracked nipples:

---

*Human milk has also been used in some cultures very successfully as eye drops in cases of bacterial ophthalmitis.

1. Examine the breast, nipple, and nursing scene.
2. Conduct prefeeding manual expression.
3. Carefully position infant on breast.
4. Nurse on unaffected breast first with affected side exposed to air.
5. Apply expressed breast milk to nipples and let dry on between feedings.
6. Apply dry heat 20 minutes, four times a day with a 60-watt bulb, 18 inches (45 cm) away, or with a hair dryer on low setting.
7. If necessary, use nipple shield while nursing.
8. Rarely, temporarily stopping the nursing on affected side, replacing it with manual expressing or pumping, may be indicated.
9. If necessary, give aspirin or codeine in short-acting preparation just before nursing (Chapter 11).

The infant in the hospital

FEEDING CHARACTERISTICS.   Infants have been aptly classified by their feeding characteristics by Barnes and colleagues[9] as barracudas, excited ineffectives, procrastinators, gourmets or mouthers, and resters.

These descriptions serve to demonstrate the fact that infants are different and the management of the nursing experience will vary accordingly. Therein lies the secret to appropriate counseling—recognizing the differences among infants and responding to them.

Barracudas.   When put to the breast, barracudas vigorously and promptly grasp the nipple and suck energetically for 10 to 20 minutes. There is no dallying. Occasionally, this type of infant puts too much vigor into his nursing and hurts the nipple.

Excited ineffectives.   Excited ineffective infants become so excited and active at the breast that they alternately grasp and lose the breast. They then start screaming. It is often necessary for the nurse or mother to pick up the infant and quiet him first, and then put him back to the breast. After a few days the mother and infant usually become adjusted.

Procrastinators.   Procrastinators often seem to put off until the fourth or fifth postpartum day what they could just as well have done from the start. They wait until the milk comes in. They show no particular interest or ability in sucking in the first few days. It is important not to prod or force these infants when they seem disinclined. They do well once they start.

Gourmets or mouthers.   Gourmets insist on mouthing the nipple, tasting a little milk and then smacking their lips before starting to nurse. If the infant is hurried or prodded, he will become furious and start to scream. Otherwise, after a few minutes of mouthing he settles down and nurses very well.

Resters.   Resters prefer to nurse a few minutes and then rest a few minutes. If left alone, they often nurse well, although the entire procedure will take much longer. They cannot be hurried.

WEIGHT LOSS.   Newborns usually lose some weight, and it tends to be a function of whether they are appropriate, large, or small for gestational age as well as how many kilocalories are ingested in the first few days. The infants of multiparas who are breast-feeding often lose little weight because the milk comes in so quickly. On the other hand, the normal primipara may not have a full supply for 72 to 96 hours. If the weight loss is over 5% (150 g in a 3 kg infant), evaluate the process to identify any problems before they become serious. A 10% weight loss is acceptable if all else is going well and the physical examination is negative, but it should be justified in the record, and the infant should be seen shortly after discharge from the hospital to assure resolution of the problem. Weighing before and after feedings is successful only in producing tremendous anxiety in the mother and affords little information because it is so inaccurate. It is therefore almost never indicated.

Weighing has been improved by the introduction of electronic digital read-out scales that are accurate to 1 g and are especially helpful in the intensive care nursery for infants under 1000 g.[16] Because of the cost and the sensitivity (fragility) of the equipment, these scales are not practical for home or office use yet. Their accuracy in before-and-after weighings has been verified by a number of investigators using comparison techniques.[72] When ordinary scales are used, the margin of error has been shown to be greatest with the smaller volumes and is 20% in amounts less than 60 ml.

VOMITING BLOOD.   A breastfed baby who vomits blood should have the blood evaluated for fetal or adult hemoglobin by the Apt test. (Suspend blood in a small amount of saline solution, and add an equal amount of 10% NaOH. Adult hemoglobin turns brown; fetal hemoglobin stays pink.) If it is adult hemoglobin, the nipple may be bleeding. Sometimes this bleeding is painless and unknown to the mother, and sometimes she is afraid to report it.

LET-DOWN REFLEX.   The most important single function that affects the success of breastfeeding is the let-down reflex. Any mother can produce the milk, but if she does not excrete it, further production is suppressed. Much has been written on this single reflex by physiologists, endocrinologists, biochemists, pathologists, anatomists, psychologists, psychiatrists, obstetricians, and pediatricians. Indeed, it is a complex function that depends on hormones, nerves, and glands, which can be inhibited most easily by psychologic block.

The hormonal mechanism of milk ejection is described in Chapter 3. The reflex stimulation of milk ejection has been meticulously studied by Caldeyro-Barcia[18] while he studied intramammary pressures. The more efficient stimulus for the milk-ejection reflex is suckling of the nipple. The frequency of suckling is 70 to 120 strokes/min, and the mean pressure is between −50 and −150 mm Hg. The maximum recorded was −220 mm Hg. Within 1 minute of the onset of suckling, the first contraction of the mammary myoepithelium is recorded, but it may take 2 or more total minutes for full response. Further research by Cobo[20] has shown that, as in other species, the human response is undulating or spurtlike in release, although the level of oxytocin tends to reach a peak and plateau at 6 to 10 minutes during a feeding.[71] Some studies show no episodic secretion. When oxytocin levels are measured before the feeding, there is a response to the baby's crying or other anticipation of feeding. There is no prolactin response before actual suckling. A second release of oxytocin occurs when suckling begins.[25] There is not a direct correlation between levels of oxytocin and the volume of milk release at a given feeding.[53] The average pituitary gland contains 1000 mU of oxytocin and only 0.5 U is required for the let-down reflex.

Uterine contractions are also stimulated by suckling. Amplitude and frequency may increase over time during nursing. Mechanical stimulation of the nipple can produce the same effect on the breast and uterus. The milk-ejection reflex is inhibited centrally by cold, pain, and emotional stress. Ejection response can be elicited by seeing the infant or hearing him cry.

The milk-ejection reflex can be at least partially blocked by alcohol, which seems to have a central effect preventing the release of oxytocin, since the mammary gland and uterine response to injected oxytocin are not changed by alcohol. Studies on mothers with diabetes insipidus suggest that the patient retains the ability to synthesize and release oxytocin despite the fact that she is unable to produce ADH (vasopressin) in response to stimuli. Artificial cervical dilation postpartum will also cause milk ejection. Vaginal stimulus also initiates let-down in all species.

Injection of oxytocin reproduces the effect of suckling. A rapid series of injections of 1 to 10 mU intravenously will simulate suckling. A continuous drip is less effective. Use of Pitocin as a snuff or nasal spray is the best method for home use of oxytocin to initiate let-down.

The oxytocin concentration in the blood rises with suckling, which supports the hypothesis that suckling elicits the release of oxytocin.

The data on the question of ADH release during suckling are confused but it would seem release of oxytocin and of ADH are independent.

The mammary myoepithelium is stimulated to contraction by oxytocin, and the milk-ejection reflex results in the contraction of the myoepithelium and the release, or let-down, of milk (Fig. 8-11). In the first weeks of lactation, the threshold dose of oxytocin is very low, averaging 0.65 mU from the fifth day. Thirty days after weaning it is 100 mU. Vasopressin is not as effective and requires 100 times the dosage of oxytocin to produce the same effect during lactation. Deaminooxytocin is 1.5 times as potent as oxytocin on the third postpartum day, but the difference disappears over time, probably because of the rapid breakdown of natural oxytocin by oxytocinase early in the postpartum period. Prostaglandins have been shown to have a number of physiologic effects, including an effect on mammary epithelium to increase mammary duct pressure.[70] In a blind crossover study, oxytocin, intravenous prostaglandin, and nasal prostaglandin were given and the intraductal pressures measured. The most effective intravenous pros-

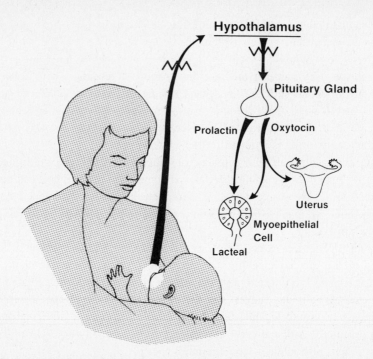

Fig. 8-11. Diagrammatic outline of ejection reflex arc. When infant suckles breast, he stimulates mechanoreceptors in nipple and areola that send stimulus along nerve pathways to hypothalamus, which stimulates the posterior pituitary to release oxytocin. It is carried via bloodstream to breast and uterus. Oxytocin stimulates myoepithelial cell in breast to contract and eject milk from alveolus. Prolactin is responsible for milk production in alveolus. It is secreted by anterior pituitary gland in response to suckling. Stress such as pain and anxiety can inhibit let-down reflex. The sight or cry of infant can stimulate it.

taglandins were 16-phenoxy-PGE_2 and $PGF_{2\alpha}$, that were then tried nasally, but only $PGF_{2\alpha}$ was effective nasally. The potential for nasal $PGF_{2\alpha}$ treatment in engorgement and failure of let-down is possible but is as yet unexplored clinically.

PRACTICAL ASPECTS OF THE MILK-EJECTION REFLEX. When the nipple is stimulated, the receptors at the nipple and areola are stimulated and nervous impulses are transmitted to the hypothalamus via the somatic afferent nerves. The hypothalamus stimulates the pituitary gland to secrete prolactin, which induces the alveoli in the breast to secrete milk. The cell membranes release fat globules and protein into the lumen. This produces the hindmilk, which has a higher protein and fat content. Foremilk has been present since the previous nursing and is released first. It is a more dilute, less fatty solution that empties into the lactiferous sinuses awaiting the next suckling. The ejection reflex induces the holocrine excretion of milk from the cells. The posterior pituitary gland secretes oxytocin, which stimulates the myoepithelial cells to contract and eject the milk from the ducts.

Newton and Newton[54] have studied the ejection reflex and clearly show the effect

Table 8-4.   Ejection reflex*

Maternal disturbance	Mean amount of milk obtained by infant (g)
No distractions (no injection)	168
Distraction (saline injection)	99
Distraction (oxytocin injection)	153

Modified from Newton, M., and Newton, N.: J. Pediatr. **91**:1, 1977.
*Interrupted milk flow can be restarted with hormone injection.

of distraction to the let-down effect. Distractions included immersing feet in ice water (reported to be the worst), being asked mathematical questions in rapid series, which resulted in electric shock if a wrong answer was given, or having painful traction on the big toe (Table 8-4). In practice, for some mothers pain, stress, and mental anguish interfere with let-down. When simple adjustments such as making the mother more comfortable, playing soft music, or leaving the mother in a quiet room do not work, other techniques should be tried.

Gentle stroking of the breast may help to decrease anxiety. Tactile warmth as opposed to cold may improve release. Since it is recommended by some that ice can be used to make the nipple erect, be sure this is not interfering with let-down, because cold experimentally interrupts the reflex.

The most direct therapy is oxytocin. When simple supportive measures fail, this can be prescribed at home as a nasal spray, most readily available as synthetic oxytocin (Syntocinon). It is packaged in 2 and 5 ml spray bottles. A mother almost never needs a second bottle. A bottle contains 40 USP units (IU) of synthetic oxytocin, a polypeptide hormone of the posterior pituitary gland, per milliliter of spray. (A prescription is required.) It is destroyed in the gastrointestinal tract; therefore, it must be sprayed nasally, where it is rapidly absorbed. One spray into one or both nostrils 2 to 3 minutes before putting the infant to the breast (or before pumping, in the case of collecting for an infant unable to nurse at the breast) is sufficient.

It has been suggested by Aono and colleagues[3] that sulpiride be given orally to mothers who produce less than 50 ml of total milk yield in first 48 hours of lactation. Sulpiride is known to stimulate secretion of prolactin. In a control study of 96 normal primiparas and multiparas with poor lactation, half were given 50 mg sulpiride twice daily from the fourth to the seventh day postpartum and half received a placebo. There was no difference in milk production in the multiparas but there was a significant difference in the primiparas, who had higher milk yield, higher prolactin levels, and higher percentage still breastfeeding at 1 month in the treated group.

POSTNATAL, OR POSTHOSPITAL, PERIOD

When the family makes the transition from hospital to home, it can be stressful. The parents hear the infant who has been passive and content wake up and cry for the first time. Because of all the procedures necessary to discharge an infant from the hospital (discharge physicals, blood tests, etc.), the well-planned discharge is often delayed and everyone is frantic, including the infant. The mother should be reassured about this and not be alarmed if she has to feed the infant frequently the first day at home.

Feeding frequency

Many hospital schedules are on a 4-hour feeding program, based on the feedings of bottle fed infants whose slow emptying time of the stomach with cow's milk formulas requires 4 hours. The emptying time for breast milk is about 1½ hours; thus frequent feedings are not unusual. Pediatric textbooks at the turn of the century described 10 to 12 feedings a day as normal. Comparison of mammalian care patterns and composition of their milk shows an inverse relationship between protein content and frequency of feedings. From this it might be deduced that the human infant might well need to be fed more frequently than every 4 hours (Table 8-5).[51] Infants who sleep 5 to 6 hours at a stretch at night may make up for skipped feedings during the day. A mother should be advised to use both breasts during each feeding (Fig. 8-12).

The pattern of intake during a feeding is different between breastfed and bottle fed infants.[44] A bottle feeding infant sucks steadily in a linear pattern, receiving 81% of the feed in 10 minutes. A breastfed infant has a biphasic pattern, which includes the first 4 minutes on the first breast and the first 4 minutes on the second breast (between 15 and 19 minutes into the feed). He receives 84% of the total volume in those 8 minutes. In another study, 50% of the feed on each breast was consumed in 2 minutes and 80% to 90% by 5 minutes. Milk flow was minimal during the last 5 minutes. All these observations were made on the fifth to seventh day.

Switch nursing is often suggested to increase total intake of an infant when milk production needs stimulating, especially if the infant is not gaining adequately. When mothers fed 10 minutes on each breast (10 × 10), they produced the same amount of milk as they did nursing 5 minutes on a side and switching back (5 × 5 × 5 × 5). The suckling-induced prolactin is similar with both patterns as well. The infants do not nurse for a full 20 minutes in some cases and the nutritive feeding time was under 15 minutes. It is suggested that the duration of the feeding should be determined by the infant's response and not by time.

New mothers are often most insecure and most concerned about lack of scheduling, especially if an ad lib program of feeding has been suggested. Other mothers seem to thrive on random scheduling. When a mother expresses concerns about frequent feedings and worries about the adequacy of her milk (she is often disturbed that it looks so thin and blue after the luxurious color of colostrum), Jackson would suggest she keep a record of feeding times and duration, as well as sleep and wakeful times. A chart was provided (Appendix B). The mother was usually surprised to find how quickly her infant developed a schedule. Often the infant was sleeping longer than she thought. The chart

Table 8-5. Mammalian care patterns and composition of species milk

				Species of mammal				
	Pinnipedia seal sea lion	Tree shrew	Rabbit	Rat	Black rhino*	Chimpanzee	Human
Infant care pattern	Return to ocean after birth	—	Cache	Carry, hibernate	—	Carry	?
Feeding interval	Once a week	48 hr	24 hr	Continuous	—	Continuous	?
Composition of milk							
Total Solids (%)	62-65	20	33-40	21	8.1	11.9	12.4
Protein (%)	8-14	11	14-23	10	0.0	3.7	3.8
Fat (%)	53	6.5	18	8	1.4	1.2	1.2
CHO (%)	0-0.90	3.2	2.0	2.6	6.1	7.0	7.0

*The rhino has an anatomic variation in the stomach that provides four pouches that fill during a feeding and provide a constant trickle of milk to the central groove leading to the small intestine, thus creating a constant feed.

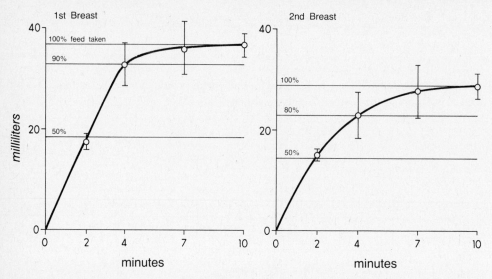

Fig. 8-12. Mother-infant pattern of milk flow. (From Lucas, A., Lucas, P.J., and Baum, J.D.: Lancet 2:57, 1979.)

is also reassuring to the physician, especially if weight gain is marginal. In some cases it will highlight a problem not previously identified, such as a poor gainer who sleeps all night, missing several feedings.

Adequate rest

If nursing is not going well, the most likely cause of problems is fatigue on the part of the mother. She may need to be ordered by her physician to nap and rest. She will have to learn to nap when the infant is napping. This becomes more difficult when there are other young children, but a simultaneous nap for all the little ones and mother may have to be engineered. Otherwise she may have to go to bed with the children at night and just concentrate on resting and feeding the infant. When the need for rest is acute, the father should be assigned infant care, with the possible inclusion of a bottle feeding, while the mother sleeps undisturbed.

Sore breasts—caked breasts

Tender lumps in the breasts in a mother who is otherwise well are probably due to plugging of a collecting duct. The best treatment is to continue nursing. Manually massaging the area to initiate and assure complete drainage should be recommended. Hot packs before feedings may help. If the breast is especially tender, initiating nursing on the opposite breast first permits the affected breast to let-down without the pressure of suckling. The affected breast should be completely emptied by nursing or manual expression. One should be sure the brassiere is not cutting off an alveolus with the undue pressure of a narrow strap. Changing the infant's position may help also.

REPEATED "CAKING." When repeated caking is recurrent, one needs to look for a major cause such as exhaustion and fatigue. Several women have come to my attention who have had repeated lumps in their breasts with poor flow of milk, often as if the ducts were plugged. The condition responded fairly well to manual expression before each feeding, often with the expulsion of small plugs. The condition dramatically improved by limiting the mother to polyunsaturated fats and adding lecithin to the diet. It was also necessary but effective for subsequent pregnancies as well in all three cases.

Galactocele

Milk-retention cysts are uncommon and when found are almost exculsively in lactating women. The contents at first are pure milk. Owing to absorption of the fluid they later contain thick creamy, cheesy, or oily material. The swelling is smooth and rounded, and compression of it may cause milky fluid to exude from the nipple. Galactoceles are believed to be caused by the blockage of a milk duct. The cyst may be aspirated to avoid surgery but will fill up again. It can be removed surgically under local anesthesia without stopping the breastfeeding. Its presence does not require cessation of the lactation. A firm diagnosis can be made by ultrasound; a cyst and milk will appear the same and a tumor will be distinguishable (Figs. 8-13 and 8-14).

Breast rejection

Infants have been observed to reject the breast intermittently, most often at 3 to 4 months, and then, to go back after several feedings or a day or so. A bottle can be substituted. Total rejection of both breasts may be due to the return of menstruation. A mother will notice the infant will reject the breast for a day or so with each period. Other infants seem unaffected. Strong foods in the diet may cause rejection of milk. It usually occurs 8 to 12 hours after ingestion and disappears by 24 hours after ingestion.

UNILATERAL BREAST REJECTION. Some infants prefer one breast and even refuse the other. When this occurs, manual expression or softening the nipple for easier grasp may help, thus enticing the infant to suckle. Holding the infant in the same position (i.e., on same side in same direction, so-called football hold) for the other breast may lead the infant to take the second breast. Sometimes applying syrup to the rejected nipple or using a breast shield will help. Unilateral breastfeeding is a custom in some parts of China. Sodium and chloride levels may rise in milk after mastitis. It is wise to taste the milk or have SMA_6 done on milk from both breasts if the problem persists, to be sure there is not a reason for the rejection.

Goldsmith[36] reported five cases of lactating women whose infants suddenly rejected a single breast. Weeks or months later a mass was noted by the mother and biopsy revealed malignancy. It would be wise to examine any patient who complains of unilateral breast rejection that does not respond to simple measures to rule out a tumor. Ultrasound followed by a mammogram, if necessary, can be performed without discontinuing lactation.

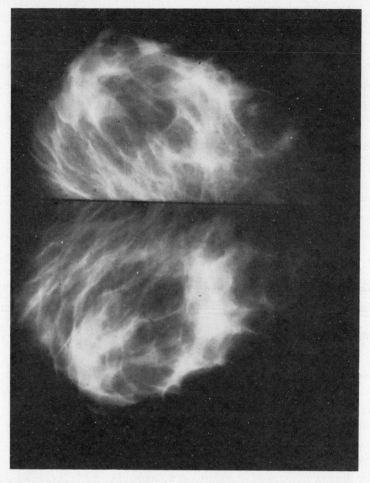

Fig. 8-13. Normal breast tissue by mammography. Tissue is one-third fat and appears cystic in nature. (Courtesy Dr. Wende Logan.)

Mastitis

Mastitis is an infectious process in the breast, producing localized tenderness, redness, and heat, together with systemic reactions of fever, malaise, and sometimes nausea and vomiting. It no longer occurs in epidemics as seen in hospitals at one time before the common use of antibiotics and when hospital stays were prolonged for normal childbirth. The infection, however, may be hospital acquired if the mother or infant is colonized with a virulent bacteria before leaving the hospital.

Little appears in the medical literature about mastitis because women are rarely hospitalized for the problem and are treated at home and, in some cases, over the

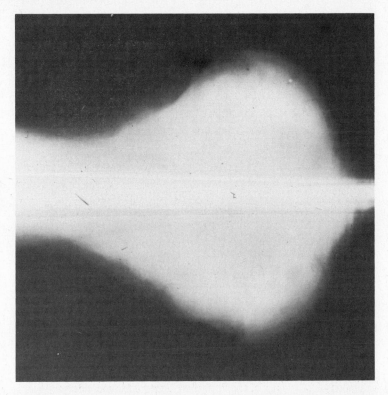

Fig. 8-14. Breast tissue during pregnancy and lactation by mammography. Fat is replaced by lactation tissue and presents solid appearance. Tumor would be easily distinguished by this procedure in lactating breast. It is a safe, noninvasive technique that does not interfere with nursing. (Courtesy Dr. Wende Logan.)

telephone. When staphylococcal disease was a major problem on postpartum wards, lactating and nonlactating women alike developed mastitis; thus the differentiation of two types was suggested by Gibbard in 1953:[34] acute puerperal mammary cellulitis, a nonepidemic mastitis involving interlobular connective tissue, and acute puerperal mammary adenitis, which was epidemic, associated with an outbreak of skin infections in infants, and involved the lactiferous ducts and lobes of the gland. Gunther later (1956)[38] simplified this differentiation to superficial and intramammary. The current definition includes fever of 38.5° C or more, chills, flulike aching, systemic illness, and pink, tender, hot, swollen, wedge-shaped area of the breast (Fig. 8-15). The significant differential points between mastitis and engorgement and plugged duct are listed in Table 8-6.

The portal of entry of the disease is through the lactiferous ducts to a secreting lobule, through a nipple fissure to periductal lymphatics, or through hematogenous spread. The common organisms involved include *Staphylococcus aureus, Escherichia coli,* and (rarely) *Streptococcus*.

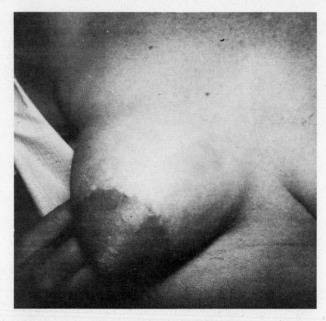

Fig. 8-15. Mastitis in medial upper quadrant. (From Marshall, B.R. JAMA 233:1377, 1975. Copyright 1975, American Medical Association.)

Table 8-6.   Comparison of findings of engorgement, plugged duct, and mastitis

Characteristics	Engorgement	Plugged duct	Mastitis
Onset	Gradual, immediately postpartum	Gradual, after feedings	Sudden, after 10 days
Site	Bilateral	Unilateral	Usually unilateral
Swelling and heat	Generalized	May shift/little or no heat	Localized, red, hot, and swollen
Pain	Generalized	Mild but localized	Intense but localized
Body temperature	<38.4° C	<38.4° C	>38.4° C
Systemic symptoms	Feels well	Feels well	Flulike symptoms

Factors predisposing the patient to mastitis include poor drainage of a duct and then of an alveolus, presence of an organism, and lowered maternal defenses such as those associated with stress and fatigue. Insufficient emptying and obstruction of ducts by tight clothing cause plugged ducts, which can be prevented from becoming mastitis if identified early and treated vigorously with local massage, moist heat, and rest. Missing a feeding or having the infant suddenly sleep through the night may cause engorgement, plugging, and then mastitis.[64] Cracked or painful nipples may herald a problem, more because mother avoids complete emptying on the painful side than because bacteria suddenly gain access.

Devereux[27] describes 20 years of experience with 53 lactating patients who experienced 71 acute attacks of mastitis. The highest incidence was in the second and third weeks postpartum. No infant was weaned because of the mastitis. No infants were sick in association with the mastitis. All but five mothers nursed subsequent infants. Six patients had mastitis with other pregnancies. Eight of 71 patients (11.1%) developed abscesses, six of which required incision and drainage. The bacterial cause was not stated. When treatment was delayed beyond 24 hours, the abscess rate increased.

Another series of 65 cases of mastitis, reported by Marshall et al.,[52] showed a 2.5% incidence of the disease among a population of 2534 lactating women. *S. aureus* was the offending organism in 23 of the 48 infected breasts that were cultured. In 19 normal lactating women, only one grew this organism. Forty-one of the sixty-five women continued to nurse without difficulty for an average of 13 weeks longer. There were three breast abscesses for a rate of 4.6%, all in women who chose to wean. Onset was 5½ weeks postpartum (5 days to 1 year range). Of the sixty-five, 9 had missed feedings or acutely weaned, 8 women had noticed a fissured nipple before the infection, and the others were unanticipated. Treatment included 41 with penicillin V, 12 with ampicillin, and 8 with other antibiotics. Mastitis recurred in four of the women who continued to nurse.

The clinician should be sure to inform his patients of the need to contact him if any unusual symptoms occur so that proper management can be initiated early, since prevention is the most effective treatment. Inappropriately or inadequately treated cases of mastitis predispose the patient to chronic mastitis, which may last for months and require more antibiotics than would have been required initially. A mother should be instructed to contact her physician if there is local pain, heat, and redness, or whenever there is a fever while lactating. When proper treatment is initiated promptly, the course of the disease is usually brief; if it is delayed, antibiotics will become necessary.

The management regimen that has been most successful at the University of Rochester is as follows:

1. Continue to nurse on both breasts, but start the infant on the unafffected side while the affected side "lets down." Be sure to empty the affected side by feeding or pumping.
2. Insist on bed rest (mandatory). The mother can take the infant to bed and obtain assistance for the care of the rest of the family.
3. Choose an antibiotic that can be tolerated by the infant as well as the mother (avoid sulfa drugs when the infant is under 1 month). The decision should be based on local sensitivities and length of time since delivery or exposure to resistant flora. In florid staphylococcal disease, amoxicillin, dicloxacillin, and nafcillin may be the drugs of choice. In streptococcal disease, penicillin is usually preferable. In uncomplicated mastitis after 1 month postpartum, penicillin, ampicillin, or erythromycin is preferable initially. Regardless of the course of the disease, the antibiotic should be given for at least 10 days. Shorter courses are associated with relapses.

4. Apply ice packs or warm packs to the breast, whichever provides the most comfort. Experience indicates that heat is better.
5. Provide plenty of fluids for the mother.
6. Give an analgesic such as aspirin.
7. The mother should wear a supporting brassiere that does not cause painful pressure.

Recurrent or chronic mastitis

Recurrent mastitis is usually caused by delayed or inadequate treatment of the initial disease. If antibiotics are initially started, they should be continued for a minimum of 10 days. Often, because the mother feels better, she discontinues them on her own. At the first recurrence, cultures should be sent of the breast and the infant's nasopharynx and oropharynx. The patient should be seen and the circumstances completely reviewed. An aggressive course of rest, nourishment, stress management, and complete drainage of the breast should be initiated. The antibiotics should be carefully selected and maintained for 2 weeks. Fluids should be increased. Failure of the second treatment is usually due to failure to complete the entire treatment, which may mean failure to get adequate rest and build up maternal resistance.

A secondary complication of recurrent mastitis is invasion of the breast by yeast or fungus such as *Candida albicans* (Chapter 15), as is frequently seen postantibiotic treatment. Mothers describe incredible pain when the infant nurses, pain they describe as feeling like hot cords burning in their chest wall. This is usually fungal infection of the ducts. The best treatment is to massage nystatin cream (Mycostatin) into the nipple and areola after each feeding. The infant should also be given oral nystatin simultaneously or the mother will be reinfected. If the mother is known to have a recurrent vulvovaginitis, initiation of nystatin prophylactically should be considered when the antibiotics are begun.

Abscess formation

Abscess can also be a complication of mastitis and is usually the result of delayed or inadequate treatment. A true abscess will require surgical drainage but should be treated with antibiotics, rest, warm soaks, and complete emptying of the breast at least every few hours. The milk will remain clean unless the abscess ruptures into the ductal system. Usually it drains to the outside. Nursing can be maintained when the breast is surgically drained as long as the incision and drainage tube are sufficiently far from the areola so that they are not involved in feeding. In any event, the breast should be manually drained frequently to maintain the milk supply until feeding can resume (usually sufficient healing takes place in 4 days).

LABORATORY FINDINGS.   Cultures of the breast milk, when indicated, should be done after the breast has been cleaned with water and the mother's hands have been thoroughly washed. The milk stream should be initiated by manual expression and the first 3 ml discarded to get a midstream clean-catch specimen. It has been suggested that antibody coating be looked for in the bacteria found in the milk to confirm its relationship to the disease.[69] It is important to remember that the normal cell count of normal uninfected human milk is 1000/mm^3 to 4000/mm^3. The presence of cells should not automatically be construed as infection.

The levels of sodium and chloride in milk from mastitic breasts have been reported in the literature to be extremely elevated (Na $\geq$100 mEq/L, Cl $\geq$80 mEq/L, K $\leq$10).[21] Usually, electrolyte abnormalities are associated with recurrent mastitis or chronic subclinical mastitis. The quickest screen for the problem is for the mother to compare the tastes of milk from each side.

Supplementary feedings

Many physicians suggest to mothers that a supplementary bottle can be added any time. Actually, when lactation is going well it is not needed, and when it is not going well, a bottle may aggravate the problem. During hospitalization, giving a substitute bottle may confuse a new infant, who may be having trouble sucking at first. Infants who are given water or glucose water in the hospital do less well and usually lose more weight. There is a significant relationship between supplements in the hospital and early discontinuation of breastfeeding. It is a marker of impending trouble and of insufficient milk production, which is best treated with frequent feedings at the breast and some intervention from an experienced support person.

Use of complementary bottles, that is, those given after a breastfeeding to top off the feeding, is the beginning of a downhill course that may doom lactation to failure. It would be better to take the infant to breast more often or switch back to the first breast if the baby is hungry. If it is necessary for the mother to be away at feeding time, she can pump a feeding ahead of time and save it in the refrigerator or freezer for someone else to give by bottle. If this is not practical, a bottle of formula can be given. It can be made up from a formula powder more economically one feeding at a time, and there is no waste. Powder preparations have a long shelf life even when open and are better tolerated by the infant because lower temperatures are required to manufacture powders; thus there is no carmelizing of the sugars or denaturing of the proteins. A powder goes quickly into solution if the water is warm when mixing is attempted. (Prepare formula powder as follows: one scoop of powder to 2 oz of water gives 20 kcal/oz).

Solid foods

Successfully nursing mothers are rarely impatient to start the baby on solid foods, as bottle feeding mothers frequently are. Milk, and especially human milk, supplies the appropriate nutrients. (Some physicians, however, prescribe additional fluorine, 0.5 mg, and vitamin D, 200 units [Chapter 9].) At about 6 months a normal infant begins to use his iron stores and that is probably an appropriate time to start solid foods, especially iron-containing ones. This permits the entire process of weaning to cup and solid foods to be a gradual one. An infant does not need teeth to eat baby food and, conversely, he does not have to be weaned from the breast because teeth have erupted. By 6 months the number of feedings usually has decreased, and the timing and volume are beginning to cycle to a schedule that resembles three meals a day and some snacks. A breastfed infant should have started some solids by 6 months of age.

Colic

Colic by definition is spasmodic contractions of smooth muscle, causing pain and discomfort. It can be experienced in many organs, such as the gastrointestinal or genitourinary tract, and at all ages. When the term *colic* is used in reference to infants it usually means a syndrome in which the young infant cries for a prolonged period of time, often at the same time of day, in the early months of life. The infant usually draws his legs up as if in pain. There are a myriad of remedies directed at various possible causes, including allergy, hypertonicity, and hormone withdrawal.

The infant-feeding survey conducted on the Isle of Wight among all infants under 1 year in 1977 was studied to determine the prevalence of infant colic[41]; 16% of the 843 infants had colic, all but 10 of the 135 cases developing before 6 weeks of age. Almost half were free of symptoms by 3 months of age. Only 12% persisted after 6 months of age. Surprisingly, only 20% occurred most commonly in the evening. Colic occurred equally among breastfed and bottle fed infants but was more common if solid foods were started under 3 months of age. The authors found no relationship to parental allergies or feeding methods, but only to social class: 23% of the professional group, 16% of the skilled group, and only 7% of the unskilled group complained of colic in their infants. Pediatricians have made this observation for generations, but it may be a matter of parenting style and expectations that brings a parent to complain about colic. Colic does occur in premature infants but usually not until they reach 42 weeks gestation.

Although colic is less common in the breastfed infant, it does occur. Characteristically, the infant will cry and scream as if in pain from 3 to 4 hours at a stretch, usually between 6 PM and 10 PM at night. The infant will nurse frequently, then scream and pull away from the breast as if in pain, only to cry out a few minutes later. Sometimes the infant can be comforted by another adult such as his father or grandmother. The infant will respond to gentle rocking when held against a warm shoulder. If the infant is put down, the screaming starts up again. If the nursing mother holds the infant, he is frantic unless nursed and yet does not need to be fed. This may disturb a new mother who wonders why she cannot console her infant (Is her milk weak? Does it disagree with her infant? Is she an inadequate mother?). None of these options is true, but the fact that the infant smells her milk makes him behave as if he needs to nurse. Anyone who is not nursing can quickly quiet the infant. Picking the infant up does not spoil him, and rocking and cuddling are appropriate.

A carefully taken history and physical examination are always in order to rule out other pathologic conditions such as otitis media, anal fissure, or hernia before a diagnosis of colic is made. If true colic is diagnosed because of the consistency of the screaming for several hours each day at the same time, treatment is in order. Elixir of diphenhydramine (Benadryl) or pyribenzamine (1 to 2 tsp immediately and every 4 hours as necessary) is usually very effective. If the medication is given 30 minutes before the anticipated colic begins, it works best. The elixir is sedating as well as having an "antiallergic" component. Spiritus fermenti or other forms of alcohol, such as 5 drops of whiskey in 1 tsp of warm water, may help the colic. When wine or beer is suggested to the mother as an aperitif before dinner, it may serve to relax the frantic mother as well as the colicky infant. It is recognized that excessive alcohol while nursing can produce failure to thrive and hypoglycemia in the neonate, but when used in moderate dosage it may be very effective.

Influence of cow's milk in maternal diet

The literature is not straightforward on the issue of the effect of cow's milk in the maternal diet and infantile colic. Talbot[68] first published information on congenital sensitization to food (especially eggs and cow's milk) in humans in 1918, which was manifested as clinical allergy in the breastfed infant. Research techniques are far superior today and information is accumulating. Gerrard and Shenassa[33] report sensitization caused by substances in breast milk thought to be due to two types of food allergy; one is IgE-mediated and triggered by trace amounts of antigen, and the other is not IgE-mediated and is triggered by large amounts of antigen. Gastrointestinal transport of macromolecules in the pathogenesis of food allergy is under investigation as is T cell–mediated immunity in food allergy. However, the present state of scientific knowledge has not resolved the issue of colic and cow's milk for the clinician.

Clinical studies have been done to test the association of dairy products in the mother with colic in some breastfed babies. Jakobsson and Lindberg[45] described a cause-and-effect relationship in a group of 18 mothers in 1978, which was criticized because it was not a double-blind study. Evans et al.[30] then reported that they found no such relationship when they did a double-blind crossover study in which mothers received cow's milk protein for 2 days and then a placebo for 2 days. Jakobsson and Lindberg[46] have repeated their work using a double-blind crossover study design in the mother-baby pairs in which the infants had colic; 35% of the infants improved on maternal diets free of cow's milk. A torrent of mail to the journals confirmed these conclusions in small clinical practice trials as well.

In the face of a clinical picture of colic, a history of allergy in the family, especially to cow's milk, is suggestive. A trial of a diet free of cow's milk should be tried in any severe colic for at least a week (2 days rarely produces significant improvement). Usually a mother eliminates drinking milk, and for some babies that is enough. If not, all milk products are then eliminated. For the group of infants who have a cow's milk allergy, the treatment is impressive. Not all colic is due to cow's milk. It may be associated with other dietary items such as eggs or chocolate, or it may be totally unrelated to maternal food intake.

Acute 24-hour colic in a breastfed infant may be due to something in the maternal diet. When a strong vegetable like beans, onions, garlic, or rhubarb is taken for the first time and the infant starts to cry within a few hours and continues for 20 to 24 hours, this may be transient colic. This colic is self-limited and does not need any treatment. The colic-inducing foods are different for different infants. Some infants have no trouble. During the period of colic the infant may need frequent small feedings and much cuddling. Sometimes the infants overfeed, then vomit and settle down and go quietly to sleep, just as an overfed bottle infant does.

The distress or discomfort may be due to tension, and "colic" has been noted to be more common in the first infants of high-strung mothers. Colic has been associated with hormone withdrawal and has been treated with progesterone. In the breastfed baby this is a less likely cause because of the presence of hormones in breast milk. Allergy to cow's milk can be manifest by bouts of pain and crying, and switching to hypoallergenic milk may help the bottle fed infant. The breastfed infant may be reacting to something in the mother's diet, which can be easily eliminated after it is identified by association. Colicky breastfed infants who are weaned to formula are usually much worse. Weaning is not an appropriate treatment for the colicky breastfed infant in most cases. Colic usually diminishes in the third month of life, when the infant's gastrointestinal tract matures.

REFERENCES

1. Amado, A., Lawrence, R.A., and Roghman, K. Perinatal home care: a report on a Blue Cross and Home Care Effort, Caring 2:27, 1983.
2. Anderson, G.C., et al.: Development of sucking in term infants from birth to four hours post birth, Res. Nurs. Health 5:21, 1982.
3. Aono, T., et al.: Effect of sulpiride on poor puerperal lactation, Am. J. Obstet. Gynecol. 143:927, 1982.
4. Aono, T., et al.: The initiation of human lactation and prolactin response to suckling, J. Clin. Endocrinol. Metab. 44:1101, 1977.
5. Applebaum, R.M.: The modern management of successful breast feeding, Pediatr. Clin. North Am. 17:203, 1970.
6. Ardran, G.M., Kemp, F.H., and Lind, J.: A cineradiographic study of bottle feeding, Br. J. Radiol. 31:11, 1958.
7. Ardran, G.M., Kemp, F.H., and Lind, J.: A cineradiographic study of breast feeding, Br. J. Radiol. 31:156, 1958.
8. Bacon, C.J., and Wylie, J.M.: Mothers' attitudes to infant feeding at Newcastle General Hospital in summer 1975, Br. Med. J. 1:308, 1976.
9. Barnes, G.R., et al.: Management of breast feeding, JAMA 151:192, 1953.
10. Bentovim, A.: Shame and other anxieties associated with breast feeding: a systems theory and psychodynamic approach. In Ciba Foundation Symposium no. 45, Breast feeding and the mother, Amsterdam, 1976, Elsevier Scientific Publishing Co.
11. Blass, E.M., and Teicher, M.H.: Suckling, Science 210:15, 1980.
12. Bowen-Jones, A., Thompson, C., and Drewett, R.F.: Milk flow and sucking rates during breast-feeding, Dev. Med. Child. Neurol. 24:626, 1982.
13. Brazelton, T.B.: Effect of maternal medication on the neonate and his behavior, J. Pediatr. 58:513, 1961.
14. Brenman, H.S., et al.: Multisensor nipple recording oral variables, J. Appl. Physiol. 26:494, 1969.
15. Brown, M.S. and Hurlock, J.T.: Preparation of

the breast for breastfeeding, Nurs. Res. **24:**448, 1975.

16. Bulte, N.F., et al.: Evaluation of the deuterium dilution technique against the test-weighing procedure for the determination of breast milk intake, Am. J. Clin. Nutr. **37:**996, 1983.

17. Burke, P.M.: Swallowing and the organization of sucking in the human newborn, Child Dev. **48:**523, 1977.

18. Caldeyro-Barcia, R.: Milk ejection in women. In Reynolds, M., and Folley, S.J., editors: Lactogenesis, Philadelphia, 1969, University of Pennsylvania Press.

19. Christensen, S., Dubignon, J., and Campbell, D.: Variations in intra-oral stimulation and nutritive sucking, Child Dev. **47:**539, 1976.

20. Cobo, E., et al.: Neurohypophyseal hormone release in the human. II. Experimental study during lactation, Am. J. Obstet. Gynecol. **97:**519, 1967.

21. Conner, A.E.: Elevated levels of sodium and chloride in milk from mastitic breast, Pediatrics **63:**910, 1979.

22. Countryman, B.A.: Breast care in the early puerperium, J. Obstet. Gynecol. Nurs. **2:**36, 1973.

23. Cross, B.A.: Comparative physiology of milk removal, Symp. Zool. Soc. **41:**193, 1977.

24. Davis, H.V., et al.: Effects of cup, bottle, and breast feeding on oral activities of newborn infants, Pediatrics **2:**549, 1948.

25. Dawood, M.Y., et al.: Oxytocin release and plasma anterior pituitary and gonadal hormones in women during lactation, J. Clin. Endocrinol. Metab. **52:**678, 1981.

26. Deem, H., and McGeorge, M.: Breastfeeding, N.Z. Med. J. **57:**539, 1958.

27. Devereux, W.P.: Acute puerperal mastitis, Am. J. Obstet. Gynecol. **108:**78, 1970.

28. Drewett, R.F.: Returning to the suckled breast: a further test of Hall's hypothesis, Early Hum. Dev. **6:**161, 1982.

29. Elder, M.S.: The effects of temperature and position on the sucking pressure of newborn infants, Child. Dev. **41:**95, 1970.

30. Evans, R.W., et al.: Maternal diet and infantile colic in breast-fed infants, Lancet **1:**1340, 1981.

31. Fisher, S.E., Painter, M., and Milmor, G.: Swallowing disorders in infancy: Symposium on pediatric otolaryngology, Pediatr. Clin. North Am. **28:**845, 1981.

32. Frantz, K.: Techniques for successfully managing nipple problems and the reluctant nurser in the early postpartum period. In Freier, S., and Eidelman, A., editors: Human milk: its biological and social value, Excerpta Medica, 1980.

33. Gerrard, J.W., and Shenassa, M.: Sensitization to substances in breast milk: recognition, management and significance, Ann. Allergy **51:**1300, 1983.

34. Gibbard, G.F.: Sporadic and epidemic puerperal breast infections, Am. J. Obstet. Gynecol. **65:**1038, 1953.

35. Goldfarb, J., and Tibbetts, E.: Breastfeeding handbook, Hillside, N.J., 1980, Enslow Publishers.

36. Goldsmith, H.S.: Milk-rejection sign of breast cancer, Am. J. Surg. **127:**280, 1974.

37. Gunther, M.: Sore nipples: causes and prevention, Lancet **2:**590, 1945.

38. Gunther, M.: Acute mastitis, Lancet **1:**175, 1956.

39. Hall, B.: Changing composition of human milk and early development of an appetite control, Lancet **1:**779, 1975.

40. Hauben, D.J., and Mahler, D.: A simple method for the correction of the inverted nipple, Plast. Reconstr. Surg. **71:**556, 1983.

41. Hide, D.W., and Guyer, B.M.: Prevalence of infant colic, Arch. Dis. Child. **57:**559, 1982.

42. Hoffman, J.B.: A suggested treatment for inverted nipples, Am. J. Obstet. Gynecol. **66:**346, 1953.

43. Horowitz, M., et al.: Effect of modification of fluid intake on puerperium on serum prolactin levels and lactation, Med. J. Aust. **2:**625, 1980.

44. Howie, P.W., et al.: The relationship between suckling-induced prolactin response and lactogenesis, J. Clin. Endocrinol. Metab. **50:**670, 1980.

45. Jakobsson, I., and Lindberg, T.: Cow's milk as a cause of infantile colic in breast-fed infants, Lancet **2:**437, 1978.

46. Jakobsson, I., and Lindberg, T.: Cow's milk proteins cause infantile colic in breast-fed infants: a double-blind crossover study, Pediatrics **71:**268, 1983.

47. Johnson, P., and Salisbury, D.M.: Breathing and sucking during feeding in the newborn. In Bosma, J.F., and Showacre, J., editors: Development of upper respiratory anatomy and function, Bethesda, 1975, National Institutes of Health.

48. Kron, R.E., Stein, M., and Goddard, K.E.: Newborn sucking behavior affected by obstetric sedation, Pediatrics **37:**1012, 1966.

49. Leonard, E.L., Trykowski, L.E., and Kirkpatrick, B.V.: Nutritive sucking in high-risk neonates after perioral stimulation, Phys. Ther. **60:**299, 1980.

50. L'Esperance, C.M.: Pain or pleasure: the dilemma of early breastfeeding, Birth Fam. J. **7:**21, 1980.

51. Lozoff, B., et al.: The mother-newborn relationship: limits of adaptability, J. Pediatr. **91:**1, 1977.

52. Marshall, B.R., Hepper, J.K., and Zirbel, C.C.: Sporadic Puerperal Mastitis, JAMA **233:**1377, 1975.

53. McNeilly, A.S., et al.: Release of oxytocin and prolactin in response to suckling, Br. Med. J. **286:**257, 1983.

54. Newton, M., and Newton, N.: The let-down reflex in human lactation, J. Pediatr. **33:**698, 1948.

55. Newton, M., and Newton, N.: The normal course and management of lactation, Clin. Obstet. Gynecol. **5:**44, 1962.

56. Newton, N.: Nipple pain and nipple damage problems in the management of breast feeding, J. Pediatr. **41:**411, 1952.

57. Newton, N., and Newton, M.: Relationship of ability to breast feed and maternal attitudes toward breast feeding, Pediatrics **5:**869, 1950.

58. Noel, G.L., Suh, H.K., and Frantz, A.G.: Prolactin release during nursing and breast stimulation, J. Clin. Endocrinol. Metab. **38:**413, 1974.

59. Nowlis, G.H., and Kessen, W.: Human newborns differentiate differing concentrations of sucrose and glucose, Science **191:**865, 1976.

60. Nysenbaum, A.N., and Smart, J.L.: Sucking behavior and milk intake of neonates in relation to milk fat content, Early Hum. Dev. **6:**205, 1982.

61. Pollitt, E., Consolazio, B., and Goodkin, F.: Changes in nutritive sucking during a feed in two-day and thirty-day-old infants, Early Hum. Dev. **5:**201, 1981.

62. Raphael, D.: The tender gift: breast feeding, New York, 1976, Schocken Books, Inc.

63. Rayner, C.R.: The correction of permanently inverted nipples, Br. J. Plast. Surg. **33:**413, 1980.

64. Riordan, J: A practical guide to breastfeeding. St. Louis, 1983, The C.V. Mosby Co.

65. Salisbury, D.M.: Bottle-feeding: influence of teat hole size on suck volume, Lancet **1:**655, 1975.

66. Skoog, T., Surgical correction of inverted nipples, J. Am. Med. Wom. Assoc. **20:**931, 1965.

67. Süsswein, J.: Zur Physiologie des Trinkens beim Säugling, Arch. Kinder. Heilkd. **40:**68, 1905.

68. Talbot, F.B.: Eczema in childhood, Med. Clin. North Am. **1:**985, 1918.

69. Thomsen, A.C.: Infectious mastitis and occurrence of antibody-coated bacteria in milk, Am. J. Obstet. Gynecol. **144:**350, 1982.

70. Toppozada, M.K., El-Rahman, H.A., and Soliman, A.Y.: Prostaglandins as milk ejectors: the nose as a new route of administration, Adv. Prost. Thrombox. Leukotr. Res. **12:**449, 1983.

71. Weitzman, R.E., et al.: The effect of nursing on neurohypophyseal hormone and prolactin secretion in human subjects, J. Clin. Endocrinol. Metab. **51:**836, 1980.

72. Whitfield, M.E., Kay, R., and Stevens, S.: Validity of routine clinical test weighing as a measure of the intake of breast-fed infants, Arch. Dis. Child. **56:**919, 1981.

73. Whitley, N.: Preparation for breastfeeding: a one-year followup of 34 nursing mothers, J.O.G.N. **7:**44, 1975.

74. Wolff, P.H.: Sucking patterns of infant mammals, Brain Behav. Evol. **1:**354, 1968.

75. Wolff, P.H.: The serial organization of sucking in the young infant, Pediatrics **42:**943, 1968.

76. Woolridge, M.W., Baum, J.D., and Drewett, R.F.: Does a change in the composition of human milk affect sucking patterns and milk intake, Lancet **2:**1292, 1980.

77. Woolridge, M.W., Baum, J.D., and Drewett, R.F.: Effect of a traditional and of a new nipple shield on sucking patterns and milk flow, Early Hum. Dev. **4:**357, 1980.

78. Woolridge, M.W., et al.: The continuous measurement of milk intake at a feed in breast-fed babies, Early Hum. Dev. **6:**365, 1982.

79. Young, D.: Personal communication, 1978.

Diet and dietary supplements for the mother and infant

9

The Committee on Recommended Dietary Allowances of the Food and Nutrition Board considers the question of diet for the lactating mother fully answered by saying the diet should supply somewhat more of each nutrient, except vitamin D, than that recommended for the nonpregnant female. Most writings for the nursing mother make the sweeping statement that maternal diet during lactation should be simple and well balanced with several glasses of milk and extra calories. All over the world women produce adequate and even abundant milk on very inadequate diets.[27] Women in primitive cultures with modest but adequate diets produce milk without any obvious detriment to themselves and none of the fatigue and loss of well-being that some well-fed Western mothers seem to experience.

IMPACT OF MATERNAL DIET ON MILK PRODUCTION

Much can be learned from the study of the diets of lactating women of different cultures[28] about critical dietary differences. Accepting the limitations imposed by the methods of sampling and the variations inherent in pumping samples (associated with time of day and length of lactation), there are some important observations.

Volume

The volume of milk produced by mothers has been measured in many studies and in many countries. Malnutrition does seem to have an effect on the total volume of milk produced. In the extreme, when famine occurs the milk supply dwindles and ceases, with ultimate starvation of the infant. The classic study in our time is the report of Smith[41] on the effects of maternal undernutrition on the newborn infant in the Hunger Winter in Holland in 1944 to 1945. It was reported that the volume of milk was slightly diminished but the duration of lactation was not affected. The latter is a testimony of courage rather than diet. Analysis of milk produced showed no significant deviations from normal chemical structure. Milk was produced at the expense of maternal tissue.

In countries where foods supplied vary with the season, milk supplies drop 1 dl/day during periods of increased food shortage. Studies continue on lactation performance of poorly nourished women around the world including Burma, The Gambia, New Guinea, and Ethiopia as well as among the Navajo. Results continue to reflect an impact on quantity, not quality, of milk.[7,11,15,31,33,39]

When food is supplemented, the volume output and protein content increase (Table 9-1). Edozien et al.[13] showed in a Nigerian village that the ultimate result of supplementing maternal diet with protein and kilocalories was an increased rate of weight gain in the infant. Sosa et al.[42] have shown a dramatic increase in milk volume by supplementing maternal diets in Guatemala (Fig. 9-1, A). The weight gain in these infants is shown in Figure 9-1, B. Thus an inadequate diet seemed to affect volume and not the composition because the breast depleted the maternal stores of nutrients to maintain the proper composition of milk.

Of great concern, however, is the report of dietary supplementation of Gambian nursing mothers in which the lactational performance was not affected by increased calories (700 kcal/day).[36] The supplement produced a slight initial improvement in maternal body weight and subcutaneous fat, but not in milk output. Whether the mothers utilized the increased energy to work harder farming or whether the infants did not stimulate increased milk production is unresolved. These observations suggest that other

Table 9-1. Effect of maternal dietary supplementation with protein on the volume and protein content of breast milk and weight gained by baby (Nigeria)*

	Daily protein intake					
	50 g (initially, mean ± SD)	100 g (mean ± SD)	P	25 g (initially, mean ± SD)	100 g (mean ± SD)	P
Number of subjects	7	7		3	3	
Total milk solids (g/100 ml)	13.8 ± 1.3	13.4 ± 0.9		12.0 ± 0.6	11.9 ± 0.5	
Milk protein (g/100 ml)	1.61 ± 0.15	1.57 ± 0.19		1.20 ± 0.21	1.25 ± 0.23	
Milk lactose (g/100 ml)	8.1 ± 0.9	7.9 ± 1.0		7.3 ± 1.4	8.0 ± 1.8	
Milk produced (ml/day)	742 ± 16	872 ± 32	<0.05	817 ± 59	1059 ± 63	<0.05
Milk consumed (ml/day)	617 ± 15	719 ± 10	<0.05	777 ± 38	996 ± 74	<0.05
Weight gained by infant (g/day)	30.4 ± 3.6	45.7 ± 2.0	<0.05	10.5 ± 3.6	32.2 ± 10.1	<0.05

From Edozien, J.C., Rahim-Khan, M.A., and Waslien, C.I.: J. Nutr. 106:312, 1976, copyright © American Institute of Nutrition.
*Subjects were fed the initial diets for the first 14 days and then a diet providing 100 g protein/day for the next 14 days. Results for each subject represent the mean values for milk samples collected during days 8 to 14 (for initial diet) and days 21 to 28 (for diet providing 100 g protein/day). Duration of lactation for all subjects was between 30 and 90 days.

assessments are necessary before conclusions about supplementation are revised. The Committee on Nutrition of the Academy of Pediatrics suggests that the data in support of the value of protein supplements justify a recommendation that malnourished mothers receive their additional supplements.[9]

Protein content

Since the recent work of Hambraeus et al. has reestablished the norms for protein in human milk to be 0.8 to 0.9 g/100 ml in well-nourished mothers, figures from previous studies will have to be recalculated to consider the fact that all nitrogen in human milk is not protein (25% of the nitrogen is nonprotein nitrogen [NPN] in human milk, and 5% of the nitrogen is NPN in bovine milk). The protein content of milk from poorly nourished mothers is surprisingly high.[34] An increase in dietary protein increases volume but not overall protein content, given the normal variations seen in healthy well-nourished women.

Observations made over a 20-month period of continued lactation showed that milk quality did not change although the quantity decreased slightly, which Von Mural[44] attributed to the decreasing demand of a child who is receiving other nourishment. Therefore, the total protein available with the decreased volume of milk and increased weight of the child decreased from 2.2 g/kg of body weight to 0.45 g/kg. The need for additional protein sources for the child after 1 year of age becomes obvious (Table 9-2).

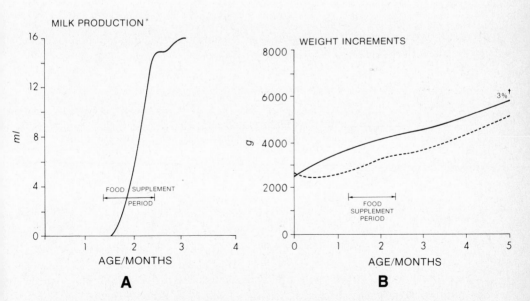

Fig. 9-1. A, Increments in milk production during maternal supplementation period. *Milliliters of milk obtained 1 hour after milk production. B, Weight increments of infants during maternal supplementation and follow-up period. †Boston growth curves. (From Sosa, R., Klaus, M., and Urrutia, J.J.: J. Pediatr. **88:**668, 1976.)

Table 9-2. Constituents of maternal milk in areas of socioeconomic deprivation compared to average figures from the Western world

Constituent	Western world	India, New Guinea, and Pakistan
Protein (g/100 ml of milk)	1.16	0.9
Total lipids (g/100 ml of milk)	4.78	2.5
Lactose (g/100 ml of milk)	6.95	6.20
Phospholipids (mg/100 ml of milk)	2.3	1.11
Cholesterol (mg/100 ml of milk)	18.8	21.1
Calcium (mg/100 ml of milk)	30.9	28.4

Modified from Jelliffe, D.B., and Jelliffe, E.F.P.: Human milk in the modern world, New York, 1978, Oxford University Press.

Table 9-3. The nutritional state of healthy and malnourished mothers

Factors	Apparently healthy		Clinically malnourished	
	Range	Mean	Range	Mean
Arm circumference (cm)	20-40	32.9	16-22	19.3
Weight (% of predicted)	80-168	121.4	76-96	85.1
Serum albumin (g/100 ml)	2.8-5.9	3.81	1.6-3.2	2.53
Urea N/Creatine N	6-44	22.1	2-26	11.3
NSIM*	82.5-152.5	116.3	50-95	71.5

Modified from Hanafy, M.M., et al.: J. Trop. Pediatr. 18:188, 1972.
*Nutritional state index of mothers.

A very painstaking study by Hanafy et al.[24] comparing maternal nutrition and lactation performance demonstrates what most clinicians have believed must be true: the well-fed lactating mother is more likely to produce a healthy infant. The investigators compared two groups of urban mothers of a moderate to poor socioeconomic standard in Egypt. The groups were similar except for the state of nutrition that was assessed (Table 9-3). The comparison of their milks is presented in Table 9-4. The ultimate goal of lactation is a healthy, growing infant. One must recognize that the foundation for good nutrition in any infant is established in utero. Nonetheless, significant differences in growth were shown by the two groups (Table 9-5).

The effect of very low-protein (8% of energy) and very high-protein (20% of energy) diets on the protein and nitrogen composition of breast milk in three healthy Swedish women "in full lactation" was significant.[20] High-protein diets produced higher production and greater concentrations of total nitrogen, true protein, and NPN. The increased NPN was due to increased urea levels and free amino acids. The 24-hour outputs of lactoferrin, lactalbumin, and serum albumin were not significantly higher. The practical significance, except as related to fad diets, of these results is limited because the diets were extreme and were maintained for only 4 days. The impact on human nutritional physiology, however, is significant.

Table 9-4. Comparison of the milks of healthy and malnourished mothers

Factors	Apparently healthy		Clinically malnourished	
	Range	Mean	Range	Mean
Protein (g/100 ml)	0.95-1.36	1.09	0.76-1.32	0.93
Lactose (g/100 ml)	5.58-7.95	6.65	4.08-8.29	6.48
Fat (g/100 ml)	2.8-6.8	4.43	2.8-6.2	4.01
Calories (kcal/100 ml)	61-92	70.8	48-78	65.8
Amount (ml/day)	450-1290	922	180-1770	723
Protein (g/day)	4.3-15.0	10.02	1.6-14.9	6.65
Calories (kcal/day)	310-900	648	100-1080	475

Modified from Hanafy, M.M., et al.: J. Trop. Pediatr. 18:188, 1972.

Table 9-5. Comparison of the infants of healthy and malnourished mothers

Factors	Apparently healthy		Clinically malnourished	
	Range	Mean	Range	Mean
Age (mo)	1-10	5.0	1-12	4.7
Arm circumference (% of predicted)*	43-133	72	43-102	70
Weight (% of predicted)*	60-139	102	43-120	86
Height (% of predicted)*	87-106	94	76-106	93
Serum albumin (g/100 ml)	1.8-4.6	3.11	1.2-3.7	2.50
NSII†	55-119	83	45-101	70

Modified from Hanafy, M.M., et al.: J. Trop. Pediatr. 18:189, 1972.
*Percent of predicted value.
†Nutritional state index of infants.

Fat and cholesterol

Considerable interest has been focused on the impact of dietary fat and cholesterol on the composition of human milk. Fat is the main source of kilocalories in human milk for the infant. The concern about fat composition in terms of the polyunsaturated fatty acid (PUFA) to saturated fatty acid ratio (P/S ratio) and the high level of cholesterol normally found in breast milk have led to monitoring of mothers on altered lipid intakes. Potter and Neste[35] studied lactating women who were placed on one of two experimental diets after a period of a study of their normal Australian diet, which includes 400 to 600 mg of cholesterol/day and fat that is rich in saturated fatty acids. Following this baseline study, the mothers were either given diet A, with 580 mg cholesterol and a high level of saturated fats, or diet B, with 110 mg cholesterol and a higher level of polyunsaturated fats from vegetable oils. A second study was carried out with the two diets high in either saturated or unsaturated fats, but the cholesterol remained the same, 345 to 380 mg/day.

The low-cholesterol diets lowered the maternal blood cholesterol but not the triglyceride levels. The cholesterol level of the milk, however, was unaffected in any diet combination. The increase in PUFA in the diet rapidly increased the levels of linoleate in the milk to twice the previous level at the expense of myristate and palmitate. Protein levels remained the same in the milk throughout the study. Infant plasma cholesterol levels decreased in response to an increase in the concentration of linoleate in the milk. The significant dietary change seemed to depend on the consumption of high PUFA and low cholesterol to alter the levels in the milk and thus in the infant's plasma (Table 9-6).

The synthesis of fatty acids up to the carbon number of 16, as well as the direct desaturation of stearic acid into oleic acid, can take place in the mammary gland, while longer chain fatty acids come directly from plasma triglycerides (see Chapter 4). The intake of both carbohydrate and fat must be taken into account when evaluating maternal diet, because high-carbohydrate diets increase lauric acid and myristic acid and moderate levels of carbohydrate influence linoleic acid.

When serum lipids are measured in African women, accustomed to a low fat intake, the levels are relatively low and the women are virtually free of coronary heart disease.[2] Among long-lactating (1-2 years minimum) African mothers, the amount of fat in their daily milk is of the same order as that ingested in their habitual diet. In spite of this, they are not significantly hypolipidemic when compared with nonlactators.

Guthrie and associates[22] have provided data on the fatty acid patterns of human milk in correlation with the current American diet, which has a high P/S ratio. Compared with previous studies in 1953, 1958, and 1967, there was a shift toward higher levels of $C_{18:2}$ fatty acids, linoleic acid, and $C_{18:3}$, linolenic acid. Depot fat reflects dietary fatty acid patterns and thus the pool for mammary gland synthesis of milk fats. The mammary gland can dehydrogenate saturated and monosaturated fatty acids.

The habitual diet of healthy primiparas in Finland was associated with breast milk containing 3.8% fat.[45] Their diet was 16% protein, 39% fat, and 45% carbohydrate. Half the fatty acids of the diet and the milk were saturated and one third were monoenoic. PUFAs were 15% of the diet and 13% of the breast milk, with a P/S ratio of 0.3 for both. The maternal diet had no effect on total fat content of the milk except for the low level of oleic acid, which is apparently peculiar to Finnish breast milk.

A word of caution on the lowering of fats in the diet inordinately—evaluation of the effects of a low-fat maternal diet on neonatal rats by Sinclair and Crawford[40] is pertinent. They made the distinction between two types of lipid in animals: storage and structural. This is correlated with histologic findings of visible and invisible fats. Visible

Table 9-6. Lipid concentrations of mature human milk

Study	Plan	Diet		Lipid concentration in milk		
		Saturation of fat*	Cholesterol (mg/day)	Cholesterol (mg/100 ml)	Triglyceride (g/100 ml)	Phospholipid (mg P/100 ml)
I (n = 7)	A	S	580	18.1 ± 2.7†	3.42 ± 0.61	4.04 ± 0.71
	B	P	110	19.3 ± 3.6	3.57 ± 0.82	4,18 ± 0.91
II (n = 3)	C	S	380	23.3 ± 2.3	4.11 ± 0.42	
	D	P	345	21.3 ± 2.4	4.12 ± 0.56	

From Potter, J.M., and Nestel, P.J.: Am. J. Clin. Nutr. **29:**54, 1976.
*S, rich in saturated fatty acids (P/S ~ 0.07); P, rich in polyunsaturated fatty acids (P/S ~ 1.3).
†Mean ± SEM.

fats are triglycerides found in body depots. Invisible or structural fats include phospho-glycerides, sphingolipids, and some neutral lipids, including cholesterol. The structural fats are key constituents of cellular membranes, certain enzymes, and myelin. The brain contains more structural lipids than protein.

Sinclair and Crawford[40] found that neonatal rats born to mothers raised on low-fat diets had a higher mortality, and survivors had smaller body, brain, and liver weights than controls. The lipid content of the body, brain, and liver was significantly less than controls. During life, the rat pups had depended entirely on their mother's milk for nutrition.

Lactose

The lactose level is recognized as being reasonably stable in human milk, which may be a function of the fact that lactose is a determinant of volume. Changes in the carbohydrate levels in the diet have been studied by Morrison[32] and reported by Hytten and Thomson.[26] Comparison of mothers on diets with three different levels of carbo-hydrate shows that the amounts of protein, fat, and carbohydrate in their milk are similar (Table 9-7).

Water

There are no data to support the assumption that increasing fluid intake will increase milk volume. Conversely, restricting fluids has not been shown to decrease milk vol-ume, according to Hytten and Thomson.[26] From a practical standpoint, mothers have an increased thirst, which usually maintains a need for added fluid intake. When fluids are restricted, mothers will experience a decrease in urine output, not in milk. From a management standpoint, sharply decreasing fluids to prevent engorgement in the mother who is not lactating is ineffectual and only adds another inconvenience and discomfort.

Kilocalories

The caloric content, sample by sample, of milk from well-nourished mothers does vary somewhat but averages about 75 kcal/100 ml. Since fat is the chief source of kilocalories, the fat content has the greatest impact on total kilocalories, with lactose

Table 9-7. Effect of various carbohydrate diets on milk composition

Milk components	Carbohydrate level in diet (g/kg of body weight)		
	5-6	6-7	7-8
Protein (g/100 ml)	1.168	1.146	1.177
Fat (g/100 ml)	4.09	4.40	4.67
Lactose (g/100 ml)	7.30	7.38	7.38

Modified from Hytten, F.E., and Thomson, A.M.: Nutrition of the lactating woman. In Kon, S.K., and Cowie, A.T., editors: Milk: the mammary gland and its secretion, vol. II, New York, 1961, Academic Press, Inc.; and Morrison, S.D.: Technical communication bulletin no. 18, London, 1952, Commonwealth Bureau of Animal Nutiriton.

and protein also contributing to the total. Thus, in malnourished mothers, the caloric content may be reduced.

Body fat increases during pregnancy and decreases during lactation. Changes in the adipose depot are primarily due to change in fat cell size, not number. Adipose tissue fatty acid synthesis remains low throughout lactation, as does lipoprotein lipase activity. Mammary lipoprotein lipase activity, on the other hand, increases and remains high during lactation.[43]

How does this correlate with the caloric needs of the mother to produce the milk? The calculations for energy requirement have been made by comparing the energy intakes of nursing mothers and nonnursing mothers who were matched for other variables. English and Hitchcock[15] found that nursing mothers consumed 2460 kcal daily and nonnursing mothers consumed 1880 kcal, a net difference of 580 kcal (Tables 9-8 and 9-9).

Lactation will not produce a net drain on the mother if the amount of energy available and the requirement of any given nutrient are replaced in the diet. There is an energy cost of milk production because the breast does not work at 100% efficiency. During pregnancy, fat and other nutrients are stored for the fetus and in preparation for lactation. Lactation is subsidized, as is fetal growth, by maternal stores, even though the diet on any given day may be relatively deficient in a specific nutrient. This can be clarified by Fig. 9-2, which shows that diet and stores are available for milk, as well as for maintenance of the mother.

The energy requirement can be calculated by determining the caloric content of the milk itself, plus an allowance for the energy cost of production. Using this formula, if there is 850 ml of milk with 600 kcal and the production efficiency is estimated at 60%,

Table 9-8. Average daily intake of nutrients by 20 Australian women during the second and third trimesters of pregnancy*

	Second trimester	Third trimester
Weight (kg)	58.7 ± 1.53	63.5 ± 1.42
Height (cm)	163.1 ± 1.38	163.1 ± 1.38
Age (yr)	25 ± 1.0	25 ± 1.0
Protein (g)	75.5 ± 2.98	70.7 ± 2.63
Fat (g)	95.0 ± 3.41	85.8 ± 4.40
Calories (kcal)	2150 ± 64	2030 ± 80
Calcium (mg)	1097 ± 90	1072 ± 70
Iron (mg)	11.3 ± 0.28	10.1 ± 0.36
Vitamin A value (IU)	8467 ± 940	8750 ± 857
Thiamin (mg)	1.1 ± 0.05	1.0 ± 0.05
Riboflavin (mg)	2.1 ± 0.14	2.0 ± 0.13
Nicotinic acid equivalent (mg)	24 ± 0.7	22 ± 0.8
Ascorbic acid (mg)	101 ± 9.1	97 ± 7.0
Calories (kcal/kg of body weight)	36.6	32.0

From English, R.M., and Hitchcock, N.E.: Br. J. Nutr. 22:15, 1968.
*Mean values with their standard errors.

Table 9-9. Weight changes of Australian women related to physical activity, calorie intake, appetite, and dietary advice

Group	Weight (kg)*	Physical activity	Calorie intake (kcal)*	Appetite	Dietary advice
Breastfeeders					
Nonpregnant	54.5 ± 1.92 (recall)	Grade 1†	—	Normal	None
Third trimester of pregnancy	62.3 ± 2.11	Between grade 0† and grade 1†	2090 ± 78	Decrease noted by 10 subjects (62%)	Restrict calorie intake
6-8 weeks postpartum	55.4 ± 1.77	Grade 1†	2460 ± 111	Increase noted by 6 subjects (38%)	None
6 months postpartum or after cessation of breastfeeding	54.1 ± 2.06	Grade 1†	2260 ± 95	Normal	None
Nonbreastfeeders					
Nonpregnant	52.6 ± 1.89 (recall)	Grade 1†	—	Normal	None
Third trimester of pregnancy	62.3 ± 1.44	Between grade 0† and grade 1†	1910 ± 110	Decrease noted by 6 subjects (60%)	Restrict calorie intake
6-8 weeks postpartum	54.5 ± 1.98	Grade 1†	1880 ± 161	Normal	None
6 months postpartum	53.0 ± 2.06	Grade 1†	1980 ± 193	Normal	None

From English, R.M., and Hitchcock, N.E.: Br. J. Nutr. 22:16, 1968.
*Mean values with their standard errors; ± SE.
†National Health and Medical Research Council: Nutrition Committee (1965).

ENERGY UTILIZATION
IN LACTATION

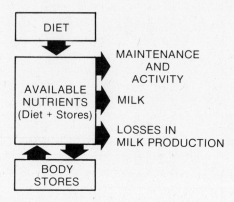

Fig. 9-2. Energy utilization in lactation, showing availability of body stores and dietary sources.

then the additional caloric need each day will be 1000 kcal. English and Hitchcock[15] collected their data between days 6 and 8 postpartum, when milk production is adequate for a newborn and the mother may be less active. If one assumes a production efficiency of 90%, as stated by Worthington[47] then, indeed, the added caloric requirement to produce 850 ml of milk is less (945 kcal).

Vitamins

WATER-SOLUBLE VITAMINS.   Water-soluble vitamins move with ease from serum to milk; thus, their dietary fluctuation is more apparent. Levels of water-soluble vitamins in milk are raised or lowered by change in the maternal diet. Vitamin C levels reflect ingestion of vitamin C–laden beverages within 30 minutes. It has been pointed out by Anderson et al.[3] that the body's requirement for vitamin C increases under stress, including lactation. Furthermore, the vitamin C content of human organs at autopsy is much higher in the neonate than at any other time of life. This is true of all the major organs, including the brain.

The level of B vitamins, also water soluble, reflects dietary intake. The levels are affected acutely by maternal diet. Infantile beriberi is not unheard of in seemingly normal infants nursed by apparently well-nourished mothers with thiamin-deficient diets. The influence of maternal diet has been pointed out dramatically in the recently reported case of megaloblastic anemia and methylmalonic aciduria and homocystinuria in the breastfed infant of a strict vegetarian. Vitamin B_{12} exists in all animal protein but not in vegetable protein. A strict vegetarian would require B_{12} supplements during pregnancy and lactation. B_{12} deficiency in infants has also been seen in New Delhi, where mothers had B_{12}-deficient milk. These infants also had megaloblastic anemia.

Riboflavin (B_2) requirements of lactating women in The Gambia in a controlled study showed the minimum to be 2.5 mg/day to maintain normal biochemical status in the mother and adequate levels of B_2 in her milk.[6] This level is higher than that recommended in the United States and the United Kingdom. The pantothenic acid content of human milk does not vary appreciably with dietary variations in well-nourished mothers but the overall intake over time does influence milk levels.[29]

Pyridoxine (B_6) intake and milk levels were studied in healthy lactating women by West and Kirksey.[46] There were marked diurnal variations of B_6 levels, with peaks occurring in those mothers taking supplements 3 to 5 hours after a dose. Intakes of two to five times the recommended allowances did not increase the B_6 in the milk. Those taking less than 2.5 mg/day had much lower milk levels (129 μg/L), however.

Deodhar and Ramakrishnan[11] studied the effect of the stage of lactation on levels of vitamins B_1, B_2, B_3, B_{12}, and ascorbic acid. The values remained fairly constant throughout, except for those of B_3, which increased slightly over time. The relationship to socioeconomic group showed an increase in B_3 and B_6 levels with increased status. B_1 was higher in poorer mothers. The effect of diet on vitamin levels in maternal milk is summarized in Tables 9-10 and 9-11.

FAT-SOLUBLE VITAMINS. The concentration of fat-soluble vitamins is of concern because the levels in human milk are less easily improved by dietary changes. The low concentration of vitamin A in human milk is influenced by dietary inadequacies in this country as well as the developing countries. Levels may be marginal, and they may well vary seasonally. Since the levels of vitamin D in human milk appear to be marginal, maternal intake should be closely watched. Vitamin D and vitamin E levels in human milk are not raised by increasing their levels in the maternal diet. Vitamin E is in high levels in human milk, but vitamin D levels are thought to be low. Additional vitamin D has been identified in the aqueous fraction, but whether the aqueous levels are influenced by diet is yet to be determined.

Dark-skinned infants reared in climates where sunlight is minimal may be at significant risk for rickets when breastfed unless attention is given to the possible need for supplements of vitamin D.[5]

Minerals

CALCIUM. Calcium has been associated with bone growth, and concern has been expressed because the total calcium in breast milk is low. The available information is inadequate to determine the requirement for lactation. Studies with radioactive calcium in the nonpregnant adult have shown that there are losses into the gut and through the kidney. Absorption and retention also depend on the reserves in the body. Long-term shortage causes economy of utilization and the apparent requirement is lower. In lacta-

Table 9-10.   Water-soluble vitamins in human milk

| Vitamin | Recognizable clinical deficiency | Effect of maternal supplements | | Effect of dietary intake on milk content |
		In malnourished	In well nourished	
Ascorbic acid	Rare	Yes	No	Yes
Thiamin	Yes	Yes	Yes	Yes
Riboflavin	Unknown	Yes	Yes	Yes
Niacin	Unknown	Yes	Yes	Yes
Pantothenic acid	Unknown	Yes	No	Yes
Pyridoxine	Unknown	Yes	Yes	Unknown
Biotin	Yes	Yes	No	Unknown
Folate	Unknown	Yes	No*	No
Cyanocobalamin	Rare	Yes	Yes	Yes

From the committee on Nutrition, American Academy of Pediatrics: Nutrition and lactation, Pediatrics 68:435, 1981, copyright American Academy of Pediatrics, 1981.
*Thomas, M.R., et al.: unpublished data, 1981.

Table 9-11.   Fat-soluble vitamins in human milk

| Vitamin | Recognizable clinical deficiency | Effect of maternal supplements | | Effect of dietary intake on milk content |
		In malnourished	In well nourished	
D	Yes	Yes	Unknown	Unknown
K	Yes	Unknown	None	None
A	Unknown	Unknown	Yes	Yes
E	Unknown	Unknown	Yes	Unknown

From the Committee on Nutrition, American Academy of Pediatrics: Nutrition and lactation, Pediatrics 68:435, 1981, copyright American Academy of Pediatrics, 1981.

tion, the absorption and retention are greater but not as great as during pregnancy. Atkinson and West[4] showed by scanning transmission techniques that lactating women mobilize about 2% of their skeletal calcium over 100 days of nursing. The calcium content of milk appears to be maintained despite markedly deficient intake, probably because of skeletal stores. The milk calcium levels are the same in mothers of rachitic and nonrachitic infants.

The additional requirement for calcium in the lactating women's diet is 400 mg daily over normal or 1200 mg totally, which is not easily achieved without milk products and may require special attention on the part of the physician.[34]

SODIUM.   The sodium content of milk depends on dietary intake, but unless there is a deliberately low sodium intake, values do not vary significantly with modest restriction.

IRON.   The iron content of milk is not readily affected by the iron content of the diet or the maternal serum iron level. Increases in dietary iron that increase serum levels do not increase iron in the milk, according to Hytten and Thomson.[26] It is important, however, for the mother to replace her iron stores postpartum.

PHOSPHORUS, MAGNESIUM, ZINC, POTASSIUM, AND COPPER.   Phosphorus, magnesium, zinc, potassium, and copper levels in milk are not affected by dietary administration of

Table 9-12. Minerals in human milk

Mineral	Concentration throughout lactation	Facilitated bioavailability	Effect of maternal mineral intake on milk content
Sodium	Declines	Unknown	None (unpublished)
Calcium	Unchanged	Unknown	None
Iron	Unchanged	Facilitated	None
Zinc	Declines	Facilitated	None
Copper	Unchanged	Unknown	None
Manganese	Declines	Unknown	Yes
Selenium	Unknown	Unknown	Unknown
Iodine	Declines	Unknown	Yes
Fluoride	Unknown	Unknown	None

From The Committee on Nutrition, American Academy of Pediatrics: Nutrition and lactation, Pediatrics **68:**435, 1981, copyright American Academy of Pediatrics, 1981.

these elements. Again, however, it is important for the mother to replenish her stores. Dietary potassium may influence milk potassium more significantly. With increasing numbers of women with cardiac and renal disease wishing to lactate, potassium levels in the diet would be of significance in addition to concerns about necessary medications.[30]

IODINE.   Iodine in milk does depend on dietary content. The breast is able to raise the concentration of iodine in the milk above that in the blood, and thus there is an increased danger in giving radioactive iodine to the lactating woman.

FLUORINE.   The data are conflicting as to the impact of dietary fluorine on milk levels.[1,16] Fluorine levels are low in milk, although it has been suggested that fluorine content may be higher than is reflected by present measuring techniques. Fluorine excretion in milk can be increased by giving sodium fluoride by mouth, but the rise is small relative to the dose, according to Hodge and Smith.[25] Milk products in particular have been cited as decreasing the bioavailability of fluorine in adults when administered by sodium fluoride tablet. Thus the use of fluoride medication in the mother is not an effective means of assuring adequate fluorine available in her milk.[14]

The effects of diet on mineral levels in maternal milk are summarized in Table 9-12.

RECOMMENDATIONS FOR NUTRITIONAL SUPPORT DURING LACTATION _____

In the previous section it was noted that the quantity, protein content, and calcium content of milk are relatively independent of maternal nutritional status and diet. Amino acids, lysine and methionine, certain fatty acids, and water-soluble vitamin contents vary with intake. It is important to point out that stores of calcium, minerals, and fat-soluble vitamins need to be replenished. Much of the data collected have varied depending on the method used in collection. The daily intakes believed necessary for infants were determined by feeding infants processed human milk in a bottle, which is not a physiologic standard. It is known, for example, that putting the entire sample in one container removes the natural variation in fat from beginning to end of the feeding.

The Committee on Recommended Dietary Allowances of the Food and Nutrition Board[19] has recommended a balanced diet comparable to one for the nonlactating postpartum patient, with a few additions (Table 9-13). Although the calculated caloric cost of producing 1 L of milk is 940 kcal, it should be noted that during pregnancy most women store 2 to 4 kg of extra tissue in the physiologic preparation for lactation. It is probably necessary, therefore, to add only 500 kcal to the diet, except in women with known high metabolic rates.

Table 9-13.   Components of the average weight gained in normal pregnancy

Component	Amount (g) gained			
	10 wk	20 wk	30 wk	40 wk
Total gain of body weight	650	4000	8500	12500
Fetus	5	300	1500	3300
Placenta	20	170	430	650
Amniotic fluid	30	250	600	800
Increase of:				
Uterus	135	585	819	900
Mammary gland	34	180	360	405
Maternal blood	100	600	1300	1250
Total (rounded)	320	2100	5000	7300
Weight not accounted for	330	1900	3500	5200

Reproduced from Committee on Maternal Nutrition, Food and Nutrition Board, National Research Council: Maternal nutrition and the course of pregnancy, Washington, D.C., 1970, Government Printing Office, p. 64, with the permission of the National Academy of Sciences.

Table 9-14.   Recommended dietary allowances for adult women (ages 23 to 50 years)

	Nonpregnant	Pregnant
Energy (kcal)	2000	2300
Protein (g)	46	76
Vitamin A		
RE*	800	1000
IU	4000	5000
Vitamin D (IU)	200-400	400-600
Vitamin E (αTE)	8	10
Vitamin C (ascorbic acid) (mg)	60	80
Folic acid (μg)	400	800
Niacin (mg)	13	15
Riboflavin (mg)	1.2	1.5
Thiamin (mg)	1.1	1.5
Vitamin B_6 (mg)	2.0	2.6
Vitamin B_{12} (μg)	3.0	4.0
Calcium (mg)	800	1200
Phosphorus (mg)	800	1200
Iodine (μg)	150	175
Iron (mg)	18	18+
Magnesium (mg)	300	450
Zinc (mg)	15	20

Reproduced from Food and Nutrition Board, National Research Council: Recommended daily allowances, ed. 8, Washington, D.C., 1974, Government Printing Office, with the permission of the National Academy of Sciences.
*RE (retinol equivalent) replaces IU (international unit) as the standard measure of vitamin A activity.

Preparation for lactation begins in pregnancy, if not before. The average gains in weight during pregnancy in various organs are noted in Table 9-13.

The recommended dietary allowances (RDA) for pregnancy are compared to the recommendations for an adult woman in Table 9-14. The major daily increases for pregnancy are 300 kcal, 20 g of protein, a 20% increase in all vitamins and minerals except folic acid, which is doubled, and a 33% increase in calcium, phosphorus, and magnesium. The RDA for lactation have been prepared for various age groups and are listed in Table 9-15. It should be noted in comparing the RDA for 19- to 22-year-old lactating women to nonlacting adult women that the increases suggested should provide ample nutrition and replace stores (Table 9-16).

When dietary supplements are suggested, there is concern about increased costs. Cost increases are modest for the standard diet and minimal for the low-budget diet, as demonstrated by Worthington.[47] The cost figures have been adjusted for 1984 levels

Table 9-15.   Recommended dietary allowances for lactation

	Age			
	11-14 years	15-18 years	19-22 years	23-50 years
Body size				
Weight (kg)	46	55	55	55
(lb)	101	120	120	120
Height (cm)	157	163	163	163
(in)	62	64	64	64
Nutrients				
Energy (kcal)	2700	2600	2600	2500
Protein (gm)	66	66	64	64
Vitamin A (RE*)	1200	1200	1200	1200
Vitamin D (μg)	15	15	12.5	10
Vitamin E activity (mg αTE†)	13	13	13	13
Ascorbic acid (mg)	90	100	100	100
Folacin (μg)	500	500	500	500
Niacin (mg‡)	20	19	19	18
Riboflavin (mg)	1.8	1.8	1.8	1.7
Thiamin (mg)	1.6	1.6	1.6	1.5
Vitamin B_6 (mg)	2.3	2.5	2.5	2.5
Vitamin B_{12} (μg)	4.0	4.0	4.0	4.0
Calcium (mg)	1600	1600	1200	1200
Phosphorus (mg)	1600	1600	1200	1200
Iodine (μg)	200	200	200	200
Iron (mg)	18§	18§	18§	18§
Magnesium (mg)	450	450	450	450
Zinc (mg)	25	25	25	25

From Worthington, B.S.: Lactation, human milk, and nutritional considerations. In Worthington, B.S., Vermeersch, J., and Williams, S.R., editors: Nutrition in pregnancy and lactation, 2nd ed., St. Louis, 1981, The C.V. Mosby Co.; modified from Food and Nutrition Board, National Research Council, National Academy of Sciences: Recommended dietary allowances, ed. 9, Washington, D.C., 1980, U.S. Government Printing Office.
*RE = Retinol equivalent.
†α-Tocopherol equivalents; 1 mg d-α-tocopherol = 1 αTE.
‡Although allowances are expressed as niacin, it is recognized that on the average, 1 mg of niacin is derived from each 60 mg of dietary tryptophan.
§Iron needs during lactation are not substantially different from those of nonpregnant women but continued supplementation of the mother for 2 to 3 months after parturition is advisable in order to replenish stores depleted by pregnancy.

Table 9-16. Dietary increases for lactation

	Increase required
Kilocalories	600
Protein (g)	20
Vitamin A (RI)	400
Vitamin D (μg)	5
Vitamin E (mg αTE)	3
Vitamin C (mg)	40
Folacin (μg)	100
Niacin (mg NE)	5
Riboflavin (mg)	0.5
Thiamin (mg)	0.5
B_6 (mg)	0.14
B_{12} (μg)	1.0
Calcium (mg)	400
Phosphorus (mg)	400
Iodine (ug)	50
Iron (mg)	0*
Magnesium (mg)	150
Zinc (mg)	10

*All postpartum women are considered to need 30-60 mg elemental iron for 2 to 3 months to replenish stores.

Table 9-17. Nutrients, amounts, and estimated cost of foods needed to meet additional nutritional requirements of a lactating woman: standard (nonbudget) plan

Suggested foods	Amount	Cost*	Kilo-cal-ories	Pro-tein	Vitamins					Cal-cium	Iron
					A	C	B_1	B_2	B_3		
Milk, fresh, 2%	2 cups	0.25	290	18	700		0.14	0.82	0.4	576	
Meat (round steak)	2 oz	0.45	150	13	35		0.04	0.11	2.8	6	1.7
Vegetable, dark green or yellow, cooked (broccoli)	½ cup ¾ cup	0.15	20	2.5	1990	70	0.07	0.15	0.6	68	0.6
Other vegetable or fruit (grapefruit)	½	0.20	45	1	10	44	0.05	0.02	0.2	19	0.5
Citrus fruit (orange juice)	½ cup	0.10	60	1	275	60	0.11	0.01	0.5	12	0.1
Enriched (or whole-grain) bread	1 slice	0.08	65	3			0.09	0.03	0.8	24	0.8
TOTAL		$1.23	630	38.5	3010	174	0.50	1.14	5.3	705	3.7

Modified from Worthington, B.S.: Lactation, human milk, and nutritional considerations. In Worthington, B.S., Vermeersch, J., and Williams, S.R., editors: Nutrition in pregnancy and lactation, ed. 2, St. Louis, 1981, The C.V. Mosby Co.
*Costs as of Jan. 1984, Rochester, N.Y.

(Tables 9-17 and 9-18). Although one rarely chooses breastfeeding or bottle feeding on the basis of cost, one really needs to consider far more than the price of a few extra maternal kilocalories, and the cost of formula feeding makes a reassuring comparison. Hypoallergenic formulas are even more costly (Table 9-19).

Malnutrition

SPECIAL SUPPLEMENTATION FOR THE LACTATING WOMAN. It has been suggested that supplementing the diet of malnourished mothers with a special formula would be the

Table 9-18. Nutrients, amounts, and estimated cost of food needed to meet additional nutritional requirements of a lactating woman: budget plan

| Suggested foods | Amount | Cost* | Kilo-cal-ories | Pro-tein | Vitamins | | | | | Cal-cium | Iron |
					A	C	B₁	B₂	B₃		
Nonfat dry milk (prepared for drinking)	2 cups	0.14	180	18	20		0.18	0.88	0.40	592	
Peanut butter	2 oz	0.12	190	8			0.04	0.04	4.8	18	0.6
Vegetable, dark green or yellow, cooked (carrots)	½ cup ¾ cup	0.09	25	0.5	7610	4.5	0.04	0.03	0.04	24	0.45
Citrus fruit (tomato juice)	½ cup	0.07	25	1	970	20	0.06	0.04	0.95	86	1.1
Enriched (or whole grain) bread	2 slices	0.15	130	6			0.18	0.06	1.6	48	1.6
TOTAL		$0.57	550	33.5	8600	24.5	0.50	1.05	7.79	768	3.75

Modified from Worthington, B.S.: Lactation, human milk, and nutritional considerations. In Worthington, B.S., Vermeeroch, J., and Williams, S.R., editors: Nutrition in pregnancy and lactation, ed. 2, St. Louis, 1981, The C.V. Mosby Co.
*Costs as of Jan. 1984, Rochester, N.Y.

Table 9-19. Cost per day of the most commonly used prepared formulas, basic equipment, and fuel

Formula	Cost*		Average cost per day	
Formula, 13 oz can, double strength (formula, ready-to-feed, 1 qt)	$0.89	($1.19)	$0.89	($1.19)
12 unbreakable bottles with nipples	9.48		0.06	0.06
12 nipples at 60 cents each	7.20		0.04	0.04
Energy, electricity			0.04	0.04
TOTAL COST			$1.03 to	1.33

Modified from Worthington, B.S.: Lactation, human milk, and nutritional considerations. In Worthington, B.S., Vermeersch, J., and Williams, S.R., editors: Nutrition in pregnancy and lactation, ed. 2, St. Louis, 1981, The C.V. Mosby Co.
*Costs as of Jan. 1984, Rochester, N.Y.

best way to achieve nourishment for mother and child. The infant will then gain the additional advantages of human milk, such as protection against infection. Such formulas have been devised. Sosa et al.[42] have tried this approach in Guatemala.

With the ready availability of well-balanced nutrition supplements today in both supermarkets and drugstores in the form of stable powders, it should not be difficult to initiate a high-protein, vitamin-enriched diet supplementation that is also palatable for the occasional mother who is at nutritional risk. With the inclusion of breastfeeding as a goal in the Women, Infants, and Children (WIC) Program, dietary counseling and supplementation are available for mothers at poverty level to encourage these mothers to breastfeed.

Allergy

In families with a strong history of allergy, a hypoallergenic diet avoiding the common allergens such as wheat and eggs should be recommended. Further details are described in Chapter 15. An allergy prophylaxis scheme is described in Appendix M.

Vegetarian diet

The growing interest in vegetarianism has necessitated the clinician's having a better understanding of the several types of diets and their potential for adequate nutrients and growth as well as the motivation for these diets (Table 9-20). In general, serious vegetarians usually have a greater knowledge of and commitment to good nutrition.[8] Reports of malnutrition among breastfed infants of vegetarians usually focus on the very strict groups such as vegans and those on macrobiotic diets. The dietary risks involved are chiefly with the B vitamins because these vitamins are usually associated with protein, which is also proportionally lower from vegetable sources. An additional concern is the availability of various amino acids in specific concentrations in order to utilize them for protein synthesis. The net protein utilization (NPU) of a food may be considerably lower than total protein content; therefore, it is important when using vegetable sources of protein to use foods with "complementary protein" at the same meal. Vegetarian cookbooks emphasize this.[37] Throughout history, culturally traditional meals have assured complementary proteins.

B_{12} deficiency has been described in vegans because of the absence of animal protein.[48] It is advisable in these cases to supplement diets of the pregnant or lactating woman, as well as of an infant or growing child, with up to 4 mg/day of B_{12}. It has been shown that fermented soybean foods do contain B_{12} as do the single-cell proteins such as yeast.

Reports of growth curves in vegetarian children over the first few years show them to be shorter and leaner than standard, with the greatest effect among the most restricted diets.[12] Breastfed vegetarian infants are usually on the norms for growth with the exception of those receiving minimal vitamin D and calcium as reported in dark-skinned

Table 9-20. Vegetarianism and associated risks

Type of vegetarian	Diet includes	Diet avoids	Risks
Semi-vegetarian	Vegetables, milk products, seafood, poultry	Red meat	Minerals*
Ovo-lacto-vegetarian	Vegetables, milk products, eggs	Flesh foods (meat, seafood, poultry)	Minerals* esp. zinc
Lacto-vegetarian	Vegetables, milk products	Flesh foods, eggs	Minerals* esp. zinc and protein†
Ovo-vegetarian	Vegetables, eggs	Flesh foods, milk products	Minerals* esp. iron and zinc, protein,† riboflavin, vitamin D, B_{12}
Vegan	Only vegetables	Flesh foods, milk products, eggs	Minerals,* protein,† riboflavin, vitamin D, B_{12}
Macrobiotic	Gradual progression to a diet of only cereals		Advanced stage nutritionally inadequate

*Excessive dietary phytates and dietary fiber inhibit absorption of minerals such as iron, zinc, and calcium. Phytates are organic chemicals present in many vegetables and unleavened bread that bind with minerals.
†Diets not using complementary proteins may be deficient in net protein because the NPU is low.

mothers in cloudy climates. Among 34 breastfed infants at 7 months in the Tufts study, three infants were below the tenth percentile for height and weight, one had low weight for length, and three had high weight for length, whereas of the 51 who were not breastfed, six were below the tenth percentile, two had low weight for length, and four had high weight for length.[21]

General recommendations for lactating vegetarian women are as follows:
1. Supplement with soy flour, molasses, and nuts.
2. Use complementary protein combinations.
3. Avoid excessive phytates and bran.
4. Watch protein, iron, calcium, vitamins D, B_{12} and riboflavin to assure adequate intake.

Supplementing the breastfed infant's diet

For the newborn infant, human milk is the ideal food containing all the necessary nutrients. In establishing dietary norms for infants fed cow's milk, many nutrients identified as being needed in the diet were found to exist in greater amounts in cow's milk than in human milk. This does not consider the probability that the nutrient may be in a more bioavailable form in human milk. The specific items in question are protein, sodium, iron, vitamin D, and fluorine.

The Committee on Nutrition of the Academy of Pediatrics[9] has noted that iron deficiency is rare in breastfed infants and attributes this to increased absorption and the absence of microscopic blood loss into the gastrointestinal tract, which is seen in bottle fed infants. The committee recommends a source of iron in solid foods (fortified infant cereal) by 4 to 6 months of age for breastfed infants.

Since rickets have been described in breastfed infants, consideration should be given to the maternal intake of vitamin D and the exposure of the infant to sunshine. Fomon[17] cautions, however, against reliance on sunshine in the first year of life and advises providing infants with 400 IU of vitamin D. Individual discretion is appropriate, since infants of healthy mothers have not been observed to have rickets.

Fomon has stated that fluorine levels in breast milk are not adequate and therefore supplementation should be given. He provides the following dosage scale based on amounts of fluorine in the drinking water.

Fluorine concentration (ppm)	Dosage of fluorine (mg/day)
<0.3	0.25
0.3 to 0.7	0.25
0.8 to 1.1	0.25
>1.1	0

Many breastfed infants have done without fluorine supplementation and have had no adverse dental problems, but the decision should be based on individual determinants, including family dental history.

Dieting while breastfeeding

If one eats a balanced diet of nutritious food, one need not gain weight while nursing. If 940 kcal are used to nourish an average 3-month-old infant, then a mother could lose weight while nursing by not increasing her caloric intake. Weight loss by this method would require attention to selecting nourishing foods and avoiding junk food. With elimination of the "empty calorie" part of a diet, the infant will be provided with adequate nutrients. Fad diets are inappropriate. The high-protein low-carbohydrate diet is apt to increase a mother's blood urea nitrogen level, which would be passed into the milk. Since dieting involves mobilizing fat stores, it should not be pursued if there is a chance there are PBCs, DDT, or any other environmental toxin stored in the fat.

Foods to avoid

The concern about gassy foods causing gas in the breastfed baby has no scientific basis. The normal intestinal flora produces gas from the action on fiber in the intestinal tract. Neither the fiber nor the gas is absorbed from the intestinal tract, or do they enter the milk even though they may afford the mother some discomfort. The acid content of the maternal diet does not affect the milk either because it does not change the pH of the maternal plasma. There are essential oils in such foods as garlic, and some spices that have characteristic odors and flavors may indeed pass into the milk, and an occasional infant objects to their presence.

Some infants do not tolerate certain foods in the mother's diet, predominantly specific vegetables and fruits. Garlic and onions may cause colic in some infants. Cabbage, turnips, broccoli, or beans may also bother others, making them colicky for 24 hours. The same has been said of rhubarb, apricots, and prunes. If a mother questions the effect of a food, she should avoid it or document its effect carefully by watching for colic in the 24 hours following ingestion. In the summer, a heavy diet of melons, peaches, and other fresh fruits may cause colic and diarrhea in the infant. Chocolate rarely lives up to its reputation and can be consumed in moderation without causing colic, diarrhea, or constipation.

Color of milk and maternal diet

Although the color of mature human milk is bluish white and the color of colostrum is yellow to yellow-orange, mothers will occasionally report changes in the color of their milk. Most of these reports can be traced to pigments consumed in the diet. The infant's urine may also turn color.

PINK OR PINK-ORANGE MILK.   Pink-orange was traced to Sunkist orange soda, which contains red and yellow dyes. A case of a breastfed infant with pink to orange urine was reported by Roseman.[38] This combination of food dyes is also used in other brands of soda, fruit drinks, and gelatin desserts.

GREEN MILK.   Several cases of green milk have been reported to us. A careful search of the diet for the offending substance was made in each case. The effect of ingestion of the identified culprit and avoidance of it were then tested to confirm the association with the color in the milk. Several items have been clearly identified. Gatorade (the green beverage), kelp and other forms of seaweed, especially in tablet form, and natural vitamins from health-food sources each have been associated with one or more cases of green milk and usually green urine.

REFERENCES

1. Adair, S.M., and Wei, S.H.Y.: Supplemental fluoride recommendations for infants based on dietary fluoride intake, Caries Res. **12:**76, 1978.
2. Alexander, R.P., et al.: Serum lipids in long-lactating African mothers habituated to a low-fat intake, Atherosclerosis **44:**175, 1982.
3. Anderson, T.W., et al.: To dose or megadose: a debate about vitamin C, Nutr. Today **13:**6, 1978.
4. Atkinson, P.J., and West, R.R.: Loss of skeletal calcium in lactating women, J. Obstet. Gynecol. Br. Commonwealth **77:**555, 1970.
5. Bachrach, S., Fisher, J., and Parks, J.S.: An outbreak of vitamin D-deficiency rickets in a susceptible population, Pediatrics **64:**871, 1979.
6. Bates, C.J., et al.: Riboflavin requirements of lactating Gambian women: a controlled supplementation trial, Am. J. Clin. Nutr. **135:**701, 1982.
7. Butte, N.F., Calloway, D.H., and Van Dozen, J.L.: Nutritional assessment of pregnant and lactating Navajo women, Am. J. Clin. Nutr. **34:**2216, 1981.
8. Christoffer, K.: A pediatric perspective on vegetarian nutrition, Clin. Pediatr. **20:**632, 1981.
9. Committee on Nutrition, Academy of Pediatrics: Iron supplementation for infants, Pediatrics **58:**765, 1976.
10. Committee on Nutrition, Academy of Pediatrics: Nutrition and lactation, Pediatrics **68:**435, 1981.
11. Deodhar, A.D., and Ramakrishnan, C.V.: Studies on human lactation, part II. Effect of socioeconomic status on vitamin content of human milk, Indian J. Med. Res.**47:**352, 1959.
12. Dwyer, J.T., et al.: Preschoolers on alternate lifestyle diets, J. Am. Diet. Assoc. **72:**264, 1978.
13. Edozien, J.C., Khan, M.A.R., and Waslien, C.I.: Human protein deficiency: results of a Nigerian village study, J. Nutr. **106:**312, 1976.
14. Ekstrand, J., and Ehrnebo, M.: Influence of milk products on fluoride bioavailability in man, Eur. J. Clin. Pharmacol. **16:**211, 1979.
15. English, R.M., and Hitchcock, N.E.: Nutrient intakes during pregnancy, lactation and after the cessation of lactation in a group of Australian women, Br. J. Nutr. **22:**615, 1968.
16. Ericsson, Y.: Fluoride excretion in human saliva and milk, Caries Res. **3:**159, 1969.
17. Fomon, S.J.: Infant nutrition, ed. 2, Philadelphia, 1974, W.B. Saunders Co.
18. Fomon, S.J., and Wei, S.H.Y.: Prevention of dental caries in nutritional disorders of children: screening, follow-up, and prevention. Washington, D.C., 1976, Department of Health, Education and Welfare.
19. Food and Nutrition Board, National Research Council: Recommended dietary allowances, ed. 9, Washington, D.C., 1984, National Academy of Sciences.
20. Forsum, E., and Lonnerdal, B.: Effect of protein intake on protein and nitrogen composition of breast milk, Am. J. Clin. Nutr. **33:**1809, 1980.
21. Fulton, J.R., Hutton, C.W., and Sitt., K.R.: Preschool vegetarian children, J. Am. Diet. Assoc. **76:**260, 1980.
22. Guthrie, H.A., Picciano, M.F., and Sheehe, D.: Fatty acid patterns of human milk, J. Pediatr. **90:**39, 1977.
23. Hambraeus, L.: Proprietary milk versus human breast milk in infant feeding: a critical approach from the nutritional point of view. In Neumann, C.G., and Jelliffe, D.B., editors: Symposium on nutrition in pediatrics, Pediatr. Clin. North Am. **24:**17, 1977.
24. Hanafy, M.M., et al.: Maternal nutrition and lactation performance, J. Trop. Pediatr. **18:**187, 1972.
25. Hodge, H.C., and Smith, F.A.: Some public health aspects of water fluoridation. In Shaw, J.H., editor: Fluoridation as a public health measure, Washington, D.C., 1954, American Association for the Advancement of Science.
26. Hytten, F.E., and Thomson, A.M.: Nutrition of the lactating women. In Kon, S.K., and Cowie, A.T., editors: Milk: the mammary gland and its

secretion, vol. II, New York, 1961, Academic Press, Inc.

27. Jelliffe, D.B., and Jelliffe, E.F.P.: Human milk in the modern world, New York, 1978, Oxford University Press.

28. Jelliffe, E.F.P.: Maternal nutrition and lactation. In Ciba Foundation Symposium no. 45, Breast feeding and the mother, Amsterdam, 1976, Elsevier Scientific Publ. Co.

29. Johnston, L., Vaughn, L., and Fox, H.M.: Pantothenic acid content of human milk, Am. J. Clin. Nutr. **34:**2205, 1981.

30. Keenan, B.S., et al: Diurnal and longitudinal variations in human milk sodium and potassium: Implications for nutrition and physiology, Am. J. Clin. Nutr. **35:**527, 1982.

31. Khin-Maung-Naing, Tin-Tin-Oo, Kywe-Thein, and Nwe-New-Hlaing: Study on lactation performance of Burnese mothers, Am. J. Clin. Nutr. **33:**2665, 1980.

32. Morrison, S.D.: Technical communication bulletin no. 18, London, 1952, Commonwealth Bureau of Animal Nutrition.

33. Paul, A.A., Muller, E.M., and Whitehead, R.G.: The quantitative effects of maternal dietary energy intake on pregnancy and lactation in rural Gambian women. Trans. Roy. Soc. Trop. Med. Hygiene **73:**686, 1979.

34. Pitkin, R.M.: Nutritional support in obstetrics and gynecology, Clin. Obstet. Gynecol. **19:**489, 1976.

35. Potter, J.M., and Nestel, P.J.: The effects of dietary fatty acids and cholesterol on the milk lipids of lactating women and the plasma cholesterol of breast-fed infants, Am. J. Clin. Nutr. **29:**54, 1976.

36. Prentice, A.M., et al.: Dietary supplementation of Gambian nursing mothers and lactational performance, Lancet **2:**886, 1980.

37. Robertson, L., Flinders, C., and Godfrey, B.: Laurel's kitchen: a handbook for vegetarian cookery and nutrition, Petaluma, Calif. 1976, Nilgiri Press. 1976.

38. Roseman, B.D.: Sunkissed urine (letter to the editor), Pediatrics **67:**443, 1981.

39. Schutz, Y., Lechtig, A., and Bradfield, R.B.: Energy expenditures and food intakes of lactating women in Guatemala, Am. J. Clin. Nutr. **33:**892, 1980.

40. Sinclair, A.J., and Crawford, M.A.: The effect of a low-fat maternal diet on neonatal rats, Br. J. Nutr. **29:**127, 1973.

41. Smith, C.A.: Effects of maternal undernutrition upon newborn infants in Holland (1944–1945), J. Pediatr. **30:**229, 1947.

42. Sosa, R., Klaus, M., and Urrutia, J.J.: Feed the nursing mother, thereby the infant, J. Pediatr. **88:**668, 1976.

43. Steingrimsdottir, L., Brasel, J.A., and Greenwood, M.R.C.: Diet, pregnancy, and lactation: effects on adipose tissue, lipoprotein lipase, and fat cell size, Metabolism **29:**837, 1980.

44. Von Muralt, A.: Maternal nutrition and lactation. In Ciba Foundation Symposium no. 45, Breast feeding and the mother, Amsterdam, 1976, Elsevier Scientific Publ. Co.

45. Vuori, E., et al.: Maternal diet and fatty acid pattern of breast milk, Acta Paediatr. Scand. **71:**959, 1982.

46. West, K.D., and Kirksey, A.: Influence of vitamin B_6 intake on the content of the vitamin in human milk, Am. J. Clin. Nutr. **29:**961, 1976.

47. Worthington, B.S.: Lactation, human milk, and nutritional considerations. In Worthington, B.S., Vermeersch, J., and Williams, S.R., editors: Nutrition in pregnancy and lactation, ed. 2, St. Louis, 1981, The C.V. Mosby Co.

48. Zmora, E., Gorodescher, R., and Bar-Ziv, J.: Multiple nutritional deficiencies in infants from a strict vegetarian community, Am. J. Dis. Child. **133:**141, 1979.

Weaning

10

What does *weaning* mean? The textbooks on pediatrics and the mother's manuals all imply that it is the process by which one changes from one method of feeding to another. Raphael[15] states that the very first introduction of solid foods is the true beginning of weaning. If one consults the dictionary, however, one learns that to wean is to transfer the young of any animal from dependence on its mother's milk to another form of nourishment or to estrange from former habits or associations. A weanling is a child or animal who is newly weaned.

INFANT'S NEED

When discussing the process of weaning the human infant, one might say it is the transfer of the infant from dependence on mother's milk to other sources of nourishment. If one were to determine the appropriate time for this to take place, it would be based on nutritional needs and developmental goals. The observations made among other mammals suggests achievement of a degree of maturity that allows the pup to forage for himself. When weaning time is correlated with birth weight in placental mammals, a ratio of 3:1 is noted, that is, weaning takes place when birth weight has been tripled. As a general rule, the smaller the animal the shorter the time required for both gestation and maturation of the young. The weaning process is a gradual one, terminating after a time approximately equal to the period of gestation. The elephant's gestational period is 20 to 21 months and the young are totally weaned at about 2 years of age. Other species gradually introduce other foods and teach their offspring how to obtain them on their own. Usually the mother of most species makes the determination for final termination and no longer permits the young to nurse. Studies on the milk borne factors that might cue the initiation of weaning in other species have not shown any cause and effect.

Among humans there are many cultural influences that mandate weaning time and process. Public and social pressure have influenced weaning for some families in industrialized society. There are very few societies that wean under 1 year.

Nutritionally, it is appropriate to begin iron-containing foods at 6 months, since that is the time the stores from birth are being diminished. The requirement at this age exceeds that supplied by human milk. An additional source of protein becomes necessary toward the end of the first year of life because the grams of protein per kilogram of body weight supplied by milk drop as the infant grows heavier. The content of protein in the milk begins to drop slightly after 9 months of lactation. A human infant also needs bulk, or roughage, in the diet. The exact time this need becomes apparent is not known, but it is certainly by the end of the first year. Developmentally, he is ready to learn to chew solids instead of suckle liquids at about 6 months. Chewing is an entirely different motion of the tongue and mouth from sucking. The sucking fat pads in the cheeks begin to disappear at the end of the first year. The rooting reflex has been lost. Even though the teeth are not all in, the development of good dentition requires chewing exercise.

In summary, the infant is ready to explore new feeding experiences around 6 months. Feeding is an important social as well as nutritional encounter. Eating solids and learning to drink from a cup are important social achievements as well. That does not mean the infant is taken from the breast, but his diet is expanded and now includes solid foods, other liquids, and breast milk.

Introduction of solids

The Academy of Pediatrics Committee on Nutrition[4] made recommendations on the feeding of supplemental foods to infants. They described three overlapping stages of infant feeding: the nursing period, during which breast milk or infant formula is the source of nutrition; a transitional period, during which solid foods are introduced; and the modified adult period, during which most of the nutrition is similar to the family's. They further stated that no nutritional advantage results from the introduction of supplemental foods prior to 4 to 6 months of age.

MOTHER'S RIGHTS

In practice, mothers are often the determinants of weaning time. Some mothers want to nurse for a few weeks and wean to a bottle to go to work. Other mothers wean at 3 months to be free again. Certainly any time spent breastfeeding is to the infant's advantage. The critical point in weaning is to make it a gradual adjustment for both the mother and infant.

WEANING PROCESS

Gradually replacing one feeding at a time with solids or a bottle or cup, depending on the infant's age and stage of development, is usually preferable.[1] After the adjustment has been made to one substitute feeding, then a second feeding is replaced with a substitute, usually at the opposite time of day. This process is continued until only the morning and night feedings remain. Then these two are stopped. The morning and night feedings can be maintained for some months and often an infant may be nursed beyond the second year, especially at these times. Mothers who wish to wean partially as early as 3 months may continue the morning and night nursing. This is especially suited to the working mother. The decline in lactation and the regression of the mammary gland occur slowly with gradual weaning.

The composition of milk during abrupt weaning, carefully analyzed by Hartmann and Kulski,[9] revealed that the secretory capability of the mammary gland of women changed dramatically after complete cessation of breastfeeding but that the involuting gland remained partially functional for 45 days. After termination that occurred in one day, sample collections were attempted for each breast by manual expression at the same time on days 1, 2, 4, 8, 16, 21, 31, 42, and 45. The concentrations of lactose and potassium decreased, while sodium, chloride, fat, and total protein increased progressively over 42 days. The increase in protein was related to increases in the concentrations of lactoferrin, IgA, IgG, IgM, albumin, and lactalbumin, and casein. Concentrations from each breast were similar throughout. One woman in the study breastfed for 39 days; six women fully lactated an average of 332 days (251 to 443 range).

The involution in other species is rapid. There is complete resorption in 7 days in cows for instance. The threshold dose of oxytocin required to elicit milk ejection was shown by Caldeyro-Barcia[7] to increase progressively for at least 30 days after termination of breastfeeding. It is believed that a psychologic nursing stimulus contributes to this effect in humans because they continue contact with their infants, whereas other species are separated. Experimental animals given oxytocin postweaning also show a delay in involution.

Emergency weaning

Occasionally there is a need for sudden weaning because of severe illness in the mother or some prolonged separation of mother and infant. (Sudden illness in the infant does not require weaning and, in fact, weaning would be contraindicated.) This is difficult for both. After abrupt weaning, the mammary glands remain partially functional for over a month.

Depending on the age of the infant and his flexibility, it may take a patient surrogate mother a feeding or two to switch the infant to a bottle. In other cases the infant may take only solids and refuse other liquids for days. The mother may have considerable discomfort. Engorgement may be significant if it is only 4 to 6 weeks postpartum. The mother may experience milk fever at any time there is abrupt weaning. This illness is characterized by fever, chills, and malaise, resembling a flulike syndrome. It is believed to be due to the sudden resorption of milk products into the system. Milk fever usually lasts 3 to 4 days and should not be confused with more serious illness.

The hormonal change resulting from sudden weaning early in lactation is more definitive because the prolactin levels from suckling are higher immediately postpartum (Chapter 3). The hormone-withdrawal syndrome may be more marked with early weaning. Prolactin has been associated with a feeling of well-being; thus its decrease may be associated with relative depression. Patients with psychiatric disorders have been observed to cope by compensation postpartum until they wean the infant from the breast. It is important to provide an adequate support system during weaning for the mother who is prone to depression.

The normal, well-adjusted mother may experience some depression and sadness at the reality of the last feeding. It may be very difficult to face this experience. It is important to recognize this as a physiologic phenomenon as well as an emotional one. If a mother is forced by circumstances beyond her control to wean early, she may need a lot of understanding and encouragement to cope with the disappointment. If she has had pressure from friends or relatives to breastfeed, she may need to face what she considers failure and recognize that one can bottle feed and still mother very well.

Historically, weaning has varied from strict to permissive schedules with cultural styles. Rigid feeding schedules were associated with early weaning. Weaning has varied from early denial to slow and gentle withdrawal. In this century, the time considered proper for weaning has gradually shortened from as much as 2 or 3 years to as little as 6 to 8 months, or less. Public opinion has overlooked the infant's needs in favor of what are considered the mother's rights. It is not necessary to have clearly in mind a specific plan for weaning in the early weeks of nursing unless there are some constraints on the mother's time. Weaning should be done with the infant's needs as a guide. If an infant under 1 year of age rejects the breast, it is unusual but not abnormal and should not be considered by the mother as a personal rejection. Some bottle fed infants throw down the bottle at 9 months also.

Studies of weaning practices are few. Most observations are done on duration of feeding when the success rate is low. Jackson and associates[14] studied weaning times in mothers participating in the rooming-in project from 1942 to 1951 as compared with mothers who received traditional postpartum care at the New Haven Hospital during the same period. Rooming-in meant mother and infant were together in a special unit designed to accommodate both mothers and infants and managed as a pair by the same nursing staff. Infants were with their mothers as much as each mother wished. The rooming-in mothers nursed significantly longer.[13] They averaged 3.5 to 3.8 months, whereas the controls weaned at 1.8 to 2.5 months postpartum. The incidence of breastfeeding decreased as the difficulty of the delivery increased. The number who breastfed their infants did not differ by age, education, or race. Older mothers, better-educated mothers, and black mothers who breastfed, however, nursed longer.

The reasons given why women in Dunedin, New Zealand elected to wean their infants early included concern about their milk supply and other maternal problems.[12] One of the most significant factors in lactation termination was mismanagement of breastfeeding by health professionals, according to the authors. A similar study in Swe-

Table 10-1. Main reasons for premature weaning

Reason	Number	Percentage
Not enough, inadequate, or "weak" milk	307	30.9
Child refused breast	177	17.8
Illness of child	159	16.0
Mother needed to go to work	149	15.0
"Correct age for bottle feeding"	139	14.0
Other reasons	64	6.3
TOTAL	995	100.0

Table 10-2. Reasons for "milk inadequacy"

Reason	Number	Percentage
Milk is weak, thin, translucent	189	61.0
Infant cries after being breastfed	59	18.7
Infant needs to be fed very often	35	11.2
Breast not adequately full	24	9.1
TOTAL	307	100.0

den reported that 66% of the mothers weaned because they thought their milk was drying up.[16]

The patterns of weaning were studied in southern Brazil by Sousa et al.[17] Brazil was also experiencing a decline in breastfeeding. The study was undertaken to understand the causes of early weaning to develop better means of encouraging longer breastfeeding and delaying weaning. The bottle was introduced at birth by 24%, by 2 months by 72.6%, and by 6 months by 88.0%. The main reasons given for weaning are shown in Table 10-1. A third of the mothers believed their milk was weak. The reasons the mothers thought their milk was thin are shown in Table 10-2. The researchers believed these data supported the hypothesis that the mothers did not understand the value of human milk and were influenced by advertisements about formulas and therefore compared their milk with formulas. In general most studies of weaning practices indicated that most weaning is mother initiated, most commonly because she thinks her milk is no longer adequate. Those who breastfeed longer tend to be older than 25 years, be well-educated middle class, and enjoy breastfeeding.

Infant-initiated weaning

Infant-initiated weaning the first year of life was investigated by Clarke and Harmon,[3] who studied 50 healthy breastfed infants who were totally weaned; 46% of the group of infants initiated the weaning. This is often mistakenly referred to as self-weaning. The onset was usually between 5 to 9 months of age with a median age of 6 months. Mothers described the behavior as an increased interest in exploring the environment and in other foods with a decreased interest in the breastfeeding. Brazelton described a similar phenomenon and reported that there are three ages in the first year during which the infant exhibits a lagging interest in breastfeeding as a direct or indirect result of developmental events. These times are 4 to 5 months, 7 months, and 9 to 12 months.

The duration of the infant-initiated weaning is about 1 month and is an interactive process that requires "at a minimum maternal complicity."[6] It can lead to relatively easy mutual weaning.

Refusal to breastfeed: "nursing strike"

Sudden onset of refusal to nurse can occur at any time and often is taken as a personal rejection by the mother, who promptly follows through by weaning completely. Often these mothers consider it to mean that they do not have enough milk or that something is wrong with their milk. This behavior has been called "nursing strike" and has been noted to be temporary.[10] The various causes associated with this abrupt behavior include the following:
1. Onset of menses in the mother
2. Dietary indiscretion by the mother
3. Change in maternal soap, perfume, or deodorant
4. Stress in the mother
5. Earache or nasal obstruction in the infant
6. Teething
7. Episode of biting with startle and pain reaction of mother

If a reason is identified that is possibly associated and it can be changed, nursing will resume. It may take extra effort to reestablish the relationship. Suggestions that may be made to the mother include the following:
1. Make feeding special and quiet, with no distractions and no other people.
2. Increase amount of cuddling, stroking, and soothing the baby.
3. Offer the breast when the infant is very sleepy.
4. Do not starve the child into submission.
5. If simple remedial steps do not result in a return to nursing, the physician should see the child to rule out otitis media, fever, infection, thrush, and so on.

Weanling diarrhea

Most writings on weaning refer to the problems in underdeveloped countries when infants are weaned early to overdiluted cow's milk or formulas that cost money but do not contain the anti-infective properties of human milk for the human infant. Weanling diarrhea is well described by Gordon and Ingalls[8] as the clinical syndrome (weanling diarrhea is a collection of diseases) associated with weaning from the breast. In 1900 in New York City, the death rate from dysentery, diarrhea, and enteritis in children in the first year of life was 5603/100,000 infants. This was largely attributed to weaning from the breast. Diarrheas are strongly associated with weaning not only because of the introduction of other foods, but also because of the loss of the protective properties of human milk. The diarrheas themselves contribute to the malnutrition seen in underdeveloped countries because of the resultant lack of appetite and increased metabolic losses. In Third World countries morbidity and mortality in infancy rise sharply at the time of weaning from human milk because of the rapid onset of infections. In well-nourished mothers and their infants, diarrhea does not occur from controlled gradual weaning unless there is a milk allergy or metabolic disorder in the infant.

Changes in milk composition during gradual weaning

Changes in the nutrient composition of human milk during gradual weaning were studied by Garza et al.[5] in six fully lactating women recruited at 5 to 7 months postpartum (Table 10-3). The weaning consisted of decreasing the frequency and duration of breastfeeding by one third each month for a period of three months. Milk was collected at 2-week intervals. Volume decreased to 67%, 40%, and 20% of baseline each month. The concentrations of protein and sodium were increased to 142% and 220% of baseline respectively by the twelfth week of weaning. Changes in fat composition were linear through the tenth week, but at the twelfth week were similar to baseline. Iron was increased 172%, calcium was unchanged, and zinc fell to 58%. Similar observations have been made in bovine milk. Milk produced during either rapid or gradual weaning is characterized by a decreasing concentration of lactose. Fat accounts for an increasing percentage of calories up 80% and protein a stable 6% of calories.

The immunologic components in human milk were also measured and the concentrations of certain components of the immunologic system are maintained during gradual weaning.[7] The effect of gradual weaning differs from that of abrupt weaning, in which the concentrations of all components rise dramatically. Measurements at 4 weeks, 8 weeks, and 12 weeks showed a decrease in the milk volume of 67%, 40%, and 20% as the levels of IgA and secretory IgA rose slightly. Lysozyme and lactoferrin rose slightly.

Studies in other species suggest that gut maturation observed at normal weaning time is not dependent on components in the milk but is triggered by thyroxine and corticosterone in the plasma of the offspring.[11] The anatomic changes in the breast during weaning are discussed in Chapter 2.

The physician's role in weaning

The physician's responsibility is the initiation of the appropriate solid foods, which probably should begin at 6 months of age.

Table 10-3. Nutrient density (mg/100 kcal) of milk during weaning

	Week								
	0	2	4	6	8	10	12	PTM*	R†
Protein	1.5	1.2	1.3	1.0	1.3	1.2	1.9	1.8	2.7
Na	24.0	17.0	20.0	13.0	24.0	25.0	46.0	25.0	53.0
Ca	38.0	30.0	33.0	21.0	30.0	26.0	38.0	34.5	140.0
Zn	0.21	0.17	0.19	0.09	0.10	0.10	0.11	3.8	0.5

From Garza, C., et al.: Am. J. Clin. Nutr. 37:61, 1983.
*Nutrient densities of milk from delivering premature infants (17).
†Nutrient densities calculated to achieve intrauterine growth rates assuming that the caloric requirements of low birth weight infants is 130 kcal/kg (18).

Introduction of a cup as a developmental step should usually begin by 7 months.

Eating finger foods and learning to feed himself are the next steps for the child to be taught.

None of the above means the termination of breastfeeding, but rather the gradual developmental progression of feeding. As other foods are introduced and feeding begins to cluster into three meals and some "snacks," breastfeedings will be decreased eventually in number to two or three per day.

The nourishment value is not a key issue after 1 year if other foods are adequate. The physician's role is to assure adequate nutrition.

There is no known detriment to nursing and some indication that nursing a few times a day or during times of stress is beneficial to the mother-infant relationship when the child is over a year of age. The objections raised are usually based on custom or personal taste. It is important for the clinician to avoid judgmental counseling based only on personal biases. There are lay publications that may help the mother who is nursing a toddler.

The physician may need to help the mother work through her own feelings about nursing her infant beyond the first year. Many women have been overwhelmed by friendly advice from lay experts about the infant who nurses for several years. Beyond a year, weaning is rarely child initiated until age 4. The child may not lose interest, so that the final steps in termination may require maternal intervention. A mother is not a poor parent if she begins to feel resentful toward nursing. Planning appropriate alternatives to the breastfeeding session that is to be eliminated is helpful in turning the child's attention toward the new event instead of toward the loss of an old and cherished one, a feeding at the breast. The mother may need to be helped to see how to avoid situations that easily predispose to nursing. She needs to know that it is acceptable to set some rules and to have some limitations and control over the breastfeeding.

If mother becomes pregnant, she will want to decide when she wishes to wean or whether she will continue to nurse right through pregnancy and then tandem nurse the new baby (see Chapter 17). For the child, it is important to avoid abrupt weaning or weaning to make room for the new baby who will now take his place. Weaning well before delivery is usually less traumatic for the child.

WEANING AND THE WORKING MOTHER

There are mothers who will return to work. Whether the reason is money, career, or personal satisfaction is not relevant to management. It takes tremendous commitment to work and breastfeed, but it can be done, it has been done, and it will be done. Usually the biggest problem a mother faces is coping with people who do not understand why she bothers. An understanding physician who provides the reassurance and support necessary to manage is a great asset. A mother may go home for a feeding in the middle of the day, pump milk to leave for the infant to have from a bottle, or give a substitute bottle. If there are occasional bottles of formula, the powder preparations are more economical and require only warming the water before adding the powder to assure rapid solution. Suggestions for collecting milk are in Chapter 19. Some infants quickly learn the mother's schedule and will sleep while she is away and feed more frequently during the evening and night to make up for it. It takes some personal adjustment to plan ahead and a baby-sitter who is patient and cooperative. A mother needs to be alert to the infant's needs as well and may need to leave feedings ready when she is away even if she had hoped the infant would sleep through the day. If a mother works long hours or an inflexible schedule, it may be necessary to wean the infant to morning and night feedings at the breast. However, this arrangement still provides the special benefits of human milk as well as the closeness that an infant needs; thus it is worth the effort. Employment is discussed in Chapter 13.

REFERENCES

1. Barnes, G.R., et al.: Management of breast feeding, JAMA **151**:192, 1953.
2. Caldeyro-Barcia, R.: Milk ejection in women. In Reynolds, M., and Folley, S.J., editors: Lactogenesis: the initiation of milk secretion at parturition, Philadelphia, 1969, University of Pennsylvania Press.
3. Clarke, S.K., and Harmon, R.J.: Infant-initiated weaning from the breast in the first year, Early Hum. Dev. **8**:151, 1983.
4. Committee on Nutrition, American Academy of Pediatrics: On the feeding of supplemental foods to infants, Pediatrics **65**:1178, 1980.
5. Garza, C., et al.: Changes in the nutrient composition of human milk during gradual weaning, Am. J. Clin. Nutr. **37**:61, 1983.
6. Goldfarb, J., and Tibbetts, E.: Breastfeeding handbook, Hillside, N.J., 1980, Enslow Publishers.
7. Goldman, et al.: Immunologic components in human milk during weaning, Acta Paediatr. Scand. **72**:133, 1983.
8. Gordon, J.E., and Ingalls, T.H.: Weaning diarrhea, Am. J. Med. Sci. Prev. Med. Epidemiol. **245**:345, 1963.
9. Hartman, P.E., and Kulski, J.K.: Changes in the composition of the mammary secretion of women after the abrupt termination of breast-feeding, J. Physiol. **275**:1, 1978.
10. Helsing, E., King, F.S.: Breast-feeding practice, New York, 1980, Oxford University Press.
11. Henning, S.J.: Role of milk-borne factors in weaning and intestinal development, Biol. Neonate **41**:265, 1982.
12. Hood, L.U., et al.: Breast feeding and some reasons for electing to wean the infant: a report from the Dunedin Multidisciplinary Child Development Study, N.Z. Med. J. **88**:273, 1978.
13. Jackson, E.B.: Pediatric and psychiatric aspects of the Yale Rooming-In Project, Conn. State Med. J. **14**:616, 1950.
14. Jackson, E.B., Wilkins, L.C., and Auerbach, H.: Statistical report on incidence and duration of breast feeding in relation to personal-social and hospital maternity factors, Pediatrics **17**:700, 1956.
15. Raphael, D.: The tender gift: breastfeeding, New York, 1976, Schocken Books.
16. Sjölen, S., Hofvander, Y., and Hillervik, G.: Factors related to early termination of breast feeding, Acta Paediatr. Scand. **66**:505, 1977.
17. Sousa, P.L.R., et al.: Patterns of weaning in South Brazil, J. Trop. Pediatr. **21**:210, 1975.

Drugs in breast milk

11

Does a given drug pass into the breast milk? Can a patient take certain medications and still nurse her infant? Physicians are constantly perplexed by these questions because the data are meager and conflicting. In an analysis of 100 consecutive medical consultations about breastfeeding in Rochester, 70 were about medications needed for the mother, 15 were about infants who were not thriving, 10 were about sore or cracked nipples or mastitis, and 5 were miscellaneous in nature.

There are a number of general reviews of drugs in breast milk and dozens of articles about the effect of a specific medication in a particular infant.* The Committee on Drugs of the American Academy of Pediatrics[14] has published a list of drugs and other chemicals that transfer into human breast milk. The list is divided into those that are contraindicated, those that require temporary interruption of breastfeeding, and those that are compatible with breastfeeding. Concern about this issue of drugs in breast milk has spread. The Department of Health and Human Services and the Food and Drug Administration have proposed a standard warning on all nonprescription drugs that are absorbed by the body. The warning states, "As with any drug, if you are pregnant or nursing a baby, seek professional advice before using this product." Since studies of pregnant women have shown that they take five to eight medications on their own during pregnancy and postpartum, the education by the clinician of these patients needs to continue. It is not appropriate to substitute wishful thinking for specific knowledge, yet it is equally inappropriate to discontinue breastfeeding when it is not medically necessary.

Consideration of some of the pharmacokinetics will contribute to the understanding of the problems involved. Some of the data reported have been extrapolated from experiments performed on cows, goats, and rodents. Bovine experiments have been con-

---

*See references 2, 7, 8, 10, 21, 26, 35, 36, 50, 64, 69.

ducted using continuous infusions, which provide data on the passage of a drug into milk under certain circumstances of pH and plasma level.

Factors that influence the passage of a drug into the milk in humans include the size of the molecule, its solubility in lipids and water, whether it binds to protein, the drug's pH, and diffusion rates. Following is a summary of these factors:

I. Drug
    A. Route of administration: oral, IM, or IV
    B. Absorption rate
    C. Half-life
    D. Dissociation constant
II. Size of molecule
III. Degree of ionization
IV. pH of substrate (plasma 7.4, milk 6.8)
V.   Solubility
    A. In water
    B. In lipids
VI. Protein binding more to plasma than to milk protein

Passive diffusion is the principal factor in the passage of a drug from plasma into milk. The drug may appear in an active form or as an inactive metabolite. The route of administration to the mother, the drug's half-life, and drug dissociation constants are also to be considered. Finally, a factor that has received relatively little attention is the infant. Will the infant absorb the chemical from the intestinal tract? If the infant absorbs the chemical, can the infant detoxify and excrete it or will minimal amounts in the milk build in the infant's system? Is the drug a material that could be safely given to an infant directly and at what risk? What dosages and blood levels are safe? These latter two questions are more critical than the pharmacokinetic theory. The ultimate question faced by the physician is, "Can this infant be safely exposed to this chemical as it appears in breast milk without a risk that exceeds the tremendous benefits of being breastfed?" Almost any drug present in mother's blood will appear to some degree in her milk.

CHARACTERISTICS OF THE DRUG
Protein binding

Drugs entering the circulation become protein bound or remain free in the circulation. The protein-bound component of the drug serves as an inactive reservoir of the drug that is in equilibrium with the free drug. Most drugs enter the mammary alveolar cells in the unbound form. Only those drug molecules that are free in solution can pass through the endothelial pores, either by diffusion or by reversed pinocytosis. Pinocytosis is the process whereby drug molecules that are dissolved in the interstitial fluid attach to receptors located at the surface of the cell membrane.[51,52] The cell membrane invaginates at the site of the drug attachment, bringing the drug into the cell. The membrane is pinched off, and the drug, surrounded by membrane, remains in the cell. Then the membrane is dissolved, leaving the drug molecule free in the cell. Reverse pinocytosis or apocrine secretion is the process by which the apical membrane evaginates after fusion of the intracellular membrane-bound secretion granules with the plasma membrane. The granules include lipids, proteins, lactose, drug molecules, and other cellular constituents. The evagination of the plasma membrane is pinched off and released into the alveolar lumen. Within the extravascular space, the drug may be bound to proteins in the interstitial fluid. Some agents in free solution can pass into the alveolar milk directly by way of the spaces between the mammary alveolar cells. These paracellular areas account for a major portion of the fluid changes across the epithelium. These spaces between adjacent alveolar cells serve to carry water-soluble drugs from the tissue into the milk.

Ionization

Drugs that are nonionized are excreted in the milk in greater amounts than are ionized compounds. Depending on the pH of the solvent and the drug dissociation constant (pk_a), many weak electrolytes are more or less ionized in solution. Blood plasma and interstitial fluid are slightly alkaline (pH 7.4). Drugs that are weak acids are ionized to a greater extent in alkaline solution and are more extensively bound to protein. The amount of drug excreted from plasma (pH 7.4) to milk (pH 6.8 to 7.3, average 7.0) depends on the pH of the compound. Thus a weakly acidic compound has a higher concentration in plasma than in milk. Conversely, weakly alkaline compounds are in equal or higher levels in the milk than in the plasma (Table 11-1). The degree of drug ionization changes with the pH of the plasma and milk. Weak bases become more ionized with decreasing pH; thus the ionized component will increase in milk. The concentration in plasma and milk for the nonionized fraction will be the same, but the total amount of drug in the milk will be greater than in plasma. The sulfonamides demonstrate the effect of the pK_a on the concentration of drug that reaches the milk. Sulfacetamide, with a low pK_a, has a low milk/plasma (M/P) ratio, whereas sulfanilamide has a pK_a of 10.4 and an M/P ratio of 1.00 (Table 11-2).

The studies done in cows and goats with constant infusions demonstrate this principle more dramatically because the pH of bovine plasma is 7.4 to 7.5 and of bovine milk 6.5. Under normal circumstances, however, concentrations of drugs are rarely constant, and there is a delay in achieving a new equilibrium. During periods of rapidly decreasing blood levels there is some back diffusion into the plasma, according to Catz and Giacoia.[10]

Molecular weight

The passage of molecules into the milk also depends on the size of the molecule, or the molecular weight (mol wt). Water-filled membranal pores permit the movement of

Table 11-1. Concentration of various drugs in maternal blood and breast milk under normal pH conditions

| Drug administered (therapeutic dosage) | Drug levels (unit/100 ml) | | Administered drug appearing in milk (% day) |
	Plasma or serum (pH 7.4)	Milk (ph 7.0)	
Aspirin	1-5 mg	1-3 mg	0.5
Bishydroxycoumarin	11-16.5 mg	0.2 mg	0.5
Chloral hydrate	0-3 mg	0-1.5 mg	0.6
Chloramphenicol	2.5-5 mg	1.5-2.5 mg	1.3
Chlorpromazine	0.1 mg	0.03 mg	0.07
Colistin sulfate	0.3-0.5 mg	0.05-0.09 mg	0.07
Cycloserine	1.5-2 mg	1-1.5 mg	0.6
Erythromycin	0.1-0.2 mg	0.3-0.5 mg	0.1
Ethanol	50-80 mg	50-80 mg	0.25
Ethyl biscoumacetate	2.7-14.5 mg	0-0.17 mg	0.1
Folic acid	3 μg	0.07 μg	0.1
^{131}I	0.002 μCi	0.13μCi	2.5
Imipramine hydrochloride	0.2-1.3 mg	0.1 mg	0.1
Isoniazid	0.6-1.2 mg	0.6-1.2 mg	0.75
Kanamycin sulfate	0.5-3.5 mg	0.2 mg	0.05
Lincomycin	0.3-1.5 mg	0.05-0.2 mg	0.025
Lithium carbonate	0.2-1.1 mg	0.07-0.4 mg	0.12
Meperidine hydrochloride	0.07-0.1 mg	trace (<0.1 mg)	<0.1
Methotrexate	3 μg	0.3 μg	0.01
Nalidixic acid	3-5 mg	0.4 mg	0.05
Novobiocin	1.2-5.2 mg	0.3-0.5 mg	0.15
Penicillin	6-120 μg	1.2-3.6 μg	0.03
Phenobarbital	0.6-1.8 mg	0.1-0.5 mg	1.5
Phenylbutazone	2-5 mg	0.2-0.6 mg	0.4
Phenytoin	0.3-4.5 mg	0.6-1.8 mg	1.4
Pyrilamine maleate	—	0.2 mg	0.6
Pyrimethamine	0.7-1.5 mg	0.3 mg	0.3
Quinine sulfate	0.7 mg	0.1 mg	0.05
Rifampin	0.5 mg	0.1-0.3 mg	0.05
Streptomycin sulfate	2-3 mg	1-3 mg	0.5
Sulfapyridine	3-13 mg	3-13 mg	0.12
Tetracycline hydrochloride	80-320 μg	50-260 μg	0.03
Thiouracil	3-4 mg	9-12 mg	5

From Vorherr, H.: Postgrad. Med. **56:**98, 1974.

Table 11-2. Association between milk/plasma ratios and pK_a of sulfonamides

Sulfonamide	Milk/plasma ratio	pK_a
Sulfacetamide	0.08	5.4
Sulfadiazine	0.21	6.5
Sulfathiazole	0.43	7.1
Sulfamethazine	0.51	7.4
Sulfapyridine	0.85	8.4
Sulfanilamide	1.00	10.4

Modified from Lein, E.J., Kuwahara, J., and Koda, R.T., from Gaginella, T.S.: U.S. Pharm. 3:39, 1978.

molecules of less than 200 mol wt. Owing to action similar to the limitation of transport of certain large molecular chemicals across the placenta, insulin and heparin are not found in human milk, presumably because of the size of the molecule.

Solubility of the drug

The passage of drugs from the perialveolar interstitium into the milk has been likened by Vorherr[64] to the manner in which drugs penetrate the intestinal mucosa and reach the bloodstream. The alveolar epithelium is a lipid barrier that is most permeable in the first few days of lactation, when colostrum is being produced. The solubility of a compound in water and in lipid is a determining factor in its transfer. Un-ionized drugs, which are lipid soluble, usually dissolve and descend in the lipid phase of the membrane. The solubility is closely linked to the manner in which the drug crosses the membranes (Table 11-3). The membrane of the alveolar epithelial cells is composed of lipoprotein, glycolipid, phospholipid, and free lipids, as described in Chapter 3. The transfer of water-soluble drugs and ions is inhibited by this hydrophobic barrier. Water-soluble materials pass through pores in the basement membrane and paracellular spaces. Low lipid solubility of an un-ionized compound will diminish its excretion into milk.

Mechanisms of transport

Drugs pass into milk by simple diffusion, carrier-mediated diffusion, or active transport. Following is a summary of the methods of transport:
Simple diffusion—concentration gradient decreases
Carrier-mediated diffusion—concentration gradient decreases
Active transport—concentration gradient increases
Pinocytosis
Reverse pinocytosis (apocrine secretion)
Pharmacokinetic principles relate to the specific variation with time of the drug concentration in the blood or plasma as a result of its absorption, distribution, and elimination. Ultimately, by extrapolation of these factors, one determines the effect of the drug. The most elementary kinetic model is based on the body as a single compartment.

Table 11-3. Predicted distribution ratios of drug concentrations in milk and plasma

	Milk/plasma ratio
Highly lipid-soluble drugs	~1
Small (mol wt <200) water-soluble drugs	~1
Weak acids	≤1
Weak bases	≥1
Actively transported drugs	>1

From Gaginella, T.S.: U.S. Pharm. 3:39, 1978

Distribution of the drug in the compartment is assumed to be uniform and rapidly equilibrated. In the single-compartment model, the volume of distribution of a drug is considered to be the same as that of the plasma, assuming a rapid uniform distribution.[22] The volume of distribution is

$$V_d = \frac{\text{Total amount of drug in body}}{\text{Concentration of drug in plasma}}$$

The absorption and elimination are considered to be exponential or first-order kinetics. A two-compartment model of drug kinetics takes into account the phase of decreasing drug concentration as drug distributes into the tissues. There is an initial rapid fall in concentrations as the drug distributes; then first-order elimination follows. When considering the pharmacokinetics of drugs in breast milk, one has to consider also that elimination in the breast is then by two potential routes: one excreted with the milk to the infant and the other by back diffusion into the plasma to reequilibrate with the falling level in the plasma. Wilson[69] has proposed a model that involves a deep compartment, a third compartment: the breast. When the infant is feeding, the rate constant is zero-order kinetics and when there is no milk being removed, drug accumulates in the deep compartment and begins to transfer back.

With access to the volume of distribution of the drug in question, the amount of the dose, and the weight of the mother, the concentration of drug in breast milk could be theoretically calculated:

$$\text{Concentration in breast milk} = \frac{\text{Dose}}{\text{Volume of distribution}}$$

The average total body store of drug at the plateau is approximately equal to 1.5 times the amount administered per one-half time of elimination. The effect of a single dose of the drug is characterized by latency, time of peak effect, magnitude of peak effect, and duration. As dosage is increased, latency is reduced, and peak effect is increased without changing the timing. Repeated dosage is usually calculated on one-half times of elimination, assuming four half-times are required for complete elimination. When the drug is given in less time, then the drug accumulates. Accumulation continues, in first-order kinetics, until the rate of elimination equals the rate of administration. A constant fraction of the drug is eliminated per unit of time. In general terms, maximal accumulation occurs after four half-times, and at this time the rate of elimination is equal to the rate of administration.

The concentration of the drug in the circulation of the mother depends on the mode of administration (oral, intramuscular, or intravenous) and the distribution, protein binding, and metabolism of the drug by the mother. Nonelectrolytes such as ethanol, urea, and antipyrine enter the milk by diffusion through the lipid membrane barrier and may reach the same concentrations in the milk as in the plasma, irrespective of the pH. The main entrance site of molecules is at the basement laminal membrane, where water-soluble materials pass through the alveolar pores. Un-ionized drugs cross the membrane more easily than ionized ones because of the structure of the membrane. The un-ionized drugs pass through the membrane by diffusion. When simple diffusion takes place, the ratio between the concentration in the milk and in the plasma (the M/P ratio) is 1.0. Passive diffusion provides the same ratio regardless of the plasma concentrations of the drug or the volume of milk secreted. Different M/P ratios depend on the binding to protein and are a measure of the protein-free fraction. The dissimilar ratios for the sulfa drugs (Table 11-2) are due to the difference in protein binding.

Large molecules depend on their lipid solubility and ionization to cross the membrane, since they pass in a lipid-soluble nonionized form. The M/P ratio is determined when there is equilibrium in the amount of un-ionized drug in the aqueous phase on both sides of the membrane. When drugs are only partially ionized, it is the un-ionized fraction that determines the concentration that crosses the membrane. The drugs whose un-ionized fraction is not very lipid soluble will pass only in limited degree into breast milk.

Passive drug transport may occur in the form of facilitated diffusion. The active compound is transported across the cell membrane by a carrier enzyme or protein. The gradient is toward a lesser or equal concentration in both simple diffusion and facilitated diffusion and is controlled by chemical activity gradients. Facilitated diffusion usually involves a water-soluble substance too large to pass through the membrane pores.

Active transport mechanisms provide a process whereby the gradient is "uphill," or higher, in the milk. The process is similar to facilitated diffusion except that metabolic energy is required to overcome the gradient. Examples of substances actively transported include glucose, amino acids, calcium, magnesium, and sodium. Pinocytosis and reverse pinocytosis, as described previously, are involved in the transport of very large molecules and proteins. Chloride ions are secreted into milk via an active apical membrane pump, whereas sodium and potassium are diffused by electrical gradient. Since the level of sodium is kept low, there may be an active return of sodium into the plasma.

A summary of the steps in the passage of drugs into breast milk follows[65]:

1. Mammary alveolar epithelium represents a lipid barrier with water-filled pores and is most permeable for drugs during colostral phase of milk secretion (first week postpartum).
2. Drug excretion into milk depends on the drug's degree of ionization, molecular weight, solubility in fat and water, and relation of pH of plasma (7.4) to pH of milk (7.0).
3. Drugs preferably enter mammary cells basally in the un-ionized, non-protein-bound form by diffusion or active transport.
4. Water-soluble drugs of mol wt below 200 pass through water-filled membranal pores.
5. Drugs leave mammary alveolar cells apically by diffusion, active transport, and apocrine secretion.

6. Drugs may enter milk via spaces between mammary alveolar cells.
7. Most ingested drugs appear in milk; drug levels in milk usually do not exceed 1% of ingested dosage and are independent of milk volume.
8. Drugs are bound much less to milk proteins than to plasma proteins.
9. Drug-metabolizing capacity of mammary epithelium is not understood.

EFFECT ON THE NURSING INFANT
Absorption from the gastrointestinal tract

Although there is concern about the amount of a given agent in the breast milk, of greater importance is the amount that is absorbed into the infant's bloodstream. There is no accurate way to measure this because other factors also affect the level in the infant's bloodstream. The tolerance of the chemical to the pH of the stomach and the enzymatic activity of the intestinal tract is significant. The volume of milk consumed is a factor as well.

Infant's ability to detoxify and excrete the agent

Any drug that is given to an infant by any route has to be evaluated according to the infant's ability to detoxify or conjugate the chemical in the liver and/or excrete it in the urine or stool. Some compounds that appear in milk in very low levels are not well excreted by the infant and therefore accumulate in the infant's system to the point of toxicity.

Drugs that depend on the liver for conjugation, such as acetaminophen, are theoretic risks because of the limited reserve of the neonatal hepatic detoxification system. When actual measurements have been made of neonates given acetaminophen, they handle it well because they conjugate it in the sulfhydral system as an alternative pathway used only to a small extent in adult metabolism of acetaminophen. When a single dose of a drug is given to a mother and the level is measured in her milk and in her infant, it does not give a clear picture of the potential for accumulation in the infant's system. The competition for binding of a drug to protein is also important. Some drugs such as sulfadiazine compete for binding sites that might normally bind bilirubin in the first week or so of life. This puts the infant in jeopardy of kernicterus at a given bilirubin level because of an increase in the fraction of unbound bilirubin even though the indirect bilirubin level appears to be below the dangerous level. Some other compounds that displace bilirubin from albumin-binding sites include salicylic acid (aspirin or acetylsalicylic acid breaks down to salicylic acid), furosemide, and phenylbutazone.

The chronologic age of the infant and the infant's gestational age play a part in the interpretation of risks. An infant who is premature handles some drugs well but may have immature activity of liver enzymes and other mechanisms that normally detoxify, inactivate, or excrete such agents. Premature infants also have lower albumin levels, and thus have fewer available binding sites in protein.

The age of the infant makes a difference in the total volume of milk consumed, and in the older child there are other items in the diet so that milk does not comprise the total intake. Age makes a difference because the more mature infant can metabolize drugs more effectively; thus sulfa drugs, for instance, can be given to infants after the first month of life.

If the agent is fat soluble, the fat content of the milk may be significant. The fat content at any feeding increases over time; thus the so-called foremilk is low in fat and the hindmilk is four to five times richer in fat toward the end of a feeding. The total amount of fat in a given feeding is less in the morning, peaks at midday, and drops off in the evening even though the total amount of fat will be about the same each 24-hour period. The coefficient of lipid solubility for an un-ionized drug determines both its penetration of the biologic membrane to gain entrance to milk and its concentration in milk fat, according to Wilson.[69] Sulfonamides with low fat solubility are in the aqueous and protein fraction of milk, whereas many barbiturates are in the lipid fraction. There is an inverse relationship between a drug's lipid solubility and the amount that appears in the skim fraction. The concentrations in fat differ for each member of the barbital family. Pentobarbital and secobarbital are found in the lipid phase, whereas phenobarbital is found in the aqueous phase.

The agent may appear in low levels in a mother's serum, but mammary blood flow during lactation is 500 ml/minute and a mother produces about 60 ml of milk/hour. The agent that appears in minimal concentrations in the milk may present a significant problem when one considers that 1000 ml of milk may be consumed in a day by an infant. During the colostral phase of lactation, the breast is more permeable to drugs.

EVALUATING THE DATA ABOUT A GIVEN DRUG

The paucity of carefully controlled studies done on large enough samples to validate the results when such a large number of variables are active has been lamented by many authors. Some of the data collected are not pharmacokinetically sound. The clinician needs to have an understanding of these variables as well as of pharmacokinetic principles so that a reasonable judgment about a given case can be made.

Although it should be theoretically possible to determine how much of a specific drug reaches the infant in his mother's milk by knowing all the properties of the drug, including its volume of distribution, pH, pK_a, lipid solubility, protein-binding activity, and rate of detoxification in the maternal system, there is sufficient variation in the levels that reach the infant and how he deals with the agent to make it necessary to have specific data about a specific drug. Thus a few simple steps in the decision-making process are helpful in determining risk.

Safety of drug for an infant

Is this a drug that can be given to the infant directly if necessary? Antibiotics such as penicillin, for instance, that one could give the infant are in this category, whereas an antibiotic such as chloramphenicol, which one would not give the infant under ordinary circumstances, should be avoided in the nursing mother. The toxicity of chloramphenicol in the infant is dose related and associated with an unpredictable accumulation of the drug. There is also an idiosyncratic reaction that occurs with chloramphenicol, which is unrelated to dose but is capable of causing pancytopenia.

If the drug in question can be given to the infant, is there any risk to the infant in the amount in the milk? Phenobarbital can be given to infants for various reasons; thus the question is whether enough will reach the infant to cause difficulty. The infant should be watched for symptoms of depression, such as a change in feeding or sleeping pattern. If the infant is sleeping long periods and feeding less than usual (specifically, fewer than five or six times a day), then the medication may be at fault. Phenobarbital is a significant drug for the mother with seizures; therefore, a careful review of the risk-to-benefit ratio to the mother as well as to the infant should be undertaken. In anepileptic dosages it has not been reported as a problem. Barbiturates vary in their effect in young infants because the newborn does not handle the short-acting barbiturates well. They are readily detoxified in the adult liver, whereas phenobarbital depends more on the kidney for excretion. If one can safely give the drug to an infant, then it is only a question of watching for any symptoms of excessive accumulation that might develop. The age of the infant is critical also.

When the drug in question is one that is not normally given to an infant of his particular age, weight, or degree of maturity, then a more difficult decision has to be made. Specific information about the amount of the drug that appears in the milk is essential in decision making. Often conflicting information is available. Many lists of drug-milk levels have perpetuated the same errors in calculation; thus, having more than one reference may not provide confirmed information.

If the medication will have to be taken for weeks or months, as is the case with the cardiovascular drugs, the drug has greater potential impact than when it will only be taken for a few days. If the drug exposure has gone on for 9 months in utero already, some feel it is less of a problem; on the other hand, it may compound the problem.

Sensitization

Is there risk of sensitization, even in the small dosages of a drug that might pass into the milk? This question arises most frequently around the use of antibiotics, and use of penicillin is most frequently questioned. Certainly if there is a strong history of drug sensitization in the family, it should be considered. In that case, however, it should be questioned for the mother as well. Whether infants are put at risk of developing resistant strains of bacteria in their systems by small amounts of antibiotic in their feedings is a serious question and, of course, is pertinent for the dairy and meat industry as well as for the humans who consume these products.

Correlation of drug safety in pregnancy and lactation

Very rarely is valid information on the appearance of a drug in milk available on the package insert, since the pharmaceutical companies usually merely indicate that it should not be taken during pregnancy and lactation. Agents that may be safe in pregnancy may not be so in lactation because during pregnancy the maternal liver and kidney are serving as detoxification and excretion resources for the fetus via the placenta, whereas during lactation the infant has to handle the drug totally on his own once it has reached his circulation. The infant in utero receives the drug in greater quantity via the circulation, whereas the nursing infant receives only what reaches the milk. One should be cautious about translating data pertaining to these two states back and forth.

MINIMIZING THE EFFECT OF MATERNAL MEDICATION

If a mother needs a specific medication and the hazards to the infant are minimal, the following important adjustments can be made to minimize the effects:
1. Do not use the long-acting form of the drug because the infant has even more difficulty in excreting such an agent, which usually requires detoxification in the liver. Accumulation in the infant is then a genuine concern.
2. Schedule the doses so the least amount possible gets into the milk. Given the usual absorption rates and peak blood levels of most drugs, having the mother take the medication immediately after a breastfeeding is the safest time for the infant.
3. Watch the infant for any unusual signs or symptoms such as change in feeding pattern or sleeping habits, fussiness, or rash.
4. When possible, choose the drug that produces the least amount in the milk (Table 11-2).

SPECIFIC DRUG GROUPS

The information that is available about specific individual drugs has been provided in Appendix F. It is hoped that the increase in the incidence of breastfeeding will be accompanied by an increase in information and specific data about such factors as the appearance of a drug in milk. Considerably more information is needed to provide proper insight into the question than that obtained by giving a single specific dose of a medication to a mother and measuring the level in her milk without also measuring her serum level and identifying the peak level and half-life in her serum and milk and in her infant.

Analgesics

Drugs such as heroin have been known for decades to appear in milk, and at one time withdrawal symptoms in the neonate were prevented or treated by breastfeeding and then gradual weaning. Codeine, meperidine (Demerol), and pentazocine (Talwin) appear in milk at low levels. Individual variation is common, and neonates can be depressed by the medication; therefore care should be taken to monitor the infant carefully. For example, a breastfed newborn was transferred to the special-care nursery at

Rochester because of unusual floppiness and poor muscle tone. His mother was taking dextropropoxyphene (Darvon) every 4 hours. Temporarily stopping the nursing until the mother's drug level dropped and discontinuing use of the drug produced dramatic improvement, which persisted when the infant went back to nursing. Diazepam (Valium) has caused sleepiness, mild depression, and decreased intake in some infants and has a tendency to accumulate in the neonate, especially in the first weeks.

The dose schedule for analgesics is usually single dose, especially in the postpartum period. A mother should not be subjected to great discomfort when a dose or two of analgesics would improve her well-being. Aspirin on a single-dose schedule is quite safe, although it is known to pass into the milk. The case of metabolic acidosis reported in a nursing infant occurred when the mother took 10 grains of aspirin every 4 hours for arthritis.[12] A serum salicylate on the third day of hospitalization with no breastfeeding was still 24 mg/100 ml. This demonstrates the tendency of salicylate to accumulate in the neonate. Acetylsalicylic acid, not the metabolite salicylate, is responsible for the platelet aggregate abnormalities, so there should be no concern about aspirin in this regard, since it is the metabolite that appears in the milk.

Antibiotics

Levels in milk vary with the pH of the drugs and their pK_a. The risks vary among groups of antibiotics. Penicillins are not usually toxic but theoretically can cause sensitivity. Sulfa drugs should not be used in the first month of life because they can interfere with the binding of bilirubin to protein. The risk diminishes with age, and infants are given sulfa drugs directly at 6 to 8 weeks of age. Infants with G6PD deficiency should never receive sulfa drugs directly or via the breast milk. Chloramphenicol is contraindicated in nursing very young infants because of the risk of accumulation of the drug even from small amounts in milk and the potential for idiosyncracy. Tetracycline causes staining of teeth and abnormalities of bone growth when given directly to children for a week or more. Infants breastfed by mothers taking tetracycline for mastitis may have stained and mottled first and second teeth when therapy exceeds 10 days. The amount in milk is half that in the mother's plasma.

Erythromycin appears in higher amounts in milk than in plasma. When given intravenously to the mother, the levels are 10 times higher. When the infant is old enough to receive erythromycin directly, the mother can take it as well.

Aminoglycosides are common constituents of postpartum antibiotic therapy and are given parentally. They readily appear in the milk but, like kanamycin, are not readily absorbed from the gastrointestinal tract; therefore, under usual circumstances they pose no problem to the neonate, who will not absorb them.

Metronidazole (Flagyl) does appear in milk at levels equal to those in serum. Most researchers consider the risk to the infant to be sufficient to suggest alternative therapy for the mother. Symptoms include decreased appetite and vomiting and, occasionally, blood dyscrasia.

An alternative treatment regimen is 2 g in a single dose. When milk concentrations are measured with a 2 g dose, the highest concentrations are found at 2 and 4 hours postingestion and decline over the next 12 hours to 19.1 μg/ml and to 12.6 μg/ml at 24 hours.[19,26] The dose to the infant is calculated to be 21.8 mg over the first 24 hours and only 3.5 mg in the second 24 hours. It has been recommended that the single-dose regimen be used in nursing mothers, which necessitates that a mother pump and discard milk for only 24 hours. Metronidazole is often the only drug that works in a serious trichomoniasis, giardiasis, or amebiasis infection.[19]

Amoxicillin, cephalexin, and cefadroxil, when given orally in a single dose, peak in the milk at 4 to 6 hours.[31] Cephalothin, cephapirin, and cefotaxime, when given in a bolus IV injection, peak at 2 hours. Cefadroxil reached the highest levels (1.64 ± 0.73 μg/ml) at 6 hours. Although the levels in the milk were low and the M/P ratios were also low, no data were available on the infants' ability to absorb these compounds from the milk.

Chloroquine, oxacillin, and para-aminosalicylic acid are reported by O'Brien[50] to be safe because they are not excreted in milk.

Anticholinergics

Anticholinergic drugs include atropine, scopolamine (hyoscine), and synthetic quaternary ammonium derivatives, some of which are available in over-the-counter medications. Some atropine does enter the milk. Infants are particularly sensitive to this drug; therefore the infant involved should be watched for tachycardia and thermal changes, which are more easily measured in infants. There may be a decrease in milk secretion in the mother, and constipation and urinary retention may occur in the infant. The quaternary anticholinergics should not appear in milk in any degree because, as cations, they do not pass into the acidic milk. Mepenzolate methylbromide (Cantil) has been reported by both O'Brien[50] and Gaginella[21] not to appear in milk.

Cimetidine (Tagamet), a potent H_2-receptor antagonist is used for conditions associated with acid peptic digestion in the gastrointestinal tract. Cimetidine excretion into breast milk has resulted in concentrations higher than in the corresponding plasma sample.[59] Levels were highest at 1 hour after a single dose. Chronic-dose studies revealed variable M/P ratios, all of which were higher than the single-dose ratio. The authors suggest an active transport mechanism for this medication. The maximum amount of cimetidine ingested by an infant was calculated at 6 mg for 1 L of milk (or 1.5 mg/kg). Caution is recommended in nursing with this medication until more is known of its side effects, especially the antiandrogenic features.

Sulfasalazine treatment of ulcerative colitis and Krohn's disease during breastfeeding has been widely discussed on theoretic grounds because the compound splits to sulfapyridine and 5-aminosalicylic acid (5-ASA). The sulfapyridine is absorbed from the colon and is metabolized in the liver. The 5-ASA is partly absorbed and rapidly excreted in the urine, so serum concentrations are low. The sulfapyridine and its metabolites do appear in the milk in lower concentrations than in the serum. A dose of 2 g/day of drug to the mother would produce 4 mg/kg of sulfapyridine in the milk, about 40% of maternal levels.[30] It is felt the risk of recurrent ulcerative colitis if medication is withdrawn outweighs the risk of sulfasalazine to the infant.[33]

Anticoagulants

Heparin does not pass into milk, but it is not a drug that can be given orally to the mother or without close monitoring of prothrombin times. Anticoagulants had been reported to appear in breast milk and to prolong prothrombin times, not only in the mother, but also in the infant. Infants nursed by these mothers had been sustained with 1 mg of vitamin K daily. Because of the competition for conjugation in the glucuronidase system, extra vitamin K is not recommended in the first few weeks of life. Knowles[35] has reviewed the literature thoroughly on anticoagulant drugs and specifically bis-3':3'-(4-oxycoumarinyl) ethyl acetate (Tromexan). Although infants nursed by mothers taking the drug had been observed to hemorrhage, they had improvement of their prothrombin times. Infants given the drug directly in milk had poorer prothrombin times. It is believed the drug is altered by maternal metabolism. The drug has also been observed to cause changes in capillary resistance, especially when there has been previous vascular damage. Vitamin K has no effect on the hemorrhagic tendencies in these infants. When the mother was taking phenindione (an indanedione derivative), hemorrhaging in the nursing newborn has been associated with trauma. Ethyl biscoumacetate has also been found in mother's milk by Illingworth and Finch.[28]

Analysis of the milk of mothers using warfarin by L'E Orme et al.,[39] however, did not reveal any drug in the milks or in the infants. The infants' prothrombin times remained normal. This has been further confirmed by McKenna et al.,[45] who followed two breastfed infants whose mothers were anticoagulated prior to delivery and maintained on warfarin postpartum. They found no immediate or delayed biologic effect on coagulation in 56 and 131 days of follow-up. From this it has been suggested that warfarin is the drug of choice in the lactating mother who requires anticoagulant therapy and wishes to continue breastfeeding. If surgery is contemplated or unusual trauma occurs, a review of the coagulation status of the infant is indicated as a precautionary measure.

Antithyroid drugs

Iodide has been known for generations to pass into the milk and has been recorded to cause symptoms in infants not only when used for hyperthyroidism but also in asthma preparations and cough medicines. Iodides have been noted to be goitrogenic and to sensitize the thyroid gland to other drugs such as lithium, chlorpromazine, and methylxanthines.

Thiouracil is actively transported into the milk and appears in higher concentration in milk than in blood or urine, being reported at three to twelve times higher in milk than blood. It has the potential of causing goiter-suppressing thyroid activity or agranulocytes.

Methimazole (Tapazole) presents risks to the nursing infant similar to those seen with thiouracil, that is, thyroid suppression and goiter. Giving 0.125 grain of thyroid extract to an infant may not adequately protect him, and careful monitoring of neonatal thyroid function is mandatory. Measurement of amounts of methimazole in milk and serum when a mother received 2.5 mg every 12 hours were performed by Tegler and Lindström[63] and found to be similar. They found 7% to 16% of the maternal dose in the milk; thus a dose of 5 mg, four times daily, might provide the infant with 3 mg daily. Studies of carbimazole done using ^{35}S-labeled compound show a similar trend, with 0.47% of the dose appearing in the milk. Studies were done on a single dose of 10 mg carbimazole.

Propylthiouracil, (PTU) has been investigated by several groups and similar results have been reported, showing that little of the compound is excreted in the milk (0.025% to 0.077% of total dose) in single-dose studies.[32,44] An infant followed 5 months on maternal doses of 200 to 300 mg PTU daily showed no neonatal thyroid symptoms and normal triiodothyronine (T_3), thyroxine (T_4), and thyroid-stimulating hormone (TSH). On the strength of these reports, others have proceeded to use PTU and permit breast-feeding. The availability of microdeterminations for T_3, T_4, and TSH improve the quality of monitoring, and all infants given PTU via the milk should be followed closely.

Caffeine and other methylxanthines

Caffeine ingestion has been singled out for discussion because it is a frequent concern, yet the data provided in most reviews are misleading. Although with a given dose of caffeine that is comparable to that in a cup of coffee the level in the milk is low (1% of level in mother) and the level in the infant's plasma is also low, caffeine does accumulate in the infant. Before the availability of the laboratory test for caffeine, cases were managed on clinical symptoms alone. It had been recognized by many clinicians and documented in the Rochester series[38] of nursing mothers that wakeful, hyperactive infants were often the victims of caffeine stimulation. If a mother drank more than 6 to 8 cups of any caffeine-containing beverage in a day's time, her infant could accumulate symptomatic amounts of caffeine. It was often the soft drinks such as colas and other carbonated drinks (such as Mountain Dew) that contributed to the caffeine buildup. When the situation was identified—a wide-eyed, active, alert infant who never slept for long—it was suggested that the mother try caffeine-free beverages, both hot and cold drinks. Often the infant settled down to a reasonable sleep pattern after a few days with no caffeine. Since information on milk and plasma levels has become available, researchers[38] have identified three cases of caffeine excess in breastfed infants, one of which Rivera-Calimlin[53] reported. The infants all had measurable levels of caffeine in the plasma, which disappeared over a week's time after the caffeine was discontinued. The corresponding milk levels were as previously reported, about 1% of the mother's level, which supports the hypothesis that caffeine accumulates in the infant. The infants do not need to be hospitalized, and verification of blood caffeine levels is helpful but not mandatory, since clinical trial will suffice. Smoking has been observed to augment the caffeine effect. Caffeine added to the diet of rats in amounts comparable to current amounts consumed daily by adults caused some decrease in growth in length and weight in the lactating pups.[18]

With an increasing number of women with asthma wishing to breastfeed, a question arises about the impact of theophylline. The methylxanthines have also been used in apnea of prematurity so that information has been generated around dose, clearance, and toxicity in the neonate.[5] In addition, obtaining microdeterminations of blood levels is readily available.

Several studies of theophylline in mothers on regular doses have shown that the serum levels are lowest just before the oral dose and that M/P ratio is 0.60 to 0.73, with milk levels paralleling serum levels.[6,60,71] It has been estimated that the infant receives 1% of the maternal dose. Data on IV and oral medication are similar in terms of M/P ratio. Maximum exposure was estimated at 7 to 8 mg/24 hours.

Dyphylline is a compound introduced clinically as a bronchodilator because of its lack of side effects.[29] It is excreted renally with little biotransformation. The milk serum ratio was determined to be 2.08 ± 52 and the biologic half-life was 3.21 hours. Although this is considerably greater than theophylline, it is not yet known how this would affect the infant.

Theobromine, which occurs in chocolate and cocoa has been studied as well to evaluate its possible cumulative effects when taken with caffeine or theophylline.[5] A very small amount was detected in the milk, with a potential dose to the infant after one chocolate bar (1.2 oz) of 0.44 to 1.68 mg. No theobromine was found in the infant's urine.[6]

Herbs and herbal teas

There has been an increase in the use of herbs and herbal teas, especially among those interested in natural foods. As is well known to all students of pharmacology, many of the effective medications of today originated in these natural products. In the early part of the century many compounds were still being dispensed in their natural form, including foxglove leaves for digitalis. The natural product was unpredictable because one leaf or plant will contain more or less active principle than another, so that careful dose control was impossible and results were often unpredictable. Much of the interest in herbal teas has evolved as individuals seek a beverage that does not contain caffeine; what they get is another compound instead, often one more potent and much of the time one about which considerably less is known (Table 11-4).

There are herbal teas available that are prepared carefully, using herbs only for essence (Celestial Seasonings brand tea) and avoiding heavy doses of herbs with active principles. The strength of any tea depends on how it is made, however. An ordinary teabag with hot water run over it will contain little caffeine and theobromine; however, when it is steeped for 5 minutes the potency is increased tenfold. Some of the preparations are benign or even nutritious, such as rose hips tea, which contains a large amount

Table 11-4. Psychoactive substances used in herbal preparations

Labeled ingredient	Botanical source	Pharmacologic principle	Suggested use	Reported effects
African Yohimbe Bark; Yohimbe	*Corynanthe yohimbe*	Yohimbe	Smoke or tea as stimulant	Mild hallucinogen
Broom; Scotch Broom	*Cytisus* spp	Cytisine	Smoke for relaxation	Strong sedative-hypnotic
California Poppy	*Eschscholtzia californica*	Alkaloids & glucosides	Smoke as marihuana substitute	Mild euphoriant
Catnip	*Nepeta cataria*	Nepetalactone	Smoke or tea as marihuana substitute	Mild hallucinogen
Cinnamon	*Cinnamomum camphora*	?	Smoke with marihuana	Mild stimulant
Damiana	*Turnera diffusa*	?	Smoke as marihuana substitute	Mild stimulant
Hops	*Humulus lupulus*	Lupuline	Smoke or tea as sedative and marihuana substitute	None
Hydrangea	*Hydrangea paniculata*	Hydrangin, saponin, cyanogenes	Smoke as marihuana substitute	Stimulant
Juniper	*Juniper macropoda*	?	Smoke as hallucinogen	Strong hallucinogen
Kavakava	*Piper methysticum*	Yangonin, pyrones	Smoke or tea as marihuana substitute	Mild hallucinogen
Kola Nut; Gotu Kola	*Cola* spp	Caffeine, theobromine, kolanin	Smoke, tea, or capsules as stimulant	Stimulant
Lobelia	*Lobelia inflata*	Lobeline	Smoke or tea as marihuana substitute	Mild euphoriant
Mandrake	*Mandragora officinarum*	Scopolamine, hyoscyamine	Tea as hallucinogen	Hallucinogen
Mate	*Ilex paraguayensis*	Caffeine	Tea as stimulant	Stimulant
Mormon Tea	*Ephedra nevadensis*	Ephedrine	Tea as stimulant	Stimulant
Nutmeg	*Myristica fragrans*	Myristicin	Tea as hallucinogen	Hallucinogen
Passion Flower	*Passiflora incarnata*	Harmine alkaloids	Smoke, tea, or capsules as marihuana substitute	Mild stimulant
Periwinkle	*Catharanthus roseus*	Indole alkaloids	Smoke or tea as euphoriant	Hallucinogen
Prickly Poppy	*Argemone mexicana*	Protopine, bergerine, isoquinilines	Smoke as euphoriant	Narcotic-analgesic
Snakeroot	*Rauwolfia serpentina*	Reserpine	Smoke or tea as tobacco substitute	Tranquilizer
Thorn Apple	*Datura stramonium*	Atropine, scopolamine	Smoke or tea as tobacco substitute or hallucinogen	Strong hallucinogen
Tobacco	*Nicotiana* spp	Nicotine	Smoke as tobacco	Strong stimulant
Valerian	*Valeriana officinalis*	Chatinine, velerine alkaloids	Tea or capsules as tranquilizer	Tranquilizer
Wild Lettuce	*Lactuca sativa*	Lactucarine	Smoke as opium substitute	Mild narcotic-analgesic
Wormwood	*Artemisia absinthium*	Absinthine	Smoke or tea as relaxant	Narcotic-analgesic

From Siegel, R.K.: JAMA, **236**:473, 1976, copyright 1976, American Medical Association.

of vitamin C. Other teas are made from plants known to the toxicologist as poisonous. Isolated reports of toxicity from these preparations are appearing in the medical literature; many others probably go undiagnosed.[56] Use of these preparations is certainly an important part of a medical and dietary history.

Mother's milk tea is a blend of plants handed down for many generations as a galactagogue; it contains a mixture of fennel seeds, coriander seeds, chamomile flowers, lemongrass, borage leaves, blessed thistle leaves, star anise, comfrey leaves, and fenugreek seeds.[62] It is promoted as containing no caffeine. Some of the things it does contain are shown in Table 11-5. Although not all the constituents have pharmacologic actions, several do and these were used medicinally for centuries. These popular teas have the same potential for problems as do the common popular beverages of coffee and cola. The euphoric effects are the most prominent.

A hemorrhagic diathesis was described in a woman who drank quarts of a herbal tea that contained tonka beans, melilot (sweet clover), and woodruff, all of which contain natural coumarins.[27] She narrowly avoided gynecologic surgery for excessive hemorrhaging before the history was obtained. The tea also included hawthorn, which contains cardioglucosides that cause hypotension.

Sassafras contains an aromatic oil, safrole, which has been shown to cause cancer

Table 11-5. Ingredients and effects of mother's milk tea

Plant	Constituents	Effects	Toxicity
Fennel seed	Volatile oil, anisic acid	Weak diuretic stimulant	"Disturbs CNS"
Coriander seed	Volatile oil, coriandrol	Increases flow of saliva and gastric juice	
Chamomile flower	Volatile oil, bitter glycoside	Sudorific; antispasmodic; used to lighten hair	Vomiting and vertigo
Lemongrass	Lemon flavor		
Borage leaf	Volatile oil, tannin, mineral acids	Diuretic, sudorific, euphoric	Possible
Blessed thistle leaf	Volatile oil, bitter principle	Appertif, galactagogue, diaphoretic	Strongly emetic
Star anise	Volatile oil, anethole, resin, tannin	Stimulant, mild expectorant	
Comfrey leaf	Protein, vitamin B_{12}, tannin, allantoin, choline	Used as mucliage to knit bones, weak sedative, demulcent, astringent	
Fenugreek seed (Greek hay) (Coffee substitute and natural dye)	Mucilage, trigonelline, physterols, celery flavor		
Other beverages			
Coffee plant	Volatile oil, caffeine, tannin	Stimulant, diuretic, coloring	Insomnia, restlessness
Blue cohosh	Saponin, "glucoside that affects muscles"	Oxytocic, potent, acts on voluntary and involuntary muscles	Irritant, causes pain in fingers and toes

in mice; it is therefore no longer permitted as a commercial flavoring but it appears in herbal teas. It causes central nervous system symptoms in mice including ataxia, ptosis, and hypothermia.[56] It is also thought to interfere with the action of other medications. Belladonna alkaloids are common in some teas used to create euphoria or ease pain.

Pyrrolizidine alkaloids have been identified in an herbal tea used in the Southwest that was responsible for several deaths in children given the tea when they were ill. The alkaloid is excreted within 24 hours but symptoms may not start for several days or weeks. Death is due to liver failure.

The clinician needs to inquire about all foods and beverages when taking a history. If an excessive amount of any herbal product is being consumed, its contents should be checked. The regional poison control center may be able to identify active principles if the plant constituents of the tea are known.

Amphetamines

Reports on amphetamines have also varied; some published reports have claimed the drug does not appear in the milk, whereas others have reported measurable amounts. The symptoms reported are tremors, jitteriness, and wakefulness in the infant. If a mother is taking amphetamines for significant therapeutic reasons, then careful observation of the infant will indicate if there are problems from accumulation of the drug. The difference in observed reports may well be due to dosage, frequency of medication, and individual variation. In two identified cases when amphetamines were used for weight loss in over-the-counter diet preparations (dextroamphetamine [Dexedrine], 5 to 10 mg daily), the infants were jittery and wakeful and responded to withdrawal of the drug.

Cardiovascular drugs and diuretics

Digitalis is given to infants, but only for serious reasons. Measurements of digitalis in the milk in mothers maintained on digitalis throughout pregnancy and lactation showed concentrations of 0.825 nmol/L, which was 59% of the maternal plasma level in one study[11] and 75% in another.[20] Authors agree that digoxin levels would be low and the dosage to the infant low, but the long-range effects are not known.[11,20,43] There is sufficient experience accumulated to date to conclude that mothers taking sustaining doses of digitalis preparations may nurse their infants without any harm to the infant.

Propranolol was found in the milk of mothers but does not appear to accumulate in the infant. Thus experienced cardiologists have permitted mothers taking propranolol to nurse their infants without any ill effect observed in the infants. In 1973, Levitan and Manion[40] reported significant quantities of propranolol in breast milk. Propranolol and its major metabolites were measured in milk and found by Smith et al.[58] to provide the infant with a maximum dose of less than 0.1% of the maternal dose or approximately 7μg/100 ml. The half-life of elimination from the milk was over 6 hours.[5] β-adrenergic blockade effects have been described, including hypoglycemia, in an infant breastfed by a mother taking propranolol. Since the reports are conflicting, it would be necessary to monitor the breastfed infant carefully when the mother is taking propranolol. Monitoring plasma levels of the infant may be helpful if there is any question.

The antihypertensive drugs atenolol (Tenormin) metoprolol (Lopressor) and nadolol (Corgard, Corzide) have been evaluated in human milk.[16,17,46] Metoprolol had a peak level in the blood of 713 ng/100 ml at 1.1 hours and in the milk of 4.7 ng/100 ml at 3.8 hours. The data suggest that metoprolol appears minimally in milk and is probably safe for the breastfeeding neonate.[17] Nadolol appears in serum at 77 ng/100 ml and in milk at 357 ng/100 ml.[16] Atenolol and metoprolol levels in milk are also higher than in the maternal serum.[46] Serum levels of antenolol in one breastfed infant reached 0.16 μmol/L.

Reserpine, on the other hand, has been reported to cause nasal stuffiness, bradycardia, and respiratory difficulty with increased tracheobronchial secretion and is contraindicated in both pregnancy and lactation.

Use of diuretics requires careful observation because they have the potential for causing a diuresis in the neonate that could be markedly dehydrating. Although diuretics such as furosemide (Lasix) are given to neonates, this is done only when fluid and electrolyte levels can be followed closely. Oral diuretics were used to suppress lactation in a study by Healy[24] in 40 postpartum women who chose not to breastfeed. Bendroflumethiazide (Naturetin) was used, 5 mg twice daily for 5 days. He found it more effective than estrogens, with fewer side effects. This also points out that diuretics can suppress lactation, at least to some degree. Reports have also appeared documenting the interaction of three diuretics with bilirubin-albumin complexes.[66] Chlorothiazide presented the greatest risk for producing free bilirubin, with ethacrynic acid and furosemide producing considerably less. The latter two are clinically effective in lower doses as well. The levels of chlorothiazide and hydrochlorothiazide in milk are less than 100 ng/ml.[47,48] For most infants these are safe; however, these findings certainly suggest caution is necessary if the infant is jaundiced or very immature. Chlorthalidone (Hygroton) appears in milk.[67] A term baby might receive 180 μg per day. The half-life is 60 hours. Furosemide has been shown by several techniques not only to displace bilirubin from albumin in the newborn but also to be slowly excreted by the newborn, with only 84% excreted in 24 hours.

A mother who is lactating may actually require substantially less medication, particularly diuretics. Close monitoring of the mother during lactation to try to reduce her medications may provide a therapeutic balance that is good for the mother and safe for the infant.

Central nervous system drugs

Phenobarbital can be given to infants and is usually safe, but careful observation of the infant for variation in sleeping habits is important.

Phenytoin in the breast milk has been associated with vomiting, tremors, rash, blood dyscrasia (rarely), and methemoglobinemia, but not with drowsiness and lethargy. Many

mothers have nursed without apparent incident while taking phenobarbital and phenytoin. Phenytoin levels in milk of mothers treated for epilepsy have been measured and
levels in the infant have been calculated to provide less than 5% of the calculated
therapeutic dose for infants.[49] Valproic acid in maternal milk is low (3% of maternal
serum concentrations) but the mean half-life is 47 hours, four times that in adults, so
there is risk of accumulation.[61] Fetal hydantoin syndrome has been described; therefore
any possible correlation with further exposure during nursing should be considered.
When infant plasma level determinations are available, it might be advisable to check
the plasma level after 1 or 2 weeks of nursing, providing an opportunity to evaluate
possible accumulation.

Psychotherapeutic agents

Lithium is the one drug in the psychotherapeutic group with a clear risk of toxicity
in the neonate as well as clear evidence that it reaches the breast milk. Lithium is
contraindicated in pregnancy as well as in lactation. Infants have been reported to be
hypotonic, flaccid, and ''depressed'' when the nursing mother is taking lithium.

Chlorpromazine or phenothiazine appears in the milk in small amounts even at doses
of 1200 mg, but does not appear to accumulate. Doses of 100 mg/day do not appear to
cause symptoms in the infants. It has been the practice in Rochester to permit breastfeeding while the mother is taking phenothiazines, considering it an important part of
the treatment of the mother. All infants so nursed gained well and were not dehydrated
or unusually depressed. Diazepam (Valium) has been detected in milk and in breastfed
infants' serum and urine. It has caused depression and poor feeding with weight loss in
the infant. Chlordiazepoxide (Librium) and clorazepate (Tranxene) do reach the milk
and may cause drowsiness and poor suckling. These substances' metabolites are also
active, and therefore the half-life of therapeutic activity is prolonged. Meprobamate
(Miltown, Equanil) has an M/P ratio greater than 1 and has been identified in milk.
Infants whose mothers are taking meprobamate may become drowsy, but dosage adjustment may be indicated if the risk/benefit ratio is significant.

Tricyclic antidepressants such as imipramine have been identified in the breast
milk[35]; thus cautious use may well be appropriate.[36] Amitriptyline (Elavil) was not
found in milk according to Ayd.[3] The Committee on Drugs of the American Academy
of Pediatrics[13] has reviewed psychotropic drugs in lactation and concluded that most
drugs are found in the milk but the concentration is usually low; therefore, there is little
likelihood of an effect on the infant. The infant should be observed for overt signs of
drug effect as well as long-term effects on the developing nervous system, even with
low doses.

Pesticides and pollutants

Human milk has been known to contain insecticides. Chlorinated hydrocarbons such
as DDT and its metabolites dieldrin, aldrin, and related compounds are the best known.
The major reason these compounds appear in breast milk is that they are deposited in

body lipid stores and move with lipid. It has been pointed out that the fetus receives his greatest dose in utero and that adult body fat has approximately 30 times the concentration in milk.

Polychlorinated biphenyls (PCBs) in heavily contaminated pregnant Japanese women produced small for gestational age infants who had transient darkening of the skin ("cola babies"). Polybrominated biphenyls (PBBs) are similar compounds associated with a heavy exposure to farm animals and contaminated cattle fed in the lower Michigan Peninsula. The women in the United States who have the greatest risk of high exposure to PCBs or PBBs are those who have worked with or eaten in excess (i.e., at least once a week) fish that was caught by sports fishing in contaminated waters. Others at high risk are those who live near a waste disposal site or have been involved in environmental spills. Unless there is heavy exposure, however, there is no contraindication to breastfeeding. When there is a question, the state health department can be consulted for specific advice or to measure plasma and milk levels. The epidemiologists are usually aware of the risks in a given geographic area and whether it is necessary to measure milk levels once lactation is fully established. If this sampling is planned for in advance during the pregnancy, little time need be lost. Unless there is a unique and excessive exposure, the infant could breastfeed until levels are returned from the laboratory.

In most cases, the levels of pesticides in human milk have been less than those in cow's milk. The accumulated amounts have not usually exceeded safe allowable limits. There are several extensive reviews published about the dilemma of pollutants in human milk.[54,55,68,70] It has been suggested that the body burden at birth can be added to by exposing the infant to small levels in the milk that may indeed exceed the exposure limits allowable for daily intake set by the World Health Organization. Human milk levels are used epidemiologically as markers of human exposure in a community exposure because there is a close correlation of milk levels to the levels in the fat stores. Unselected mothers in the Great Lakes region were tested by the State of New York in 1978 and there was no chemical (PCB, PBB) in any milk in random sampling of residents. Thus, unless the circumstances are unusual, breastfeeding should not be abandoned on the basis of insecticide contamination.

Most common air pollutants are not found in human milk.

Radioactive materials

Because of the increasing number of diagnostic tests available today with radioactive materials, it is not uncommon for a nursing mother to face such a procedure.

Radioactive iodine (^{125}I and ^{131}I) passes into milk at levels as high as 5% of the dose. When this is used for diagnostic purposes, breastfeeding should be discontinued for 24 hours. The excretion by the breast may alter the validity of the test result. If radioactive iodine is to be used therapeutically, breastfeeding must be discontinued until the iodine has cleared the system, which may be 1 to 3 weeks. A carefully collected sample of milk can be tested for radioactivity so that the period that the infant is off the breast is not unnecessarily long. If more than a 30 μci dose of ^{131}I is used, nursing should not be resumed until the milk is clear. If the infant is older and getting other foods, time can be altered accordingly.

^{67}Gallium citrate appears in significant amounts in the milk. It does clear the body quickly and is relatively safe for use in patients. Breastfeeding should be discontinued for at least 72 hours.

^{99m}Technetium is reported to clear the milk in 6 to 48 hours. The stage of lactation, whether or not the breast is emptied prior to receiving the dose, and the method of clearing the breast may well be responsible for the inconsistent results. Discontinuing breastfeeding for at least 24 hours is advisable.

With the advent of ultrasound examination, CT scanning, and other techniques, occasionally there is an alternative to use of radioactive material during lactation.

The psychologic impact of a toxin in the milk

The psychologic reactions of a group of nursing mothers from the lower Michigan Peninsula whose breast milk was contaminated with a toxic fire-retardant chemical, PBB, were studied.[23] Every tenth woman who had had her milk tested for PBB was contacted for the study (a sample of 200 women); 139 responded and received a questionnaire and 97 (70%) filled out the questionnaire. The subjects knew their own level and that the range for all mothers was from undetected to 0.46 ppm with an average of 0.1 ppm. The testing was voluntary and cost $25. Of all those tested, 96% had measurable amounts.

The data were collected in a six-page questionnaire that included demographics, facts and attitudes about pregnancy and breastfeeding, what the respondent knew about PBB, why she had her milk tested, her feelings about the contamination, a section consisting of three projective tests to tap less conscious attitudes, and any medical problems that had occurred since the contamination. Two modes of coping emerged: denial and mastery. In general, the findings indicated that the greater the level of toxic contamination of PBB reported in a mother's milk, the greater the denial, to the point of not having correct information about even her own level. Those in the denial group were less able to allow unconscious conflicts about nursing to surface. The entire study group was a select group, of course, because the majority of Michigan's nursing mothers chose not to have their milk tested at all, thus electing to remain uninformed. Those who handled the PBB situation by mastery changed their breastfeeding patterns or their food buying, or even moved away. These individuals tested to be more consciously aware of what they were feeling as well as the behaviors they wished to change. This group was also more knowledgeable about the facts in general.

In response to a question about what they would advise someone else to do, they were decisive: 77% would suggest testing, 52% would suggest stopping breastfeeding, and 10% more would suggest at least shortening the breastfeeding. Ambivalence toward nursing was correlated with guilt in both groups (only 15% discontinued breastfeeding).

The "draw-a-baby" test showed an unusual amount (94%) of distortion and expressions of anguish. These findings were consistent throughout all the test modalities, thus they were not thought to be a function of personality.

The information from this study may be relevant to other situations in which a mother's milk becomes contaminated either environmentally or by self-medication. The psychologic implications of environmental contamination need further research. The clinician should be aware of the implications of contamination for patient management.

IMMUNIZATIONS
Immunizing the breastfed infant

Questions often arise as to whether a breastfed infant should be immunized on a different schedule because of the protective maternal antibodies that might interfere with the infant's response to antigen stimulation. Following are some brief guidelines on the more common situations of concern:

1. Diphtheria-pertussis-tetanus (DPT) vaccination is not altered by breastfeeding, and the regular schedule should be followed for the infant.[15]
2. Since oral poliovirus vaccine (OPV) is an oral live virus vaccine, there was concern that the maternal antibodies would inactivate the live virus. The recommendation of the Centers for Disease Control is, however, that the same schedule be followed. They state that the current scientific literature indicates that for infants older than 6 weeks (which is the earliest age of vaccination recommended), there is no indication for withholding breastfeeding in relationship to OPV administration nor is there need for extra doses of vaccine.[15]
3. Rubella, mumps, and measles vaccines should be given at the regularly scheduled times.[15]

Immunizing the nursing mother

SMALLPOX. Smallpox vaccination is inadvisable for the mother of any infant under 1 year of age, nursing or not. It is the personal contact, not the breastfeeding, that causes the risk; therefore there is no advantage to weaning if vaccination is necessary.

Rh$_0$GAM. Only rare trace amounts of anti-Rh are present in colostrum and none in mature milk of women given large doses of Rh$_0$GAM immediately postpartum. No adverse response was noted, even with these high dosages. It has been thought that any Rh antibodies in the mother's milk were inactivated by the gastric juices. Rh$_0$GAM or Rh sensitization is not a contraindication to breastfeeding.

RUBELLA. Following is the recommendation of the American College of Obstetrics and Gynecology with respect to rubella:

1. In the adult female population, approximately 85% to 90% of the individuals are thought to have a high level of naturally acquired immunity and only 10% to 15% are considered to be susceptible to rubella infection.

2. Vaccination of pregnant women is contraindicated under all circumstances.

3. No woman of childbearing age should be vaccinated without having been first tested for immunity.

4. If the test is negative, the woman may be vaccinated if there is reasonable assurance that she will not become pregnant for at least 2 months.

5. At present the duration of immunity acquired from vaccination remains in question. It is possible that adult women vaccinated in childhood may be susceptible and might acquire an active rubella infection, which may go undetected.

The rubella virus was found in the milk of 69% of the women immunized with live attenuated rubella (HPV-77 DE5 or RA 27/3 strains).[41] A virus-specific IgA antibody response was seen in milk of all the women. Infectious rubella virus or virus antigen was recovered from the nasopharynx and throat of 56% of the breastfed infants and none of the nonbreastfed infants. No infant had disease in this study, but 25% of the breastfed group had seroconversion transiently.[42]

A breastfed infant whose mother developed laboratory-confirmed rubella 8 days postpartum had virus in the pharynx at 15 days of age and serum rubella antibodies 1:64 at 2 months of age, but no clinical disease.[9] Virus has been isolated from the milk of a mother who received HPV-77 DE5 strain rubella vaccine. The mother developed a rash and nodes on day 12 and had rubella cultured from the throat.[34] Another infant whose mother was immunized with HPV-77 DE5 developed disease on the thirteenth day, although all cultures including the milk were negative for rubella.[37] Diagnosis was confirmed by serum titers. Although the attenuated virus may appear in the milk, this should not dissuade one from vaccinating a breastfeeding mother at the safest time, that is, immediately postpartum.

REFERENCES

1. Aranda, J.V., et al.: Metabolism and renal elimination of furosemide in the newborn infant, J. Pediatr. **101**:777, 1982.

2. Arena, J.M.: Drugs and breast feeding, Clin. Pediatr. **5**:472, 1966.

3. Ayd, F.: Excretion of psychotrophic drugs in human breast milk, Int. Drug Ther. Newsletter **8**:33, 1973.

4. Bauer, J.H., et al.: Propranolol in human plasma and breast milk, Am. J. Cardiol. **43**:860, 1979.

5. Berlin, C.M.: Excretion of methylxanthines in human milk, Semin. Perinatol. **5**:389, 1981.

6. Berlin, C.M., and Daniel, C.H.: Excretion of theobromine in human milk and saliva, Pediatr. Res. **15**:492, 1981.

7. Bowes, W.A., Jr.: The effect of medications on the lactating mother and her infant, Clin. Obstet. Gynecol. **23**:1073, 1980.

8. Briggs, G.G., et al., editors: Drugs in pregnancy and lactation, Baltimore, 1983, Williams & Wilkins.

9. Buimovici-Klein, E., et al.: Isolation of rubella virus in milk after postpartum immunization, J. Pediatr. **91**:939, 1977.

10. Catz, C.S., and Giacoia, G.P.: Drugs and breast milk, Pediatr. Clin. North Am. **19**:151, 1972.

11. Chan, V., Tse, T.F., and Wong, V.: Transfer of digoxin across the placenta and into breast milk, Br. J. Obstet. Gynecol. **85**:605, 1978.

12. Clark, J.H., and Wilson, W.G.: A 16-day-old breast-fed infant with metabolic acidosis caused by salicylate, Clin. Pediatr. **20**:53, 1981.

13. Committee on Drugs, American Academy of Pediatrics: Psychotropic drugs in pregnancy and lactation, Pediatrics **69**:241, 1982.

14. Committee on Drugs, American Academy of Pe-

diatrics: The transfer of drugs and other chemicals into human breast milk, Pediatrics **72:**375, 1983.

15. Committee on Infectious Disease: Report of the Committee on Infectious Disease, ed. 19, Evanston, Ill., 1982, American Academy of Pediatrics.

16. Devlin, R.G., Duchin, K.L., and Fleiss, P.M.: Nadolol in human serum and breast milk, Br. J. Clin. Pharmacol. **12:**393, 1981.

17. Devlin, R.G., and Fleiss, P.M.: Captopril in human blood and breast milk, J. Clin. Pharmacol. **21:**110, 1981.

18. Dunlap, M., and Court, J.M.: Effects of maternal caffeine ingestion on neonatal growth in rats, Biol. Neonate **39:**178, 1981.

19. Erickson, S.H., Oppenheim, G.L., and Smith, G.H.: Metronidazole in breast milk, Obstet. Gynecol. **57:**49, 1981.

20. Finley, J.P., et al.: Digoxin excretion in human milk, J. Pediatr. **94:**339, 1979.

21. Gaginella, T.S.: Drugs and the nursing mother-infant, U.S. Pharm. **3:**39, 1978.

22. Gilman, A.G., Goodman, L.S., and Gilman, A., editors: Goodman and Gilman's the pharmacological basis of therapeutics, ed. 6, New York, 1980, Macmillan Publishing Co., Inc.

23. Hatcher, S.L.: The psychological experience of nursing mothers upon learning of a toxic substance in their breast milk, Psychiatry **45:**172, 1982.

24. Healy, M.: Suppressing lactation with oral diuretics, Lancet **1:**1353, 1961.

25. Heislerberg, L., and Branebjerg, P.E.: Blood and milk concentrations of metronidazole in mothers and infants, J. Perinat. Med. **11:**114, 1983.

26. Hervada, A.R., Feit, E., and Sagraves, R.: Drugs in breast milk, Perinat. Care **2:**19, 1978.

27. Hogan, R.P., III: Hemorrhage diathesis caused by drinking an herbal tea, JAMA **249:**2679, 1983.

28. Illingworth, R.S., and Finch, E.: Ethyl discoumacetate (Tromexan) in human milk, J. Obstet. Gynecol. Br. Empire **66:**487, 1959.

29. Jarboe, C.H., et al.: Dyphylline elimination kinetics in lactating women blood to milk transfer, J. Clin. Pharmacol. **21:**405, 1981.

30. Järnerot, G., and Into-Malmberg, M.B.: Sulphasalazine treatment during breast feeding, Scand. J. Gastroenterol. **14:**869, 1979.

31. Kafetzis, D.A., et al.: Passage of cephalosporins and amoxicillin into breast milk, Acta Paediatr. Scand. **70:**285, 1981.

32. Kampmann, J.P., et al.: Propylthiouracil in human milk, Lancet **1:**736, 1980.

33. Khan, A.K.A., and Truelove, S.C.: Placental and mammary transfer of sulphasalazine, Br. Med. J. **2:**1533, 1979.

34. Klein, E.B., Byrne, T., and Cooper, L.Z.: Neonatal rubella in a breast-fed infant after postpartum maternal infection, J. Pediatr. **97:**774, 1980.

35. Knowles, J.A.: Excretion of drugs in milk: a review, J. Pediatr. **66:**1068, 1965.

36. Knowles, J.A.: Breast milk: a source of more than nutrition for the neonate, Clin. Toxicol. **7:**69, 1974.

37. Landes, R.D., et al.: Neonatal rubella following postpartum maternal immunization, J. Pediatr. **97:**465, 1980.

38. Lawrence, R.: Unpublished data.

39. L'E Orme, M., et al.: May mothers given warfarin breast-feed their infants? Br. Med. J. **1:**1564, 1977.

40. Levitan, A.A., and Manion, J.C.: Propranolol therapy during pregnancy and lactation, Am. J. Cardiol. **32:**2, 1973.

41. Losonsky, G.A., et al.: Effect of immunization against rubella on lactation products. I. Development and characterization of specific immunologic reactivity in breast milk, J. Infect. Dis. **145:**654, 1982.

42. Losonsky, G.A., et al.: Effect of immunization against rubella on lactation products. II. Maternal-neonatal interactions, J. Infect. Dis. **145:**661, 1982.

43. Loughnan, P.M.: Digoxin excretion in human breast milk, J. Pediatr. **92:**1019, 1978.

44. Low, L.C.K., Lang, J., and Alexander, W.D.: Excretion of carbimazole and propylthiouracil in breast milk, Lancet **2:**1011, 1979.

45. McKenna, R., Cole, E.R., and Vasan, V.: Is warfarin sodium contraindicated in the lactating mother? J. Pediatr. **103:**325, 1983.

46. Melander, F.A., et al.: Accumulation of atenolol and metoprolol in human breast milk, Eur. J. Clin. Pharmacol. **20:**229, 1981.

47. Miller, M.E., Cohn, R.D., and Burghart, P.H.: Hydrochlorothiazide deposition in a mother and her breast-fed infant, J. Pediatr. **101:**789, 1982.

48. Mulley, P.A., et al.: Placental transfer of chlorthalidone and its elimination in maternal milk, Eur. J. Clin. Pharmacol. **13:**129, 1978.

49. Nau, H., et al.: Valproic acid and its metabolites: Placental transfer, neonatal pharmacokinetics, transfer via mother's milk and clinical status in neonates of epileptic mothers, J. Pharmacol. Exp. Ther. **219:**768, 1981.

50. O'Brien, T.E.: Excretion of drugs in human milk, Am. J. Hosp. Pharm. **31:**844, 1974.

51. Rasmussen, F.: Mammary excretion of benzyl penicillin, erythromycin and penethamate hydriodide, Acta Pharmacol. Toxicol. (Kbh) **16:**194, 1959.

52. Rasmussen, F.: Mammary excretion of antipyryne ethanol and urea, Acta Vet. Scand. **2:**151, 1961.

53. Rivera-Calimlim, L.: Drugs in breast milk, Drug Ther. **2:**20, Dec., 1977.

54. Rogan, W.J., Bagniewska, A., and Damstra, T.: Pollutants in breast milk, N. Engl. J. Med. **302:**1450, 1980.

55. Rogan, W.J., and Gladen, B.: Monitoring breast milk contamination to detect hazards from waste disposal, Environ. Health Perspect. **48:**87, 1983.

56. Segelman, A.B., et al.: Sassafras and herb tea, JAMA **236:**477, 1976.

57. Siegel, R.K.: Herbal intoxication: psychoactive effects from herbal cigarettes, tea and capsules, JAMA **236:**473, 1976.

58. Smith, M.T., et al.: Propranolol, propranolol glucuronide, and naphthoxylactic acid in breast milk and plasma, Ther. Drug Monit. **5:**87, 1983.

59. Somogyi, A., and Cugler, R.: Cimetidine excretion into breast milk, Br. J. Clin. Pharmacol. **7:**627, 1979.

60. Stec, G.P., et al.: Kinetics of theophylline transfer to breast milk, Clin. Pharmacol. Ther. **28:**404, 1980.

61. Steen, B., et al.: Phenytoin excretion in human breast milk and plasma in nursed infants, Ther. Drug Monit. **4:**331, 1982.

62. Stuart, M., editor: The encyclopedia of herbs and herbalism, New York, 1979, Crescent Books.

63. Tegler, L., and Lindström, B.: Antithyroid drugs in milk, Lancet **2:**591, 1980.

64. Vorherr, H.: Drug excretion in breast milk, Postgrad. Med. **56:**97, 1974.

65. Vorherr, H.: The breast, morphology, physiology and lactation, New York, 1974, Academic Press, Inc.

66. Wennberg, R.P., Rasmussen, L.F., and Ahlors, C.E.: Displacement of bilirubin from human albumin by three diuretics, J. Pediatr. **90:**647, 1977.

67. Werthmann, M.W., and Krees, S.V.: Excretion of chlorothiazide in human breast milk, J. Pediatr. **81:**411, 1981.

68. Wichizer, T.M., and Brilliant, L.B.: Testing for polychlorinated biphenyls in human milk, Pediatrics **68:**411, 1981.

69. Wilson, J.T.: Drugs in breast milk, Balgowlah, Australia, 1981, Adis Press.

70. Wolff, M.S.: Occupationally derived chemicals in breast milk, Am. J. Ind. Med. **4:**259, 1983.

71. Yurchak, A.M., and Jusko, W.J.: Theophylline secreted into breast milk, Pediatrics **57:**518, 1976.

Normal growth, failure to thrive, and obesity in the breastfed infant

12

NORMAL GROWTH

Bottle fed infants gain more rapidly in weight and length during the first months of life than do breastfed infants. Therefore, evaluating an infant's physical growth by standards set by bottle fed infants predisposes one to the diagnosis of failure to thrive. Fomon et al.[12] reported a longitudinal study of breastfed and bottle fed infants during the first few months of life that demonstrated that the tenth and ninetieth percentile values for weight and length of the two groups were similar at birth, and the tenth percentile values of the two groups were similar at age 112 days. The significant difference was in the values for the ninetieth percentile, which showed the bottle fed infants to be substantially greater (Table 12-1). These differences were attributed to caloric intake rather than to the difference in composition of the diet. Similar differences have been noted by other investigators, including Mellander et al.[26] in the 1959 Norbotten study of Swedish infants. Mellander et al. recorded a weight gain of 3.34 kg for 162 breastfed infants and 3.53 kg for 143 bottle fed infants at age 4¼ months.

A study of "well-born" American infants reported by Jackson et al.[19] showed no difference between breastfed and bottle fed infants in the first 4 months of life in either weight or length. Between 4 and 6 months of life, they observed, the gain in weight and length was less rapid in the breastfed infants. Fomon et al.[13] have shown that not only did the bottle fed infant gain more in weight and length but also he gained more weight for a unit of length. This reflects the overfeeding of the bottle fed infants. Whether this contributes to subsequent obesity is an important issue.

Most studies of growth in breastfed infants have been plagued with the problem of variation in supplementation and the occurrence of partial weaning.[21] The growth of the exclusively breastfed infant was investigated by Ahn and MacLean[1] in 1980, who conducted a retrospective study of enthusiastic and successful La Leche League mothers and their babies in the Baltimore-Washington D.C. area. Mothers who had exclusively

Table 12-1. Size of breastfed infants and those fed milk-based formulas: percentile values

| Age (days) | Per-cen-tile | Weight (kg) | | | | Length (cm) | | | |
| | | Males | | Females | | Males | | Females | |
		Fed milk-based formulas (65)*	Breast-fed (58)	Fed milk-based formulas (77)	Breast-fed (46)	Fed milk-based formulas (65)	Breast-fed (58)	Fed milk-based formulas (77)	Breast-fed (46)
Birth	10	2870	2947	2816	2798				
	25	3125	3216	3135	2994				
	50	3410	3470	3350	3188				
	75	3705	3642	3615	3520				
	90	3804	3916	3964	3730				
8	10	2878	2881	2903	2746	48.9	49.5	48.8	48.5
	25	3248	3216	3274	2978	50.1	50.4	49.9	49.5
	50	3502	3459	3401	3260	51.7	51.2	51.1	50.7
	75	3688	3642	3698	3465	52.6	52.3	52.0	51.4
	90	3906	3839	4031	3555	53.4	52.8	53.2	52.2
14	10	3132	3089	3124	2990	49.8	50.6	49.4	49.7
	25	3399	3375	3426	3199	50.9	51.5	50.7	50.4
	50	3665	3681	3575	3500	52.6	52.4	52.0	51.6
	75	3876	3881	3894	3630	53.4	53.3	53.0	52.2
	90	4089	4065	4127	3698	54.1	54.2	54.1	53.4
28	10	3636	3406	3605	3511	51.6	52.0	51.5	51.6
	25	3970	3960	3824	3763	52.8	53.3	52.4	52.0
	50	4235	4271	4134	3935	54.6	54.2	53.8	53.3
	75	4470	4507	4440	4148	55.3	55.1	55.1	53.9
	90	4761	4692	4593	4230	55.9	55.7	56.0	55.0
42	10	4250	3962	4028	3930	53.0	53.8	53.0	53.2
	25	4506	4466	4275	4136	54.8	54.8	54.0	53.7
	50	4828	4808	4579	4360	56.2	56.0	55.2	54.7
	75	5080	5040	4915	4600	57.3	56.8	56.5	55.5
	90	5437	5312	5060	4692	57.7	57.5	57.6	56.6
56	10	4685	4387	4441	4243	54.3	55.2	54.6	54.6
	25	4967	4933	4603	4498	56.3	56.3	55.3	55.1
	50	5255	5250	4953	4758	57.6	57.6	56.8	56.3
	75	5599	5550	5308	4959	58.7	58.4	58.1	56.9
	90	5918	5791	5500	5161	59.3	59.4	59.2	57.7
84	10	5292	5320	5000	4707	57.8	58.3	57.0	57.2
	25	5740	5589	5388	5161	59.3	59.0	58.2	57.7
	50	5973	5955	5675	5424	60.8	59.9	59.5	58.6
	75	6501	6236	6027	5654	61.6	61.0	60.8	59.7
	90	7015	6773	6357	5800	62.6	61.9	61.7	60.2
112	10	5949	5933	5568	5282	60.1	61.1	59.6	59.7
	25	6305	6186	5976	5582	61.4	61.8	60.3	60.0
	50	6697	6482	6288	5987	63.0	62.6	61.9	60.9
	75	7253	7051	6669	6204	64.5	63.8	63.2	62.2
	90	7993	7306	7018	6428	65.4	64.2	64.0	63.1

From Fomon, S.J., et al.: Acta Paediatr. Scand. (suppl.) **223**:1, 1971.
*Values in parentheses are number of subjects.

breastfed for 6 months or longer were randomly selected and all agreed to participate. They were educated, middle-income, married women. Growth records were obtained from the mothers from their pediatrician's records. The weight and length curves of these infants remained above the fiftieth percentile of the National Center for Health Statistics through at least the sixth month. In those infants who were exclusively breastfed longer, all were above the twenty-fifth percentile through the ninth and tenth month of life. Vitamin and mineral supplements were taken by 75% of all mothers and given to 35% of the infants. This study does demonstrate that under optimal circumstances exclusive breastfeeding does indeed support growth in the first 6 months or longer. When the growth of healthy exclusively breastfed infants was evaluated in the first 6 months of life in Australia, the weight increments in the first 3 months compared favorably with standards from the Ministry of Health in Great Britain.[18] The weight increment for the second 3 months was significantly less. The data from Great Britain had been accumulated from a mixed sample of breastfed and bottle fed infants in the 1950s, when most infants were fed cow's milk with a high solute load. A study of infants in Singapore, on the other hand, showed that breastfeeding resulted in greater weight gain at 6 months for poor Indian and Chinese babies but no significant difference was found in well-to-do breastfed Chinese babies compared to formula fed infants.[27]

The growth pattern of full-term infants in the United States followed prospectively from birth showed no significant differences in mean growth measurements (weight, crown-rump length, head circumference, and skinfold thickness) between infants fully breastfed and those fed whey-predominant formula. Plasma amino acid concentrations, including those for taurine, were similar at 3 days and 2, 8, and 16 weeks of age in both groups.[32]

A group of 56 Finnish infants who were breastfed for at least 6 months were compared by Saarinen and Siimes[31] to infants weaned prior to 1 month of age. Weight, weight for height and age, and skinfold thickness were similar in the breastfed and formula fed infants but were lower than the values in infants fed cow's milk at 6 months.

In assessing the normal growth of the breastfed infant, the tables devised by Fomon et al.,[12] Jackson et al.,[19] or Mellander et al.[26] will serve better than the standard tables (Appendix A). It is appropriate to compare a breastfed infant to standards set by healthy breastfed infants. Increments of gain in weight and length per day and week can also be found in Appendix A. As more growth tables are established recording data from infants fed whey-prominent formula with reduced solute load, patterns not unlike those in healthy breastfed infants may appear.

Gain in physical growth is not as critical as gain in brain growth, but measurements of brain growth are only indirectly implied from growth of the head. In evaluating any infant's progress, head circumference is an important consideration, especially in the

Table 12-2. Increment in head circumference in various age intervals

Age interval (mo)	Percentiles	SD	Increment in head circumference (cm)	
			Males	Females
0-1		−2	1.0	0.8
	10		2.0	1.5
	25		2.5	2.6
	50		3.6	3.3
	75		4.3	4.0
	90		5.3	4.7
		+2	6.2	5.6
1-3		−2	1.9	1.9
	10		2.4	2.5
	25		2.8	2.6
	50		3.3	3.1
	75		3.7	3.4
	90		4.2	3.8
		+2	4.7	4.3
3-6		−2	1.7	1.8
	10		2.2	2.3
	25		2.6	2.5
	50		3.0	2.9
	75		3.3	3.2
	90		4.0	3.4
		+2	4.5	3.8
6-9		−2	1.1	0.9
	10		1.3	1.4
	25		1.6	1.6
	50		1.9	1.9
	75		2.1	2.2
	90		2.3	2.5
		+2	2.7	2.9
9-12		−2	0.5	0.4
	10		0.8	0.8
	25		1.0	1.0
	50		1.3	1.2
	75		1.6	1.6
	90		1.8	1.7
		+2	2.1	2.0
12-18		−2	0.6	0.4
	10		1.0	0.7
	25		1.3	1.1
	50		1.6	1.5
	75		1.8	1.7
	90		2.1	1.9
		+2	2.6	2.4
18-24		−2	0.0	0.0
	10		0.2	0.5
	25		0.6	0.7
	50		0.9	0.9
	75		1.3	1.2
	90		1.7	1.5
		+2	2.0	2.0
24-36		−2	0.0	−0.5
	10		0.5	0.5
	25		0.7	0.8
	50		1.0	1.1
	75		1.3	1.3
	90		1.5	1.6
		+2	2.0	2.7

From Fomon, S.J.: Infant nutrition, ed. 2, Philadelphia, 1974, W.B. Saunders Co. Data from Karlberg et al. (1968).

Table 12-3. Head circumference at various ages

Age (mo)	Percentiles	SD	Head circumference (cm)	
			Males	Females
1		−2	34.4	34.2
	10		35.2	35.0
	25		36.2	35.6
	50		37.0	36.2
	75		37.8	36.7
	90		38.6	37.6
		+2	39.6	38.2
3		−2	37.9	37.3
	10		38.6	37.9
	25		39.5	38.7
	50		40.3	39.5
	75		41.0	39.8
	90		41.7	40.4
		+2	42.3	41.3
6		−2	40.9	40.1
	10		41.9	40.9
	25		42.7	41.5
	50		43.3	42.2
	75		44.0	42.8
	90		44.8	43.4
		+2	45.7	44.1
9		−2	42.8	42.0
	10		43.7	42.7
	25		44.5	43.3
	50		45.0	44.0
	75		45.8	44.5
	90		46.6	45.5
		+2	47.6	46.0
12		−2	44.3	43.3
	10		45.0	44.0
	25		45.8	44.5
	50		46.5	45.3
	75		47.2	45.9
	90		47.7	46.6
		+2	48.7	47.3
18		−2	45.4	44.6
	10		46.4	45.4
	25		47.1	45.9
	50		48.1	46.7
	75		49.0	47.3
	90		49.6	48.2
		+2	50.6	48.6
24		−2	46.4	44.8
	10		47.3	46.4
	25		48.1	46.8
	50		49.0	47.8
	75		49.7	48.3
	90		50.5	49.0
		+2	51.6	50.4
36		−2	47.4	46.5
	10		48.0	47.1
	25		49.3	47.8
	50		50.0	48.8
	75		50.9	49.5
	90		51.7	50.1
		+2	52.6	50.9

From Fomon, S.J.: Infant nutrition, ed. 2, Philadelphia, 1974, W.B. Saunders Co. Data from Karlberg et al. (1968).

first year of life (Tables 12-2 and 12-3). Deceleration in the rate of increase in head circumference occurs over the first year. The head circumference increases about 3 inches in the first year of life and another 3 inches in the next 16 years of life. When growth failure includes failure of head growth, the failure is severe. Many other factors independent of body growth influence head growth, however.

Initially after birth, the normal infant loses 5% of his body weight before starting to gain, whether breastfed or bottle fed. In a study of infants at the University of Rochester, it was noted that breastfed infants who were given added water or added formula to force fluids in the first few days of life lost more weight and were less likely to start gaining prior to discharge than infants who were entirely breastfed or who were bottle fed.

The human infant requires at least 100 days to double his birth weight, whereas the calf with the high protein, ash, calcium, and phosphorus contents of cow's milk requires only 50 days. If a reference infant at the fiftieth percentile is followed, it is estimated the birth weight will double at about 110 days for the breastfed infant.

Development

More recently, cognitive development in the first 7 years of life was related to breastfeeding practices in a birth cohort of New Zealand children.[8] The researchers took into account maternal intelligence, maternal education, maternal training in child rearing, childhood experiences, family socioeconomic status, birth weight, and gestational age. The breastfed children had slightly higher test scores on the Peabody Picture Vocabulary Test, the 5-year measure on the Stanford Binet Intelligence Scale, and the 7-year measure on the Weschler Child Intelligence Scale. Measures of language development were equally influenced. This very small improvement in scores persisted when all variables were taken into account. The scores were also influenced by length of breastfeeding below and above 4 months.

Another group of children was followed in New Zealand to evaluate the effects of infant feeding, birth order, paternal occupation, and socioeconomic status on speech in 6-year-old children. Controlling for the demographic effects, the association of breastfeeding with clear speech was different for the sexes, being negligible for girls and strongly positive for boys.[33]

The relationship of infant-feeding practices and dependent variables to the subsequent cognitive abilities were reported by Young et al.[35] from the Yale Harvard Research Project in Tunisia. Within the underprivileged group they found that breastfeeding promoted not only physical growth but also sensory motor development as assessed by Bayley motor and mental scales. There were no great differences in the ability to sit alone or to take first steps, but especially among males in the lower socioeconomic group there was significant superiority of breastfed infants at 8, 14, and 16 months of age in Bayley mental scales.

FAILURE TO THRIVE
Definition

The term *failure to thrive* has been loosely used to include all infants who show some degree of growth failure. For the breastfed infant, it may be a matter of comparing a slower gainer to the excessive weight-gain patterns of the bottle fed infant. The definition offered by Fomon[11] states that "failure to thrive [should] be defined as a rate of gain in length and/or weight less than the value corresponding to two standard deviations below the mean during an interval of at least 56 days for infants less than five months of age and during an interval of at least three months for older infants." The values for 2 standard deviations (SD) below the mean in gains in length and weight for various age intervals are given in Appendix A. Fomon further suggests that infants gaining in length and weight at rates less than the tenth percentile values be suspected of failing to thrive. Certainly in managing the breastfed infant, more careful and frequent medical evaluation should be provided for the infant who drops to the tenth percentile for weight, fails to gain weight, or continues to lose after the tenth day of life, rather than waiting for 56 days to establish the trend unquestionably. For the sake of this discussion, therefore, an infant should be evaluated for possible failure to thrive or slow weight gain when he continues to lose weight after 10 days of life, does not regain birth weight by 3 weeks of age, or gains at a rate below the 10th percentile for weight gain beyond 1 month of age. Unlike the bottle fed infant, who can then be placed in the hospital where professionals can feed him, the breastfed infant needs to be evaluated in the home setting, nursing at the breast.

As more and more women breastfeed, increasing numbers of cases of failure to thrive appear in the literature, although it is a rare phenomenon. No statistical data on incidence rates are available because there has been no large prospective study. Only extreme cases are hospitalized.

Diagnosis of failure to thrive

The problem of slow or inadequate weight gain has confounded even the physicians most committed to breastfeeding. It should be approached with the same orderly diagnostic process that one uses to attack any medical problem. Thus a complete history, a physical examination of the infant, an examination of the maternal breast, observation of the feeding, and appropriate laboratory work are indicated. Organizing the data amassed by this process will help identify the facts that do appear. Fleiss and Frantz[10] have experience with a questionnaire they developed to analyze the breastfed infant who is failing to grow. The questionnaire has been modified slightly to assemble questions about the mother and the infant separately; it appears in Appendix D.

Slow gaining versus failure to thrive

There are some helpful distinctions between the breastfed infant who is slow to gain weight and the infant who is failing to thrive while breastfeeding.[10] These parameters

Table 12-4.   Parameters for evaluation of breastfed infants

Infant who is slow to gain weight	Infant with failure to thrive
Alert healthy appearance	Apathetic or crying
Good muscle tone	Poor tone
Good skin turgor	Poor turgor
At least 6 wet diapers/day	Few wet diapers
Pale dilute urine	"Strong" urine
Stools frequent, seedy (or if infrequent, large and soft)	Stools infrequent, scanty
8 or more nursings/day, lasting 15–20 minutes	Fewer than 8 feedings, often brief
Well-established let-down reflex	No signs of functioning let-down reflex
Weight gain consistent but slow	Weight erratic—may lose

should be included in the routine "well baby" evaluation of all breastfed infants, beginning with the first visit a week to 10 days after discharge home (Table 12-4).

The feeding pattern of the infant with slow weight gain is usually frequent feedings with evidence of a good suck. The mother's breasts are full before feeding and she can describe a let-down during the feeding. There are at least six wet diapers a day and urine is pale and dilute; stools are loose and seedy. Weight gain is slow but consistent. If the infant is gaining painfully slowly but is alert, bright, and responsive and developing along the appropriate level, he is a "slow gainer." In contrast the infant with true failure to thrive is usually apathetic or weakly crying with poor tone and poor turgor. There are few wet diapers (none are ever soaked) and "strong" urine. Stools are infrequent and scanty. Feedings are often by schedule but always fewer than eight per day and brief. There are no signs of a good let-down reflex. True failure to thrive is potentially serious; early recognition is essential if the integrity of both brain growth and breastfeeding is to be safely preserved.

A schema for classifying failure to thrive at the breast is suggested in Fig. 12-1. Here the causes associated with infant behavior and problems are distinguished from those due to problems in the mother. The causes in the infant can be further evaluated by looking at intake, which is the cause, in association with poor feeding, poor net intake due to additional losses, and high energy needs. The maternal causes can be divided into poor production of milk and poor release of milk. When a poor let-down reflex acts long enough, it will eventually cause a decrease in milk production. There may be several factors affecting the outcome, thus more than one management change may be indicated.

EVALUATION OF THE INFANT.   Examination of the infant should suggest any underlying physical problems such as hypothyroidism, congenital heart disease, or mechanical abnormalities of the mouth such as cleft palate, or major neurologic disturbances.[4] The infant's ability to root, suck, and coordinate swallowing should be observed. There is a greater risk today of missing subtle structural problems because infants spend much of their hospital life out of the newborn nursery away from the watchful eyes of experienced nurses and then are discharged before problems become manifest. The first office visit for breastfeeding infants should be at 1 week following discharge home or earlier and include a complete inspection whether there are complaints from the parents or not. A small number of infants will be identified with physical abnormalities that need medical attention (Table 12-5).

Small for gestational age infant.   The small for gestational age (SGA) infant will be identified if gestational age and birth weight are scrutinized. This infant is small at birth despite full gestational time in utero. The SGA infant has a large nutritional deficit to make up from his intrauterine failure to grow. The cause of his intrauterine problem should be assessed (placental insufficiency, maternal disease, toxemia, heavy smoking, or intrauterine infection such as toxoplasmosis). SGA infants are difficult to feed initially by any method and often require tube feedings for a few days. Their caloric needs parallel the needs of an infant of appropriate weight for gestation rather than their actual low weight. The SGA infant should be placed on frequent feedings, every 2 to 3 hours by day and every 4 hours at night. He should be awakened for feedings if he sleeps long periods of time. If he has not been nursing well, the breast has not been stimulated to produce to its full capability. The mother may need to express milk manually or mechanically pump milk to enhance her production. Her milk may then be given by a passive means such as a tube, a dropper, or Lact-Aid (see App. H). An infant who is

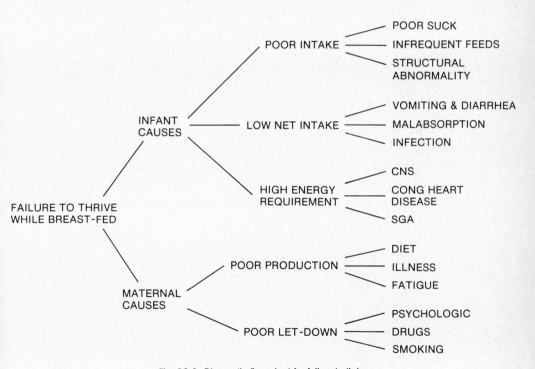

Fig. 12-1. Diagnostic flow chart for failure to thrive.

Table 12-5. Conditions associated with or causing disorders of sucking and swallowing

Absent or diminished suck	Mechanical factors interfering with sucking	Disorders of the swallowing mechanism (not including esophageal abnormalities)
Maternal anesthesia or analgesia	Macroglossia	Choanal atresia
Anoxia or hypoxia	Cleft lip	Cleft palate
Prematurity	Fusion of gums	Micrognathia
Trisomy 21	Tumors of mouth or gums	Postintubation dysphagia
Trisomy 13-15	Temporomandibular ankylosis	Palatal paralysis
Hypothyroidism	or hypoplasia	Pharyngeal tumors
Neuromuscular abnormalities		Pharyngeal diverticula
Kernicterus		Familial dysautonomia
Werdnig-Hoffmann disease		
Neonatal myasthenia gravis		
Congenital muscular dystrophy		
Infections of the CNS		
Toxoplasmosis		
Cytomegalovirus infection		
Bacterial meningitis		

Modified from Gryboski, J.: Philadelphia, 1975, W.B. Saunders Co. From Behrman, R.E., Driscoll, J.M., Jr., and Seeds, A.E., editors: Neonatal-perinatal medicine: diseases of the fetus and infant, ed. 2, St. Louis, 1977, The C.V. Mosby Co.

sufficiently starved in utero may have a degree of inanition that prevents active suckling at first, predisposing him to further starvation. The successful nursing of an SGA infant may require extended effort on the part of the mother to assure adequate growth. On the other hand, such effort is well worth the trouble if one considers the impact of intrauterine growth failure on the central nervous system (CNS). It would be to the infant's advantage to have the critical amino acids such as taurine and the lipids of human milk with which to "catch up" brain growth.

Jaundice. Hyperbilirubinemia is discussed in Chapter 13, but an infant with an elevated bilirubin level from any cause may be depressed and lethargic and therefore may not nurse well. If the infant appears jaundiced, laboratory evaluation in search of the cause and its appropriate treatment should be undertaken. When an infant is taken from the breast at 2 or 3 days of age because of jaundice, it interferes with the establishment of lactation at a critical time especially for a primipara. "Breast-milk jaundice" does not develop until the infant is 3 or more days old, so other causes must be sought. In addition, care must be taken to help the mother continue to stimulate production with manual expression or pumping to avoid inducing iatrogenic lactation failure.

Metabolic screen. Most hospitals provide, often because the law mandates it, screening for metabolic disorders including galactosemia, phenylketonuria, maple sugar urine disease, and disorders of metabolism of other amino acids. If these simple screening tests were not performed or their validity is in doubt, they should be done again. Usually the service is available in the state or county laboratory. Thyroid screening for abnormal thyroxine (T_4) and/or thyroid-stimulating hormone (TSH) should also be performed. Mass screening programs for neonatal thyroid disease have identified cases of deficiency that, even in retrospect, show none of the characteristic findings of hypothyroidism, such as thick, coarse features, hoarse cry, slow pulse, macroglossia, umbilical hernia, or jaundice. In the neonate hypothyroidism is often associated with failure to thrive, if undiagnosed.

Galactosemia.   Galactosemia, which is a hereditary disorder of the metabolism of galactose-1-phosphate, is manifested by renal disease and liver dysfunction following the ingestion of galactose. The lack of galactose-1-phosphate uridyl transferase may be relative or partial. The clinical symptoms may be fulminating with severe jaundice, hepatosplenomegaly, vomiting, and diarrhea or may be more subtle. Cataracts are not invariably present. In mild cases, failure to thrive may be the presenting symptom. A screen of the urine for reducing substances (by Clinitest and not just Dextrostix, which will only identify glucose) should be done on all infants who fail to thrive, especially if there is hepatomegaly or jaundice. The definitive diagnosis is the identification of absence or near absence of galactose-1-phosphate uridyl transferase in red blood cell hemolysates. A screen of the urine should be considered even though an initial metabolic screen for galactosemia was done on the second or third day of life by hospital routine. The treatment is a galactose-free diet, which would mandate prompt weaning from breast milk to prevent further insult to the liver and kidneys. This is one of the few indications for prompt weaning from human milk. A formula free of lactose such as Isomil or Nutramigen is indicated. (Refer to pediatric texts on neonatal metabolic disorders for a full description of the disease; see Chapter 14.)

Vomiting and diarrhea.   Vomiting and diarrhea are very unusual in a breastfed infant. Spitting up small amounts of milk after feedings is sometimes observed in otherwise normal infants and is of no consequence if it does not affect overall weight gain. Although pyloric stenosis is reportedly less common in breastfed infants, this phenomenon should be ruled out in any infant who vomits consistently after feeding, has diminished urine and stools, shows no weight gain or actually loses weight, and has reverse peristalsis. Usually these infants do well initially, and the vomiting becomes progressive.

Vomiting may be a presenting symptom for various metabolic disorders. Thus metabolic disorders should be considered in the differential diagnosis. The usual causes of vomiting, as well as the causes peculiar to breast milk, should be considered. Maternal diet should be checked for unusual foods. In families at high risk for allergy, intake by the mother of known family food allergens may cause symptoms in the infant. Diarrhea may be due to foods in the mother's diet or the use of cathartics by the mother such as phenolphthalein (Ex-Lax).

Infection.   Chronic intrauterine infection, which predisposes an SGA infant to intrauterine growth failure, may continue to cause problems of growth in the presence of adequate kilocalories.

Acute infections.   An infant who is not growing well may have an infection in the gastrointestinal tract; therefore, the nature of the stools is important. The urinary tract may be another site of infection not readily identified. If, however, the initial evaluation includes a urinalysis with microscopic evaluation and a white blood cell count and differential count, this will be ruled out.

High energy requirements.   When the metabolic rate of the infant is increased, the weight gain will be diminished or absent. When the infant is hyperactive with a strong startle reflex and sleeps poorly, consideration should be given to stimulants present in the milk as well as to neurologic disorders. When a mother drinks coffee, tea, including herbal teas, cola, or other carbonated beverages with added caffeine, the accumulated caffeine may be sufficient to make the infant very irritable and hyperactive. The best treatment is to replace the caffeine-containing beverages (Chapter 11). Some CNS disorders are associated with hyperactivity. Infants with severe congenital heart disease are constantly exercising to breathe and oxygenate and have markedly increased metabolic rates. For management of these special infants at the breast see Chapter 14.

OBSERVATION OF NURSING PROCESS.   When it has been established that there are no obvious physical or metabolic reasons for the failure to gain weight, the infant should be observed suckling at the breast. Does the infant get a good grasp and suck vigorously? If not, what interferes? A receding chin, a weak suck, lack of coordination, the breast obstructing breathing, and mouthing of the nipple or other ineffectual sucking techniques are some of the possibilities. If the problem is the suckling process, the infant may need retraining. This cause is more common with infants who have had some experience with bottles or rubber nipples or who use a pacifier. Small or slightly premature infants who were started on bottle feedings have trouble relearning the proper sucking motion with the tongue (Figs. 8-6 to 8-8). Bottle feedings and pacifiers may have to be discontinued until the infant is more experienced at the breast. This will require a program of manually expressing milk to soften the areola, having milk at the nipple to entice the infant, and gently offering the nipple and areola well compressed between two fingers. If the infant has a receding chin or a relaxed jaw, it may help to have the mother hold the lower jaw forward by supporting the angle of the jaw with her thumb.

It may be necessary to retrain both mother and baby. If the infant cannot maintain the breast in his mouth without the mother holding it there, it is an indication of improper suckling. In that situation, the infant may need to be repositioned with his ventral surface squarely facing the mother's chest.[14] The infant's lower arm should be around the mother's chest wall and the breast presented with thumb on top and fingers below breast. (See discussion in Chapter 8.) A good check of adequate let-down is to observe the opposite breast as the baby nurses to see if milk flows or to interrupt nursing abruptly. If there has been a good let-down, milk will continue to flow, at least drop by drop, for a few moments from the breast being suckled. The mother can also be trained to listen for the infant's swallowing. During proper sucking, the masseter muscle is in full view and is contracting visibly and rhythmically. There are occasional infants who do not suck vigorously at the breast but use rapid shallow sucks referred to by Frantz[14] and others as "flutter sucking." These infants can be gradually taught to suck effectively.

The most productive part of the diagnostic workup is often observation of the baby at the breast. For this reason, this critical responsibility should not be passed on to others but should be performed personally by the physician.

The five general types of nursing patterns described in Chapter 8 should be kept in mind. If the mother understands that it is acceptable for the infant to drop off to sleep and snack later, she may not hesitate to follow his lead, thus providing a more adequate feeding.

Some infants will not settle down and nurse well if there is too much activity or noise. Some need to be tightly swaddled; others fall asleep and need to be unwrapped and stimulated to provide adequate suckling time. Frequent feedings, using both breasts, may be the answer in some cases. In others there may be too many ineffective feedings, which are wearing the mother out; a change that lengthens the time between feedings but also lengthens the time at the breast may help.

MATERNAL CAUSES FOR FAILURE TO THRIVE. The special questionnaire by Fleiss and Frantz[10] includes questions about the mother's health, her dietary habits, sleep pattern, smoking habits, medication intake, the events that occur during nursing, and the psychosocial atmosphere in the home.

Poor milk production

Diets. Although it has been demonstrated that malnourished mothers can produce milk for their infants, marginal diets in Western cultures do affect some mothers' ability to nourish an infant. If the mother is restricting intake deliberately or inadvertently, she should be instructed to meet the dietary requirement for lactating women (Chapter 9). One does not have to drink milk to make milk, but the necessary dietary constituents should be in the diet through cheese, eggs, ice cream, or other sources of calcium and protein. Prescribing brewer's yeast as a dietary supplement has been observed to provide improvement in milk production beyond that accounted for by mere addition of the same nutrients. Some mothers report a feeling of well-being from taking yeast that they do not obtain from taking daily vitamins. Concern has been expressed regarding the effect of increased vitamin B_6 on prolactin production, but doses that suppress lactation are 60 times the therapeutic dose.

Maternal illness. The presence of infection or other illness in the mother may affect milk production, and the cause of the illness should be identified and treated. Urinary tract infection, endometritis, or upper respiratory infection may need treatment with antibiotics. The antibiotic prescribed should be appropriate for the infant as well, since it will pass into the milk.

Fatigue. The most common cause of inadequate milk supply is fatigue. Fatigue may be lack of sleep because the infant demands considerable attention at night, but generally it is more subtle. The pressures of the rest of the family for meals or services or the self-inflicted demands of a job, career, or social commitments may be the cause. The mother must be placed on a medically mandated strict rest regimen that is respected by family and friends. In the first month, while lactation is being established, fatigue is devastating to milk production. The infant then becomes hungry more often, cries, and demands more frequent feeding; thus the vicious cycle is established. In later months of lactation, a mother becomes quickly aware of the impact of protracted fatigue on the nursing experience and usually will take steps to increase her rest.

Poor release of milk. Interference with the let-down reflex may cause a well-nourished lactating mother to fail to satisfy her infant. The collecting ducts may be full, but if the let-down or ejection reflex is not triggered the process will be at a standstill. The infant becomes frustrated and pulls away crying or screaming. Interference with the ejection reflex is predominantly iatrogenic and rarely hormonal (Fig. 7-10).

Smoking may interfere with the let-down reflex, and if this is the case, a mother who wants to smoke while nursing should wait to light up until the infant is sucking vigorously and the ejection is well established.

Experimentally, alcohol has been shown to interfere with oxytocin release in laboratory animals, but the dosage used collates with moderate to heavy drinking in humans. Therapeutically, alcohol has been recognized as an excellent adjunct to nursing if used judiciously. A glass of wine, a mug of beer, or a cocktail, especially in the early evening when some mothers may be under tension to feed the infant and family, will provide the relaxation necessary to permit adequate let-down response to take place. In countries where wine and beer are common beverages, they have been recognized for centuries as important tonics for lactation. Alcohol's medical uses have been obscured by the concern for the disease of alcoholism, but the small amount of alcohol that would reach the milk is a sedative and muscle relaxant for the frantic infant.*

Medications that the mother may be taking should be evaluated. Although L-dopa and ergot preparations are known to inhibit prolactin release, other medications less well identified may have the same effect (see Chapter 11).

The most common cause for the failure of the ejection reflex is psychologic inhibition. In a few cases the cause of the psychologic stress may be obvious, such as a husband or mother who openly disapproves of breastfeeding, but in most cases the nursing mother has already considered this possibility and reassures the physician that she is relaxed and calm. It will require carefully taking the mother's history to "tease out" the source of stress. This is the time when a home visit by the nurse practitioner from the physician's office or an experienced public health nurse will be valuable. The nurse may observe what is overlooked by the mother: construction for a new building next door, incessant barking from the neighbor's dog, or marital discord.

NO OBVIOUS CAUSE. Even though no obvious cause for failure to thrive is identified, the treatment may have to include establishing a positive attitude. Jelliffe[20] has often referred to nursing as a "confidence game." It becomes necessary to instill confidence rather than fear in the mother. Threatening the mother with stopping breastfeeding and switching to formula does not instill confidence. The physician should prescribe a pos-

---

*An alternative treatment for colic is a few drops of alcohol in warm water or via the breast milk. An elixir is 25% alcohol, and it is often the elixir, not the drug for which it serves as the vehicle that sedates the infant. Thus elixir of phenobarbital is more sedating to the infant than the same dose of phenobarbital alone.

Table 12-6.   Normal values of human milk per 100 milliliters

	Colostrum	Transitional	Mature	Bovine
Sodium (mg)	48.0	29.0	15.0	58.0
[mEq/L]	[20-30]	[10-15]	[5-10]	[22]
Chloride (mg)	85.0	46.0	40.0	108.0
Potassium (mg)	74.0	64.0	57.0	145.0
Calcium (mg)	39.0	46.0	35.0	130.0
Phosphorus (mg)	14.0	20.0	15.0	120.0
Iron (μg)	70.0	70.0	100.0	70.0
Lactose (gm)			6.8	4.9

itive plan for number and length of feedings, suggest diet and rest for the mother, and set reachable goals for growth.

If the let-down reflex is the crux of the problem and simple adjustments have not changed the ejection quality, oxytocin as a nasal spray (Pitocin), described in Chapter 8, should be prescribed. It is available only by prescription and should be used under the physician's guidance, although it is not dangerous. It does not affect the milk or the infant. It is contraindicated only in pregnancy or hypersensitivity.

The rare infant who does not respond to this management protocol may have a malabsorption or metabolic disease as yet undiagnosed that will not become overt until cow's milk is introduced. Infants with a strong family history of cystic fibrosis, milk allergy, or malabsorption should have a careful diagnostic workup before abandoning human milk, which may be the most physiologic feeding available for the infant.

DEHYDRATION, HYPERNATREMIA, OR HYPOCHLOREMIA.   A few cases of severe disease have been reported in the literature.* These infants have been hospitalized because of dehydration and evidence of more severe metabolic disturbance. They serve to illustrate the outcome if anticipatory care or palliative home management is unsuccessful. The mothers are usually but not always primiparas, new at breastfeeding and child rearing. Often it is seen when the record is reviewed that the early danger signs were present at discharge from the hospital. There may be a history of difficult delivery or of maternal medication for pain that leads to a less vigorous baby and, secondarily, inadequate stimulus for lactation. Supplementary bottles of water or milk are initiated in the hospital instead of directing attention toward the lactation process.

As a precautionary measure, the physician should see all breastfeeding dyads at 10 days to 2 weeks of age. At this visit review of the weight, feeding history, number of wet diapers, stool pattern, and physical findings should alert the physician to impending difficulties. If, on the other hand, the patient is not seen in the office until there is significant dehydration, it is urgent that laboratory studies be obtained including sodium, chloride, potassium pH, BUN, and hematocrit (bilirubin when indicated). An assessment of the degree of dehydration should be made based on skin and tissue turgor and tone (Table 12-6). When the breastfed infant has abnormal electrolyte levels, the phy-

*See references 2, 3, 6, 15-17, 28.

sician should also obtain levels of sodium, chloride, and potassium from mother's milk, being certain to sample each breast separately. Collecting a few milliliters before and after the feeding and mixing the two samples from a single breast is a good technique. There may be occult loss of electrolyte in the infant such as that seen in abnormal renal wasting or retention, cystic fibrosis, hyperaldosteronism, or pseudohyperaldosteronism. The simplest approach is to measure milk electrolytes and infant urine levels, to rule out high milk sodium.

In the cases reported in the literature, infants with hypernatremic failure to thrive are no different at initial presentation from infants with normal sodium levels.[6,14] They may even have a negative neonatal history. At home, they develop a poor suck, sleep for long intervals, cry infrequently, and feed infrequently. When observed at the breast they may be labeled as having a sucking disorder. On examination, however, the lethargy, dehydration, and malnutrition are obvious to the skilled clinician. In the extreme, there may be cardiovascular collapse with hypothermia and hypoglycemia. Elevated serum BUN, creatinine, and hematocrit and urinary specific gravity confirm the diagnosis. Hypernatremia has been observed in approximately half the reported cases of severe dehydration.[29,30] Although milk sodium levels were not reported in all cases, several cases of elevated milk sodium are reported. Sodium, chloride, and lactose are the prime constituents that control the osmolarity of the milk. Because the sodium chloride and lactose have a reciprocal relationship, inadequate lactose production ultimately results in elevated sodium levels.

Hypernatremic dehydration is an emergency that requires hospitalization.[23,24] The mother should room-in if at all possible. Most pediatric units provide this option. It is preferable to maintain lactation in most cases. The treatment of the illness after the dehydration has been treated with intravenous fluids depends on the etiology of the hypernatremia. The sodium of the infant's serum and mother's milk should be followed until stable. In decreasing maternal output with appropriate lactation counseling, including mechanical pumping between feedings to increase volume usually normalizes the sodium. The oral feedings for the infant should be limited to the breastfeeding while the intravenous fluids are tapered. In order to provide increased caloric resources to the infant and an appropriate sodium load, the Lact-Aid supplementer may also be used (see Chapter 8 and Appendix J).

Chloride deficiency has received attention because of a highly publicized formula-manufacturing error. This syndrome is characterized by failure to thrive with anorexia, hypochloremia, and hypokalemic metabolic alkalosis. Chloride deficiency syndrome has also been reported in an infant whose mother had only 2 mEq/L chloride in her milk (normal is 8 mEq/L).[17] The mother had successfully nourished her previous five infants. The infant had done well until 3 months of age and then had gradually slipped below the third percentile for weight at 6 months. The infant was severely dehydrated and hypotonic with plasma sodium of 123 mEq/L, chloride of 72 mEq/L, potassium of 2.9 mEq/L, and blood pH of 7.61. There were no abnormal urinary losses. When there is clinical dehydration in the infant who is breastfeeding, it is important to check not only the sodium but also the chloride content of infant's serum, infant's urine, and mother's milk.

Human infants younger than 3 weeks of age do not respond to negative effects of suckling. This finding is also observed in studies in other species in which pups continue to suck when the solution is unphysiologic.[5] A natural experiment occurred in a new-born nursery in the 1960s, when six infants died of hypernatremia after receiving many feedings of formula inadvertently made from salt rather than sugar.[9] The infants who were less than 1 week old did not reject the feedings.

LACTATION FAILURE.   There are occasional situations in which the failure to thrive is actually due to lactation failure. Historically, sudden complete cessation of lactation has been described in the 1800s after coaching accidents and other great trauma. Advocates of breastfeeding have tended to dismiss this as a possibility and struggle frantically to reverse the situation. There are women who cannot make milk; some of these women have primary hypoprolactinemia, and others have secondary hypoprolactinemia as in Sheehan's disease (see Chapter 15). Because it is now possible to identify these women by obtaining prolactin levels[33] that confirm the diagnosis, when reasonable efforts at stimulation are ineffective and the mother is unable to do without the Lact-Aid providing almost a full feeding volume, evaluation of the mother is appropriate. Some mothers prefer to discontinue efforts to breastfeed before they have been totally stripped of their egos by total failure.

If one explores the animal literature, one finds a similar situation in other species. Lactation failure in nursing animals is rare because it is not a trait that is transmitted from generation to generation, since the offspring do not survive. Interferences with milk ejection can be identified and treated in other mammals. There is a syndrome in sows of agalactia associated with mastitis and metritis.[7] Mammalian lactation failure is attributed to nutritional, pharmacologic, and "emotional stress" causes in animals. Aside from gross dietary deficiency, there is depression or inhibition of the anterior pituitary gland, which is responsible for synthesis in the alveolar cells, and inhibition of transport and discharge of synthesized products from alveolar cells to the lumen. Certain plant alkaloids have been noted in other species to inhibit lactation. Ergot derivatives are best known, but colchicine, vincristine, and vinblastine are also causative. Some plant lectins such as concanavalin interfere with transport and discharge phases of milk production. Understanding of lactation failure is increasing among clinicians as the diagnostic resources expand.[33]

OBESITY

The best definition of obesity should be based on the percentage of body weight accounted for by fat. What percentage would be detrimental and how it could easily be measured is not known. Fomon[11] suggests, however, that until that is possible a clinical definition that circumvents clinical impressions would be useful. He suggests that "values greater than +2 standard deviation value for triceps and subscapsular skin-

Table 12-7.   Increments in skinfold thickness at various age intervals

Age interval (mo)	Percentiles	SD	Triceps (mm) Males	Triceps (mm) Females	Subscapular (mm) Males	Subscapular (mm) Females
1-3		-2	-0.6	-0.9	-1.8	-1.4
	10		0.7	0.1	-0.5	-0.7
	25		1.5	1.4	0.2	0.5
	50		2.5	2.5	1.4	1.6
	75		3.6	3.4	2.2	2.6
	90		4.7	4.4	3.1	3.4
		+2	5.8	5.9	4.6	4.6
3-6		-2	-1.5	-1.7	-3.3	-2.3
	10		-0.1	-0.1	-1.5	-1.2
	25		0.8	0.7	-0.7	-0.6
	50		1.8	2.1	0.2	0.2
	75		2.8	3.3	1.2	1.1
	90		3.6	4.4	2.3	2.0
		+2	5.3	5.9	3.9	2.9
6-9		-2	-3.0	-3.5	-2.9	-3.3
	10		-1.7	-2.2	-1.5	-2.0
	25		-0.7	-1.1	-0.8	-1.1
	50		0.2	-0.2	0.0	-0.2
	75		1.4	0.8	0.8	0.5
	90		2.6	1.6	1.9	1.2
		+2	3.8	3.3	3.1	2.7
9-12		-2	-3.7	-3.6	-3.2	-2.5
	10		-2.4	-2.4	-1.4	-1.6
	25		-1.5	-1.4	-0.6	-1.0
	50		0.0	-0.2	0.0	-0.3
	75		1.2	1.0	0.7	0.4
	90		2.4	2.1	1.8	1.1
		+2	3.5	3.2	3.2	1.9
12-18		-2	-3.2	-3.0	-3.3	-3.1
	10		-2.0	-2.2	-2.1	-2.1
	25		-1.0	-0.9	-1.0	-1.3
	50		-0.1	0.2	-0.4	-0.6
	75		1.4	1.3	0.4	0.2
	90		2.3	2.1	1.3	1.5
		+2	3.6	3.4	2.7	2.1
18-24		-2	-3.4	-3.0	-3.2	-2.7
	10		-2.0	-2.0	-1.7	-1.6
	25		-1.3	-0.8	-1.2	-1.1
	50		0.0	0.1	-0.5	-0.6
	75		1.2	1.2	0.2	0.2
	90		2.4	2.5	0.9	0.9
		+2	3.4	3.4	2.4	1.7
24-36		-2	-3.5	-4.2	-2.9	-3.5
	10		-2.3	-2.7	-1.9	-1.8
	25		-1.2	-1.2	-1.2	-0.9
	50		-0.2	0.3	-0.6	-0.4
	75		1.2	1.3	0.0	0.3
	90		2.3	2.3	0.4	1.2
		+2	3.3	4.2	1.5	3.3

From Fomon, S.J.: Infant nutrition, ed. 2, Philadelphia, 1974, W.B. Saunders Co.

fold thickness be considered evidence of obesity'' (Table 12-7). Fomon also recognizes the difficulty of obtaining skinfold measurements on young infants and offers as a less satisfactory alternative the relation of body weight to stature (Table 12-8). The infant with a heavy bone structure and musculature but without excessive fat may appear to be obese based on this table. Infants who are overfed also grow in height and may well be in an advanced percentile for height. The infant who is born with a weight in the eightieth percentile (weight for age) and remains there may not be obese, but the infant who is born with a weight in the fiftieth percentile and crosses percentiles over time to the eightieth percentile may be at risk for long-term obesity. Therefore, some discretion is advised when using these criteria for obesity.

There are no benefits from infantile obesity. The concern for obesity rests with the long-range outcome as an obese adult. There is a problem that obesity in infancy predisposes the child to immobility and inactivity; thus an obese infant lags on the developmental curve. The question of whether obesity in infancy predisposes the child to obesity in adult life has not been resolved satisfactorily. There are retrospective studies that support both sides of the question. A prospective study of 403 newborns in Canada was done measuring weight, length, and subcutaneous fat but an infant was considered ''breastfed'' if he received any breastfeeding for 2 months and early solids.[22] Food feeding was defined as beginning solids by 2 months of age. The authors felt they refuted the hypothesis of bottle fed obesity in their 18-month follow-up. Most students of this subject would question the population definitions. A study of adolescents retrospectively tested the question of whether breastfeeding and delayed introduction of solids protect against subsequent obesity. The author concluded that breastfeeding does protect, but delayed solids alone do not protect, against obesity.[34]

Breastfed infants are rarely obese. The usual cause of obesity in these infants is the early addition of solids. Solids often provide excessive kilocalories. The obese breastfed infant should have his diet and the feeding pattern scrutinized. If necessary, some restriction of prolonged feeding should be suggested. In the normal course of a breastfeeding, the fat content of the milk increases over time and satisfies the infant after 10 to 15 minutes of nursing.

Since there is general agreement that, once established, childhood obesity often becomes chronic and resistant to treatment,[25] it is appropriate to focus attention on prevention and early intervention. The physician can counsel a family whose breastfed infant meets the criteria for obesity (above the eighty-fifth percentile for weight for length). The routine use of skinfold measurements as part of well baby care will increase the ability to diagnose obesity as it distinguishes the constitutionally bigger body frame from the fat infant.

Recommendations that will help taper unusual weight gain include the following:
1. Limit excessive feedings that are being provided on the mistaken belief that all the infant's needs are nutritional.
2. Encourage nonnutritive cuddling. If feeding is a response to all distress signals,

Table 12-8.   Tentative definition of obesity*

Age (mo)	Males		Females	
	Length (cm) less than	Weight (kg) more than	Length (cm) less than	Weight (kg) more than
1	51.8	4.2	51.5	4.0
	53.0	4.5	52.2	4.3
	54.2	4.7	53.5	4.6
	55.2	5.1	54.6	4.8
3	58.0	6.0	57.1	5.6
	59.2	6.4	58.0	5.9
	60.2	6.9	59.2	6.2
	61.5	7.3	60.2	6.6
6	65.6	7.7	63.3	7.5
	66.5	8.2	65.2	8.0
	67.8	9.0	66.3	8.4
	69.2	9.6	67.8	8.9
9	70.0	9.1	68.2	8.9
	70.9	9.7	69.5	9.4
	72.3	10.7	71.1	9.9
	73.6	11.2	73.1	10.4
12	73.6	10.2	72.5	9.9
	74.7	10.9	73.2	10.5
	76.4	11.6	75.1	11.1
	78.0	12.5	76.9	11.6
18	80.0	11.6	78.7	11.1
	81.7	12.6	80.2	11.8
	83.2	13.3	82.0	12.7
	85.3	14.4	84.2	13.2
24	85.0	12.8	84.2	12.3
	87.3	13.9	85.8	13.1
	88.8	14.5	87.5	14.2
	90.9	16.0	90.3	14.9
36	93.4	14.8	92.1	14.3
	95.3	15.7	94.2	15.3
	97.3	16.8	96.2	17.0
	100.6	18.6	99.0	17.7

From Fomon, S.J.: Infant nutrition, ed. 2, Philadelphia, 1974, W.B. Saunders Co.
*The table is based on data of Fomon et al. (1970, 1971, 1973) for ages 1 and 3 months, and on the data of Karlberg et al. (1968) for subsequent ages. At each age, the values for length for each sex are the 10th, 25th, 50th and 75th percentiles, while the values for weight are the 50th, 75th and 90th percentiles, and the mean +2 standard deviations.

the infant may expect feeding inappropriately, causing disassociation between appetite and energy need.

3. Use exclusive breastfeeding, i.e., no solids for 4 to 6 months.

4. Increase activity and energy utilization by encouraging movement rather than containing or restricting the infant in carriers or swaddlings. For the older infant, encourage play activity and crawling and minimize sitting.

5. If there is a persistent growth excess, it is appropriate to obtain a sample of maternal milk to rule out the rare case of hyperlipidemia with a "creamatocrit." See p. 455.

REFERENCES

1. Ahn, C.H., and MacLean, W.C.: Growth of the exclusively breast-fed infant, Am. J. Clin. Nutr. **33:**183, 1980.

2. Anard, S.K., et al.: Neonatal hypernatremia associated with elevated sodium concentration of breast milk, J. Pediatr. **96:**66, 1980.

3. Asnes, R.S., et al.: The dietary chloride deficiency syndrome occurring in a breast-fed infant, J. Pediatr. **100:**923, 1982.

4. Behrman, R.E., Driscall, J.M., Jr., and Seeds, A.E., editors: Neonatal-perinatal medicine: diseases of the fetus and infant, ed. 2, St. Louis, 1977, The C.V. Mosby Co.

5. Blass, E.M., and Teicher, M.H.: Suckling, Science **210:**15, 1980.

6. Clarke, T.A., et al.: Hypernatremic dehydration resulting from inadequate breastfeeding, Pediatrics **63:**931, 1979.

7. Cowie, A.T., Forsyth, I.A., and Hart, I.C.: Hormonal control of lactation monographs on endocrinology, Heidelberg-New York, 1980, Springer-Verlag.

8. Fergusson, D.M., Beautrais, A.L., and Silva, P.A.: Breastfeeding and cognitive development in the first seven years of life, Soc. Sci. Med. **16:**1705, 1982.

9. Finberg L., Kiley J., and Luttrell C.N.: Mass accidental salt poisoning in infancy: a study of a hospital disaster, JAMA **184:**187, 1963.

10. Fleiss, P.M., and Frantz, K.B.: Management of slow gaining breast fed infants, Keeping Abreast J. (In press).

11. Fomon, S.J.: Infant nutrition, ed. 2, Philadelphia, 1974, W.B. Saunders Co.

12. Fomon, S.J., et al.: Growth and serum chemical values of normal breast fed infants, Acta Paediatr. Scand. (suppl.) **202:**1, 970.

13. Fomon, S.J., et al.: Food consumption and growth of normal infants fed milk-based formulas, Acta Paediatr. Scand. (suppl.) **223:**1, 1971.

14. Frantz, K.B., and Magnus, P.D.: Contentment in the breast-fed baby (correspondence), Arch. Dis. Child. **53:**967, 1978.

15. Gilmore, H.E., and Rowland, T.W.: Critical malnutrition in breast-fed infants, Am. J. Dis. Child. **132:**885, 1978.

16. Ghishan, F.K., and Roloff, J.S.: Malnutrition and hypernatremic dehydration in two breast-fed infants, Clin. Pediatr. **22:**592, 1983.

17. Hill, I.D., and Bowie, M.D.: Chloride deficiency syndrome due to chloride-deficient breast milk, Arch. Dis. Child. **58:**224, 1983.

18. Hitchcock, N.E., Gracey, M., and Owles, E.N.: Growth of the healthy breast-fed infants in the first six months, Lancet **2:**64, 1981.

19. Jackson, R.L., et al.: Growth of "well-born" American infants fed human and cow's milk, Pediatrics **33:**642, 1964.

20. Jelliffe, D.B., and Jelliffe, E.F.P.: Human milk in the modern world, Oxford, 1978, Oxford University Press.

21. Karlberg, P., et al.: The development of children in a Swedish urban community: a prospective longitudinal study. III. Physical growth during the first three years of life, Acta. Paediatr. Scand. (suppl.) **187:**1, 1968.

22. Kramer, M.S.: Do breast-feeding and delayed introduction of solid foods protect against subsequent obesity? J. Pediatr. **98:**883, 1981.

23. Lawrence, R.A.: Successful breastfeeding, Am. J. Dis. Child. **135:**595, 1981.

24. Lawrence, R.A.: Infant nutrition, Pediatr. Rev. **5:**133, 1983.

25. Marmot, M.G., et al.: Effect of breast-feeding on plasma cholesterol and weight in young adults, J. Epidemiol. Community Health **34:**164, 1980.

26. Mellander, O., et al.: Breast feeding and artificial feeding: a clinical, serological and biochemical study of 402 infants with survey of the literature, The Norbotten study, Acta Paediatr. Scand. **48**(suppl. 116):1, 1959.

27. Millis, J.: The influence of breastfeeding on weight gain in infants in the first year, J. Pediatr. **46:**770, 1955.

28. Paneth, N.: Hypernatremic dehydration of infancy, Am. J. Dis. Child. **134:**785, 1980.

29. Roddey, O.F., et al.: Critical weight loss and

malnutrition in breastfed infants, Am. J. Dis. Child. **135:**597, 1981.

30. Rowland, T.W., et al., Malnutrition and hypernatremic dehydration, JAMA **247:**106, 1982.
31. Saarinen, J.M., and Siimes, M.A.: Role of prolonged breastfeeding in infant growth, Acta Paediatr. Scand. **68:**245, 1979.
32. Volz, V.R., Book, L.S., and Churella, H.R.: Growth and plasma amino acid concentrations in term infants fed either whey-predominant formula or human milk, J. Pediatr. **102:**27, 1983.
33. Weichert, C.E.: Lactational reflex recovery in breast-feeding failure, Pediatrics **63:**799, 1979.
34. Yeug, D.L., et al.: Infant fatness and feeding practices: a longitudinal assessment, J. Am. Diet. Assoc. **79:**531, 1981.
35. Young, H.B., et al.: Milk and lactation: Some social and developmental correlates among 1000 infants, Pediatrics **69:**169, 1982.

Maternal employment

13

Maternal employment has been cited by many authors as the major reason for the decline in breastfeeding worldwide.[3,18] The international data do not actually support this contention. For the individual mother who wishes to return to work and breastfeed there are significant constraints, regardless of the statistical data. The physician should be knowledgeable about the principles and practice of this dual role and minimize the influence of his own biases when counseling about maternal employment. Much of the literature is plagued with personal bias, glib generalizations, and anecdotal reports.

HISTORICAL PERSPECTIVE

In modern culture there has been a stigma attached to a mother's earning money while her children are young, but no such stigma associated with leaving her children for social interaction, personal reasons, or a volunteer job. All women work when work is defined as expending energy for a purpose, but not all women are employed when it is defined as earning money for labor. Before industrialization, the working mother was the rule and not the exception. Home and work were separated by industrialization, making parenting a separate role for women. Women's work has been described by Sanday[20] as domestic or productive, public or private, traditional or modern. Domestic work, when performed for the family, is unpaid and thus is undervalued and not counted as productive work. Domestic work is performed in the private domain and productive work is associated with the public domain. Women had previously worked in agriculture and cottage industries as well as in small-scale marketing, whereas today they participate in formal work including clerical, factory, and professional jobs predominantly in urban settings.

More women are employed outside the home today than previously in this century.[23] In 1900, 20% of the labor force was women and in 1950 29% was women, whereas in 1971 43% of the work force was women, including 12.2 million mothers, which was

42% of all mothers of children 18 years of age or younger. 1980 census reports for the United States indicate that 60% of women are employed, including 55% of all mothers with children under 18 years of age, and 45% of mothers with preschool-aged children. Sixty-two percent of the women between 24 and 34 years of age, the traditional child-bearing years, have jobs. Women with children under 6 years of age, representing 6 million mothers, are the fastest growing segment of the female work force. This group tripled from 1950 to 1978, and by 1985 should reach 10 million. Three generations ago, the woman who worked violated the Victorian norms of role definition. Even when forced to work by sheer necessity, she was accused of neglecting her primary responsibility to her children. The new ethic proclaims work a cardinal virtue for the liberated woman, so that the woman who can and does stay home begins to feel inadequate.

Why women enter the work force is important to understanding the trend.[11] Before 1970 the need to earn money motivated 3 million women either because the mother was a single parent or husband-fathers were unable to earn an adequate income. For women whose husbands earned "enough" there was the need to provide a higher standard of living or provide the father with greater freedom of career choice.[27] There were few who sought careers for careers' sake because need for income was the only socially acceptable, defensible reason for a mother to work outside the home.

Since that time many women have found that the full-time care of a home leads only to higher standards of cleanliness with no greater sense of achievement or completion.[6] The exclusive investment of energy and emotion in the rearing of one to three children involves a considerable hazard not only to a mother but also to her children's ultimate achievement and ability to form a variety of responsive and satisfying personal relationships.[11,17] Women are responding to the pressures of an inflationary economy, to the costs of higher education, to the opportunities for personal fulfillment, and to the growing market for service occupations. Married women continue to carry at least 70% to 80% of the child care and household duties when both parents work.

ATTITUDES OF PROFESSIONALS TOWARDS WORKING MOTHERS

Professional[4,8] and lay books[13,21] alike on child rearing have viewed working negatively except for economic necessity, thus enhancing the working mother's guilt and providing little substantial advice. The American College of Obstetrics and Gynecology[1] has acknowledged the current trend to work throughout pregnancy and to return to work promptly after delivery by preparing a physicians guide to patient assessment and counseling. There is also a patient occupational questionnaire provided the practitioner. This forms a basis of discussion with the patient and provides an opportunity to counsel the patient and her husband about plans to maintain a healthy environment and any special needs for child care. It is stated that with few exceptions, "the normal woman with an uncomplicated pregnancy and a normal fetus in a job that presents no greater potential hazards than those encountered in normal daily life in the community may continue to work without interruption until the onset of labor and may resume working several weeks after an uncomplicated delivery.''

Pediatricians, on the other hand, have no organized resources and there were no measured attitudes of pediatricians toward mothers working outside the home until the study reported by Heins and colleagues.[7] Since attitudes tend to determine the advice given, recognition of personal bias in such a significant issue is important for the professional. A mail survey to the entire membership of the American Academy of Pediatrics was conducted by Heins et al.[7] in October 1980 and produced 5758 (31%) usable responses. Although female and younger pediatricians were slightly overrepresented, the sample was representative. The responses in general were positive toward working. The majority felt the children of working and nonworking women were similar and that the mother could return to work at any age of the child—that it did not make any difference. A large number of respondents said they never gave advice about working (Tables 13-1 and 13-2). Only half of the respondents provided special considerations (evening hours, etc.) for employed mothers.

Table 13-1.   Responses for reasons to recommend work

	Frequency	
	No.	%
Economic reasons	1709	25
Never recommend mother work	1566	22
Mother's emotional needs	1220	18
Mother's fulfillment	1059	15
Child is better off without mother	644	9
Reassure mother	270	4
Adequacy of child care	266	4
Child's age	170	2
Mother does important work	64	1
TOTAL	6964	

From Heins, M., et al.: Pediatrics 72:283, 1983. Copyright American Academy of Pediatrics 1983.

Table 13-2.   Responses for reasons to recommend against working

	Frequency	
	No.	%
Child's physical health	1724	24
Child's mental health	1445	20
Never recommend against work	1318	18
Inadequate child care	701	10
Child's age	591	8
Mother feels guilty	540	7
No economic need	459	6
Usually say "Do not work"	72	1
Other	402	6
TOTAL	7252	

From Heins, M., et al.: Pediatrics **72**:286, 1983. Copyright American Academy of Pediatrics 1983.

Bias against employed mothers did exist, however, among some respondents. Bias was related to the age and sex of the respondent and to whether the respondent's spouse worked. Those whose spouses did not work outside the home, those in older age groups, and male pediatricians in general held more traditional attitudes toward maternal employment. The researchers felt that a substantial number might give advice or cues that maternal employment might be detrimental to children, producing maternal conflict and guilt. The physician plays an important role in guiding parents with information about quality and availability of child-care facilities, as well as with advice about coping strategies.[5] As family counselor, the physician can help support mothers and fathers seeking to fulfill parental, occupational, and personal needs in a rapidly changing society.

OUTCOME OF CHILDREN WHOSE MOTHERS ARE EMPLOYED

There have been numerous studies since the early 1930s looking at the effects of maternal employment. Assessment of infant behavior, school achievement and adjustment, children's attitudes, adolescence, and delinquency have all been used as outcome measures. Annotated bibliographies covering the range of research in areas of medicine, psychology, sociology, and education are available.* The four major considerations are the variables that facilitate or impede maternal employment, the effect of maternal employment on children during the four developmental stages, the effects on the family, and the effects on society in general.

It has been emphasized that the presence of the mother in the home does not guarantee high-quality mothering.[6] It has also been shown that well-educated (college) mothers, including those who are employed, spend time with their children at the expense of their own personal needs. Because employed mothers encompass a large group of women with different educations, different reasons for working, and different opportunities for employment, it is difficult to generalize about effects. In general, literature reviews have emphasized critical factors that are more important than maternal employment, such as good substitute care, maternal role satisfaction, family stability, paternal attitude toward maternal employment, and the quality of time spent with the children.[10] Despite the abundance of research on school-age children, there is still little reported about preschoolers because there are no school records or test results available to use in large-population analysis. To date there is no direct effect of nonexclusive mothering per se. In studies of infants of adolescent mothers it has been shown that the children do better socially and academically if there are multiple caregivers instead of the adolescent alone.[14] No uniformly harmful effects on family life or on the growth and development of children have been demonstrated. Maternal employment may jeopardize family life when the conditions of the mother's employment are demeaning to self-

---

*See references 3, 6, 12, 20, 22, 23.

esteem, when others are strongly disapproving of her work away from the home, or when arrangements for child care are not adequate.[20]

BREASTFEEDING AND EMPLOYMENT

An important distinction must be made between work that separates the mother and infant for blocks of time and work that does not. In rural settings, women's work is usually compatible with all aspects of child care, including breastfeeding. Work in or around the home is usually flexible. If there are provisions for infants at the workplace, even formal urban work is compatible with child care and breastfeeding. The higher the education of the mother and the more advanced the job, the more opportunity there is for flexible arrangements that permit breastfeeding. Among the strategies available is pumping and saving milk while on the job to be fed to the baby by the baby-sitter the next day.

Dismissal from employment of nursing mothers demonstrates the unique problems for working women in certain jobs. Overall, the breastfeeding rates for working women do not show that breastfeeding and employment are mutually exclusive.[27] In Finland, the incidence of mothers breastfeeding at 1 month is 78% among nonworking and 80% among working mothers. The duration is also unaffected; 29% of nonworking and 32% of working mothers are breastfeeding at 3 months and 8% and 7% at 6 months.[24] Similar statistics are reported from Nigeria, the Philippines, and Chile.

The figures for the United States have been reported by Martinez and Dodd[15] (Table 13-3), who conducted a mail and telephone survey of new mothers in 1981, as described

Table 13-3. Percentage of infants breastfed by maternal employment status, 1981*

| | Infant age | | | |
	In hospital	2 mo	4 mo	6 mo
Full-time employment				
Breastfed alone	45.1	24.8	8.5	3.6
Breastfed with bottle	5.8	8.3	8.3	6.6
TOTAL	50.9	33.1	16.8	10.1
Milk, bottle supplementation as % of total	11.4	25.1	49.4	65.4
% still breastfeeding among those breastfeeding in hospital	100.0	65.0	33.0	19.8
Not employed				
Breastfed alone	53.4	41.1	30.8	22.9
Breastfed with bottle	6.1	6.4	6.5	6.9
TOTAL	59.5	47.4	37.3	29.8
Milk, bottle supplementation as % of total	10.3	13.5	17.4	23.2
% still breastfeeding among those breastfeeding in hospital	100.0	79.7	62.7	50.1

From Martinez, G.A. and Dodd, D.A.: Pediatrics 71:169, 1983. Copyright American Academy of Pediatrics 1983.
*Employment status was not elicited in second quarter of 1981. Data represent first, third, and fourth quarters only. Some totals do not add due to rounding.

in Chapter 1. The survey has been conducted since 1955 but data on employment were not collected until 1981, so no trends are available. When the infant was 6 months of age, 20% of the respondents were employed full time outside the home. The higher incidence of employment was among mothers who were college educated, upper income, and primiparous. The incidence of breastfeeding was not significantly influenced by employment, but the duration was negatively influenced. For every 100 mothers employed full time and breastfeeding full time in the hospital, 19.8% were still breastfeeding at 6 months, whereas 50.1% of unemployed mothers were still breastfeeding at 6 months. Working mothers also used more supplementary bottles.

When the factors influencing the duration of breastfeeding were examined by West[25] by postal questionnaire at 6 months in Edinburgh, only 5 mothers of 116 listed "return to work" as a reason for discontinuing.

A comparison by Martinez and Stahle[16] of low-income mothers who were receiving assistance from the Women's, Infants and Children's (WIC) Program showed that of the 38% who planned to work full time and left the hospital breastfeeding, only 8.8% were breastfeeding at 6 months, whereas of the 42.4% who had no plans for employment on leaving the hospital, 17.1% were still breastfeeding at 6 months.

Although work has been listed as a primary cause of early weaning, women seldom give employment as a reason for terminating breastfeeding. When Van Esterik and Greiner[24] reviewed the world literature documenting reasons for weaning, starting bottle feeding, or not initiating breastfeeding, employment was rarely mentioned. In studies of the effect of mother's employment on the nutritional status of her children, it was poverty and not mother's work that was associated with poor nutrition.

The effect of employment on the duration of breastfeeding may be influenced by the fact that breastfeeding can be carried out while the mother performs other tasks around the house so that it is easier to breastfeed when she is home.[9] Many studies have found that employment has little or no effect on the duration of breastfeeding. Other authors have reported an association with longer duration of breastfeeding in mothers who are employed, especially in higher-status jobs. It has been speculated that those women who work outside the home must schedule and plan carefully and are motivated to continue once the complex schedule is established. They also are able to anticipate and accommodate themselves to the stresses of uneven schedules and little sleep. A national study was conducted by Auerbach and Guss[2] among women who responded to an advertisement in popular parenting magazines requesting working breastfeeding women to fill out a questionnaire about their experiences. This study found a relationship between work and breastfeeding success. The timing of the return to work and the number of hours worked, not the type of work, influenced the duration of breastfeeding. Most of the respondents, however, were well educated and were motivated to respond to the advertisement and to retrospectively fill out a lengthy questionnaire. Half of the respondents provided their own milk for the missed feedings. Results showed that mothers who pumped or hand expressed (86% of the respondents) while at work continued to breastfeed longer than the small percentage who did not pump at work.

Counseling the breastfeeding mother who wishes to work

Part of the physician's counseling session before the birth of a baby should include inquiry about mother's plan to work postpartum. Open discussion about work, breast-feeding, child-care arrangements, and general stress so incurred will be helpful. Most well-educated women who plan to return to a career have thought out the entire process carefully but may wish some reassurance or alternative suggestions. The physician should know what services are available locally. It may be helpful to have a list of other working mothers who are willing to share experiences and knowledge of resources. It is often helpful for a woman to know a real person who has experienced similar career choices.

There are some women who have no experience with newborns and are totally un-realistic about the new responsibility and what it entails. The new mother needs to appreciate that there are events that occur around children that cannot be totally con-trolled. If a woman has been an efficient career woman in total control of her destiny, an infant with normal needs may be overwhelming. Women who have jobs that are rigid from the standpoint of work hours and workplace will not find a few glib remarks in a pamphlet very helpful when she wants to maintain her milk supply.

The physician may need to discuss specific issues:

Child care

1. Child-care arrangements should be sought that permit sufficient time for feeding an infant inexperienced with a bottle and sufficient time for extra cuddling an infant who is used to a closer relationship with his "feeder." The child-care specialist should be familiar with breastfeeding and sympathetic to the philoso-phy.
2. The advantages and disadvantages of child care in the infant's home, in the sitter's home, with or without the sitter's children, and with or without other children should be discussed. Is day care a good arrangement for this family, and what centers take young infants and will work with breastfeeding mothers? In spite of low cost, nursery warehousing is to be avoided.
3. Are there child-care facilities available close to the workplace so that mother could leave work on her breaks to breastfeed?

Feeding the infant while mother is working

1. Plans for feeding depend on the age of the child and his feeding pattern. If the infant is totally breastfed and under 6 months of age, feeding will be mother's milk (a) if his mother can actually breastfeed him because she can leave work and go to the infant or he can be brought to her at the workplace, (b) mother's milk in a bottle. If mother cannot leave work to nurse, then she may wish to pump her milk at work and save it for the following day. This necessitates having a reasonably sanitary place to pump, such as a lounge or clean locker room. It also necessitates having a means of storing the milk until she gets home, either

in a refrigerator at work or by placing the milk in a portable refrigerator system. Mothers have used Styrofoam containers with ice or dry ice for the container of milk. If no such arrangement for chilling can be made, the milk should be discarded. A woman who is away from her breastfeeding infant past feeding time for any reason may need to pump to maintain her milk supply or simply for comfort. Techniques for pumping and storing milk are reviewed in Chapter 19.

A mother may also anticipate the infant's needs before she returns to work and practice pumping and actually store in her home freezer a small amount daily for several weeks so that mother's milk is available.

The mother should be instructed to introduce the baby to the bottle and an alternate caregiver before the first day of work. Developing a plan of organization and practicing it prior to the first day of work may avoid initial disaster.

The pediatrician may wish to consider that if the infant is over 6 months of age, other foods can be introduced and the feeding given by the caregiver can be the solids by spoon and liquids from a cup so that no breastfeeding is actually missed. The professional can anticipate these issues and tailor feeding counseling accordingly. Some infants quickly learn the mother's schedule and may adjust their sleep pattern to allow a long stretch while mother is away. This may result in feedings during the night instead, but if the mother is informed of this phenomenon she may be less anxious if it occurs. It has been suggested in some studies that infants of mothers who work have more infections and illnesses, which is a reason to encourage a mother to continue breastfeeding, especially during the first weeks of adjustment to transient recurrent separation. Children who are cared for in a day-care setting have been thought by pediatricians to have more infections.

Maternal considerations

Counseling the breastfeeding family when the mother returns to work should also include attention to mothering the mother. Fatigue is a significant problem for all postpartum women and many nursing mothers and can easily become a major stress when the mother adds outside employment to her schedule. Any time there is a major change in anyone's schedule, there are several days or more of adjustment. If during this time the mother can be encouraged to focus on a few essential concerns—her infant, her job, and her own well-being, as opposed to the housework, fancy meals, or a social schedule—she will weather this transition without despair. The first casualty of fatigue may be breastfeeding, unless some anticipatory caution is taken. Once the schedule has been adjusted and a routine established, breastfeeding may offer tremendous satisfaction for both mother and infant in terms of a sustained relationship as well as a reaffirmation for the mother of the quality of her parenting. One of the most difficult adjustments to motherhood for an efficient career woman is the need to set priorities and eliminate some chores of lesser urgency. The counselor needs to reinforce this when the mother returns to work. If a mother continues to breastfeed, holding and cuddling her baby cannot become a lower priority.

Maternal benefits and breastfeeding

In 1919 the International Labor Organization established the Maternity Protection Convention for working women.[19] This document provided for two half-hour nursing breaks per day. It also recommended that employers provide creches or day care when more than a given number of women are employed, but few countries hold to its tenets today. Maternity benefits vary from country to country and may include maternity leave with or without pay, nursing breaks, provision of day-care facilities, and prohibition of dismissal. Physicians who care for mothers and infants should take a leadership role in ensuring that mothers can continue breastfeeding even when the mother is employed.

The physician can help support fathers and mothers alike who are faced with fulfilling the roles of parent, employee, and citizen in a rapidly changing society.

REFERENCES

1. American College of Obstetricians and Gynecologists: Guidelines on pregnancy and work, Chicago, 1977, ACOG publications.
2. Auerbach, K.G., and Guss, E.: Maternal employment and breast feeding: a study of 567 women's experience. (In press.)
3. Baden, C.: Work and family—an annotated bibliography 1978-1980, Boston, 1981, Boston Wheelock College Center for Parenting Studies.
4. Brazelton, T.B.: Toddlers and parents, New York, 1974, Delta Books.
5. Eisenberg, L.: Caring for children and working dilemmas of contemporary womanhood, Pediatrics 56:24, 1975.
6. Ginsberg, E.: The changing pattern of women's work, Am. J. Orthopsychiatr. 28:313, 1969.
7. Heins, M., et al.: Attitudes of pediatricians toward maternal employment, Pediatrics 72:283, 1983.
8. Helsing E., and King F.S.: Breast-feeding in practice: a manual for health workers, Oxford, 1982, Oxford University Press.
9. Hirschman, C., and Sweet, J.A.: Social background and breastfeeding among American mothers, Soc. Biol. 21:39, 1974.
10. Hoffman, L.: The professional woman as mother, Ann. N.Y. Acad. Sci. 208:209, 1973.
11. Howell, M.C.: Employed mothers and their families, Pediatrics 52:252, 1973.
12. Hurst, M., and Zambrana, R.E.: Determinants and consequences of maternal employment,

Washington D.C., 1981, Business and Professional Women's Foundation.
13. La Leche League: The womanly art of breastfeeding, Franklin Park, Ill., 1981, La Leche League.
14. Lawrence, R.A.: Early mothering by adolescents. In McAnarney, E.R., editor: Premature adolescent pregnancy and parenthood, New York, 1983, Grune & Stratton, Inc.
15. Martinez, G.A., and Dodd, D.A.: 1981 milk-feeding patterns in the United States during the first 12 months of life, Pediatrics 71:166, 1983.
16. Martinez, G.A., and Stahle, D.A.: The recent trend in milk feeding among WIC infants, Am. J. Public Health 72:68, 1982.
17. Mead, M.: A cultural anthropologist's approach to maternal deprivation. Public Health Papers no. 14, Deprivation of maternal care, Geneva, 1962, World Health Organization.
18. Popkin, B.M.: Time allocation of the mother and child nutrition, Ecol. Food Nutr. 9:1, 1980.
19. Richardson, J.L.: Review of the international legislation establishing nursing breaks, J. Trop. Pediatr. 21:249, 1975.
20. Sanday, P.: Female status in the public domain. In Rosaldo, M., and Lamphere, L., editors: Woman, culture and society, Stanford, 1974, Stanford University Press.
21. Spock, B.: Baby and child care, New York, 1977, Pocket Books.
22. U.S. Department of Labor: Manpower Report of

the President, Washington, D.C., 1974, U.S. Government Printing Office.

23. U.S. Department of Labor, Office of the Secretary: Facts on Women Workers, Washington, D.C., 1980, Women's Bureau.

24. Van Esterik, P., and Greiner, T.: Breastfeeding and women's work: constraints and opportunities, Stud. Fam. Plan. **12:**184, 1981.

25. West, C.P.: Factors influencing the duration of breast feeding, J. Biosoc. Sci. **12:**325, 1980.

26. Winikoff, B., and Baer, E.: The obstetrician's opportunity: translating "breast is best" from theory to practice, Am. J. Obstet. Gynecol. **138:**105, 1980.

27. Zambrana, R.E., Hurst, M., and Hite, R.L.: The working mother in contemporary perspective: a review of the literature, Pediatrics **64:**862, 1979.

14

Breastfeeding the infant with a problem

A normal full-term infant can usually be breastfed with only minor adjustment problems, even without the support of medical expertise. The infant with a medical or surgical problem presents special concerns that cannot be conquered simply by a strong-willed mother who is determined to overcome all obstacles to breastfeed her infant. An understanding of the medical problem of the infant, his special nutritional needs, and the mechanical obstacles to feeding and nutritional absorption will be necessary before a rational judgment can be made about breastfeeding. When the infant cannot nurse directly at the breast, would providing mother's milk be appropriate? What is the overall prognosis for ever feeding at the breast or, perhaps, for survival itself? Parents are so awed by the medical staff of special and intensive care nurseries that they are often afraid to bring up the subject of breastfeeding. In addition, the nursery staff may be so busy balancing electrolytes and adjusting ventilators and monitors that they have not thought to ask what plans the mother might have had for feeding before the infant developed a problem. There are absolute contraindications to breastfeeding infants with certain problems. Those problems are few in number and rare in occurrence. Each medical problem will be dealt with separately. General information on establishing a milk supply without the stimulus of the infant's suckling will be provided in Chapter 17.

LOW–BIRTH WEIGHT INFANTS

Infants who are born weighing less than average, or less than 2500 g, will be referred to as low–birth weight infants. If the infants are less than 37 weeks of gestation, they are premature; if they are full term and low birth weight, they are small for gestational age (SGA).

Premature infants

The prognosis for survival of infants who are less than 37 weeks of gestation at birth depends on the gestational age, weight, respiratory status, and presence of any other complicating factors. For instance, if the infant develops hyaline membrane disease requiring respiratory support with continuous positive airway pressure (CPAP) or a ventilator, the survival rate is decreased as compared with that of an infant of the same weight and age without hyaline membrane disease.

A 2001 to 2500 g infant without complications may be weaned from the incubator to an open crib within 24 hours. Although his suck reflex may be poor, he can usually be nipple fed. If he is vigorous enough, he can be tried at the breast. If he can stimulate the breast briefly and obtain the rich, antibody-containing, cell-filled colostrum, it will protect against infection while providing a small amount of nutrition. If the infant cannot suck and must be tube fed, any colostrum the mother can manually express or pump from the breast can be given by gavage tube along with donor milk or the prescribed formula necessary for nourishment. The value of colostrum to the infant has been thoroughly reviewed in Chapter 5. A recent study in Guatemala that was repeated in the special care nursery of the Rainbow Children's Hospital in Cleveland showed that the infection rate among sick and premature newborns was greatly diminished by providing 15 ml of human colostrum contributed by random donors daily.[72] These findings were especially dramatic in Guatemala, where the mortality from infection in the nursery is extremely high.

ANTIMICROBIAL PROPERTIES OF PRETERM BREAST MILK. The infection-protective properties of human milk have been considered a key reason to provide human milk for high-risk infants who are prone to devastating infections including necrotizing enterocolitis, sepsis, meningitis, and viral infections such as a respiratory syncytial virus (RSV) and rotavirus. The antimicrobial properties of milk produced by mothers who deliver preterm have been studied by several investigators.

The cells of preterm milk were compared to those of term milk and found to be similar in number and in capacity to phagocytose and kill staphylococci.[89] The ability of the preterm cells to produce interferon on stimulation with mitogens was marginally better than that of term cells. The cells survived 24 hours refrigerated at 4° C; at 48 hours there was a reduction in number but not function. Passing the milk through a feeding tube did not diminish the number or function of the cells. The levels of lactoferrin and lysozyme were greater in preterm milk than in term milk from the second to the twelfth week postpartum.[51] Secretory IgA (sIgA) was the predominant form of IgA and values increased from the sixth to the twelfth week in preterm milk. The increase in IgA was not dependent on method of collection, rate of flow, or time of day but the concentration varied inversely with the milk volume; thus, total production of IgA in 24 hours is thought by some investigators to be comparable for the two groups.[25,57] When preterm (31 to 36 weeks' gestation) infants were fed human milk and compared to a matched group of premature infants fed infant formula, the serum levels of IgA at 9 to

13 weeks were higher in the formula fed infants.[106] Those infants who received at least 60% of their own mothers' milk had higher IgA levels at 3 weeks of age than those receiving less than 30% of the feedings from their mothers' milk. Serum IgG levels were higher in the breast milk group, and serum IgM levels were similar in the two feeding groups. Samples of precolostrum collected from undelivered mothers was assayed and found to contain equal or greater amounts of IgA, IgG, IgM, lactoferrin, and lysozyme than mature colostrum.[77]

When the impact on actual prevention of infection among premature infants is reviewed, significantly less infection is found in infants receiving human milk as compared with those receiving formula (9 of 32 breast milk; 24 of 38 formula).[90]

PROTEIN REQUIREMENTS. The major concern of nutritionists in contemplating the use of human milk for low–birth weight infants has been based on the protein concentration.[93] Calculations made from information extrapolated from intrauterine growth curves indicate that the premature infant requires more protein than can be provided by human milk. There is no easy way to determine the availability of this protein for absorption, although it is agreed that more of the protein in human milk is utilizable than that in formulas derived from a cow's milk base. Fomon et al.[40] have provided calculations to demonstrate the needs of the premature infant and the nutrients supplied by an appropriate amount of human milk (Table 14-1).

These determinations are made by using a reference infant, who has been described for various ages and weights and the daily increment of body content of protein. Allowances are made for inevitable losses and the degree of intestinal absorption; the total of these is the requirement. For the premature infant, the body content of a fetus of his gestational age is considered ideal, and the ideal growth curve is presumed to be that achieved in normal intrauterine growth. Fomon et al. point out that for the reference fetus between 28 and 32 weeks of gestation, protein accounts for 12.2% of the weight gained. They took a 1200 g premature infant gaining 20 g/day, of which 12.2% is protein, and determined that the increment in body protein will be 2.44 g/day. There is additional protein necessary for metabolism or "nongrowth" that averages 0.5 g/kg/day. Thus the total requirement for protein absorbed by the body is 3.04 g (2.44 g +

Table 14-1. Protein, calcium, and sodium requirements by growing premature infants and composition of human milk

	Protein (g/100 kcal)	Calcium (mg/100 kcal)	Sodium (mEq/100 kcal)
Estimated requirements for hypothetical growing premature infants*	2.54	132†	2.3
Composition of banked human milk	1.50	43	0.8

From Fomon, S.J., Ziegler, E.E., and Vazquez, H.D.: Am. J. Dis. Child 131:463, 1977. Copyright 1977, American Medical Association.
*Assumed body weight is 1200 g; weight gain, 20 g/day, energy intake, 120 kcal/kg/day. The basis for estimating requirements is described in the text.
†This estimate does not apply to infants fed formulas from which calcium absorption is less than 65% of intake.

Table 14-2.   Weight gain supported by intake of 180 ml human milk/kg at selected body weights

	Weight gain (gm/day)			
	800 g	1000 g	1500 g	2000 g
Ca	4	5	6.7	8.4
P	4	5	6.8	8.7
N	10	12	16	21
Na	5	7	11	15
Mg	12	15	22	28
Cl	22	30	48	68
K	21	33	49	66

Based on data compiled by Forbes, G.B.: Nutritional adequacy of human breast milk for premature infants. In Lebenthal, E., editor: Textbook of gastroenterology and nutrition, New York, 1981, Raven Press.

[1.2 × 0.5]). If only 83% of the dietary protein ingested is absorbed, 3.66 g of protein is required in the diet. If the dietary requirement for kilocalories is 120 kcal/kg/day, then conclude Fomon and Ziegler,[38] the 1200 g infant needs 144 kcal/day from human milk, or 2.54 g of protein/100 kcal, or 216 ml of human milk (180 ml/kg). Calculations based on intrauterine growth have also been published by Forbes,[42] who expresses genuine concern about proper nutrition for the normal growth and development of the already compromised premature. He has compiled a table of weight gain supported by intake of 180 ml of human milk per kilogram at selected body weights (Table 14-2).[44] The high growth rate of the premature infant demands an intake of a milk that is richer in protein, sodium, calcium, and phosphorus than that produced even by the mother who delivers preterm.[43] The variability in the composition of "preterm milk" is also of concern. Forbes concludes: "Brain growth is rapid in late gestation, and it is generally held that such babies should grow well to insure eventual well being. Unless one assumes that the fetus *in utero* is overnourished, it is necessary to strive to meet the goal of intrauterine growth and body composition. . . . Human milk is not equal to the task. The acknowledged virtues of human milk and breastfeeding in certain spheres of child rearing should not blind us to its nutritional shortcomings for this special group of babies."[43]

MILK OF MOTHERS WHO DELIVER PREMATURELY.   Human milk was noted to differ chemically and immunologically from woman to woman but also may differ in the same woman from feeding to feeding (Chapter 4). Fresh milk from the infant's own mother may offer advantages.[41] This point was demonstrated by studies done by Atkinson et al.[12] on the nitrogen concentrations of milk from mothers of term and premature infants. The data demonstrated that for a given volume of milk, the premature would receive 20% more nitrogen than would the full-term infant if both were fed their own mother's milk. The significance of the higher nitrogen concentration in the premature infant's own mother's milk will be even greater when compared with the same volume of intake of mature breast milk from a third-party donor or pooled milks. The researchers point out that if there is a similar distribution between protein and nonprotein nitrogen in the

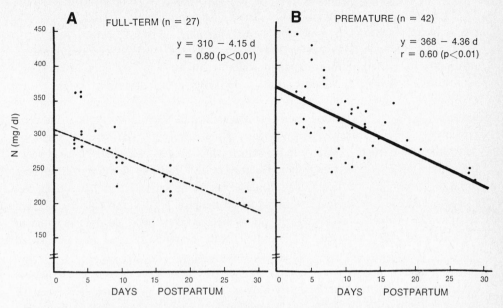

Fig. 14-1. The relationship of nitrogen concentration *(N)* in milk to day of lactation. Analysis performed to define regression lines as indicated for **A,** full-term and **B,** premature infant. (From Atkinson, S.A., Bryan, M.H., and Anderson, G.H.: J. Pediatr. **93:**67, 1978.)

Table 14-3. Comparison of mean nitrogen (N) concentration in milk from mothers of premature (PT) and full-term (FT) infants*

Milk group	Number	N concentration (mg/100 ml) Observed	N concentration (mg/100 ml) Adjusted†
FT	27	260.6 ± 8.9‡	267.5 ± 8.7
PT	42	315.5 ± 8.4	312.3 ± 8.3
FT vs PT		$P < 0.001$	$P < 0.001$

From Atkinson, S.A., Bryan, M.H., and Anderson, G.H.: J. Pediatr. **93:**67, 1978. Copyright American Academy of Pediatrics 1978.
*Adjusted values were obtained by covariance analysis to correct for effect of day and volume.
†N adj = $\bar{N}$ − day error − volume error.
‡Mean ± SE.

milk of mothers of both mature and immature infants, the premature infant would receive at least twice as much protein and utilizable nitrogen from an equal volume of his own mother's milk during early lactation (Fig. 14-1 and Table 14-3).

These initial provocative studies by Atkinson et al.[12] on the composition of milk from mothers who deliver preterm have initiated an avalanche of reports from many laboratories, some confirming, others questioning the findings.[5,58,59,107] The studies have been expanded to include many of the constituents of human milk. The expressions "preterm milk" and "term milk" have come to mean milk produced by a woman who has delivered preterm or at term respectively. They shall be so used here.

There is good general agreement that preterm milk contains higher concentrations of total nitrogen, protein nitrogen, sodium, chloride, magnesium, and iron. Preterm and term milk are similar in volume, calories, fat, fatty acids, potassium, calcium, and phosphorus.[11,27] There is disagreement about lactose, which one laboratory reports as reduced.[113] Most investigators remark on the tremendous variability among mothers, possibly partially dependent on their degree of preterm status. They also comment on variability from sample to sample in the same mother. Others note that beyond 2 weeks postpartum the difference diminishes. Guerrini et al.[60] reported significant differences in fat to be more marked in the first 10 days in preterm milk. Others have found tremendous variation in the creamatocrit across all samples.[75] They also noted fat content to vary with method of collection as noted in Chapter 18, the electric pump being associated with high fat levels.[60] The osmolality of the serum of premature infants fed human milk did not differ from those fed formula with 2.7 g/100 ml, 15.4% of total calories.[20] When infants were fed 8.5 g/kg or 21.1% of total calories, their plasma osmolality was elevated, although they were not edematous, nor did they gain excessive weight.[30] The osmolality of the gastric and duodenal contents showed a linear relationship with the osmolality of the milk with those infants fed human milk or isotonic formula being 295 mosm/kg and those with hypertonic formulas reaching 622 mosm/kg.

Mineral content of preterm milk in some studies showed slight increases in iron and magnesium for the first week or so, but levels of copper, zinc, calcium, and phosphorus were the same for term and preterm milks.

Experience feeding human milk to premature infants. Räihä and others[20,95–97] have approached the question of feeding premature infants by performing a controlled study in

---

MILK OF MOTHERS WHO DELIVER PRETERM

Level increased in preterm	Level unchanged in preterm	Estimated requirement for premature
Total nitrogen	Volume	P 2.4 g/100 kcal
Protein nitrogen	Calories	Na 2.1 mEq/100 kcal
Long-chain fatty acids	Lactose (? less)	Cl 1.8 mEq/100 kcal
Medium-chain fatty acids	Fat (?) by creamatocrit	K 1.8 mEq/100 kcal
Short-chain fatty acids	Linolenic acid	Mg 0.28 mmol
Sodium	Potassium	
Chloride	Calcium	
Magnesium (?)	Phosphorus	
Iron	Copper	
	Zinc	
	Osmolality	
	Vitamin $B_{(1-12)}$	

which a group of premature infants was fed human milk and other groups of premature infants were fed formulations of cow's milk altered to provide different ratios of casein and whey and total protein. They reported their studies in a series of four articles highlighting metabolic responses, effect on growth, effects on aliphatic amino acids and sulfur-containing amino acids, and effects on tyrosine and phenylalanine in plasma and urine. The premature infants were from one of three groups weighing less than 2100 g; T_1 was 28 to 30 weeks, T_2 was 31 to 33 weeks, and T_3 was 34 to 36 weeks. The infants were randomly assigned to one of five feeding groups including breast milk or an isocaloric formula varying in the quality and quantity of protein but not in fat or mineral content (Table 14-4). Caloric intake was 117 kcal in 150 ml/kg/day for formulas and 170 ml/kg/day for human milk (to obtain the same caloric intake per kilogram as the formulas provide).

Räihä and associates found no significant differences in rate of growth, in crown to rump length, in femoral length, in head circumference, or in rate of gain in weight from time of regaining birth weight to time of discharge at 2400 g. Their data also demonstrate that the blood urea nitrogen, urine osmolarity, total serum protein, serum albumin, and serum globulin levels varied directly with the quantity of protein in the diet. Blood ammonia concentration also varied with the quantity and quality of the protein in the diet: the more protein and the more casein, the higher the ammonia concentration. Metabolic acidosis in this study was more frequent, more severe, and more prolonged in the infant fed casein-predominant formulas than in those fed whey protein or breast milk (Figs. 14-2 to 14-5). Investigations on specific amino acids showed that the plasma amino acid concentrations of infants fed formulas high in protein and in casein had high levels of methionine and phenylalanine compared to those fed breast milk. Räihä and coworkers suggest that the human preterm infant has limited capacity to convert methionine to cystine.

Feeding prematures their mothers' "preterm" milk. Since there are data to support the concept that preterm milk is different, the critical factor is the effect on the premature infant's growth pattern. This has been investigated at a number of centers and, indeed, the premature fed his own mother's milk does grow along a curve more like intrauterine

Table 14-4. Intake of protein and calories of the formulas compared to pooled human milk

Nutrient	True protein (g/kg/day)	Calories* (kcal/kg/day)	Protein kcal ratio (g/100/kcal)	Distribution (%) of calories		
				Protein	Fat	Carbohydrate
Pooled human milk	1.63	114	1.4	6	51	43
1.5% (60:40)	2.25	118	1.9	8	50	42
3.0% (60:40)	4.5	116	3.8	17	51	32
1.5% (18:82)	2.25	118	1.9	8	50	42
3.0% (18:82)	4.5	116	3.8	17	51	32

From Räihä, N.C.R., et al.: Pediatrics **57**:661, 1976. Copyright American Academy of Pediatrics 1976.
*Caloric intake calculated on the basis of combustion fuel values of 4.4 for protein, 9.4 for fat, and 3.95 for carbohydrate.

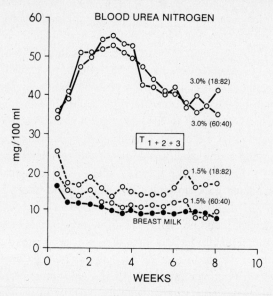

Fig. 14-2. Effect of dietary regimen on mean concentration of blood urea nitrogen. Data for all gestational age groups combined. Whey-predominant protein formulas are indicated by *1.5% (60:40)* and *3.0% (60:40)* and casein-predominant formulas by *1.5% (18:82)* and *3.0% (18:82)*. (Modified from Räihä, N.C.R., et al.: Pediatrics **57**:659, 1976.)

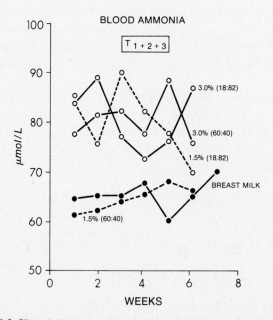

Fig. 14-3. Effect of dietary regimen on mean concentration of blood ammonia.

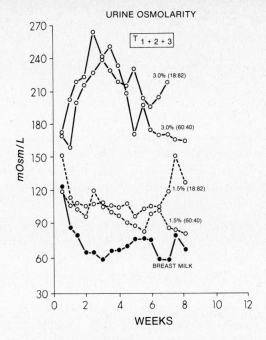

Fig. 14-4. Effect of dietary regimen on mean urine osmolarity.

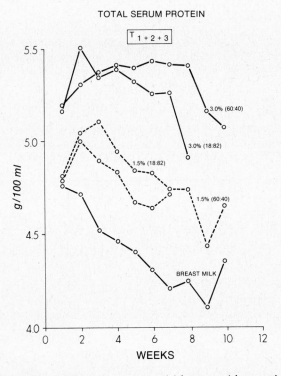

Fig. 14-5. Effect of dietary regimen on mean total serum protein concentration.

growth curves.[67,87] The growth curves of a group of infants fed their mothers' milk were compared with those fed whey-based infant formula and those fed banked human term milk. The mean number of days required to regain birth weight were similar in the preterm mother's milk group and formula, and both were significantly less than the bank milk. Rates of weight gain were greater in the preterm milk and formula groups.[56] The average increments in length and head circumference were also greater in those groups compared to the term bank milk group. The calcium and phosphorus were higher and the alkaline phosphatase lower in the formula group compared with the two groups fed human milk. The infants in the term bank milk group required more sodium supplements to maintain sodium at 133 mmol/L. Acid-base studies, BUN, and total protein were not significantly different.

Another study was performed on premature infants in which one group received bank milk supplemented with whatever the mother could provide to a total of 185 to 200 ml/kg/day and the control group received taurine- and cholesterol-supplemented formula.[66] Mothers provided approximately 45% of total intake of the group fed human milk. There was no difference in rate of gain in weight, length, or head circumference, in serum total protein, in acid-base status, or in plasma amino acid concentrations. The growth averaged 196 $\pm$ 6 g/week for human milk and 205 $\pm$ 7 g/week for formula groups compared to 207 g/week in utero. There were no metabolic problems in either group.

The metabolic rate was measured by computerized indirect calorimetry, enabling determination of the partition of energy metabolism in infants fed their mother's preterm milk and compared to intrauterine growth curves and accretion rates for comparable gestational ages.[26] The infants gained weight and grew along intrauterine curves and the accretion rates of fat and protein were comparable. The energy expenditure for metabolism was 56 kcal/kg/day and for tissue building 44 kcal/kg/day. Energy and nitrogen balance studies in growing premature infants fed their mothers' milk or formula were compared. The gross energy intake, metabolizable energy intake, nitrogen intake, and nitrogen retention were similar. Energy expenditure was significantly lower in the human milk group compared with the formula group, although the energy storage was the same. The ratio of energy storage to weight gain was significantly greater in the infants fed their mothers' milk.[120]

Metabolic differences in infants fed human milk have also been evaluated. Higher intraluminal concentrations of bile acids are present in infants fed human milk than in those fed formula. The addition of taurine to the formula did not affect synthesis or secretion of tauroconjugated bile acids. The fats of human milk were absorbed more efficiently than those of formula. The addition of taurine and cholesterol to formula did not improve fat absorption.[67]

Essential amino acids. Important exceptions to the finding that high-protein formulas producing high plasma protein levels were the findings on cystine and taurine. Taurine, which is present as a free amino acid in human milk and the milks of many mammals with the exception of the cow, was in highest concentration in infants fed human milk. Infants fed formulas low in taurine had reduced concentrations of taurine in the urine and plasma. Räihä and co-workers[95] suggested that the ability of the infant to convert cystine to taurine via cysteine sulfinic acid decarboxylase is limited. They found the enzyme in only trace amounts in fetal and mature human liver. The levels of this enzyme in the human are a small fraction of levels found in other mammals such as rat (1/1000), cat (1/10), or monkey (1/10). Infants who receive low-protein casein-predominant formulas with half the cystine of human milk and almost no taurine had urinary excretion of cystine and taurine reduced significantly in 2 weeks. The plasma taurine levels fell steadily. When fed high-protein casein-predominant formulas, they maintained cystine levels but the plasma taurine level dropped steadily. This work suggests a dietary requirement for taurine (Figs. 14-6 and 14-7). Taurine has been shown to be of special importance in the developing nervous system in the human and other mammals such as the rat, rabbit, cat, and monkey[114] (see Chapter 4).

In-depth study of tyrosine and phenylalanine by these researchers[97] provides additional evidence that the immature infant is ill-prepared to metabolize these aromatic amino acids. Plasma and urine concentrations of tyrosine and phenylalanine were higher in infants fed high-protein formulas than in infants fed breast milk. The role of high protein intakes and resultant metabolic inbalances on brain development have not yet been prospectively reported. Even the appropriate physiologic mean serum levels of tyrosine are not agreed on. It should be noted that no infant fed breast milk had a tyrosine level over 20 μmol/100 ml (Figs. 14-7 to 14-11).

Snyderman[112] considers tyrosine an essential amino acid for the low–birth weight infant and has determined that the minimum daily requirement is 50 mg/kg of body weight. Plasma levels are 1 mg/100 ml or 5.5 μmol/100 ml. Filer et al.[36] confirmed these findings. Gaull et al.[49,50] have concluded that cystine is an essential amino acid for prematures and newborns. Protein absorption and plasma amino acids in preterm infants reflect the composition of the milk ingested and fluctuate continuously. Postprandial plasma amino acid measurements are a useful means of testing an infant's ability to handle protein and amino acid loads. Present studies indicate that premature infants fed preterm milk have adequate absorption and retention of protein.[115]

SODIUM AND CALCIUM REQUIREMENTS. Nutritionally, the ash content, specifically sodium and calcium, required for the premature infant is also calculated to be greater than can be provided by human milk. According to Fomon and Ziegler,[39] for the reference fetus between 28 and 32 weeks of gestation, 617 mg of calcium is added to the body for each 100 g of weight gained. Nongrowth requirements for calcium are insignificant. Fomon and Ziegler calculated that if 65% of the calcium is absorbed from human milk, then the premature infant would require 190 mg/day or 132 mg/100 kcal/day. As noted in Table 14-1, human milk provides only 43 mg of calcium/100 kcal. Forbes[41] makes similar observations by mathematical calculations of an increase in body weight of 30 g in a 1500 g infant consuming 120 kcal/kg/day. Human milk would provide 85 mg of

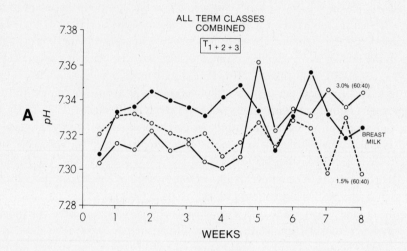

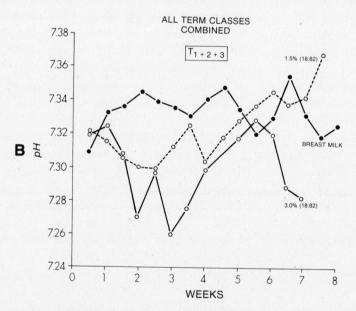

Fig. 14-6. A, Breast milk compared to 60:40 milk preparations with pH of 1.5% and 3.0%. **B,** Breast milk compared to 18:82 milk preparations with pH of 1.5% and 3.0%.

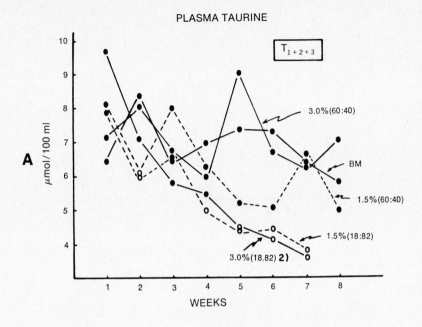

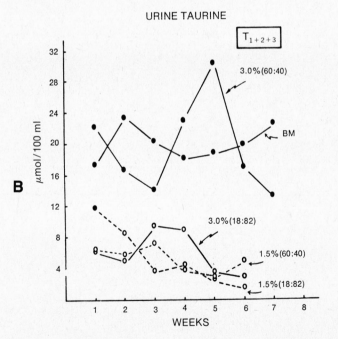

Fig. 14-7. A, Effect of dietary regimen on mean plasma concentration of taurine. **B,** Effect of dietary regimen on mean urine concentration of taurine. (From Gaull, G.E., et al.: J. Pediatr. **90:**348, 1977.)

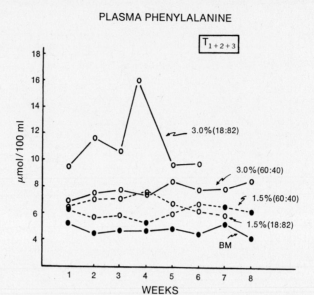

Fig. 14-8. Effect of dietary regimen on the mean plasma concentration of phenylalanine.

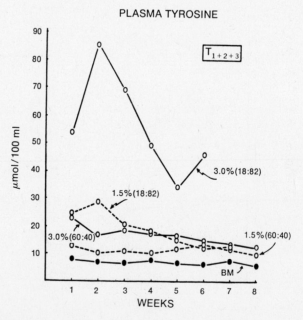

Fig. 14-9. Effect of dietary regimen on the mean plasma concentration of tyrosine.

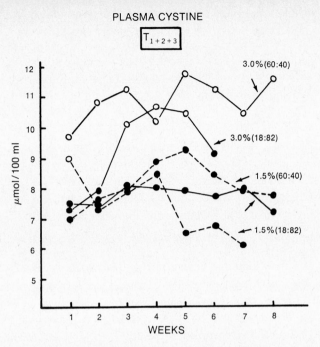

Fig. 14-10. Effect of dietary regimen on the mean plasma concentration of cystine.

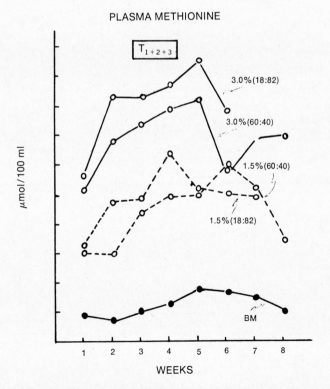

Fig. 14-11. Effect of dietary regimen on the mean plasma concentration of methionine.

calcium, whereas 250 mg is calculated to be needed. Forbes has shown the weight of the infant, regardless of gestational age, to advance on a logarithmic curve and the rate of increase in calcium to be equal to the rate of change in weight times a power of the weight (a 1000 g infant who gains 30 g needs 229 mg of calcium for proper growth during that gain).

Similar calculations have been made for sodium, demonstrating that the same reference fetus of 28 to 32 weeks has 7.4 mEq of body sodium. When 20 g/day is gained in weight, there is a retention of 1.48 mEq of sodium. Considering a urinary loss of 1.0 mEq/kg and 0.2 mEq/kg via the skin, there is a total loss of 1.44 mEq/kg/day. With 87% absorption from dietary sources, the requirement is 3.36 mEq/day or 2.3 mEq/100 kcal, according to Fomon et al.[40] Human milk provides 0.8 mEq/100 kcal.

•   •   •

Fomon et al.[40] conclude that human milk is inadequate in meeting the nutritional requirements of the small premature infant. In the larger premature infant of 1800 g or more, the requirements, except for calcium, would just barely be met by human milk, if he only gained 20 g/day (Table 14-5). A workshop was held by the Office for Maternal and Child Health of the Department of Health, Education, and Welfare to determine the benefits and risks of feeding human milk to premature infants. Representatives of the major organizations interested in infant nutrition as well as key representatives of the research in this field attended the December 1975 workshop. They concluded that it

Table 14-5. Accumulation of various components during the last trimester of pregnancy

Component	Accumulation during various stages of gestation				
	26-31 wk	31-33 wk	33-35 wk	35-38 wk	38-40 wk
Body weight (g)*	500	500	500	500	500
Water (g)	410	350	320	240	220
Fat (g)	25	65	85	175	200
Nitrogen (g)	11	12	12	6	7
Calcium (g)	4	5	5	5	5
Phosphorus (g)	2.2	2.6	2.8	3.0	3.0
Magnesium (mg)	130	110	120	120	80
Sodium (mEq)	35	25	40	40	40
Potassium (mEq)	19	24	26	20	20
Chloride (mEq)	30	24	10	20	10
Iron (mg)	36	60	60	40	20
Copper (mg)	2.1	2.4	2.0	2.0	2.0
Zinc (mg)	9.0	10.0	8.0	7.0	3.0

Modified from data of Widdowson, reproduced with permission from Heird, W.C., and Anderson, T.L.: Nutritional requirements and methods of feeding low birth weight infants. In Gluck, L., et al., editors: Current problems in pediatrics, vol. VII, no. 8, Chicago, 1977, Year Book Medical Publishers, Inc., copyright © 1977.
*Body weight of the 26-week fetus is 1000 g, that of the 40-week fetus is 3000 g.

is safe to feed human milk to human premature infants with the possible exception of fresh human milk from a donor other than the mother. Most participants believed that risk of nutritional inadequacy was small in relation to possible benefits. It was thought important to know the chemical composition of the food and to monitor the nutritional status of the infant.

MACRONUTRIENTS. Macronutrients remain a concern to investigators because nutritional hypophosphatemic rickets have been reported in prematures fed human milk.[98]

The macromineral contents of preterm and term human milk have been reported.[13,14] Sodium, chloride, potassium, magnesium, calcium, and phosphorus concentrations were similar in both milks; thus the calcium and phosphorus would not be adequate to meet the requirements of premature infants in the early weeks of life.[88] Copper, iron, and zinc were also similar in both milks so that absorption of 25% of the zinc and 35% of the copper, but 100% of the iron would be needed. Zinc deficiency has been reported in two exclusively breastfed prematures who did not have abnormal absorption. Whether iron supplements given to the infant influenced uptake or whether this was due to maternal milk deficiency is a question. Trace element content of milk from mothers in Nigeria showed higher levels of copper, zinc, and iron in preterm milk than in term milk in the first 8 weeks postdelivery.[10]

Macromineral balance studies in prematures (less than 1300 g) fed their mother's milk revealed that preterm milk provides sufficient retention of sodium, chloride, and potassium during the first four postnatal weeks. Preterm milk, term milk, and unsupplemented formula do not provide sufficient calcium for the very low–birth weight infant.[104]

The effect of early oral calcium supplementation in preterm infants was to prevent early neonatal hypocalcemia, partially through the reduction in the postnatal rise of serum immunoreactive calcitonin.[105] The exact mechanism of the developing rickets in low–birth weight infants continues under study, since rickets have been reported in infants receiving mineral and vitamin D supplements.[55,108] It has been shown that vitamin D and phosphorus supplementation in infants fed banked human milk does enhance calcium retention.[100] Most neonatologists agree that premature infants under 1500 g at birth require 150 mg/kg/day of calcium and 65 mg/kg/day of phosphorus.[74] Whether fed preterm or term human milk, the very low–birth weight infant should have the following:

1. Vitamin D supplement to provide 400 IU daily
2. Supplementation of calcium to provide total intake of 220 to 250 mg/kg/day
3. Supplementation of phosphorus to provide total intake of 120 mg/kg/day
4. Addition of active form of vitamin D ($1,25[OH]_2$-D_3) (calcitriol [Rocaltrol]) if osteopenia occurs.

HUMAN MILK ENRICHED WITH BANKED HUMAN MILK OR POWDERED FORMULA. Along a parallel track to research in preterm milk have been studies to enhance human milk to meet the calculated needs of the small infant.[81] There is general agreement that banked term human milk should not be the sole source of nutrients for the low–birth weight infant.[117]

Human milk protein supplements were added to preterm human milk and fed to prematures weighing less than 1500 g, increasing the protein intake by 0.8 g/100 ml.[117] The supplemented infants received 0.6 to 1.6 g/kg/day from 2 to 12 weeks. The unsupplemented infants developed hypoproteinemia at 8 to 12 weeks, although growth was similar in the two groups. There was no evidence of amino acid metabolic imbalance in the supplemented group although their BUNs were 15 mg/100 ml at 2 weeks of age.[99]

A similar feeding was prepared by adding to fresh mother's milk a product made from pooled human milk that had been ultrafiltrated and freeze-dried. The protein content was 3.0 to 3.5 g/kg/day with 110 kcal/kg/24 hours.[61] Growth followed intrauterine growth curves. Amino acid levels in the serum remained within normal limits. These authors also reported considerable specific sIgA activity against *Escherichia coli* O antigen. The development of another human milk "formula" has been studied, which involves taking whole human milk, human cream, separated by centrifugation, plus salt-free, lactose-free human milk protein extracted by dialysis and freeze drying.[78] It is energy-enriched human milk with extra protein and fat. Clinical trials continue with these preparations.

A commercial product is also available called human milk fortifier, which is designed so that one packet of powder weighing 0.95 g is added to 25 ml human milk. This will provide additional calories, protein, carbohydrate, calcium, phosphorus, magnesium, copper, zinc, and sodium (see Human Milk Fortifier on the opposite page). The protein is from cow's milk modified to a 60:40 whey/casein ratio.

FEEDING THE PREMATURE INFANT AT THE BREAST. Large premature infants of 36 weeks of gestation or older may be nursed at the breast if otherwise stable. Particular care should be given to assist the mother in getting the infant to suckle, especially if the breast and/or nipples are large or engorged.[15] Weight should be followed closely to prevent excessive weight loss. In our experience, infants who receive sugar water and formula supplements lose more weight than those who are nursed frequently at the breast without supplementation. If breastfeeding is going well, the infant could be discharged with his mother from the hospital as soon as he begins to gain substantially.

Feeding at the breast when the infant is under 1500 g is considered too strenuous by many neonatologists. When the feeding of 17 infants of less than 1500 g was examined by Pearce and Buchanan,[94] they found the growth of those fed at the breast was comparable to matched control infants fed expressed human milk by bottle. Breastfeeding was started when sucking movements were observed. Twelve babies started at a mean weight of 1324 g and ten were fully breastfed at 1600 g and ready for discharge. Initially they all received supplementary human milk by tube plus 800 units of vitamin D and 60 mg vitamin C daily. The authors attributed their success to unrestricted visiting of parents to the neonatal unit, an optimistic and knowledgeable attitude of the nursing staff toward breastfeeding, and the avoidance of a bottle for the infants. They also

HUMAN MILK FORTIFIER

Four packets (3.8 g) of Enfamil Human Milk Fortifier, the amount usually added to 100 ml of preterm human milk, supply the following:

Calories	14
Protein	0.7 g
Fat	0.04 g
Carbohydrate	2.7 g
Minerals (ash)	0.19 g
Calcium	60 mg
Phosphorus	33 mg
Magnesium	4 mg
Copper	40 mcg
Zinc	0.8 mg
Chloride	17.7 mg
Potassium	15.6 mg
Sodium	7 mg
Moisture	0.17 mg

Additional 60 mosm/kg H_2O gives a total osmolarity of 360 mosm/kg H_2O. Fortifier is made from corn syrup solids, whey protein concentrate, casein, calcium phosphate, potassium citrate, potassium chloride, sodium chloride, magnesium oxide, zinc sulfate, and cupric sulfate. Mead-Johnson & Co., Nutritional Division.

encouraged the expression of milk by the mothers early in the postpartum period. The main deterrent to successful breastfeeding was lack of maternal interest and commitment.

When infants weighing less than 1500 g are fed by nasogastric tube, it has been shown that offering the infant a pacifier to suck while being tube fed improves gastric emptying and weight gain. Those mothers who wish to breastfeed can put the infant to breast at the time of the tube feeding to avoid introduction of a rubber nipple. If there is concern for swallowing and aspiration of fluid, the mother can pump her breasts first and milk can be given by tube. Infants in our unit have suckled at breast while being tube fed without complications.

Small for gestational age infants

Infants who are below the tenth percentile or 2 SD in weight for their gestational age are termed small for gestational age (SGA). These infants may also be shorter in length and have smaller heads, depending on when in the gestational life the insult to their growth occurred. The more general the growth failure, the earlier the intrauterine effect. For example, rubella in the first trimester causes total growth retardation, whereas hypertension in the mother in the third trimester predominantly affects weight.

The more profound the growth retardation, the more difficult the nutritional problems.

SGA infants are prone to be hypocalcemic; however, if they can be provided with adequate breast milk early, this complication may be avoided. Other problems, including hypothermia and hypoglycemia, which lead to a vicious circle of acidosis and associated problems, can be triggered by unmonitored exposure of the infant to thermal stress in the first hours of life and failure to identify the hypoglycemia early. Thus the perinatal nursery staff may appear to be obstructive to breastfeeding when they hover over this infant or even insist on his transfer to the nursery. Initially breastfeeding at delivery is permissible if adequate external heat is provided. Testing with Dextrostix should be performed in the delivery room recovery area and the infant sent to the nursery if hypoglycemia or hypothermia cannot be controlled. Frequent breastfeeding can be initiated unless the blood sugar level is too low (below 30 mg/100 ml or unresponsive to oral treatment). It may not be possible for even an actively lactating multipara to sustain an SGA infant initially, but the infant should be put to breast at least every 3 hours and given IV glucose in addition. SGA infants often have a poor suck and poor coordination with the swallow reflex. There may be considerable mucus with gagging and spitting. A simple lavage of the stomach with a no. 8 feeding tube (or 5, if the infant weighs less than 2600 g) and warmed glucose water usually relieves the gagging. Once this SGA infant begins to eat, he will do well and will require sufficient kilocalories to meet the needs of an infant who is appropriate for gestational age. The mother may need to use a breast pump to stimulate lactation initially.

•   •   •

Infants who are less than 1800 g at birth and have to be gavaged or infants of any weight who are acutely ill present a complex problem. The mother should be instructed to express her milk manually initially and contribute any colostrum she produces. This can be given by gastric or nasojejunal tube. An Egnell pump is effective in helping a mother increase the volume produced. When the infant is born at 1000 g, requires ventilator support for days, and is not discharged for 8 weeks, it is difficult to maintain a large volume of milk by pumping. When the infant is strong enough, he may nurse at the breast while still in the hospital (see Fig. 17-3). When the infant is sent home, the breast milk may be limited in volume or the infant may refuse the breast because he has to work harder to obtain the milk after becoming accustomed to soft premature rubber nipples in the hospital. He becomes frustrated and may even turn away screaming.

A mother reported when seen in the follow-up clinic at the University of Rochester that it took her 4 days to break her premature into breastfeeding and she gave him nothing but the breast during that seige. She thought he might have to starve first! One can see that the reserves of the premature are limited if one studies the absolute and relative body composition of infants at birth (Fig. 14-12). If one considers how long it takes to starve a premature compared to a full-term infant,[63] the risks of starving a premature infant while he adapts to nursing at the breast are real (Fig. 14-13). The

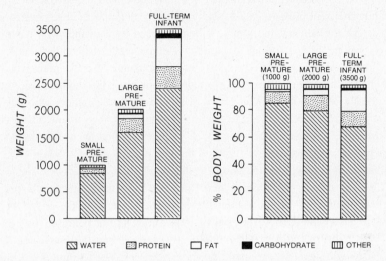

Fig. 14-12. Absolute and relative body composition of infants weighing 1000, 2000, and 3000 g at birth. (Reproduced with permission from Heird, W.C., and Anderson, T.L.: Nutritional requirements and methods of feeding low birth weight infants. In Gluck, L., et al., editors: Current problems in pediatrics, vol. VII, no. 8, Chicago, 1977, Year Book Medical Publishers, Inc., copyright © 1977.)

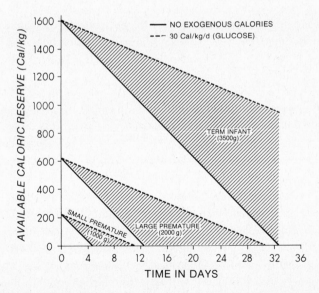

Fig. 14-13. Estimated survival of starved and semistarved infants weighing 1000, 2000, and 3500 g at birth.

solution to the problem is to provide nourishment while the infant stimulates maternal milk production by suckling at the breast. There is equipment called Lact-Aid Nursing Supplementer that will provide this set-up very effectively. It was developed to provide nourishment for the adopted infant that is being nursed by a mother who has not been pregnant or has never lactated and sustains the infant while the mother's milk supply develops. The same effect can be provided for the premature or sick infant who has not nursed at the breast since birth and needs nourishment while the mother's supply develops. Experience to date at the University of Rochester with mothers who have taken home infants 4 to 12 weeks of age to nurse has been good. The infant can continue to gain weight while stimulating the breast. The volume required from the Lact-Aid Nursing Supplementer dropped continually in all but one case so that the infants were on the breast alone after a week. In one case the infant required the Lact-Aid for a month. Chapter 17 gives details of the equipment. Lact-Aid Nursing Supplementer provides a simple means of assuring adequate nourishment while adapting to the breast. It is preferable to using supplemental bottles because the infant is not confused by the rubber nipple, which requires a different mechanism of sucking than the human nipple. Furthermore, the suckling of the human nipple provides continued stimulus for milk production.

POSTMATURE INFANTS

Postmature infants are full-grown mature infants who have stayed in utero beyond the full vigor of the placenta and began to lose weight in utero. They are usually "older looking" and look around wide eyed. Their skin is dry and peeling, and subcutaneous tissue is diminished; thus the skin appears too big. These infants have lost subcutaneous fat and lack glycogen stores. Initially they may be hypoglycemic and require early feedings to maintain blood glucose levels of 45 mg/100 ml or higher. If breastfed, the infant should go to the breast early, giving care to maintain body temperature, which is quite labile. Blood sugar levels should be followed. These infants may feed poorly initially and require considerable prodding to suckle. If the infant becomes hypoglycemic despite careful management, consideration should be given to a feeding of 10% glucose in water. In extreme cases of hypoglycemia an intravenous infusion may be necessary, and management should follow guidelines for any infant who has hypoglycemia that is resistant to routine early feedings. Calcium problems, on the other hand, although common in these infants, generally are uncommon if the infant is adequately breastfed early. This is due to the physiologic ratio of calcium and phosphorus in breast milk. Once a postmature infant begins to feed well, he is apt to catch up quickly and continue to adapt very well. Problems with hyperbilirubinemia are uncommon.

Fetal distress and hypoxia

Infants who have been compromised in utero or during delivery because of insufficient placental reserve, cord accidents, or other causes of intrauterine hypoxia have had very low Apgar scores at birth and need special treatment. An asphyxiated infant cannot be fed for at least 48 hours, and depending on associated findings it may be 96 hours or more. He will have to be maintained on intravenous fluids. If the mother is to breast-feed, her colostrum will be valuable to the infant and will be better tolerated when he can feed by the intestinal tract, which has usually suffered hypoxic damage in these circumstances. The mother will need help initiating lactation and understanding the pathophysiology of the infant's disease. These infants often have a poor suck and do not coordinate with the swallow so that nursing at breast is difficult. The mother may need to hold her breast in place and hold the infant's chin as well. These infants are especially susceptible to nipple confusion, so other means of sustaining nourishment should be sought. Weaning slowly from the intravenous fluids while breastfeeding is introduced is helpful. Using a dropper and using the Lact-Aid Nursing Supplementer are options. These infants may continue to feed poorly for neurologic reasons. They do not do better with a bottle. If the mother is taught to cope with the problem, nursing should progress satisfactorily.

MULTIPLE BIRTHS

It is possible to nurse twins and triplets. There are many case reports to support this fact. That a single mother can provide adequate nourishment for more than one infant has been documented for centuries. In the seventeenth century in France, wet nurses were allowed to nurse up to six infants at one time. Foundling homes provided wet nurses for every three to six infants. The key deterrent to nursing twins is not usually the milk supply, but time. If the mother can nurse both infants simultaneously, the time factor is minimized. Many tricks have been suggested to achieve this feat. As the infants become larger and more active, it may be difficult to keep them simultaneously nursing with only two hands to cope. If the mother has help at home to assist with feedings, it can be accomplished. The first year of life for the mother of a set of twins is an extremely busy one and really requires additional help, particularly if the mother is going to breastfeed. She will need time for adequate rest and nourishment.

Twins

The challenge of breastfeeding twins was investigated by Addy,[2] who reviewed 173 questionnaires returned by mothers who were members of the Mothers of Twins Clubs of Southern California. This is a national organization that offers help and advice to mothers of twins. No other socioeconomic information was available. Forty-one mothers (23.7%) breastfed from birth, although 30% of the infants were premature. Of those who did not breastfeed, 9% were told not to by their doctor, 11% did not think it was possible, and 11% did not think they would have enough milk for two. Of multiparas who had breastfed their first child, an equal number breastfed and bottle fed. Of those mothers who breastfed, 39 breastfed over 1 month and 12 over 6 months.

•   •   •

Mothers have also breastfed triplets, and a mother of quintuplets provided milk for her babies and nursed each of them for some of the feedings for a month!

FULL-TERM INFANTS WITH MEDICAL PROBLEMS

Infants who have self-limited acute illnesses, such as fever, upper respiratory infection, colds, diarrhea, or contagious diseases like chickenpox, do best if breastfeeding is maintained. Because of breast milk's low solute load, an infant can be kept well hydrated despite fever or other increased fluid losses. If respiratory symptoms are significant, an infant seems to nurse well at the breast and poorly with a bottle. This observation has been documented many times when nursing mothers have "roomed-in" with their sick infants in the hospital.[101] The studies of Johnson and Salisbury[71] on the synchrony of respirations in breastfeeding in contrast to the periodic breathing or gasping apnea pattern of the normal bottle fed infant may well be the underlying explanation for the phenomenon of an acutely ill infant continuing to nurse at the breast.

In addition to the appropriateness of the human milk for a sick infant, there is the added comfort of nursing because of the closeness with the mother. If the infant is suddenly weaned, psychologic trauma is added to the stress of the illness.

It may become difficult to distinguish the effect of the trauma of acute weaning from the symptoms of the primary illness, such as poor feeding or lethargy, if the acutely weaned infant fails to respond to adequate treatment. Going back to breastfeeding may be the answer because the stress of acute weaning will be removed.

It is not appropriate to give the mother medicine intended to treat the infant, especially antibiotics. This has been tried to the detriment of the child, since variable amounts of the drug reach the infant, depending on the dose, dosage schedule, and amount of milk consumed.

Gastrointestinal disease

Bouts of diarrhea and intestinal tract disease are much less common in breastfed infants than in bottle fed infants, but when they occur, the infant should be maintained on the breast if possible.[68,69] Human milk is a physiologic solution that causes neither dehydration nor hypernatremia. Occasionally an infant will have diarrhea or an intestinal upset because of something in the mother's diet. It is usually self-limited and the best treatment is to continue to nurse at the breast. If the mother has been taking a laxative that is absorbed or has been eating laxative foods such as fruits in excess, she should adjust her diet. Intractable diarrhea should be evaluated as it would be in any infant. Allergy to mother's milk is extremely rare and would require substantial evidence to support the diagnosis.

Lactase deficiency may be manifested by chronic diarrhea and failure to thrive of a marked degree. Lactose intolerance is a manifestation of a deficiency of lactase, the enzyme that digests lactose, which is in high concentration in human milk. Prematures and infants recovering from severe diarrhea have transient lactose intolerance and very rarely it occurs as an autosomal dominant trait and is more common in males than females. The only treatment is a lactose-free diet, which excludes human milk. Reports of lactose-hydrolyzed human milk are published, suggesting that banked human milk can be treated with lactase (Kerulac), which will hydrolyze the lactose (900 enzyme activity units to 200 ml breast milk degraded 82% of the lactose).[110] In one case the reason for using human milk was that the infant became infection prone when he was weaned from the breast when the initial diagnosis was made. He showed marked improvement with human milk.

Some chronic diseases are better controlled on breast milk, and symptoms become more severe with weaning.[68] Should an infant be weaned and do poorly on formula, relactation of the mother might be considered. With the availability of the Lact-Aid Nursing Supplementer, this possibility is no longer remote (Chapter 17). Childhood celiac disease is disappearing, according to Littlewood and Crollick,[79] which they attribute to increasing incidence of breastfeeding and the decreased use of straight cow's milk. They have seen a reduction in gastroenteritis. The delayed use of gluten in the diet may also be secondarily important. Infants who have been breastfed and had introduction of solids after 4 months have not been seen to have celiac disease. Induced colitis in infants is usually due to some dietary insult, such as exposure to cow's milk.[73,109] It has been reported in breastfed infants, most of whom responded to removal of cow's milk from the maternal diet. Several had been given formula at birth. The symptoms included bloody diarrhea, and sigmoidoscopy revealed focal ulcerations, edema, and increased friability of the intestinal mucosa. On relief of symptoms by dietary change, the intestinal tract biopsy returns to normal.

Botulism

Considerable justifiable concern has been expressed because of the reports of sudden infant death from botulism. Infant botulism is distinguished from food-borne botulism from improperly preserved food containing the toxin and from wound botulism from spores entering a wound. Infant botulism occurs when the spores of *Clostridium botulinum* germinate and multiply in the gut and produce the botulinal toxin in the gastrointestinal tract.[8] The toxin binds presynaptically at the neuromuscular junction, preventing acetylcholine release. The clinical picture is descending, symmetric flaccid paralysis. The gut of only some infants is susceptible, as many infants and adults are exposed. When a previously healthy infant under 6 months of age develops constipation, then weakness, and difficulty sucking, swallowing, crying, or breathing, botulism is a likely diagnosis. The organisms should be looked for in the stools; electromyography may or may not be helpful.

In a group reviewed by Arnon et al.,[9] 33 of 50 patients hospitalized in California were still being nursed at onset of the illness. A beneficial effect of human milk was observed in the difference in the mean age at onset, breastfed infants being twice as old as formula fed infants with the disease, and the breastfed infants' symptoms were milder. Breastfed infants receiving iron supplements developed disease earlier than those who were breastfed but unsupplemented. Of the cases of sudden infant death from botulism, there were no infants who were breastfed within 10 weeks of death. All were receiving iron-fortified formulas. The only known food exposure that has been implicated is honey, in not more than 35% of the world cases. It has been recommended that honey not be given to infants under 12 months of age as a result. This includes putting honey on a mother's nipples to initiate an infant's interest in suckling.

Respiratory illness

Infants who develop respiratory illnesses should be maintained at the breast. The added advantages of antibodies and anti-infective properties are valuable to the infant. A sick infant can nurse more easily than cope with a bottle. Furthermore, the comfort of having his mother nearby is important whenever the infant has a crisis, but weaning during illness may be devastating.

Otitis media in infants occurs less frequently in breastfed infants. Recurrent otitis media is associated with bottle feeding in a study of 237 children in contrast to prolonged breastfeeding, which had a long-term protective effect up to 3 years of age.[102]

Young infants who have older siblings may well be exposed to some virulent viruses and bacteria. Developing croup or chickenpox, for instance, may make the infant seriously ill. Hydration can be maintained by frequent, short breastfeedings. Studies have shown that respirations are maintained more easily when feeding on human milk than on cow's milk. Nursing at the breast permits regular respirations, whereas bottle feeding is associated with a more gasping pattern. Thus breastfed infants continue to nurse when they are ill. If the infant is hospitalized, every effort should be made to maintain the breastfeeding if he can be fed at all. One should provide rooming-in for the mother if a care-by-parent ward is not available. Neutralizing inhibitors to respiratory syncytial virus (RSV) have been demonstrated in the whey of most samples of human milk tested. Clinical studies indicating a relative protection from RSV in breastfed infants were clouded by other factors.[116] The populations were unequal because of socioeconomic factors and smoking (i.e., bottle feeding mothers were in lower socioeconomic groups and smoked more). In general, if breastfed infants become ill, they have less severe illness.

Galactosemia

Galactosemia, which is due to the deficiency of galactose-1-phosphate uridyl transferase, is a rare circumstance in which the infant is unable to metabolize galactose and must be placed on a galactose-free diet. The disease can be rapidly fatal in the severe form. The infant may have severe and/or persistent jaundice, vomiting, diarrhea, electrolyte imbalances, cerebral signs, and weight loss. This does necessitate weaning from the breast to a special formula because human milk contains high levels of lactose, which is a disaccharide that splits into glucose and galactose. The diagnosis is suspected when reducing substances are found in the urine and confirmed by measuring the enzyme uridyl transferase in the red and white blood cells.

Inborn errors of metabolism

Other metabolic deficiency syndromes are usually only apparent as mild failure to thrive syndrome until the infant is weaned from the breast and the symptoms become severe. This particularly applies to inborn errors of metabolism due to an inability to handle one or more of the essential amino acids. Infection is often a complication early in the lives of these infants with inborn errors. In the process of treating the acute infection the infant may be weaned, and the metabolic disorder then becomes apparent precipitously.

An infant in a coma was transferred to the intensive care unit of the University of Rochester Medical Center from another hospital where he had been admitted at 7 weeks of age. He had been entirely well until 3 weeks of age, when he was abruptly weaned from the breast because he developed sepsis and possible meningitis. He became acutely acidotic, then comatose with shock symptoms. On transfer he had a blood ammonia level of 1600 μmol/L. He was ultimately diagnosed postmortem, after heroic efforts to bring the ammonia to normal levels. The disease, propionic acidemia, was incompatible with life, but the parents were able to console themselves in their loss because the child had had a few apparently "healthy, happy weeks" while being breastfed.

If one refers to Table 4-9, it will be observed that there is significantly less of certain amino acids in human milk than in cow's milk, such as phenylalanine, methionine, leucine, isoleucine, and others associated with metabolic disorders. Management of an amino acid metabolic disorder while breastfeeding would depend on careful monitoring of blood and urine levels of the specific amino acids involved. Since these are essential amino acids, a certain amount is necessary in the diet of all infants, including those with the disease. An appropriate combination of breastfeeding and a milk free of the offending amino acid could be developed. The care of such infants should be in consultation with a pediatric endocrinologist. Transient neonatal tyrosinemia, which has been reported to occur in a high percentage (up to 80%) of neonates fed cow's milk, is associated with blood tyrosine levels 10 times those of adults. Wong et al.[121] have associated severe cases with learning disabilities in later years.

The most common of the amino acid metabolic disorders is phenylketonuria (PKU), in which the amino acid accumulates for lack of an enzyme. The treatment has been phenylalanine-free formula, Lofenalac (Mead Johnson, Evansville, Indiana) with added formula to provide a little phenylalanine because every infant needs a small amount. If the infant is breastfed, the mother is usually reluctant to stop. It has been demonstrated in our own hospital and elsewhere that an infant may supplement the Lofenalac with breast milk. With careful monitoring of the blood levels and control of the amount of breastfeeding, a balance can be struck that permits optimal phenylalanine levels and some breastfeeding. The infant will require some Lofenalac to provide enough calories and nutrients. There is a detailed outline of management available called *Guide to Breastfeeding the Infant with PKU* prepared by Ernest, McCabe, Neifert and O'Flynn. It is available from the Superintendent of Documents, U.S. Government Printing Office, Washington, D.C. 20402.[34]

Literature values for phenylalanine range from 29 to 64 mg/100 ml in human milk. The amount for Lofenalac and human milk for a given baby are calculated by weight, age, blood levels, and needs for growth. As an example, a 3-week-old weighing 3.7 kg whose blood level was 52.5 mg/100 ml when he was getting an estimated 570 ml of breast milk would receive 240 ml Lofenalac and 360 ml breast milk (four breastfeedings a day with before and after weighing). The details of every step of management are available in the *Guide* to assist the physician in planning treatment. Since infants with PKU are more prone to thrush infection, the mother should be alerted to watch for symptoms in the infant and the onset of sore nipples that could be due to *Candida albicans*. Treatment is nystatin for mother and baby. The other benefits of human milk make the effort to breastfeed valuable for the infant and for the mother who usually wishes to continue to contribute to her infant's nourishment. The prognosis for intellectual development is excellent if treatment is initiated early and the blood levels maintained at less than 10 mg/100 ml.

Acrodermatitis enteropathica (Danbolt-Closs syndrome)

Acrodermatitis enteropathica is a rare but unique disease in that feeding with human milk may be lifesaving. It is inherited as an autosomal recessive trait. It is characterized by a symmetric rash around the mouth, genitalia, and periphery of the extremities. The rash is an acute vesicobullous and eczematous eruption often secondarily infected with *C. albicans*. It may be seen by the third week of life or not until later in infancy and has been associated with weaning from the breast. Failure to thrive, hair loss, irritability, and chronic severe intractable diarrhea are often life threatening. The disease has been associated with extremely low plasma zinc levels. Oral zinc sulfate has produced remission of the disease.

Human milk contains less zinc than does bovine milk, with zinc concentrations of both decreasing throughout lactation. Eckhert et al.[33] studied the zinc binding in human and cow's milk and noted that the low–molecular weight binding ligand isolated from human milk may enhance absorption of zinc in these patients. Gel chromatography indicated that most of the zinc in cow's milk was associated with high–molecular weight fractions, whereas zinc in human milk was associated with low–molecular weight fractions. The copper/zinc ratio may also be of significance, since the ratio is lower in cow's milk.

The zinc binding ligand from human milk was further identified as prostaglandin E by chromatography, ultrafiltration, and infrared spectroscopy by Evans and Johnson.[35] These patients have low arachidonic acid levels. Arachidonic acid is a precursor of prostaglandin. The efficacy of human milk in the treatment of acrodermatitis enteropathica results from the presence of the zinc-prostaglandin complex.

The clinical significance of the relationship of human milk to onset of the disease and its treatment is in developing lactation in the mother of such an infant, rare as the disease may be. Delayed lactation or relactation is possible and should be offered as an option to the mother of such an infant (Chapter 17).

Several reports of isolated cases of zinc deficiency during breastfeeding have appeared in the literature.[3,4,10,88] In some cases, zinc levels in the milk were low; in others, they were not measured.[123] One child had a classic "zinc-deficient" rash that responded to oral zinc therapy. It is advisable to keep in mind that any deficiency is possible and consider intake deficiency when symptoms occur in the breastfed infant.

Down's syndrome

Infants with Down's syndrome or other trisomies are usually difficult to feed. When they are breastfed, it takes patience on the part of the mother to teach the infant to suck with sufficient vigor to initiate the let-down reflex and to stimulate adequate production of milk. Using manual expression to start flow and holding the breast firmly for the infant so that the nipple does not drop out of the mouth when the infant stops suckling will assist the process.

The birth of an infant with a major genetic abnormality is a shock, even to the strongest parents. If the mother wants to breastfeed, she should be offered all the encouragement and support necessary. Usually she needs to talk with someone just to express her anguish about the infant, not the feeding per se. A sympathetic nurse practitioner can be invaluable in providing the support as well as the expertise necessary to help with the management problems. A number of mothers in the Rochester area and elsewhere have successfully nursed infants with a trisomy.

It is especially important that these infants be breastfed if possible because they are particularly prone to infection. Before the advent of antibiotics, they often died of overwhelming infection and rarely survived past 20 years of age. These infants and most other infants with developmental disorders do better with stimulation and affection, so the body contact and communication while at the breast is especially important. Those who have associated cardiac lesions not only can suckle, swallow, and breathe with less effort at the breast but receive a fluid more physiologic to their needs. Breastfed or bottle fed, these infants gain poorly; thus, switching to a bottle does not solve the problem. The recommendation that the Down's child receive extra vitamins was tested in a controlled study in children 5 to 13 years of age and there was no sustained improvement in the children's appearance, growth, behavior, or development.[18]

Hypothyroidism

It has been reported by Bode et al.[22] that an infant with congenital cretinism was spared the severe effects of the disease because he was breastfed. This was attributed to significant quantities of thyroid hormone in the milk. In a prospective study of 12 cases of hypothyroidism in breastfed infants, Letarte et al.[76] found no protective effect on the disease, nor was the onset of the disease delayed. Anthropometric measurements, biochemical values, and psychologic testing at 1 year of age did not differ from those in the 33 bottle fed hypothyroid infants. Successful diagnosis of congenital hypothyroidism in four breastfed neonates was also reported by Abbassi and Steinour.[1] Sack et al.[103] measured thyroxine (T_4) concentrations in human milk and found it to be present in significant amounts. Varma et al.[118] have reported the study of thyroxine (T_4), triiodothyronine (T_3), and reverse triiodothyroxine (rT_3) concentrations in human milk in 77 healthy euthyroid mothers from the day of delivery to 148 days postpartum. They calculated from their data that if an infant recieved 900 to 1200 ml of milk/day, he would receive 2.1 to 2.6 µg of T_4/day, based on 238.1 ng/100 ml of milk after the first week. This amount of T_4 is much less than the recommended dose for the treatment of hypothyroidism (18.8 to 25 µg/day of levo-triiodothyronine). T_3 in human milk may partially alleviate or mask hyperthyroidism in some infants. T_4 was essentially unmeasurable in the milk sampled. In another study, however, comparing 22 breastfed and 25 formula fed infants who were 2 to 3 weeks old, the levels of T_3 and T_4 were significantly higher in the breastfed infants.[62] No definite relationship between the levels of T_3 and rT_3 could be found. It is therefore suggested that neonatal screening for thyroid disease may be even more urgent if the clinical symptoms are apt to be masked in a breastfed infant. There is no contraindication to breastfeeding when the infant is hypothyroid, and it may well be beneficial. Appropriate therapy should also be instituted.

Adrenal hyperplasia

In an analysis of 32 infants presenting with salt-losing congenital adrenal hyperplasia in adrenal crisis, 8 had been breastfed, 5 had been breastfed with formula supplements, and 19 had been formula fed.[28] Infants who were breastfed were admitted to the hospital later than the formula fed infants, although the breastfed infants had lower serum sodium levels on admission. The breastfed infants did not vomit and remained stable longer, although they all had severe failure to thrive. Weaning initiated vomiting and precipitated crises in the breastfed infants. The authors suggest that congenital adrenal hyperplasia should be considered in failure to thrive in a breastfed infant. Electrolytes should be obtained before weaning to make the diagnosis and avoid precipitating a crisis.[28]

Neonatal breasts and nipple discharge

It is not uncommon for the newborn to have swelling of the breasts for the first few days of life, whether male or female; this is unrelated to being breastfed. If the breast is squeezed, milk can be obtained. This has been called witch's milk. The constituents of neonatal milk were studied by McKiernan and Hull[86] who measured electrolyte, lactose, total protein, and lipid concentrations in the milks of 18 normal newborns and infants with sepsis, adrenal hyperplasia, cystic fibrosis, and meconium ileus. Electrolyte values were similar to those in adult women in all the infants except one with a mastitis, in which the sodium was elevated and the potassium decreased. Total protein and lactose were also similar to those in adult women. The fat was different, increasing with postnatal age and being higher in short-chain fatty acids. It was indeed true milk.

Two infants, one female and one male, were reported to have bilateral bloody discharge from the nipples at 6 weeks of age. Cultures and smears were unrevealing.[19] No biopsy was done. The female infant's swelling and discharge cleared after 5 months; the male's was still present at 10 weeks, when he was lost to follow-up. Galactorrhea or persistent neonatal milk has been reported in association with neonatal hypothyroidism. In another report, a 21-day-old infant female was seen because of a goiter and galactorrhea. The infant had 50% 24-hour ^{131}I uptake and elevated prolactin levels, which slowly responded to Lugol's solution treatment for hypothyroidism.[84]

Hyperbilirubinemia and jaundice

Jaundice in the newborn has become a source of considerable misinformation, confusion, and anxiety in recent years. There is a higher incidence of jaundice in full-term infants than a decade ago. More physicians are paying attention to the development of hyperbilirubinemia in newborns. These two factors serve to increase the frequency of the question of the role of breastfeeding in the development of hyperbilirubinemia. Some of the confusion and inconsistencies associated with the management can be attributed to the indecisive terminology. An attempt will be made to clarify the issues and outline the causes and effects of hyperbilirubinemia.

WHY THE CONCERN ABOUT JAUNDICE. Bilirubin is a cell toxin, as can be demonstrated dramatically by adding a little bilirubin to a tissue culture, which will be quickly destroyed. Excessive bilirubin causes concern because when there is free, unbound, unconjugated bilirubin in the system it can be deposited in various tissues, ultimately causing necrosis of the cells. The brain and brain cells, if destroyed by bilirubin deposits, do not regenerate. The full-blown end result is bilirubin encephalopathy or kernicterus, which is essentially a pathologic diagnosis that depends on identifying the yellow pigmentation and necrosis in the brain, especially the basal ganglion, hippocampal cortex, and subthalamic nuclei. About 50% of the infants with kernicterus at autopsy also have other lesions due to bilirubin toxicity. There may be necrosis of the renal tubular cells, intestinal mucosa, or pancreatic cells or associated gastrointestinal hemorrhage. The classic clinical manifestations of bilirubin encephalopathy are characterized by progressive lethargy, rigidity, opisthotonos, high-pitched cry, fever, and convulsions. The mortality rate is 50%. Survivors usually have choreoathetoid cerebral palsy, high-frequency deafness, and mental retardation. Premature infants are particularly susceptible to bilirubin-related brain damage and may have kernicterus at autopsy without the typical clinical syndrome. Classic full-blown kernicterus rarely occurs today, but what may well develop are mild effects on the brain that will be manifested clinically in later life as incoordination, hypertonicity, and mental retardation or perhaps learning disabilities, symptoms sometimes collectively called minimal brain damage.

MECHANISM OF BILIRUBIN PRODUCTION IN THE NEONATE. The normal full-term infant has a hematocrit in utero of 50% to 65%. Because of the low oxygen tension delivered to the fetus via the placenta, the fetus requires more hemoglobin to carry the oxygen. As soon as the infant is born and begins to breathe room air, the need is gone. The infant bone marrow does not make more cells, and excess cells are destroyed and not replaced. The life span of a fetal red blood cell is 70 to 90 days instead of the adult's 120 days. Normally when red cells are destroyed, the released hemoglobin is broken down to heme in the reticuloendothelial system (RES). The reticuloendothelial cells contain a microsomal enzyme, heme oxygenase, which is capable of oxidizing the alpha-methene bridge carbon of the heme molecule after the loss of the iron and the globin to form biliverdin, a green pigment, according to Gartner and Lee.[48] Biliverdin is water soluble and is rapidly degraded to bilirubin. A gram of hemoglobulin will produce 34 mg of bilirubin.

The reticuloendothelial cell releases the bilirubin into the circulation, where it is rapidly bound to albumin. Bilirubin is essentially insoluble (less than 0.01 mg/100 ml soluble). Adult albumin can bind two molecules of bilirubin, the first more tightly than the second. Newborn albumin has reduced molar binding capacities.

Unconjugated bilirubin is removed from the circulation by the hepatocyte, which converts it by conjugation of each molecule of bilirubin with two molecules of glucuronic acid into direct bilirubin. Direct bilirubin is water soluble and is excreted via the bile to the stools. The balance between hepatic cell uptake of bilirubin and the rate of bilirubin production determines the serum unconjugated bilirubin concentration.

EVALUATION AND MANAGEMENT. Normal full-term newborns have serial bilirubin tests to determine the range of values. Many have observed that the cord bilirubin level may be as high as 2.0 mg/100 ml and rise over the first 72 hours to 5 to 6 mg/100 ml, which is barely in the visible range, and gradually tapers off, assuming adult levels of 1.0 mg/100 ml after 10 days. Fewer than 50% of normal infants are visibly jaundiced in the first week of life. Why any normal infant is visibly jaundiced is not known, although it has been suggested by Gartner and Lee[48] that it is due to insufficient enzyme synthesis, inhibition of enzymatic activity by naturally occurring substances, deficient synthesis of the glucuronide donor UDPGA, or a combination of factors. This would suggest the jaundice is idiopathic, not physiologic. The acceptable level of bilirubin depends on a number of factors. In some premature infants, even bilirubin levels under 10 mg/100 ml may be of concern.

Factors that influence significance. For a given level of bilirubin, several associated factors may need to be considered. If there has been acidosis, anoxia, asphyxia, hypothermia, hypoglycemia, or infection, even lower levels of bilirubin may have a significant risk of causing deposition in the brain cells. These factors increase the susceptibility of the brain to bilirubin deposition: prematurity, asphyxia, hypoxia, hypoglycemia, hypothermia, acidosis, and infection. There is an increased incidence of elevated bilirubin levels in certain races and populations. Asian populations, including Chinese, Japanese, and Korean, and American Indians may have bilirubin levels averaging between 10 and 14 mg/100 ml. There is also a higher incidence of autopsy-identified kernicterus. It does not seem to be related to G6PD deficiency, which is also common in these groups.

Determination of cause of jaundice. If one follows the chain of events from the red cell and its destruction in the newborn through to the final excretion of conjugated bilirubin in the stools, it simplifies understanding the cause of a specific case of jaundice. Causes include (1) increased destruction of red cells, (2) decreased conjugation in the glucuronidase system, (3) decreased albumin binding, and (4) increased reabsorption from the gastrointestinal tract. Conditions associated with increased destruction of red cells can be outlined as follows:

   I. Isoimmunization
      A. Rh incompatibility
      B. ABO incompatibility
      C. Subgroup and private antigen incompatibility
  II. Elevated hematocrit levels
      A. Chronic intrauterine hypoxia
      B. Maternal smoking
      C. Twin-to-twin transfusion
      D. Intrauterine growth failure
      E. Cord stripping
 III. Sequestered blood
      A. Cephalohematomas, scalp hemorrhage, subdural hematomas
      B. Ecchymoses, especially in breech delivery
      C. Extensive hemangiomas
  IV. Red cell defects
      A. G6PD deficiency
      B. Pyruvate kinase deficiency
      C. Hexokinase deficiency
      D. Congenital erythropoietic porphyria
   V. Structural abnormalities of red cells
      A. Hereditary spherocytosis
      B. Hereditary elliptocytosis
      C. Pyknocytosis
  VI. Infection
      A. Bacterial (sepsis, meningitis)
      B. Viral (cytomegalovirus)
      C. Protozoal (toxoplasmosis)

Causes of decreased conjugation of bilirubin in the hepatic cells are as follows:

  I. Inherited defects
    A. Glucuronyltransferase deficiency, type I (Crigler-Najjar syndrome)
    B. Gilbert's syndrome
    C. Glucuronyltransferase deficiency, type II
  II. Transient familial neonatal hyperbilirubinemia
  III. Drugs that compete in the conjugation system (such as vitamin K and novobiocin)
  IV. Prematurity (and therefore prematurity of the liver and its enzyme systems)
  V. Breast-milk jaundice

When albumin binding is altered, the visibility of the jaundice is not affected. The bilirubin level may not be very high, but the substance is not bound to albumin and is available at lower levels to pass into the brain cells. Premature infants have much lower albumin levels and thus have fewer binding sites. Drugs that also bind to albumin compete for binding sites. These drugs include aspirin and sulfadiazine, for instance. A lower level of bilirubin puts the infant who has these medications in his system at risk because the bilirubin is unbound and available to enter tissue cells, including brain cells.

Reabsorption from the gastrointestinal tract can increase the bilirubin level. This occurs when the conjugated bilirubin that was excreted into the colon is unconjugated by the action of intestinal bacteria and reabsorbed, which happens when stools are decreased or slowed in passage. Poor feedings, pyloric stenosis, and other forms of intestinal obstruction are common causes. Some bacteria are more apt than others to have this effect on conjugated bilirubin.

Safe levels of bilirubin. Safe levels of bilirubin depend on a number of factors noted previously, including acidosis, hypoxia or anoxia, and sepsis. A handy rule of thumb is the correlation of birth weight in the premature infant and the indirect bilirubin level, using a value 2 to 3 mg lower when the infant has multiple problems (Table 14-6).

Any value of 20 mg/100 ml or over warrants treatment. Phototherapy is generally used when the bilirubin is roughly 5 mg/ml below the exchange level. Jaundice that is visible under 24 hours of age is of special concern because it is usually associated with an incompatibility or infection. Rapidly rising bilirubin levels are also of concern, and a 0.5 mg/100 ml rise/hour is also an indication for treatment, usually an exchange transfusion.

Table 14-6. Correlation of weight to safe peak indirect bilirubin levels

Weight (g)	Indirect bilirubin level (mg/100 ml)
2500	20
2000	20
1500	15
1200	12
1100	11
1000	10

Treatment. Treatment depends on identifying the cause. Blood incompatibilities should be treated by exchange transfusion if severe enough (i.e., bilirubin 20 mg/100 ml or rising at 0.5 mg/100 ml/hour or dropping hematocrit). The exchange transfusion removes affected red blood cells (RBC) and antibodies and improves excessive bilirubin levels. If the cause is sepsis, the infection should be treated as well as the bilirubin problem. About half the cases of jaundice will not have an identified cause and may be classified as idiopathic rather than physiologic jaundice. Refer to standard texts of pediatrics and neonatology for more extensive discussions of neonatal hyperbilirubinemia.

BREAST-MILK JAUNDICE. A small group of infants estimated by Gartner and Lee[48] to be less than 1 in 200 breastfed infants will develop jaundice directly associated with breast milk. Drew[32] reported only one case of proven breast-milk jaundice in a review of 13,102 consecutively born infants; 878 (6.7%) of these infants had pathologic jaundice.

The pattern of this jaundice is distinctly different. Normally idiopathic jaundice peaks on the third day and then begins to drop. Breast-milk jaundice, however, becomes apparent or continues to rise after the third day, and bilirubin levels may peak any time from the seventh to the tenth day, with untreated cases being reported to peak as late as the fifteenth day. Values have ranged from 10 to 27 mg/100 ml during this time. There is no correlation with weight loss or gain, and stools are normal.

The syndrome of breast-milk jaundice had been attributed by Arias et al.[6,7] to a substance in the milk of some mothers that inhibits the hepatic enzyme glucuronyltransferase, preventing the conjugation of bilirubin. The substance has been identified as 5β-pregnane-3α,20β-diol, a breakdown product of progesterone and an isomer of pregnanediol that is not usually found in milk but occurs normally in about 10% of the lactating population. It has no other known significance, and these females are not discernible in any other way.

Arias and Gartner[6] administered 5β-pregnane-3α,20β-diol to full-term newborns and produced unconjugated hyperbilirubinemia that subsided as soon as the material was discontinued. Older infants and an adult given the same material did not become jaundiced.[122] It did demonstrate that unconjugated hyperbilirubinemia can be produced in very young full-term infants by oral doses of 5β-pregnane-3α,20β-diol in amounts equivalent to that isolated from inhibitory human milk. Although this material had also been isolated from the milk and serum of mothers whose infants were jaundiced, this work has not been duplicated. Foliot et al.,[37] on the other hand, showed that pathologic breast milk from mothers of jaundiced infants will inhibit bromsulphalein (BSP)-Z protein binding only when stored under conditions that also cause the appearance of the capacity to inhibit bilirubin conjugation in vitro, as well as cause the liberation of nonesterified fatty acids. They conclude that the appearance of this inhibitory capacity in vitro seems linked to the lipolytic activity peculiar to pathologic milks.

It has been reported by Luzeau et al.[82,83] that milks with inhibitory activity contain increased concentrations of free fatty acids. These simple forms of fat are presumed to be derived by the enzymatic breakdown of the triglycerides normally present in milk, suggesting a greater lipase activity. Some type of synergistic effect between pregnanediol and free fatty acids may be responsible for the clinical syndrome of breast-milk jaundice.

As research continues, there is evidence to suggest that excessive jaundice in the neonate is associated with inadequate caloric intake in the first week of life akin to starvation in the laboratory animal. It is probably not a single-cause mechanism, however, according to Gartner,[46] who further makes a distinction between late-onset breast-milk jaundice and early-onset breastfeeding-related jaundice. Late-onset breast-milk jaundice is rare but persistent, will usually occur in all breastfed siblings, and may last for weeks or months. This type may be related to maternal milk lipase. Early-onset breastfeeding-related jaundice, which Gartner associates with relative starvation in early lactation, is usually aggravated by hospital policies that interfere with the establishment of lactation. Treatment should focus on increasing feeds by increasing milk production.

Diagnosis depends on circumstantial evidence, since there is no easy rapid laboratory test. All other causes, including infection, should be ruled out in the usual manner and a thorough history taken, including medications and family history. If the mother has nursed other infants, were they jaundiced? Usually 70% of the previous children of a given mother whose infant has breast-milk jaundice have been jaundiced. The difference may be related to the greater maturity of the liver of a given infant who then is able to handle the increased demands on the glucuronyltransferase system. If the mother had a previous infant who was jaundiced but bottle fed, this should raise a question about the diagnosis of breast-milk jaundice. To establish the diagnosis firmly, and this is necessary when the bilirubin level is above 15 mg/100 ml for more than 24 hours, a bilirubin reading should be obtained 2 hours after a breastfeeding and then breastfeeding discontinued for at least 12 hours.[47] The infant must be fed fluids and calories, preferably a 60:40 lactalbumin/casein milk. In some cases, a mother of a nonjaundiced infant is available to nurse the child or provide breast milk. The infant's mother should be assisted in pumping her breasts to maintain her supply. Even more urgent is providing the mother with a sympathetic explanation of the problem and the process. After at least 12 hours without mother's milk, the bilirubin level should be measured. If there is a significant drop of more than 2 mg/100 ml, then the infant can be put to the breast. Bilirubin levels should be obtained to determine if the bilirubin rises again and, if so, how much. In most cases, in the time not breastfeeding the infant's body equilibrates the levels sufficiently, so there is only a slight increase in bilirubin on return to breastfeeding followed by a slow but steady drop. If that is the case, breastfeeding can continue. The bilirubin level should be checked at 10 days and 14 days to be certain the bilirubin is truly clearing.

If the bilirubin has not dropped significantly after 12 hours off the breast, the time off the breast should be extended to 18 to 24 hours, measuring bilirubin levels every 4 to 6 hours. If the bilirubin rises while the infant is off the breast, the cause of jaundice is clearly not the breast milk; breastfeeding should be resumed and other causes for the jaundice be reevaluated.

Phototherapy and breast-milk jaundice.   Phototherapy is the use of light energy from a fluorescent light source, which provides light in the white to blue range of the photo spectrum. Fluorescent lamps (20W), daylight, cool white, or blue, are usually used and provide 420 to 500 nm. A fluorescent bulb provides this light energy for only about 400 hours of its usual 14,000-hour life. Standard lamps are available for use with Plexiglas screens to filter out the small amount of ultraviolet light and protect the infant should the bulb break. They should be at least 16 inches (40 cm) from the unclothed infant. Phototherapy can destroy the retina in 12 hours; thus protecting the eyes with opaque eye covers is mandatory. Lights should be turned off to collect blood samples. The infant should be fed with the lights and eye covers off to provide a cycle of light and dark for the establishment of normal circadian rhythms. For discussion of the ''bronze baby'' syndrome, congenital erythropoietic porphyria, and other complications of phototherapy, refer to standard neonatology texts.

If one is attempting to establish the diagnosis of breast-milk jaundice, phototherapy should not be used while breast milk is being discontinued. If establishing the diagnosis is not necessary (perhaps because of the same diagnosis in older siblings), phototherapy can be used to bring the values to a more acceptable range, that is, under 12 mg/100 ml. When phototherapy is discontinued, it is more important to establish that there is no rebound hyperbilirubinemia. In addition, it will be important to follow the infant at home after discharge through at least 14 days of life, or longer if the values are not below 12 mg/100 ml. It should not be assumed that the diagnosis is breast-milk jaundice when breastfeeding has been stopped and phototherapy initiated simultaneously.

Late diagnosis of breast-milk jaundice.   With the frequency of early discharge from the hospital, especially for families enjoying the birthing center concept, breastfed infants are often discharged before jaundice for any reason has developed. Since breast-milk jaundice is apt to be delayed to the fourth or fifth day, peaking at 10 to 14 days of age, most normal infants are already home. Occasionally an infant is observed in the pediatrician's office at 10 days of age or older with a bilirubin level over 20 mg/100 ml, often 23 to 25 mg/100 ml (highest, 27 mg/100 ml). This is a medical emergency. It necessitates the admission of this infant to the hospital for a complete bilirubin workup. It is important to recognize that other causes of hyperbilirubinemia must be ruled out, including blood type incompatibilities. At this age it is also necessary to rule out biliary obstruction and hepatitis, which might have a high direct or conjugated bilirubin level. There is conflicting opinion as to whether it is appropriate to perform an immediate exchange transfusion or to discontinue breast milk and use phototherapy for 4 to 6 hours to establish whether this therapy will be effective in dropping the level sufficiently. It has been our approach to stop breastfeeding and start phototherapy immediately on admission while the diagnostic workup is being performed. (The bilirubin level should be obtained first, but the result need not be reported before initiating therapy if the infant is 7 days or older as long as an exchange transfusion for a blood type incompatibility is not omitted because of the temporary effect of phototherapy.) It usually takes about 4 hours to do the diagnostic workup and prepare compatible blood for an exchange transfusion, thus no time is actually lost. Only in one family have we had to do an exchange transfusion in what appeared to be a "breast-milk jaundice" infant; all three siblings required treatment.

Persistent jaundice in the breastfed infant. It has been acknowledged that breast-milk jaundice is extremely rare but in that rare case, the infant will be observed to maintain a bilirubin level over 12 mg/100 ml if breastfed. Pediatricians[54] in Rochester have reported that this persists beyond 6 weeks of age and is altered only by giving one or two feedings of formula a day to dilute the effect of the breast milk or by discontinuing breastfeeding altogether. There are no prospective studies of a 7-year long-range nature to confirm that this is a benign condition. It has been the policy to give enough formula feeding to keep the bilirubin level under 12 mg/100 ml (preferably 10 mg/100 ml), which is actually arbitrarily selected. Occasionally levels will hover at 15 mg/100 ml or higher with some formula feeding, at which point breastfeeding is discontinued (two cases in 5 years). An exchange transfusion might be an alternative to drop the bilirubin significantly and continue breastfeeding. The physician needs to weigh the advantages and risks with the family and document the final care plan. Rechecking the direct bilirubin level and the color of the urine and stools to rule out hepatitis and biliary obstruction is also appropriate. Phenobarbital has not been effective in the postnatal period.

BREASTFEEDING AND HYPERBILIRUBINEMIA. Not all breastfed infants who are jaundiced have breast-milk jaundice. When the bilirubin curves of bottle fed and breastfed infants are compared, it should be observed that the bilirubin levels are the same in the first 3 days of life. It has been suggested that the breastfed infant is dehydrated and that is why the bilirubin is elevated, but the hematocrit, urine volume, and urine specific gravity are within normal range. In a study by Dahms et al.[29] of 199 breastfed and bottle fed infants followed for the first 4 days of life, the mean bilirubin values were found to be similar, regardless of the feeding regimen. They observed an 8% mean weight loss in infants breastfed without supplements compared to a 4% weight loss in all other infants. Hyperbilirubinemia was not related to weight loss. The percentage of infants having serum bilirubin concentrations greater than 15 mg/100 ml was the same for both breastfed and bottle fed infants. The hematocrit was stable for any given infant even when the weight changed significantly. The reticulocyte count was between 7% and 8% at 48 hours.

The researchers concluded that breastfeeding per se is not associated with hyperbilirubinemia. Previous literature has been divided on this point, but no series of statistics shows a clear-cut difference. This study points out that the demand feeding group of breastfed infants lost more weight than controls and 12% of the group developed low-grade fever that responded to feeding of water or formula. Fever, however, was not associated with hyperbilirubinemia. A retrospective study of 200 infants in Rochester who were chart screened for weight loss, intake, bilirubin, and body temperature showed that breastfed infants who were supplemented with water did less well, lost more weight than those who were not supplemented, and had more problems nursing beyond 4 days of life.

Full-term breastfed infants who were receiving water or dextrose supplements had higher serum bilirubin levels on the sixth day of life than bottle fed babies in a study by Nicoll et al.[92] Supplementation with water or dextrose did not reduce hyperbilirubinemia that had developed. When the number of feedings at the breast in the first 3 days of life was related to bilirubin levels, DeCarvalho et al.[31] were able to display a significant relationship. The greater the number of breastfeedings, the lower the bilirubin. These authors also found that water and dextrose supplements were associated with higher bilirubin levels.

INFANTS WITH PROBLEMS REQUIRING SURGERY
The immediate neonatal period

FIRST ARCH DISORDERS.   Feeding of any sort may be greatly hindered by abnormalities of the jaw, nose, and mouth. A receding chin may be a minor problem and require only positioning the jaw forward. A mother can hook the angle of the jaw with her finger and draw it forward. If the tongue is too large for the jaw, the infant will actually nurse better at the breast than at the bottle because the human nipple fits into the mouth with less bulk. Infants with first arch abnormalities usually require considerable help in feeding. A cleft palate may also be present. It may be necessary to insert semipermanent nasal tubes so that the infant can be fed orally until he is older; definitive surgery may be necessary later. Once the nasal tubes are in place the infant can manage at the breast. Feeding by any technique, however, is never easy.

CLEFT LIP.   A solitary cleft lip is usually repaired in the first few weeks of life. Prior to surgery the infant will need some help, but he can nurse at the breast if a seal around the areola can be developed. Actually the breast may fill the defect, and suckling will go well. It is important to encourage the infant to suck to strengthen the tongue and jaw muscles. If all else fails, a breast shield can be tried, affixing a special cleft lip nipple to the shield.

The mother may have to express or pump milk and offer it by dropper or other means if sucking is ineffective. The pediatrician, plastic surgeon, and parents should work together as a team from the time of birth to determine a coordinated plan of treatment.[91] Some surgeons have special protocols before and after surgery to assure optimal healing. It is important to make all plans for feeding around the surgical plan. There are reports in the literature of individual mothers' experiences nursing infants with lip defects. The major caution in sharing these experiences is to consider that the supportive surgical approach may differ from those reported in the cases in the literature.[64]

CLEFT PALATE.   The prognosis for successful feeding of an infant with a cleft palate depends on the size and position of the defect (soft palate, hard palate) as well as the associated lesions. Lubit[80] recommends the application of an orthopedic appliance to the neonatal maxilla to close the gap, thus aiding nursing, stimulating orofacial development, developing the palatal shelves, preventing tongue distortions, preventing nasal septum irritation, and decreasing the number of ear infections. This will aid the plastic surgeon and help the mother psychologically as well. Lubit further relates that a cleft involving the secondary palate can interfere with normal nursing. For the infant to suckle, the nose must be sealed off from the mouth, creating a negative pressure in the oral cavity. The milk may also run out the nose. The absence of the palatal tissue can prevent expulsion of milk from the nipple. The orthopedic appliance prosthetically restores the anatomy of the palate, permitting normal suckling.

Since the purpose of the negative pressure in the mouth is to hold the nipple and areola in place and not to extract milk from the breast, a seal is needed to keep the pressure. One mother was able to perform the positioning task by holding the breast to her infant's mouth firmly between two fingers, as in Fig. 8-10.[119] The infant was then able to milk the areola and nipple with the tongue pressing it against the roof of the mouth, even with the cleft. The breast had to be held in position much as a bottle would be held throughout the feeding.[52,53]

It has been noted in this chapter that breastfed infants have fewer bouts with otitis media, which has been attributed to the position of the infant while feeding at the breast as well as the anti-infective properties of the milk. It is certainly an important consideration in infants with cleft palates, who have been identified as having more ear infections in general than other infants.

Children with cleft palates may also fail to thrive, not only as a function of their feeding difficulty but also because there may be an underlying increased metabolic need. In a study of 37 children with cleft palates and no other anomalies it was seen that the median birth weight was at the thirtieth percentile.[16] By 1 to 2 months, weights had dropped to the twentieth percentile and did not recover to the thirtieth until 6 months.

Feeding infants with oral defects requires extra effort.[17] Each infant is slightly different. Usually mothers learn to feed their own infants more effectively, even when bottle feeding, than the skilled professional can. This amplifies the fact that it requires a special patience and knack. Breastfeeding can be successful. Infants with cleft lip or palate should be managed as normal infants. They should be brought to the mother to feed and for rooming-in, as with any infant. Reinforcing the fact that the infant is normal and merely needs some reconstructive surgery is important in helping the parents adjust. Here parent-to-parent programs are most helpful.

INTESTINAL TRACT DISORDERS. Infants with anomalies of the gastrointestinal tract that cause obstruction develop symptoms that depend on the location of the problem in the intestinal tract.

Tracheoesophageal fistula. Tracheoesophageal (T-E) fistula is apparent early and, depending on the exact anatomy of the lesions, shows respiratory symptoms and signs of obstruction. This is a surgical emergency. If no feedings have been given or no milk has been aspirated, surgery can be done as soon as possible. If pneumonia intervenes, the course is protracted and the infant may have to be maintained on peripheral venous alimentation until surgery can be done and healing takes place.

A mother who wishes to breastfeed an infant with a T-E fistula can manually express milk or pump, saving all samples in the freezer until the infant can take oral milk feedings. If the infant has a gastrostomy tube in place, small feedings may be started fairly early postoperatively, and human milk is ideal if available because of its easy digestibility and anti-infective properties. If there is initially a need to partially supplement the milk with intravenous fluids, the fluids can be calculated to make up the difference between needs and nutrients supplied by breast milk taken by tube. As nutrition progresses, if supply does not keep up with requirements, feedings can be supplemented with other nutrients. When ready for oral feedings, a full-term or large premature infant can nurse at the breast. Unless the mother is able to spend most of the day and night at the hospital, the infant will have to receive bottle feedings as well. If the mother has been able to store up enough milk, the infant may be able to fulfill his needs from breast milk. Once the infant is discharged and begins to nurse at the breast every feeding for a few days, the supply will increase immediately. If there is concern for nutritional lag between needs and production, the Lact-Aid device can be used briefly to stimulate the breast without starving and exhausting the infant (Chapter 17).

Pyloric stenosis. Pyloric stenosis occurs in about 2 to 5/1000 live births. There is a family tendency, but the disease is more common in first-born males. Usually it occurs between the second and sixth weeks of life, although it can occur anytime after birth. Vomiting is characteristic. It is intermittent at first and progresses to include every feeding and is often projectile. These infants are eager feeders and go back for more milk until the weight loss and dehydration make them anxious and irritable. In the investigation of vomiting, it is important to keep in mind that overfeeding can cause spitting and vomiting, even projectile vomiting, but it is not associated with weight loss, decreased urine and stools, and dehydration. Therapy consists of pyloromyotomy following correction of the dehydration and associated electrolyte abnormalities. If the procedure is uncomplicated, the infant can go back to the breast in 6 to 8 hours after a trial of water at 4 hours shows the infant is alert and sucking well. The breastfed infant may be discharged in 24 hours if nursing has gone well. If the duodenum is entered at the time of surgery, gastric decompression and intravenous fluids will be necessary and oral feeding delayed several days until signs of healing occur. A breastfed infant may resume nursing earlier than a bottle fed infant returns to formula because of the rapid emptying time of the stomach and the zero curd tension of the milk.

Disorders of the small intestine. Disorders of the small intestine, including duodenal obstruction, malrotation, jejunoileal obstruction, and duplications, require surgery. Depending on the extent of the lesion, whether or not the bowel wall is opened, whether bowel segments are removed, and whether there are associated lesions such as annular pancreas, the infant will need postoperative maintenance on intravenous fluids and possibly alimentation. The mother who wishes to breastfeed may or may not have ever nursed the infant, depending on the time of onset of symptoms and their severity. The mother should be counseled about the prognosis and encouraged to manually express and pump if it appears feasible for her to breastfeed eventually. The decision should be made among the parents, surgeon, neonatologist, and pediatrician. Frequently infants with atresias are also small or premature.

Disorders of the colon.   Disorders of the colon occur more commonly in full-term infants. Hirschsprung's disease or congenital aganglionic megacolon is the most common lesion. There is usually delayed passage of meconium; however, only 10% to 15% of all children with delayed passage of meconium have Hirschsprung's disease. Constipation and abdominal distention are the most frequent initial symptoms. They may begin during the first few days of life and gradually progress to include bilious vomiting. The clinical picture may be indistinguishable from meconium ileus, ileal atresia, or large bowel obstruction. In any infant with perforation of the colon, ileum, or appendix, Hirschsprung's disease should be considered. The breastfed infant may have milder symptoms and delayed onset of real stress because the breast milk stools are normally loose and seedy and easily passed. The pH and flora of the intestinal tract are also different, leading to less distention. Enterocolitis may occur at any age and is the major cause of death. No data have been located to distinguish the incidence of this complication in breastfed and bottle fed infants, although an argument could be mounted regarding the projected value of sIgA and intestinal flora of the breastfed infant. The treatment depends on the symptoms, x-ray findings, and results of biopsy for the identification of the aganglionic segment. Usually colostomy is done at the time of diagnosis and definitive surgery is done later in the first year of life. Feedings can be resumed as soon as the infant is stable, after the colostomy has healed sufficiently to permit bowel activity. Human milk has the same advantages for early postoperative feeding in this disease as well because of its anti-infective properties and easy digestibility.

Meconium plug syndrome and meconium ileus.   Meconium plug syndrome and meconium ileus are less common and less severe in breastfed infants who have received a full measure of colostrum. Colostrum has a cathartic effect and stimulates the passage of meconium. Should either disorder be diagnosed, the infant should continue to nurse in addition to any other treatment.

Necrotizing enterocolitis.   Although necrotizing enterocolitis (NEC) has been known of for 100 years, it has only been since 1960 that it has been identified with any frequency, which suggests an iatrogenic component. It is most common in premature infants and infants compromised by asphyxia. It has been associated with umbilical catheters, exchange transfusions, polycythemia, hyperosmolar feedings, and infection. Its cause is not clear. Work with animals has suggested that human breast milk, specifically colostrum, provides protection against the disease. A good control study to evaluate this in human infants has not been reported. A "dose or two" of human milk may not be enough. There are cases of NEC reported that have occurred so early in life that no feedings were given. Present regimens of treatment call for cessation of all oral feedings and use of oral and systemic gentamicin, gastric decompression, plasma or blood transfusions, and rigorous monitoring for progression or perforation with serial x-ray studies as well as a septic workup. Further study is necessary to determine cause and possible prevention and the role colostrum or breast milk might play.

The organisms generally associated with NEC are gram-negative organisms such as *Bacteroides, E. coli,* and especially *Klebsiella.* Brown et al.[24] reported that 89% of the infants with NEC had received cow's milk formulas and that gram-negative bacteria and endotoxins were present in the stool. Colonization of breastfed infants with *Klebsiella* does not occur, and *Lactobacillus bifidus* predominates, according to Mata and Urrutia.[85] The uncommon occurrence of NEC in Helsinki, at the University of Helsinki Children's Hospital intensive care nursery, is remarkable. Jelliffe and Jelliffe[70] report that all the premature infants are routinely fed with colostrum and breast milk in Helsinki.

Imperforate anus. Defects in the rectum and anal sphincter are usually diagnosed in the first few hours on physical examination or because a rectal thermometer cannot be passed. When the blind pouch is more generous, diagnosis may depend on the evaluation of failure to stool. Depending on associated lesions and fistulas to bladder or vagina, the surgical decompression can be performed. Until this time, oral feedings are withheld. High lesions require an immediate colostomy with later final repair, whereas low lesions may be repaired at the primary procedure through a perineal approach. Infants may be breastfed as soon as any bowel activity can be permitted, often 2 to 3 days postoperatively.

Gastrointestinal bleeding. The most common cause of vomiting blood or passing blood via the rectum in a breastfed infant is a bleeding nipple in the mother, which may or may not be painful. Any time fresh blood is found in the vomitus or stool of any newborn, the blood should be tested for adult or fetal hemoglobin. If it is adult hemoglobin, it indicates the source is maternal. This is done by a qualitative test, the Apt test. (Mix blood with 2 to 3 ml normal saline solution, add 2 to 3 ml of 10% NaOH [0.25M]. Mix gently. Observe for color change. Fetal hemoglobin is stable in alkali and will remain pink, whereas adult hemoglobin turns brown. Use a known adult sample as a color control.) If the blood is adult hemoglobin in a breastfed infant, the possibility of a cracked and bleeding nipple should be ruled out by inspection of the maternal breast (see Chapter 8).

If the blood is fetal hemoglobin, the differential diagnosis for bleeding in any neonate should be followed. Breastfeeding can be maintained meanwhile, unless a lesion requiring surgery is identified. More than 50% of the cases of gastrointestinal bleeding in the neonate go undiagnosed. Anorectal fissure is uncommon as a cause in breastfed infants. Allergy to human milk is unreported as a cause of intestinal bleeding. The distribution of causes of intestinal bleeding in the neonate, without selection for type of feeding are idiopathic, 50%; hemorrhagic disorders, 20%; swallowed maternal blood, 10%; anorectal fissures, 10%; intestinal ischemia, 5%; and colitis, 5%.

MALFORMATIONS OF THE CENTRAL NERVOUS SYSTEM.   Malformations of the central nervous system (CNS) that are diagnosed at birth include the clinical spectrum from anencephaly and complete craniorachischisis to dermal sinuses. Defects of the spinal column run from complete spinal rachischisis to spina bifida occulta. Those that are incompatible with life or are inoperable present the additional problem to the mother who had planned to breastfeed of coping with her desire to nurse her infant. If the infant is to be given normal newborn care and the mother desires to nurse this infant, breastfeeding should be discussed by the pediatrician and parents together. It has been well demonstrated that parents grieve more physiologically if they have contact with their abnormal infants, but their imaginations are more vicious than some abnormalities of development. The professional's personal bias as to how to deal with this infant should not overshadow the discussion with the parents. If the mother chooses to nurse the infant who has no life expectancy and the infant is to be fed at all by mouth, she should have that choice.

Infants with CNS abnormalities requiring surgery can be breastfed until the operation and postoperatively as soon as oral intake is permitted. In these cases in which the gastrointestinal tract is not involved, breastfeeding can be initiated 6 to 8 hours postoperatively, at the surgeon's discretion. The risk of lung irritation from breast milk is minimal. The rapid emptying time of the stomach and other anti-infective factors serve as advantages in the postoperative course.

Surgery or rehospitalization beyond the neonatal period

The infant who requires surgery or rehospitalization can and should be breastfed postoperatively in most cases. The gravity of the surgery and the length of the recovery phase will determine the time necessary for the mother to pump and manually express her milk to keep her supply available. The infant who is hospitalized is already traumatized by the separation, the strange surroundings and people, and the underlying discomfort of the disease process itself. If he is to be fed orally, it should be at the breast as much as possible. If the mother can room-in or the hospital has a care-by-parent ward, this works out well. If obligations to other family members make it impossible for mother to stay around the clock, she can pump her milk and bring it in fresh day by day or frozen if the time interval between visits is longer than a day. Freezing will destroy the cellular content, but that is not a major problem beyond the immediate neonatal period. The infant should not be subjected to the added trauma of being weaned from the breast when he needs the security and intimacy of nursing most unless it is absolutely unavoidable.

The medical profession needs to be aware of this infant and mother and their special needs for support. An opportunity to discuss the breastfeeding aspect of the infant's management should be offered by the physician. The parents should not have to fight for the right to maintain breastfeeding. Plans for pumping and saving milk should be discussed and provided for. If the infant is housed in an open ward or even a room with other infants and their parents without adequate privacy, a separate room should be provided for the mother to nurse or pump her milk. This room should be clean, neat, adequately illuminated, and equipped with a sink for washing hands. If a mechanical pump is to be used, it should be kept clean, sterile, and operable. Storerooms, broom closets, and staff dressing rooms are inappropriate.

Arrangements for providing sterile containers for collecting milk and storing it should be discussed (Chapter 19). Occasionally a mother may become so concerned about the adequacy of her milk for her infant that she may nurse far too frequently. Actually her child will need much more nonnutritive cuddling and holding than usual. The physician may need to reassure the mother when pointing this out. The father should also be encouraged to understand all the tubes, bandages, and appliances the infant may have attached. He is an important member of the parenting team and should provide some of the cuddling and soothing as well.

Nursing bottle caries in breastfed infants

The development of rampant dental caries can occur in breastfed infants and is reported in the literature.[23] Usually the children have been nursed for 2 to 3 years, spending long stretches at the breast. One infant had early signs at 9 months, and by 18 months she required full mouth reconstruction.

The physician should be alert to the potential for dental decay when infants nurse frequently, especially through the night. Family history of dental enamel problems is worth investigating. Certainly these children were candidates for fluoride treatment.

REFERENCES

1. Abbassi, V., and Steinour, T.A.: Successful diagnosis of congenital hypothyroidism in four breast-fed neonates, J. Pediatr. **97:**259, 1980.
2. Addy, H.A.: The breast feeding of twins, Environ. Child Health **21:**231, 1975.
3. Aggett, P.J., et al.: Symptomatic zinc deficiency in a breast-fed preterm infant, Arch. Dis. Child. **55:**547, 1980.
4. Ahmed, S., and Blair, A.W.: Symptomatic zinc deficiency in a breast-fed infant, Arch. Dis. Child. **56:**315, 1981.
5. Anderson, D.M., et al.: Length of gestation and nutritional composition of human milk, Am. J. Clin. Nutr. **37:**810, 1983.
6. Arias, I.M., and Gartner, L.M.: Production of unconjugated hyperbilirubinemia in full term newborn infants following administration of pregnane-3α,20β-diol, Nature **203:**1292, 1964.
7. Arias, I.M., et al.: Prolonged neonatal unconjugated hyperbilirubinemia associated with breast feeding and steroid pregnane-3α,20β-diol in maternal milk that inhibits glucuronide formation in vitro, J. Clin. Invest. **43:**2037, 1964.
8. Arnon, S.S.: Infant botulism, Ann. Rev. Med. **31:**541, 1980.
9. Arnon, S.S., et al.: Protective role of human milk against sudden death from infant botulism, J. Pediatr. **100:**568, 1982.
10. Atinmo, T., and Omololu, A.: Trace element content of breast milk from mothers of preterm infants in Nigeria, Early Hum. Dev. **6:**309, 1982.
11. Atkinson, S.A., Anderson, G.H., and Bryan, M.H.: Human milk: comparison of the nitrogen composition in milk from mothers of premature

and full-term infants, Am. J. Clin. Nutr. **33:**811, 1980.

12. Atkinson, S.A., Bryan, M.H., and Anderson, G.H.: Human milk: differences in nitrogen concentration in milk from mothers of term and premature infants, J. Pediatr. **93:**67, 1978.

13. Atkinson, S.A., Radde, I.C., and Anderson, G.H.: Macromineral balances in premature infants fed on their own mother's milk or formula, J. Pediatr. **102:**99, 1983.

14. Atkinson, S.A., et al.: Macro-mineral content of milk obtained during early lactation from mothers of premature infants, Early Hum. Dev. **4:**5, 1980.

15. Auerbach, K.G., et al.: A symposium: breast feeding the premature infant, Keeping Abreast J. **2:**98, 1977.

16. Avedian, L.V., and Ruberg, R.L.: Impaired weight gain in cleft palate infants, Cleft Palate J. **17:**24, 1980.

17. Beck, F.: Breast feeding the baby with a cleft lip, Keeping Abreast J. **3:**122, 1978.

18. Bennett, F.C., et al.: Vitamin and mineral supplementation in Down's syndrome, Pediatrics **72:**707, 1983.

19. Berkowitz, C.D., and Inkelis, S.H.: Bloody nipple discharge in infancy, J. Pediatr. **103:**755, 1983.

20. Billeaud, C., Senterre, J., and Rigo, J.: Osmolality of the gastric and duodenal contents in low birth weight infants fed human milk or various formulae, Acta Paediatr. Scand. **71:**799, 1982.

21. Bitman, J., et al.: Comparison of the lipid composition of breast milk from mothers of term and preterm infants, Am. J. Clin. Nutr. **38:**300, 1983.

22. Bode, H.H., Vanjonack, W.J., and Crawford, J.D.: Mitigation of cretinism by breast feeding, Pediatr. Res. **11:**423, 1977.

23. Brams, M., and Maloney, J.: "Nursing bottle caries" in breast-fed children, J. Pediatr. **103:**415, 1983.

24. Brown, E.G., Ainbender, E., and Sweet, A.Y.: Effect of feeding stool endotoxins: possible relationship to necrotizing enterocolitis, Pediatr. Res. **10:**352, 1976.

25. Chandra, R.K.: Immunoglobulin and protein levels in breast milk produced by mothers of preterm infants, Nutr. Res. **2:**27, 1982.

26. Chessex, P., et al.: Quality of growth in premature infants fed on their own mother's milk, J. Pediatr. **102:**107, 1983.

27. Conde, C., DeFrias, E.C., and Moro, M.: Essential fatty acids in phosphoglycerides of human milk, Acta Paediatr. Scand. **72:**255, 1983.

28. Curtis, J.A., and Bailey, J.D.: Influence of breast feeding on the clinical features of salt-losing congenital adrenal hyperplasia, Arch. Dis. Child. **58:**71, 1983.

29. Dahms, B.B., et al.: Breast feeding and serum bilirubin values during the first 4 days of life, J. Pediatr. **83:**1049, 1973.

30. Davies, D.P.: Plasma osmolality and protein intake in premature infants, Arch. Dis. Child. **48:**575, 1973.

31. DeCarvalho, M., Klaus, M., and Merkatz, R.B.: Frequency of breast-feeding and serum bilirubin concentration, Am. J. Dis. Child. **136:**737, 1982.

32. Drew, J.H.: Breast feeding and jaundice. II. Infant feeding and jaundice, Keeping Abreast J. **3:**53, 1978.

33. Eckhert, C.D., et al.: Zinc binding: a difference between human and bovine milk, Science **195:**789, 1977.

34. Ernest, A.E., et al.: Guide to breast feeding the infant with PKU, Washington, D.C., 1980, U.S. Government Printing Office.

35. Evans, G.W., and Johnson, P.E.: Defective prostaglandin synthesis is acrodermatitis enteropathica, Lancet **1:**52, 1977.

36. Filer, L.J., Stegink, L.D., and Chandramouli, B.: Effect of diet on plasma aminograms of low birth weight infants, Am. J. Clin. Nutr. **30:**1036, 1977.

37. Foliot, A., et al.: Breast milk jaundice: in vitro inhibition of rat liver bilirubin-uridine diphosphate glucuronyltransferase activity and Z protein-bromosulfophthalein binding by human breast milk, Pediatr. Res. **10:**594, 1976.

38. Fomon, S.J., and Ziegler, E.E.: Protein intake of premature infants: Interpretation of data (editor's column), J. Pediatr. **90:**504, 1977.

39. Fomon, S.J., and Ziegler, E.E.: Milk of the premature infant's mother: Interpretation of data (editorial), J. Pediatr. **93:**164, 1978.

40. Fomon, S.J., Ziegler, E.E., and Vazquez, H.D.: Human milk and the small premature infant, Am. J. Dis. Child. **131:**463, 1977.

41. Forbes, G.B.: Is human milk the best food for low birth weight babies (Abstract), Pediatr. Res. **12:**434, 1978.

42. Forbes, G.B.: Nutritional adequacy of human breast milk for premature infants. In Lebenthal,

E., editor: Textbook of gastroenterology and nutrition, New York, 1981, Raven Press.

43. Forbes, G.B.: Human milk and the small baby, Am. J. Dis. Child. **136**:577, 1982.

44. Forbes, G.B.: Fetal growth and body composition: implications for the premature infant, J. Pediatr. Gastroenterol. Nutr. **2**(suppl.):552, 1983.

45. Ford, J.E., et al.: Comparison of the B vitamin composition of milk from mothers of preterm and term babies, Arch. Dis. Child. **58**:367, 1983.

46. Gartner, L.M.: Disorders of bilirubin metabolism. In Nathan, D.G., and Oski, F.A., editors: Hematology of infancy and childhood, Philadelphia, 1981, W.B. Saunders Co.

47. Gartner, L.M., and Arias, I.M.: Temporary discontinuation of breast feeding in infants with jaundice, JAMA **225**:532, 1973.

48. Gartner, L.M., and Lee, K-S.: Jaundice and liver disease. In Behrman, R.E., Driscoll, J.M., Jr., and Seeds, A.E., editors: Neonatal-perinatal medicine diseases of the fetus and infant, ed. 2, St. Louis, 1977, The C.V. Mosby Co.

49. Gaull, G.E., Rassin, D.K., and Räihä, N.C.R.: Protein intake of premature infants: A reply, J. Pediatr. **90**:507, 1977.

50. Gaull, G.E., et al.: Milk protein quantity and quality in low-birth-weight infants. III. Effects on sulfur amino acids in plasma and urine, J. Pediatr. **90**:348, 1977.

51. Goldman, A.S., et al.: Effects of prematurity on the immunologic system in human milk, J. Pediatr. **101**:901, 1982.

52. Grady, E.: Breastfeeding the baby with a cleft of the soft palate: success and its benefits, Clin. Pediatr. **16**:978, 1977.

53. Grady, E.: Breast feeding the baby with a cleft of the soft palate, Keeping Abreast J. **3**:126, 1978.

54. Greenberg, J., Nazarian, L., and Green, J.: Personal communications, 1976 to 1978.

55. Greer, F.R., Steichen, J.J., and Tsang, R.C.: Calcium and phosphate supplements in breast-milk-related rickets, Am. J. Dis. Child. **136**:581, 1982.

56. Gross, S.J.: Growth and biochemical response of protein infants fed human milk or modified infant formula, N. Engl. J. Med. **308**:237, 1983.

57. Gross, S.J., et al.: Elevated IgA concentration in milk produced by mothers delivered of preterm infants, J. Pediatr. **99**:389, 1981.

58. Gross, S.J., et al.: Nutritional composition of milk produced by mothers delivering preterm, J. Pediatr. **96**:641, 1980.

59. Gross, S.J., Geller, J., and Tomarelli, R.M.: Composition of breast milk from mothers of preterm infants, Pediatrics **68**:490, 1981.

60. Guerrini, P., et al.: Human milk: relationship of fat content with gestational age, Early Hum. Dev. **5**:187, 1981.

61. Hagelberg, S., et al.: The protein tolerance of very low birth weight infants fed human milk protein enriched mother's milk, Acta Paediatr. Scand. **71**:597, 1982.

62. Hahn, H.B., et al.: Thyroid function tests in neonates fed human milk, Am. J. Dis. Child. **137**:220, 1983.

63. Heird, W.C., and Anderson, T.L.: Nutritional requirements and methods of feeding low birth weight infants. In Gluck, L., editor: Current problems in pedriatrics, vol. VII, no. 8, Chicago, 1977, Year Book Medical Publishers, Inc.

64. Hemmingway, L.: Breastfeeding a cleft-palate baby, Med. J. Aust. **2**:626, 1972.

65. Hibberd, C.M., et al.: Variations in the composition of breast milk during the first 5 weeks of lactation: implications for the feeding of preterm infants, Arch. Dis. Child. **57**:658, 1982.

66. Järvendää, A.L.: Feeding the low-birth-weight infant. IV. Fat absorption as a function of diet and duodenal bile acids, Pediatrics **72**:684, 1983.

67. Järvendää, A.L., et al.: Preterm infants fed human milk attain intrauterine weight gain, Acta Paediatr. Scand. **72**:239, 1983.

68. Jelliffe, E.F.P.: Infant feeding practices: Associated diseases. In Neumann, C.G., and Jelliffe, D.B., editors: Symposium on nutrition in pediatrics, Pediatr. Clin. North Am. **24**:1, 1977.

69. Jelliffe, E.F.P.: Infant feeding practices: associated iatrogenic and commerciogenic diseases. In Neumann, C.G., and Jelliffe, D.B., editors: Symposium on nutrition in pediatrics, Pediatr. Clin. North Am. **24**:49, 1977.

70. Jelliffe, D.B., and Jelliffe, E.F.P.: Human milk in the modern world, Oxford, 1976, Oxford University Press.

71. Johnson, P., and Salisbury, D.M.: Breathing and sucking during feeding in the newborn. In Hofer, M.A., editor: Ciba Foundation Symposium no. 33, Parent-infant interaction, Amsterdam, 1975, Elsevier Scientific Pub. Co.

72. Kennell, J.H., et al.: Early neonatal contact: effect on growth, breast feeding and infection in the first year of life, Pediatr. Res. **10**:426, 1976.

73. Lake, A.M., Whitington, P.F., and Hamilton, S.R.: Dietary protein-induced colitis in breast-fed infants, J. Pediatr. **101**:906, 1982.

74. Lawrence, R.A.: Infant nutrition, Pediatr. Rev. **5**:133, 1983.

75. Lemons, J.A., et al.: Differences in composition of preterm and term human milk during early lactation, Pediatr. Res. **16**:113, 1982.

76. Letarte, J., et al.: Lack of protective effect of breast-feeding in congenital hypothyroidism: report of 12 cases, Pediatrics **65**:703, 1980.

77. Lewis-Jones, D.I., and Reynolds, G.J.: A suggested role for precolostrum in preterm and sick newborn infants, Acta Paediatr. Scand. **72**:13, 1983.

78. Lindblad, B.S., Hagelberg, S., and Lundsjö, A.: Blood levels of critical amino acids in very low birth-weight infants on a high human milk protein intake, Acta Paediatr. Scand. (Suppl.) **296**:24, 1982.

79. Littlewood, J.M., and Crollick, A.J.: Childhood coeliac disease is disappearing, Lancet **2**:1359, 1980.

80. Lubit, E.C.: Cleft palate orthodontics: why, when, how, Am. J. Orthod. **69**:562, 1976.

81. Lucas, A., et al.: A human milk formula, Early Hum. Dev. **4**:15, 1980.

82. Luzeau, R., et al.: Demonstration of a lipolytic activity in human milk that inhibits the glucurono-conjugation of bilirubin, Biomedicine **21**:258, 1974.

83. Luzeau, R., et al.: Activity of lipoprotein lipase in human milk: inhibition of glucuro-conjugation of bilirubin, Clin. Chim. Acta **59**:133, 1975.

84. Macaron, C.: Galactorrhea and neonatal hypothyroidism, J. Pediatr. **101**:576, 1982.

85. Mata, L.J., and Urrutia, J.J.: Intestinal colonization of breast fed children in a rural area of low socio-economic level, Ann. N.Y. Acad. Sci. **93**:1976, 1971.

86. McKiernan, J., and Hull, D.: The constituents of neonatal milk, Pediatr. Res. **16**:60, 1982.

87. Meberg, A., Willgraff, S., and Sande, H.A.: High potential for breast feeding among mothers giving birth to pre-term infants, Acta Paediatr. Scand. **71**:661, 1982.

88. Mendelson, R.A., Anderson, G.H., and Bryan, M.H.: Zinc, copper and iron content of milk from mothers of preterm and fullterm infants, Early Hum. Dev. **6**:145, 1982.

89. Murphy, J.F., Neale, M.L., and Mathews, N.: Antimicrobial properties of preterm breast milk cells, Arch. Dis. Child. **58**:198, 1983.

90. Narayanan, I., et al.: Partial supplementation with expressed breast-milk for prevention of infection in low-birth-weight infants, Lancet **2**:561, 1980.

91. Nau, J.: When a baby has surgery: an interview, Keeping Abreast J. **1**:38, 1976.

92. Nicoll, A., Ginsburg, R., and Tripp, J.H.: Supplementary feeding and jaundice newborns, Acta Paediatr. Scand. **71**:759, 1982.

93. Office for Maternal and Child Health, HEW, sponsor: Human milk in premature infant feeding: summary of a workshop, Pediatrics **57**:741, 1976.

94. Pearce, J.L., and Buchanan, L.F.: Breast milk and breast feeding in very low birth weight infants, Br. Med. J. **1**:897, 1980.

95. Räihä, N.C.R., et al.: Milk protein quantity and quality in low-birth-weight infants. I. Metabolic responses and effects on growth, Pediatrics **57**:659, 1976.

96. Rassin, D.K., et al.: Milk protein quantity and quality in low-birth-weight infants. II. Effects on aliphatic amino acids in plasma and urine, Pediatrics **59**:407, 1977.

97. Rassin, D.K., et al.: Milk protein quantity and quality in low-birth-weight infants. IV. Effects on tyrosine and phenylalanine in plasma and urine, J. Pediatr. **90**:356, 1977.

98. Reichman, B., et al.: Dietary composition and macronutrient storage in preterm infants, Pediatrics **72**:322, 1983.

99. Rönnholm, K.A.R., Sipilä, I., and Siimes, M.A.: Human milk protein supplementation for the prevention of hypoproteinemia without metabolic imbalance in breast milk-fed, very low-birth-weight infants, J. Pediatr. **101**:243, 1982.

100. Rowe, J.C., et al.: Nutritional hypophosphatemic rickets in a premature infant fed breast milk, N. Engl. J. Med. **300**:293, 1979.

101. Russell, G., and Feather, E.A.: Effects of feeding on respiratory mechanics of healthy newborn infants, Arch. Dis. Child. **45**:325, 1970.

102. Saarinen, U.M.: Prolonged breast feeding as prophylaxis for recurrent otitis media, Acta Paediatr. Scand. **71**:567, 1982.

103. Sack, J., Amado, O., and Lunenfeld, B.: Thyroxine concentration in human milk, J. Clin. Endocrinol. Metab. **45**:171, 1977.

104. Sann, L., et al.: Comparison of the composition of breast milk from mothers of term and preterm infants, Acta Paediatr. Scand. **70**:115, 1981.

105. Sann, L., et al.: Effect of early oral calcium supplementation on serum calcium and immunoreactive calcitonin concentration in preterm infants, Arch. Dis. Child. **55**:611, 1980.

106. Savilahti, E., Järvenpää, A.L., and Räihä, N.C.R.: Serum immunoglobulins in preterm infants: comparison of human milk and formula feeding, Pediatrics **72**:312, 1983.

107. Schanler, R.J., and Oh, W.: Composition of breast milk obtained from mothers of premature infants as compared to breast milk obtained from donors, J. Pediatr. **96**:679, 1980.

108. Senterre, J., et al.: Effects of vitamin D and phosphorus supplementation on calcium retention in preterm infants fed banked human milk, J. Pediatr. **103**:305, 1983.

109. Shmerling, D.H.: Dietary protein-induced colitis in breast-fed infants, J. Pediatr. **103**:500, 1983.

110. Similä, S., Kokkonen, J., and Kouvalainen, K.: Use of lactose-hydrolyzed human milk in congenital lactase deficiency, J. Pediatr. **101**:584, 1982.

111. Simkins, T.: Feeding the premature infant: More questions than answers, Perinatol. Neonatal. **2**:30, 1978.

112. Snyderman, S.E.: The protein and amino acid requirements of the premature infant. In Jonxis, J.H.P., Visser, H.K.A., and Troelstra, J.A., editors: Nutricia symposium: metabolic process in the foetus and newborn infant, Rotterdam, 1971, Stenfort, Kroesse, Leider.

113. Spencer, S.A., and Hull, D.: Fat content of expressed breast milk: a case for quality control, Br. Med. J. **282**:99, 1981.

114. Sturman, J.A., Rassin, D.K., and Gaull, G.E.: A mini review: taurine in development, Life Sci. **21**:1, 1977.

115. Tikanoja, T., et al.: Plasma amino acids in preterm infants after a feed of human milk or formula, J. Pediatr. **101**:248, 1982.

116. Toms, G.L., et al.: Secretion of respiratory syncytial virus inhibitors and antibody in human milk through lactation, J. Med. Virol. **5**:351, 1980.

117. Tyson, J.E., et al.: Growth, metabolic response, and development in very low birth weight infants fed banked human milk or enriched formula. I. Neonatal findings, J. Pediatr. **103**:95, 1983.

118. Varma, S.K., et al.: Thyroxine, tri-iodothyronine, and reverse tri-iodothyronine concentrations in human milk, J. Pediatr. **93**:803, 1978.

119. Weatherly-White, R.C.A.: Guest comment: breastfeeding the baby with a cleft lip, Keeping Abreast J. **3**:125, 1978.

120. Whyte, R.K., et al.: Energy balance and nitrogen balance in growing low birth weight infants fed human milk or formula, Pediatr. Res. **17**:891, 1983.

121. Wong, P.W.K., Lambert, A.M., and Komrowe, G.M.: Tyrosinaemia and tyrosluria in infancy, Dev. Med. Child. Neurol. **9**:551, 1967.

122. Wong, Y.K., and Wood, B.S.B.: Breast milk jaundice and oral contraceptives, Br. Med. J., **4**:403, 1971.

123. Zimmerman, A.W., et al.: Acrodermatitis in breast-fed premature infants: evidence for a defect of mammary gland zinc secretion, Pediatrics **69**:176, 1982.

15

Medical complications of the mother

OBSTETRIC COMPLICATIONS

Cesarean section

When delivery takes place by cesarean section, the mother becomes a surgical patient with all the inherent risks and problems. If the section is anticipated because of a previous section, cephalopelvic disproportion, or some other identifiable reason, a mother can prepare herself psychologically for the event and usually tolerates the process better. When the section is unplanned and done during the process of labor, it is psychologically more traumatic, and the mother tends to feel as if she has failed in her female role. In addition to this unexpected disappointment, there may be medical emergencies that also have an impact on the mother's well-being, such as a long hard labor, abruptio placentae, blood loss, toxemia, or infection.

The mother who plans to breastfeed following a cesarean section should be able to do so provided the infant is well enough. The method of delivery makes no significant difference to the timing of the milk coming in or the changes in the concentration the major milk constituents in the first 7 days postpartum.[30] Depending on the type of anesthesia and the associated circumstances, the mother may feel alert enough to put the infant to breast within the first 12 hours. Mothers have nursed in the first hour after the surgery is over.

Bupivacaine is being used for epidural block for cesarean section or for vaginal delivery because it does not show the decrease in muscle tone and strength reported in neonates whose mothers have received lidocaine or mepivacaine.[35,51] There is a rapid distribution of the drug, and elimination appears to be well developed at birth.

Regional anesthesia permits the mother to remain awake, and she may be ready to nurse as soon as the intravenous lines and urinary catheter are all stabilized. The mother will need considerable help from the nursing staff. She should remain flat if she has had a spinal anesthetic to prevent developing a spinal headache. She can turn to one side and offer the nipple by placing the infant on his side and stroking the infant's perioral area with the nipple. If he is a normal full-term infant and has not been depressed by maternal medication, he should do well. If the mother can be turned to the other side, the infant should nurse on both sides. The bedside rails will help the mother turn as well as provide safety for her.

Fluids and medications in the first 48 hours postoperatively should not affect the infant adversely.[68] Pain medication is required usually for 72 hours or so. It is best given immediately after breastfeeding to permit the level to peak before the next feeding. The medication used should be limited to short-acting drugs that the adult eliminates quickly (i.e., within 4 hours) and that the newborn is able to excrete also. Aspirin, for instance, is in that category despite the theoretical risk of decreased platelet aggregation because it is readily excreted by both adult and infant. Codeine is also acceptable (Chapter 11). Low-grade fever is not uncommon and should not interrupt lactation.

There are some very positive factors associated with breastfeeding for the mother who has had a cesarean section. Lactation is advantageous to the postoperative uterus in that the oxytocin production stimulated by suckling will assist in the involution of the uterus. In addition, the traumatized psyche of a mother whose delivery did not occur naturally as planned is more quickly healed when she can demonstrate her maternal capabilities by breastfeeding.

Whether breastfeeding can be introduced early or must await stabilization of medical problems in the mother or infant, it is a reasonable goal for the mother to seek, in most cases. Supportive nursing care will be critical to establishing successful lactation. But none of this can take place unless the physician has carefully assessed the condition of the mother and the infant in light of the advantages and disadvantages of breastfeeding to both.

The management should include the following:

1. A postoperative care plan must include sufficient rest. Most postpartum wards are not scheduled to include adequate rest for postoperative patients.
2. The family must be instructed on the needs for rest at home and assistance with the household chores.
3. The infant should be considered, when possible, in writing medication orders.
4. If the infant cannot be breastfed, arrangements should be made to pump the mother's breasts on a regular basis.

Toxemia

Toxemia presents a problem in management anytime it occurs. The clinical onset is insidious and may be accompanied by a variety of subtle symptoms but the diagnosis depends on the presence of hypertension and proteinuria.[5] It usually begins after the thirty-second week of gestation and has been observed to occur 24 to 48 hours or later postpartum. Convulsions, renal disease, and cerebral hemorrhage in the mother are all complications to be prevented by careful management. Because serious toxicity in the mother may necessitate delivery of a premature infant or an infant compromised by a poorly profused placenta or maternal medications, there are a number of contraindications to breastfeeding in the immediate postpartum period. Initial treatment of the preeclamptic patient includes bed rest, preferably lying on her side in a room that is darkened to prevent photic stimuli. Blood pressure and proteinuria are to be carefully watched. Sedation with phenobarbital or diazepam (Valium), salt restriction, and possibly diuretics such as thiazide or furosemide are used. Hydralazine (Apresoline) and methyldopa (Aldomet) may be indicated as well, to bring down the blood pressure. Magnesium sulfate may also be used. Many patients recover quickly once the infant and placenta are delivered, requiring only 24 to 48 hours of postpartum sedation. Often the infant is small for gestational age or premature and may require special or intensive care; therefore the decision to breastfeed depends on the infant's condition. If the infant is full term and well, then the breastfeeding is initiated when toxemia precautions are discontinued and when the mother's phenobarbital intake has been tapered off to about 180 mg/day or less, calculating that initially the amount of milk obtained is not so great as to provide a large dose of drug to the infant. Careful observation should be made to be sure the infant is not depressed by the accumulation of phenobarbital, however. Phenobarbital is a drug that can be and is given to newborns for several indications and therefore is of low risk. It is preferable to wait until the other medications can be discontinued, especially the diuretics, hydralazine, and methyldopa. Once the risk of convulsions is past, some attention can be given to manual expression or pumping even if the infant cannot be nursed yet. If medications are a problem temporarily, the milk will have to be discarded, but the expression of milk will serve to stimulate the breast and initiate lactation. Diminution of stress is a critical factor in toxemia therapy so that anxiety of the mother about being able to nurse must be managed with open discussion of the overall plan and where nursing fits in. On the other hand, the stress of early feedings that do not go well because the infant has been confused by initial bottle feedings may also present a hazard in the course of management of toxemia. The single most important element in every case is communication with the patient about her expectations or needs regarding breastfeeding. The physician's therapeutic management design can put this in appropriate perspective.

Retention of the placenta and lactation failure

Three cases of failure of the onset of lactation were reported by Neifert et al.[42] Although the original references to the association of the placenta with delayed lactation were made at the turn of the century, most reports of retained placenta merely discuss persistent hemorrhage as a recognized symptom. In each of these cases the failure of breast engorgement and leakage of milk was evident from the time of delivery, but the hemorrhage and emergency curettage occurred at 1 week, 3 weeks, and 4 weeks postpartum respectively. In each case spontaneous milk began immediately postoperatively, after the removal of placental fragments. The authors suggest that failure of lactogenesis may be an early sign of retained placenta that should not be ignored.

Venous thrombosis and pulmonary embolism

Venous thrombosis and pulmonary embolism are the most common serious vascular diseases associated with pregnancy and the postpartum period.[6] Pulmonary embolism has assumed relatively greater importance because of the decline in morbidity and mortality from sepsis and eclampsia. Varicose veins also present more problems during pregnancy than at any other time. These diseases all represent common features in vein physiology as associated with the perinatal period.

The major concerns during lactation, in addition to the well-being of the mother, include the diagnostic procedures that might be necessary to establish the diagnosis and the systemic medications necessary for treatment that could have an impact on the nursing infant via the milk. Accurate diagnosis is urgent and is far more complex than therapy. Besides the health of the mother in this life-threatening state, any program of contraception after childbirth is fundamentally affected by the established diagnosis of thromboembolism. Thus the diagnosis must be accurate.

DIAGNOSIS. Laboratory procedures such as evaluation of arterial blood gases, liver function studies, and fibrin/fibrinogen derivatives are not a problem to nursing. It might be noted that the absence of fibrin split products in plasma and serum virtually excludes the diagnosis of embolism, although their presence does not confirm it. The most definitive diagnosis is made with radioactive scanning procedures and angiography. At present, computed tomography and ultrasound are effective in major arterial aneurysms only. Radioactive materials vary in their half-lives and disappearance time from breast milk. They all appear in breast milk (Chapter 11).

TREATMENT. Anticoagulant therapy is the treatment of choice for established venous thrombosis with or without embolism. Heparin can be given parenterally, since this large molecule does not cross the placenta or appear in breast milk. This therapy is adequate for the hospitalized patient, in whom constant monitoring of coagulation is possible. An alternative, self-administered subcutaneous heparin, has been reported by Kakkar et al.[24] The cost of heparin and the patient's ability to learn self-administration are considerations. Warfarin has been considered the best replacement for heparin but it is secreted in the breast milk (Chapter 11 and Appendix F). The amount transmitted is miniscule and it is considered safe to breastfeed while taking warfarin.

MATERNAL INFECTIONS
Bacterial infections

URINARY TRACT INFECTION. Urinary tract infections are the most common of the postpartum bacterial infections. Any apparent infection is of concern because of the risk to the infant. Urinary tract infections, however, are "closed infections" and do not constitute a hazard except when the infection is due to β-hemolytic streptococci. The mother should be reminded to wash her hands thoroughly before handling the infant. The choice of medication is important when the mother is breastfeeding, since the majority of antibiotics reach the milk in some concentration. The medication should be one that could also be given to the infant, such as penicillin, ampicillin, and gentamicin. Under 1 month postpartum, sulfadiazine and sulfa-containing medications should not be given, since the hazard of interfering with bilirubin binding to albumin is significant. Beyond 1 month of age sulfa drugs are actually given to infants directly. Tetracycline and chloramphenicol should not be used. Forcing fluids and acidifying the urine via the diet are always helpful.

BREAST ABSCESSES IN STAPHYLOCOCCAL EPIDEMICS.   Breast abscesses can occur in both mothers and infants in nursery epidemics with a virulent staphylococcus. Transmission does not always go from infant to mother, since breast abscess has been seen in women who have delivered stillborn infants.

According to reports,[56] during a nursery epidemic, the colonized mothers who were nursing developed abscesses, whereas the ones not nursing did not. Both groups of infants were free of the disease but had positive nasal cultures for *Staphylococcus aureus,* phage type 80/81. Shinefeld[56] states that, in his view, in times of epidemics with virulent strains of staphylococci, infants colonized with the epidemic organism should not be breastfed. Breast abscesses should be looked for carefully in the mother and diagnosed by culturing the secretion from the nipple, since the skin and external nipple may well be colonized with the epidemic organism. The treatment is systemic antibiotics, careful drainage of the breast by massage or pump at intervals, and drainage of the abscess when surgically indicated.

Bacterial infections due to streptococci, staphylococci, or other transmissible organisms may cause skin lesions, pharyngitis, pneumonia, or endometritis. These should be treated promptly with antibiotics, and the infant permitted to breastfeed as soon as a therapeutic level of medications has been established for at least 12 hours. Usually infants who are bottle fed are separated from their mothers longer, but they will not receive the valuable anti-infective properties of human milk. Often the question of isolation from the mother and interruption of feeding at the breast comes when symptoms of fever, pain, or malaise first develop in the mother and the diagnosis is still in question. A clinical judgment must be made as to the organ infected, whether bacteria are being actively extruded from the infected source, and the estimated virulence of the organism. A draining incision that appears to show that the infection is streptococcal in origin suggests early isolation and a conservative approach, whereas a low-grade fever within 24 hours of delivery with no localizing signs might warrant continuing active breastfeeding.*

---

*It should be pointed out that engorgement may be associated with a low-grade fever. The patient should be evaluated as to other possible causes, but if none is identified the probable diagnosis is engorgement. The best treatment is to nurse the infant as often as possible and see that the breasts are gently expressed to assure proper drainage of all alveoli.

Staphylococcal infections may be passed back and forth between the mother and infant. Identification of the infection and the etiologic agent is important so that appropriate treatment may be initiated. Not all staphylococci are pathologic, and removing this flora may permit growth of real pathogens. A mother and nursing infant with non-epidemic staphylococcal disease under medication need not be separated from each other. They should be isolated from other mothers and infants. Sometimes the best plan when the symptoms are mild is to discharge the nursing couple to prevent spread in the hospital and permit freedom of contact at home, with reasonable precautions (Table 15-1).

TOXIC SHOCK SYNDROME.   A postpartum woman developed toxic shock syndrome 22 hours after delivery and coagulase-positive staphylococcus was recovered from the vagina. Breast milk specimens collected on days 5, 8, and 11 contained staphylococcal enterotoxin. The mother and infant lacked significant antibody in their sera. This case, reported by Vergeront et al.,[66] represents the first isolation of staphylococcal enterotoxin from a body fluid from a patient with toxic shock syndrome.

GROUP B β-HEMOLYTIC STREPTOCOCCAL INFECTION.   Group B β-hemolytic streptococcal infection in the neonate is not normally associated with maternal vaginal colonization. It is usually of late-onset occurring meningitis. It is thought to be nosocomial or environmental in most cases. Two cases associated with group B β-hemolytic streptococci in the maternal milk were reported by Schreiner et al.[53] and one by Kenny.[27] It is not clear yet whether the transmission is mother to baby or the reverse. When a breastfed infant becomes infected, it is appropriate to culture the milk.

TUBERCULOUS MASTITIS.   Mastitis due to the tuberculous tubercle has occurred in third-world countries; it is usually found in association with tuberculosis of the tonsils in the neonate. With the migration to industrial communities, this should always be kept in mind when mastitis progresses to abscess in spite of antibiotic therapy.

GONORRHEA.   When gonorrhea is specifically diagnosed by identification of bacteria in the cervical smear or culture prior to delivery, antibiotics should be started immediately; the mother may handle and/or feed her infant 24 hours after the initiation of therapy. Because of the occasional occurrence of established infection in the neonate despite use of silver nitrate in the eyes at birth, it is appropriate to isolate the infant from the rest of the nursery population, although the infant need not be isolated from his mother once her treatment has been established. The Credé method of eye prophylaxis may fail because it is improperly done or the infection was established prior to birth because of prematurely ruptured membranes or the development of inclusion conjunctivitis.

SYPHILIS.   A mother with positive syphilis serum reaction, which indicates a primary infection, should be treated immediately. If there are primary or secondary lesions that could contain the treponeme, the infant should be isolated from the mother as well as from other infants. The infant should have a diagnostic workup for congenital syphilis and treatment instituted when appropriate. If there are lesions around the breast and nipple, nursing is contraindicated until treatment is complete and the lesions are clear. Following is an outline of the therapeutic decisions in relation to the syphilis VDRL antigen status of the infant.[21]

I. Negative VDRL
   A. No disease: no treatment required
   B. Early disease
      1. Symptomatic: treat
      2. Asymptomatic: follow and repeat VDRL
II. Positive VDRL
   A. Symptomatic
      1. Hydrops fetalis: treat
      2. Hepatosplenomegaly, jaundice: treat
      3. Mucocutaneous manifestations: treat
      4. Hematologic manifestations: treat
      5. Nephrotic syndrome: treat
   B. Asymptomatic
      1. Perform quantitative VDRL on mother and infant
         a. If infant titer is fourfold higher: treat
      2. Perform quantitative immunoglobulin test
         a. If cord IgM is elevated ($\geqq$ 21 mg/100 ml): treat
      3. Perform hematologic studies (hemoglobin, hematocrit, reticulocyte count, platelet count, smear)
         a. If abnormal: treat
      4. Perform bone radiography
         a. If abnormal: treat
      5. Perform lumbar puncture
         a. If abnormal: treat
      6. If mother unreliable: treat

One of the most frequently sexually transmitted pathogens is *Chlamydia trachomatis,* which causes urethritis and epididymitis in men and cervicitis and salpingitis in women. Infants may be infected during delivery and develop conjunctivitis and pneumonitis. Diagnosis is made by culture and serology. Specific *Chlamydia* colostral IgA was present in the milk of a group of postpartum women who were seropositive.[58] Chlamydial-specific IgA was also found in the milk of 5 out of 6 women who had positive vaginal cultures. There are no data available on the role milk antibodies play in protection against infection in the infant.

Staphylococcal infections may be passed back and forth between the mother and infant. Identification of the infection and the etiologic agent is important so that appropriate treatment may be initiated. Not all staphylococci are pathologic, and removing this flora may permit growth of real pathogens. A mother and nursing infant with non-

Table 15-1.   Management of infectious disease

Organism	Condition	Isolate from mother	Mother can visit nursery	Mother can breastfeed	Immediate treatment	Contact with pregnant women allowed
Bacteria	Premature rupture of membranes; longer than 24 hr without fever					
	Full-term infant	No	Yes	Yes	Observe	Yes
	Premature infant	No	Yes	Yes	Treat with antibiotics	Yes
	Maternal fever greater than 38° C twice, 4 hr apart, 24 hr before to 24 after delivery, or endometriosis; full-term or premature infant	Yes, until mother afebrile 24 hr	No, until mother afebrile 24 hr	No, until mother afebrile 24 hr	Treat with antibiotics	Yes
Salmonella, Shigella		No	Yes, if culture negative	Yes, if culture negative	In most cases	Yes
Staphylococcus		No	Yes	Yes	Yes	Yes
Group B β-streptococcus	Mother with possible cervical culture but otherwise negative obstetrical history	No	Yes	Yes		Yes
	Mother with possible cervical culture and obstetrical history of fever, premature rupture of membranes >24 hr, fetal distress, meconium, low Apgar score, any symptoms of prematurity Infant with surface colonizing	No	Yes	Yes, after treatment	Treat with antibiotics	Yes

Condition					
Group A streptococcus					
Negative history and physical examination	No	Yes	Yes	Observe	Yes
With premature rupture of membrane or maternal infection	No	Yes	Yes	Treat with penicillin	Yes
Mother with infection	Yes	Not in acute stage	Not in acute stage; after 24 hr treatment	Prophylactic penicillin for 10 days	Yes
Gonorrhea					
Mother with positive smear or culture; infant well	No	Yes, after treatment	Yes, after treatment	$AgNO_3$ to the eyes, once in delivery room and once in nursery	Yes
Infant with conjunctivitis	No	Yes, after treatment	Yes, after treatment	Penicillin IM or IV, plus chloramphenicol drops topically	Yes
Syphilis					
Mother with positive VDRL test or clinical disease not treated	Only if mother with second-degree disease or with skin lesions	No, if skin lesions; yes, otherwise	Yes	Penicillin IM or IV after workup done; follow-up after discharge	Yes
Tuberculosis					
Mother treated	No	Yes	Yes		Yes
Mother with inactive disease	No	Yes	Yes	Consider BCG if follow-up in doubt	Yes
Hepatitis					
Mother had in first trimester, well at delivery	No	Yes	Yes		Yes
Mother with active hepatitis at delivery or in third trimester	No, may room-in after good handwash technique followed	No	No	Pooled globulin or hyperimmune if available and immunization	Yes
Mother is chronic carrier	No	Yes, not kiss other infants	Ask for infectious disease opinion	Immunization	Yes
Protozoa					
Toxoplasma					
Toxoplasmosis	No	Yes	Yes		No

epidemic staphylococcal disease under medication need not be separated from each other. They should be isolated from other mothers and infants. Sometimes the best plan when the symptoms are mild is to discharge the nursing couple to prevent spread in the hospital and permit freedom of contact at home, with reasonable precautions (Table 15-1).

TUBERCULOSIS.   Controversy exists around the management of tuberculosis during pregnancy and lactation. All mothers with positive tuberculin test reaction but no radiologic evidence of tuberculosis are considered by Huber[20] to be infected but not diseased. Recent tuberculin conversion, which represents a state of undetermined activity, should be distinguished from well-contained tuberculosis. Dates and results of previous skin tests and recent exposure to active cases are important parts of the history. Because of the hazard that tuberculosis presents to the newborn, careful family studies, including tuberculin skin testing and chest x-ray examinations should be performed on contacts of both the mother and the infant. Huber[20] states that all mothers with a newly positive skin test and negative chest film should be started on a course of isoniazid at the beginning of the third trimester of pregnancy. Dosage is 5 mg/kg of body weight each day as a single dose. Therapy is continued for a year postpartum. If no active cases are identified in the household, no special precautions are indicated to protect the newborn. At one time, however, approximately half the neonates born to tuberculin-positive but bacteriological-negative mothers later became infected with tuberculosis. Since the advent of antituberculous drugs in recent years, however, breastfeeding has been permitted without difficulty in these cases.

When the mother has a positive tuberculin test and a positive chest film, considerable effort should be made to identify the organism in the sputum or gastric washings. If the mother is bacteriologically positive, she should receive triple therapy of isoniazid (INH), 300 mg/day, para-aminosalicylic acid, 12 g/day, and pyridoxine, 50 mg/day, regardless of the time in pregnancy. If she is bacteriologically negative, she should receive isoniazid in the third trimester. Minimum active tuberculosis is defined as parenchymal involvement without cavities. The pregnant woman with minimum active tuberculosis should be hospitalized for evaluation. Sputum sampling and gastric washings should be done and triple treatment begun immediately. It has been shown these patients are no longer infective to others as soon as therapy is initiated. Therapy should continue for 2 years. It is important to reassure the mother that if she is given triple treatment, there is no reason to believe the newborn will have the disease at birth. The controversy arises on postpartum management and separation of mother and infant.

When maternal pulmonary tuberculosis has been treated for at least a week, and if compliance with regard to maternal therapy is assured, infant and maternal contact can be permitted, provided the infant is receiving INH prophylaxis. The INH prophylaxis (30 mg/kg/day in two doses) is always indicated when the mother has any disease requiring triple therapy, even without any contact. If the mother has been treated during pregnancy and cultures are negative, 10 mg of INH/kg/day is indicated for the infant, and no period of separation is necessary.

If it is safe for the mother to be in contact with her infant, then it is safe to breast-feed except for consideration regarding the medications. Since both mother and infant will be taking INH, it would be a matter of assuring that the accumulation in the infant is not excessive because INH does pass into the breast milk. Dosages for infants range from 10 to 20 mg/kg/day. Hepatotoxicity is possible in either the mother or infant, which can be monitored with serial serum glutamic-oxaloacetic transaminase (SGOT) tests. INH is relatively safe for children. Para-aminosalicylic acid (PAS) readily crosses the placenta, yet is reported by O'Brien[45] not to cross into breast milk; this is conflicting information. A drug that readily crosses the placenta is usually found in breast milk. PAS is not recommended, nor is it used to treat newborns. Streptomycin or kanamycin is used instead as the second drug. Jelliffe and Jelliffe[22] point out that in technically undeveloped countries, maternal pulmonary tuberculosis is not a contraindication to breastfeeding. Active treatment is given the mother, while the infant receives INH or BCG vaccine with an INH-resistant strain. In these countries the risk to the infant of not being breastfed far outweighs any risk of drug-related toxicity. That risk/benefit ratio is different in the Western world. In some populations, however, in which infant death from various infections is a major consideration, breastfeeding may be significant to survival. The isolated populations of the American Indian are such a group. Meticulous care must be given to assure that both mother and infant receive proper medication and vaccination against tuberculosis. Newborns and young infants are the most vulnerable group with the highest rate of complication.

LEPROSY. Leprosy is not a contraindication to breastfeeding, according to Jelliffe and Jelliffe.[22] The urgency of breastfeeding is recognized in leprosariums, where the infant and mother are treated with diaminodiphenylsulfone by mouth. No mother-infant contact is permitted except to breastfeed.

LISTERIOSIS. Listeriosis has been identified as the infecting organism in neonatal sepsis and meningitis in recent years and can result in neonatal death. *Listeria,* causing abortion, stillbirth, prematurity, and neonatal death, was described in the 1930s under various titles, including argyrophilic septicemia and pseudotuberculosis of the newborn. The early infection frequently is not recognized and is confused with aspiration pneumonia because of the respiratory symptoms. Examination of the meconium, placenta, and maternal lochia may locate the chief sources of the bacteria, since the symptom complex is not pathognomonic. Symptoms in the mother may be flulike or similar to those of infectious mononucleosis. The manifestations in the adult are protean and in the pregnant woman may lead to an early delivery of an infected infant. Otherwise the infection in adults may be mild and unrecognized, except in retrospect.

The outcome of listeriosis in the neonate depends on early and effective antibiotic therapy, since untreated infants usually do not survive over 4 days. Both mother and infant should be treated. At present, ampicillin plus an aminoglycoside is the treatment of choice and should be maintained pending culture sensitivities in the newborn through the fourth week of life. Treatment in the mother should be maintained 6 to 8 days after symptoms have cleared or cultures are negative. If the mother's symptoms were mild and/or brief, and she is well postpartum, she can breastfeed as soon as the infant is well enough to be fed. Usually such infants require intravenous fluids and nutrition, at least briefly. Once the mother has had adequate medication to show negative cultures, her colostrum or milk can be expressed and given to the infant. The management of lactation and feeding in listeriosis is conducted supportively as it is in any situation in which the infant is extremely ill. Hospitalization is usually required for 4 weeks.

Because of the risk to the neonate it has been suggested that cultures for *Listeria* be done in the third trimester for all women when cultures are being done for gonococcus and herpes. It is certainly important to do such cultures when there is a flulike syndrome in the mother during the second half of pregnancy.

BACTERIAL DIARRHEA. Neonatal diarrhea due to various bacteria, but especially *Escherichia coli,* is best managed by breastfeeding. Diarrhea in the mother due to infection is not a contraindication. Although infections of the gastrointestinal tract are among the principal causes of illness and death in infants in more than 85% of the world, death usually does not occur until after 4 months of age because of the incidence of early breastfeeding in other countries. Even when a diagnosis of infectious diarrhea is made in the mother, it is appropriate to treat with antibiotics that are also safe for the neonate and to start or continue breastfeeding. One should also obtain a culture from the infant without symptoms and treat accordingly. If this is a hospital-acquired disease, then the rigors of establishing the source of the outbreak are to be instituted. Epidemiologic investigation and management of cases and contacts should be initiated. A surveillance system should be established for those in the cohort who are at home.

In developing countries where diarrheal disease has significant morbidity and mortality, many mothers have demonstrable breast milk antibodies against *E. coli* and *Vibrio cholerae*. A prospective study to measure the protective value of these antibodies against disease was done by Glass et al.[16] There were no differences in antibody levels in the milk received by infants who became colonized in an epidemic and those who did not. Among those who were colonized, however, the children who developed symptoms had received milk with lower levels of antibodies than the asymptomatic infants. Apparently the antibodies do not prevent colonization but do protect against disease.

Antibodies against *Shigella, Salmonella,* and enteropathogenic *E. coli* have all been found in breast milk. Parenteral vaccination of lactating women in epidemic areas with killed cholera vaccine or with cholera toxoid vaccine have produced a booster effect on specific milk antibody levels.[36]

Viral infections

RUBELLA. Rubella can produce a variety of effects on the newborn in intrauterine infections from a classic constellation of defects to no apparent effect. Silent infections in the young infant are much more common than symptomatic ones. Schiff et al.[52] prospectively examined over 4000 infants born after the 1964 rubella epidemic using virologic and serologic techniques for the detection of infections in the newborn. The overall rate of congenital rubella was in excess of 2% during the epidemic, whereas it is usually 0.1% in endemic years. During the neonatal period 68% of the infected newborns in that study had subclinical infection; 71% of this group of neonates developed evidence of disease in the first 5 years of life. The infant who is shedding virus is contagious; he should be isolated until the presence or absence of infection can be established. The mother's virus is not considered contagious once the placenta is delivered. The infant can be breastfed. Isolation of the infant should not interfere with breastfeeding except for its inherent inconveniences. If the infant is clinically well, the mother and infant can be discharged, even without all the laboratory results reported. At home they can nurse without restriction. Regardless of method of feeding, the family should protect pregnant women from contact with the infant until the rubella status is determined.

Rubella infection in the mother postpartum will be spread to the neonate long before it is identified. If there is breastfeeding, it should be continued. A sick breastfed infant does better when breastfeeding is maintained.

HERPESVIRUS

Cytomegalovirus.   Cytomegalovirus (CMV) is one of four known herpesviruses in the human. In addition to *Herpesvirus hominis* (herpes simplex), *Herpesvirus varicellae* (varicella-zoster, V-Z), and Epstein-Barr virus (EBV), CMV has also been found to have ultrastructure and physiochemical properties of a herpesvirus.[17] CMV, EBV, and V-Z are believed to be antigenically related on the basis of cross-reactions observed in indirect fluorescent antibody tests. Herpes simplex and V-Z have antigenic similarities in cross-neutralization tests. Two or more subgroups are believed to exist in the CMV group.

The significance for the newborn who does or does not have the virus is whether or not it can be obtained by contact with his infected mother. If it can be picked up from extrauterine maternal contact, what are the risks of infection? Seroepidemiologic studies suggest that usually the infection is acquired in early infancy. A second rise in seroconversion rates occurs after puberty, suggesting venereal transmission at that time. CMV has been demonstrated in semen and cervical swabs. CMV cervicitis increases with gestational time during pregnancy. CMV has been isolated from the saliva and may well be transmitted by kissing.

Various studies[17,40] have detected that 3% to 28% of pregnant women have CMV

Table 15-2.   Incidence of CMV in human milk of seropositive women

Postpartum day	Number tested	Number positive	Percent positive
1-6 days	37	4	10.8
1-13 weeks	26	13	50.0

From Hayes, K.: N. Engl. J. Med. **287:**177, 1972. Reprinted by, permission. From the New England Journal of Medicine.

in cervical cultures; 4% to 5% have CMV in their urine. CMV was found in the milk of seropositive women by Hayes et al.[18] The data on these women with CMV-complement fixing (CF) antibody are shown in Table 15-2.

The time at which the virus gains access to the fetus may be an important determinant in the prognosis. Women who seroconvert early in pregnancy are more apt to have symptomatic infants, whereas infants born to mothers who seroconvert late in pregnancy are born with silent infections. It has been suggested that patients with periventricular calcifications acquire CMV encephalitis in the third or fourth month of gestation because this is the time that the subependymal matrix is most susceptible to damage by viruses. It has been observed that many infants are exposed to CMV during the descent through the birth canal because infections of the cervix at birth are not uncommon. This type of exposure is not associated with disease. Numazaki et al.[44] found 60% of Japanese infants to excrete virus in the urine or upper respiratory tract at 5 to 6 months of age. Some of the infections presumably occurred during passage through the birth canal, whereas others could have been transmitted through ingestion of the virus in mother's milk. In both instances, IgG antibody should have been present in the maternal serum, according to Hanshaw,[17] and have been transferred to the fetus prior to birth. It may well be that specific IgA is also transmitted. The newborn infant may be exposed to the virus at a time when he has received the passive transfer of antibodies from this mother. The lack of infection in the neonatal period may well be due to this passive and active transfer protection. These data provide evidence that infected mothers who are seropositive can breastfeed their infants safely.

In random study of postpartum women, 39% had CMV in their milk, vaginal secretions, urine, and saliva.[13] Of the infants receiving this milk, 69% developed infections; although there were specific antibodies in the milk, they prevented neither shedding nor transmission. There were, however, no sequelae in any of these infants, although they continued to shed virus. Two preterm infants, however, developed meningitis. The risk to milk-bank recipients is major, since they would not have immunity and are already at high risk for serious disease.[59]

Herpes simplex.   Herpes simplex virus (HSV) infection in the neonatal period is often fatal or severely debilitating. Reviews spanning a 39-year period, including 276 patients, have been reported by Nahmias et al.[41] The mode of transmission has been a critical question in management. Transplacental infections have been diagnosed because of the presence of HSV lesions at birth, recovery of the virus from the placenta or cord blood, demonstration of histologic changes or the virus itself in the placenta, detection of elevated IgM levels in the cord blood, presence of typical congenital malformations, or presence of HSV viremia. Because the risk of exposure of the newborn to individuals has not been fully determined, the question of removing personnel with herpetic lesions or subclinical infections from the nursery is still unsettled.

A report of the combined deliberations of the Committee on the Fetus and Newborn and the Committee on Infectious Disease[7] regarding perinatal HSV infections has recommended that with careful attention to hygiene measures a mother and infant need not be separated when the mother has genital lesions. Breastfeeding is acceptable if there are no herpetic lesions on the breast and the lesions that are present are adequately covered. This precaution of handwashing, clean covering, and no fondling or kissing of the infant pertains at home too until all the lesions are dried.[48]

A cause of disseminated herpes simplex type 1 (HSV-1) was reported to have been acquired postnatally in an infant, and the only source of the virus was the mother's milk.[12] The infant survived with significant residual CNS symptoms. Two separate cases of fatal herpes infection has been reported. In one case the infant developed oral lesions and then fulminating disease, and he died on the eighth day.[60] The mother developed lesions of both breasts, which were positive for herpes simplex type 2 (HSV-2), as were the vulva and the cervix cultures and all the infant tissue cultures including the oral lesions. Another fatal case was reported in an infant breastfed from birth.[48] The mother developed a skin sore on the areola of the left breast on the third day. On the fourth day the infant developed lesions in the corner of the mouth and on the chin. The mother had no other lesions. All infant and maternal breast lesions grew HSV-1 with the same profile. Antibody titers in mother and infant were 1:4 and, later, 1:16. A history of oral breast contact 3 weeks prior to the birth was obtained from the father who had a history of recurrent oral-labial herpes.

Two cases of areola lesions diagnosed as being due to herpes, although cultures are not reported, are discussed by Riordan.[50] Both women had extreme pain on nursing. One infant was 5 months old and continued to nurse uneventfully. The second infant was 17 months old and was weaned but remained well. No antibody titers were obtained on either mothers or babies, but it is possible that there was sufficient antibody protection by 5 months of age. It would also be important to know the mother's history of oral and genital lesions.

It is significant that infants with generalized herpes reported in the literature were 3 weeks old or less at the time of onset.[71] It is equally interesting that the presence or absence of antibodies did not correlate with the outcome. Mouth lesions were the most common site, second to skin lesions. In an extensive review of adults, no mention is made of lesions on the breast.[9]

Herpesvirus cultures are easily obtained and the virus grows in a few days; smears of secretions and the cervix are also readily available, as are serum antibody titers. Thus the clinician can obtain a definitive diagnosis when there are suspicious lesions.

Chickenpox.   Chickenpox ranks as one of the most communicable diseases, in a class with measles and smallpox. The incidence is reported at 5 cases/10,000 pregnancies.[73] There is no known reservoir of V-Z. Transfer is believed to be by respiratory droplet; contact infection from the lesions is also possible. In pregnancy, V-Z may be transmitted across the placenta, resulting in congenital or neonatal chickenpox. Most mothers and hospital personnel have had the disease and are not at risk. When chickenpox occurs in pregnancy, it is a highly lethal disease for the mother with death, when it occurs,

Table 15-3.   Fetal deaths in relation to gestational age following selected virus infections during pregnancy

Infection	Weeks of gestation	Number of cases	Number of fetal deaths	Percent
Mumps	0-11	33	9	27.3
	12-27	51	1	2.0
	> 28	43	0	-
Measles	0-11	19	3	15.8
	12-27	29	1	3.4
	> 28	17	1	5.9
Chickenpox	0-11	32	5	15.6
	12-27	60	4	4.7
	> 28	52	0	—
Controls	0-11	1010*	131	13.0
	12-27	392†	15	3.8
	> 28	152†	1	0.7

Modified from Siegel, M., Fuerst, H.T., and Peress, N.S.: N. Engl. J. Med. **274:**768, 1966; from Young, N.A.: Chickenpox, measles, and mumps. In Remington J.S., and Klein, J.O. editors: Infectious disease of the fetus and newborn infant, Philadelphia, 1976, W.B. Saunders Co.
*Subjects attending prenatal clinic in first trimester without virus infection.
†Controls matched for age, race, and parity of the mother and type of obstetric service.

usually resulting from varicella pneumonia, although there may be a bias of selective reporting (Table 15-3).

Perinatal chickenpox.   Postnatally acquired chickenpox usually begins at 10 to 28 days of age and is more common than the congenitally acquired form but generally mild. Transmission in neonates is of a low order. Congenital chickenpox by definition occurs in infants less than 10 days of age. The attack rate is about 24% when the mother has the disease within 17 days of delivery. V-Z does not readily cross the placenta. Congenital chickenpox is associated with significant mortality. The case/fatality ratio is only 5%; that is, 95% will either not get the disease or will not die. When the disease occurs more than a week before delivery, antibody titers in maternal and cord blood are the same. When the disease occurs within 4 days of delivery, maternal titers are positive and cord blood tests are negative. The greatest risk of nosocomial chickenpox exists when the mother develops lesions within 6 days of delivery. If the infant has lesions, he should be isolated with his mother and discharged as soon as his condition permits. This infant should be allowed to breastfeed if the mother is well enough (Table 15-4).

When maternal chickenpox occurs within 6 days of delivery or immediately post-partum and no lesions are present in the neonate, mother and infant should be isolated separately. Only half the infants born to mothers who developed the disease 7 to 15 days before delivery will develop the disease. They should receive zoster immune globulin (ZIG) if available. If no lesions develop by the time the mother is noninfectious, they may be sent home together. When the mother and infant can be together, the child can be breastfed (Table 15-1).

MEASLES.   Measles is a highly communicable childhood disease that is more severe

Table 15-4.   Guidelines for preventive measures after exposure to chickenpox in the nursery or maternity ward

Types of exposure or disease	Locale of chickenpox lesions		Disposition
	Mother	Neonate	
A. Siblings at home have chickenpox when neonate and mother are ready for discharge from hospital	No	No	1. Neonate: protective isolation indicated. 2. Mother: with history of previous chickenpox, she may either remain with neonate or return to older children. Without previous history, she should remain with neonate until older siblings are no longer infectious.
B. Mother with no history of chickenpox exposed during period 6-20 days antepartum*	No	No	1. Exposed mother and infant: send home at earliest date unless siblings at home have communicable chickenpox. 2. Other mothers and infants: no special management indicated. 3. Physicians and nurses in delivery room and nursery: no precautions indicated if there is a history of previous chickenpox or zoster. In absence of history, immediate serologic testing† is indicated to determine immune status. Nonimmune personnel should be excluded from patient contact for 20 days.
C. Onset of maternal chickenpox antepartum‡ or postpartum	Yes	Yes	1. Infected mother and infant: isolate together until clinically stable, then send home. 2. Other mothers and infants: send home at earlier date. ZIG§ or immune serum globulin may be given to exposed neonates. 3. Hospital personnel: same as B-3.

From Young, N.A.: Chickenpox, measles, and mumps. In Remington, J.S., and Klein, J.O., editors: Infectious disease of fetus and newborn infant, Philadelphia, 1976, W.B. Saunders Co.
*If exposure occurred less than 6 days antepartum, mother would not be potentially infectious until at least 72 hours postpartum.
†Send serum to virus diagnostic laboratory for determination of complement-fixing (CF) antibodies or, preferably, indirect fluorescent antibodies. Personnel may continue to work for period of 9 days after exposure pending serologic results, since they are not potentially infectious during this period. CF antibodies to V-Z virus $> 1:2$ probably are indicative of immunity in the absence of recent infection caused by herpes simplex virus.
‡Considered noninfectious when no new vesicles have appeared for 72 hours, and all lesions have progressed to the stage of crusts.
§ZIG (zoster immune globulin) is available from Centers for Disease Control. Atlanta, Georgia, or from regional consultants.

Continued.

Table 15-4. Guidelines for preventive measures after exposure to chickenpox in the nursery or maternity ward—cont'd

Types of exposure or disease	Locale of chickenpox lesions		Disposition
	Mother	Neonate	
D. Onset of maternal chickenpox antepartum‡ or postpartum	Yes	No	1. Infected mother: isolate until no longer infectious.‡ 2. Infected mother's infant: administer ZIG and isolate separately from mother. Send home with mother if no lesions develop by the time mother is noninfectious. 3. Other mothers and infants: same as C-2. 4. Hospital personnel: same as B-3.
E. Congenital chickenpox	No	Yes	1. Infected infant and its mother: same as C-1. 2. Other mothers and infants: same as C-2. 3. Hospital personnel: same as B-3.

in adult life or in the neonatal period. Measles is also a disease that can be prevented by immunization. The disease is contagious from the onset of the rash. Incidence of the disease in pregnancy prior to immunization is low, 0.4/10,000 pregnancies, because most adults are immune.[72] Perinatal measles includes transplacental infection as well as disease acquired postnatally by the respiratory route. Measles acquired in the first 10 days of life may be considered transplacental. When measles occurs after 14 days, it is due to extrauterine exposure. The course of extrauterine exposure is mild. A case is described in which an infant developed the disease on the fourteenth day of age, and it had a very benign course. The infant had been nursed at the breast by his mother in whom the prodromata of measles occurred on the first day postpartum. Since secretory antibodies occur within 48 hours of onset, it is possible that the disease was mitigated by the presence of measles-specific IgA in the mother's milk.[29]

As with chickenpox, the incidence of disease postpartum is minimal. The same precautions noted in the discussion of varicella are appropriate. If the mother is exposed just before delivery, mother and infant should be isolated separately, since only half the infants will acquire the disease. If the mother and infant can be isolated together because the infant has the disease, he can be breastfed. Since specific antibodies are present in the milk in 48 hours, the value of the antibodies after that time would outweigh any theoretic risk (Tables 15-1 and 15-3). The incidence of measles in the generation just reaching the childbearing years should diminish, since they should have been immunized during childhood. Epidemics still occur where there are pockets of unimmunized individuals.

MUMPS. Mumps is also an acute generalized communicable disease. It is characterized by parotid gland swelling and involvement of other glands. It is also preventable by immunization. It is less contagious, thus more adults are still susceptible. Incidence in pregnancy is from 0.8 to 10 cases/10,000 pregnancies.[72] Mumps in pregnancy, however, is generally benign. Mumps virus has been isolated on the third postpartum day from the milk of a woman who developed parotitis 2 days antepartum.[28] She did not breastfeed, and her infant did not develop clinical mumps (Table 15-3).

Mumps is not a major hazard in newborn nurseries. A mother with the disease should be isolated from the other patients but need not be separated from her infant. Clinically apparent mumps with parotitis during the first year of life tends to be very mild. Although mastitis is a rare complication of mumps in any mature female, no data are available to suggest that the incidence is greater in lactating women. Should mumps occur, breastfeeding should continue because the exposure has already occurred during the prodromata and the IgA in the breast milk may help to mitigate the symptoms in the infant.

HEPATITIS.   The two major types of hepatitis are hepatitis A virus (HAV) and hepatitis B virus (HBV). HAV is defined as the virus that causes the short incubation form of viral hepatitis; it has also been referred to as infectious hepatitis. Its virus has not yet been isolated, although electron microscopy has identified probable virus particles.

There is no indication for use of immunoglobulin or for withholding breastfeeding in HAV. In the rare circumstance in which the mother is in an active phase of the disease with jaundice, breastfeeding might be postponed temporarily.

HBV is the virus that causes the long-incubation form of viral hepatitis. This form has also been called serum hepatitis and Australian antigen hepatitis. Most of the information available on epidemiology, immunology, mode of transmission, pathogenesis, and clinical disease is about HBV, mainly because its virus has been isolated. HAV and the immune reactions to it are considered distinct from those of HBV [11]

Transmission

Carrier state in mothers.   The chief concern here is the mode of transmission of the virus from mother to infant. The transmission of HBV from mothers whose blood contains hepatitis B surface antigen HBsAg to their infants has been described. This is called vertical transmission. It may occur transplacentally in utero, at the time of delivery, or shortly after delivery. The transmission between any two individuals who may be close contacts is termed horizontal transmission. Work in Taiwan, where hepatitis occurs in 5% to 20% of the cases (one of the highest rates in the world), showed that 51 infants of 158 carrier mothers developed antigenemia within 6 months of life. This high frequency has not been observed in other populations. When the mother had a prenatal CF titer in her serum of 1:64 for HBsAg, over 90% of the infants were positive. This appears to be vertical transmission. The high incidence of transmission of HBV in Taiwan and Japan from carrier mothers to infants suggests that the virus passes the placental barrier easily. In other countries, there has been almost no evidence (0% to 8.3%) of transplacental transmission carrier mothers with infants remaining negative (Table 15–5).

Table 15-5. Transmission of HBV from HBsAg-carrier mothers to neonates in various geographic areas

Investigator	Location	Patients studied	Number infants HBsAg-positive	Vertical transmission* (%)
Stevens (1975)	Taiwan	158	63	40
Okada (1975)	Japan	11†	8	73
Schweitzer (1973)	United States	21	1	4.8
Schweitzer (1975)	United States	36	3	8.3
Skinhoj (1972)	Denmark	36	0	0
Papaevangelou (1973)	Greece	12	1	8.3
Punyagupata (1973)	Thailand	14	0	0
Ariz (1973)	Pakistan	26	1	3.8

From Crumpacker, C.S.: Hepatitis. In Remington, J.S., and Klein, J.O., editors: Infectious disease of fetus and newborn infant, Philadelphia, 1976, W.B. Saunders Co.
*Vertical transmission means transmission from mother to infant and may occur in utero, at the time of delivery, or shortly after delivery.
†One hundred thirty-nine HBsAg-positive carrier mothers were studied, but only 11 infants participated in follow-up.

Table 15-6. Transmission of HBV from mothers with acute hepatitis B during or after pregnancy

	Investigator		
	Cossart (1974)	Merrill (1972)	Schweitzer (1973)
Acute hepatitis B during 1st and 2nd trimester			
No. of mothers	1	1	10
No. of infants	0	0	1
Transmission (%)	0	0	10
Acute hepatitis B during 3rd trimester or within 2 months postpartum			
No. of mothers	4	4	21
No. of infants	2	4	16
Transmission (%)	50	100	76

From Crumpacker, C.S.: Hepatitis. In Remington, J.S., and Klein, J.O., editors: Infectious disease of fetus and newborn infant, Philadelphia, 1976, W.B. Saunders Co.

Mothers with acute hepatitis B in pregnancy. Infants born to mothers who have acute HBsAg-positive hepatitis during the perinatal period are at greater risk for transmission (Table 15-6). Studies in the United States by Schweitzer and coworkers[54,55] on a series of mothers who developed hepatitis within 2 months of delivery suggested that three newborns developed disease transplacentally (they had positive cord bloods), but the majority were infected at birth (eight infants of seventeen mothers). None of the HBsAg-positive infants were breastfed; this excluded mother's milk as a mode of transmission in these cases. Schweitzer et al.[55] further demonstrated that the frequency of HBV transmission from mother to infant is high (76%) when the disease occurs in the third trimester or early in the postpartum period. Transmission is only 10% when the disease occurs in the first two trimesters. These data and other studies suggest that the neonate becomes infected primarily during the birth process itself. Antibody levels in the mother and cord blood are comparable. Thus it appears that the antibody crosses the placenta more easily than the virus.

Transmission via postpartum fecal-oral route.   Transmission via the fecal-oral route can occur. Hepatitis is highly contagious. HBsAg has been isolated from saliva, stool, urine, prostatic fluid, and seminal fluid. The incidence by this route, however, is small, as is demonstrated by the fact that few infants have a positive reaction when the mothers have the disease at delivery and the cord blood is negative.

Transmission via colostrum or breast milk.   HBsAg is found in breast milk, therefore transmission via the milk is possible. As noted earlier, infants of mothers with the virus in their milk but who did not breastfeed them developed virus and antibodies anyway.

Clinical management.   There is a high incidence of prematurity (35%) in infants born to mothers with hepatitis, regardless of the infection in the infant. The long-term effects of chronic neonatal HBV infections are not known. Fatal cases of neonatal hepatitis are rare (only five cases reported in the literature, all occurring in infants of carriers, with two in each of two families). Specific-antibody prophylaxis of infants born to mothers with acute HGsAg-positive hepatitis at the time of delivery appears to be effective in preventing neonatal HBV infection. Both infants of carriers and those with acute hepatitis should receive high-titer hepatitis B–immune globulin (0.25 ml of a 16% solution) or standard immune globulin (2.0 ml) given immediately after delivery.

Because HBV is highly contagious, an HBsAg-positive infant should be isolated and all secretions, excretions, and instruments handled with adequate precautions. There is a diversity of opinion regarding isolation and breastfeeding in infants or HBsAg-positive mothers. The Committee on Infectious Disease,[8] in the *1982 Red Book,* has stated that hepatitis carriers who do not have active disease at the time of birth may breastfeed their infants. Immunization is now available and should also be initiated.

There is a minority report of the committee that says that in the United States, where the risk of hepatitis is minimal, the newborn should not be jeopardized by being breastfed. In third-world countries, the risks are reversed and breastfeeding is of tremendous value to these infants.[57] The clinician will need to discuss the alternatives with the patients and make an informed decision. With hepatitis B immunoglobulin and human vaccine for hepatitis available, the risks may change in the next decade.

Toxoplasmosis

Toxoplasmosis is one of the most common infections of humans throughout the world.[49] The protozoan organism is ubiquitous in nature and is the cause of a variety of illnesses that were previously thought to be due to other agents or unknown causes. The normal host is the cat. In humans, prevalence of positive serologic test titers increases with age, indicating past exposure, and there is equal distribution in males and females in the United States, but not in Norway, El Salvador, or Poland. The risk to the fetus is related to the time when the maternal infection occurs. In the last months of pregnancy, the protozoa are most frequently transmitted to the fetus but the infection is subclinical in the newborn. Early in pregnancy, the transmission to the fetus occurs less often but does result in severe disease. Once the placenta has been infected, it remains so throughout pregnancy. *Toxoplasma gondii* have been isolated from the milk, menstrual fluid, placenta, lochia, amniotic fluid, embryo, and fetal brain in 33% of the subjects in one series.

In various animal models, the toxoplasmas have been transmitted via the milk to the suckling young. They have been isolated from colostrum as well. The newborn animals became asymptomatically infected when nursed by an infected mother when her colostrum contained *T. gondii*. Three of eighteen women were reported by Langer[31] to have *T. gondii* in their milk. Two of these mothers had negative dye tests and complement. His results have been questioned because of the inadvertent presence of pollen grains in the preparation and the confusion between specimens.

Transmission during breastfeeding in humans has not been demonstrated. It is possible that unpasteurized cow's milk could be a vehicle of transmission. The human mother, however, would provide appropriate antibodies via her milk. From this information it appears there is no evidence to support depriving the neonate of his mother's milk when the mother is known to be infected with *T. gondii*[49] (Tables 15-1 and 15-7).

Vulvovaginitis

Normally during pregnancy there is an increase in cervical and vaginal secretions. Only about 1% of women have symptomatic vulvovaginitis.[6] The normal flora of the vagina at a pH of 4.5 includes predominantly Döderlein's bacilli with some bacteroides, enterococci, group B β-hemolytic streptococci, diphtheroid organisms, or coliform bacteria. Vaginitis is identified when there is inflammation and discharge associated with an alkaline pH and absence of Döderlein's bacilli. The usual pathogens are *Trichomonas vaginalis* and *Candida albicans*.

MONILIAL VULVOVAGINITIS. Monilial vulvovaginitis is usually bothersome but be-

Table 15-7. Outcome of 180 pregnancies in which maternal toxoplasmosis was acquired during gestation: incidence of symptomatic congenital toxoplasmosis among offspring surviving the early newborn period

Newborn	Number (%)	Percentage of total newborns
Not infected	110	61
Infected	64	36
Clinically normal	46* (72)	26
Clinically abnormal	18 (28)	10
Mild disease	11† (17)	6
Severe disease	7‡ (11)	4
Neonatal deaths	6§	3

Adapted from Desmonts, G., and Couvreur, J.: Bull. N.Y. Acad. Med. **50:**146, 1974; from Remington, J.S., and Desmonts, G.: Toxoplasmosis. In Remington, J.S., and Klein, J.O., editors: Infectious disease of fetus and newborn infant, Philadelphia, 1976, W.B. Saunders Co.
*Seven not examined until 14 to 45 months postpartum.
†Ten with isolated ocular lesions discovered during systematic fundus examinations; one had isolated intracranial calcifications.
‡Five with involvement of eye and central nervous system present at birth; two with delayed onset of disease.
§Two had generalized toxoplasmosis; four fetuses were lost to examination.

nign, except during pregnancy and lactation, when it is difficult to treat. The infant may become infected coming through the birth canal. The infection is manifested in the newborn as an oral infection, or thrush. The breastfed infant may transmit the oral infection to the breast and then the infection is passed back and forth unless both mother and infant are adequately treated. *C. albicans,* the causative organism, is a fungus, which thrives on milk in the breast or in the mouth. Early lesions in a newborn who is bottle fed can be treated by rinsing the mouth with water after each feeding so there are no curds on which the fungi can thrive. Water treatment is effective in early mild cases. Sodium bicarbonate should not be recommended because of the risk of hypernatremia. Sodium bicarbonate is not more effective than plain water. Furthermore, solutions mixed at home tend to be supersaturated, which further predisposes the infant to increased sodium intake. When the infant is breastfed, however, it is important to be vigorous with treatment immediately in an effort to avoid a chronic *Candida* infection of the breast.

The recommended treatment for the infant is rinsing his mouth with water after each feeding and giving 1 ml of nystatin (Mycostatin) suspension carefully by dropper onto the oral lesions. This treatment should be used for 2 weeks, even if the mouth appears to have cleared before the fourteenth day. The major reason for apparent relapse is that therapy is terminated as soon as the caseous plaques seem to disappear. Simultaneous treatment of the mother should include the use of nystatin ointment to both nipple and areola areas after each feeding and appropriate washing each day. The absorbent pads the mother uses in her nursing brassiere should be changed with each feeding and be of the disposable variety.

If this infant also is given a rubber nipple or uses a pacifier, these should be boiled daily for 20 minutes and discarded after a week of therapy and new ones used. Reseeding can occur from other articles that are placed in the mouth. Properly treated, thrush should not be a cause for weaning from the breast.

TRICHOMONAS VAGINALIS INFECTION.   A common cause of vaginitis is the parasite, *T. vaginalis,* which usually causes an asymptomatic infection in both male and female. The parasite is found in 10% to 25% of women in the childbearing years. It is transmitted predominantly by sexual intercourse. Symptoms are common in pregnancy when the infection is more difficult to cure. There is some evidence that growth of the parasite is enhanced by estrogens. It is more difficult to treat in women taking oral contraceptives. The difficulty encountered in lactation stems from the fact that the drugs of choice are contraindicated for the infant during lactation. The organism has not been identified as a particular threat to the neonate who is otherwise healthy. The treatment of choice is metronidazole (Flagyl). Metronidazole, however, does appear in the breast milk with milk levels paralleling serum levels. Severe systemic reactions occur, including headache, nausea, vomiting, and diarrhea, when metronidazole is taken in conjunction with alcohol. Leukopenia and neurologic symptoms have been described in adults who take metronidazole. Concern has been expressed because of the tumorgenicity in laboratory animals. On the other hand, metronidazole is given to children with serious infections with sensitive parasites such as amebiasis. It is recommended, therefore, that the use of metronidazole be limited to those patients in whom local palliative treatment has been inadequate. The peak serum levels occur about 1 hour after oral ingestion; therefore therapy, which is usually given three times a day, should be timed so that the peak serum levels occur between nursings. Roughly, three times a day would be after alternate feedings. An alternative approach would be to pump the breasts for the week of therapy. It should be pointed out again that the infant who is solely breastfed is at greater risk than the older infant who is getting other nourishment (Chapter 11). Thus the older infant (over 6 months of age) may not get much drug when doses are carefully timed.

Parasites

Information is emerging on the protective qualities of human milk in the face of parasitic infections in the mother. Parasites have been a serious problem in underdeveloped countries because they cause debilitation in any victim and growth failure in the young. Actually parasitic disease is increasing in industrial countries. *Giardia lamblia* is one of the more frequent infestations and is the cause of some diarrheas and malabsorption syndromes. It has been shown by Gillin[15] that human milk from uninfected donors has antiparasitic activity and this activity is not from specific antibodies but from lipase enzymatic activity, which acts in the presence of bile salts to destroy the trophozoites as they emerge from their cysts in the intestinal tract.

Giardia have also been reported to appear in mother's milk, and the parasite has been transmitted to newborns via that route. The interrelationships of the parasite and the breastfed host continue to be studied.

MATERNAL PROBLEMS
Pituitary disorders

PERSISTENT LACTATION DUE TO HYPERPITUITARY ACTIVITY. After an infant stops breastfeeding it is not unusual for the mother to be able to express milk from the breasts for many weeks, although spontaneous flow ceases in 14 to 21 days. Postlactation milk is partially a function of the length of established lactation. When spontaneous lactation persists for more than 3 months after the infant has stopped nursing, some thought should be given to the cause. The physician should evaluate the mother to make a specific diagnosis. Galactorrhea is characterized by spontaneous milky, multiple-duct, bilateral nipple discharge. It is thought to be due to increased prolactin production, either by the pituitary or by removal of hypothalamic inhibition.[67] Pituitary adenomas are not an uncommon cause. Galactorrhea can occur with normal ovulatory function for 1 or more years postpartum if everything else appears normal. More complex disorders are rare and are usually named for the physician who first described them.

Some drugs can cause galactorrhea. These include phenothiazines, tricyclic antidepressants, rauwolfia alkaloids, theophylline, amphetamines, methyldopa, and even some contraceptives.

Chiari-Frommel syndrome.   Patients with persistent postpartum or postlactation lactation extending over months or years should be evaluated for Chiari-Frommel syndrome, especially if there are abnormal menses. Often there will have been irregular menses before the pregnancy as well. The galactorrhea will occur whether the mother breastfeeds or does not breastfeed. The clinical manifestations of Chiari-Frommel syndrome are not only persistent lactation with possible breast engorgement, but also oligomenorrhea or amenorrhea, obesity, uterine and ovarian failure, and in some cases hypothyroidism. Spontaneous remission within 5 years occurs in 40% of cases.

Other possible causes of galactorrhea include other hypothalamoadenohypophyseal disorders including infection and trauma, ectopic production of lactogenic hormone as in hypernephroma, or end-organ hypersensitivity to prolactin.

Hyperprolactinemic women do not respond to breast stimulation with a rise in prolactin as breastfeeding women do. The hyperprolactinemic patient has no acute response to suckling in her growth hormone levels either, indicating that the central dopaminergic tonus was not altered but shows regulatory dysfunction.

SHEEHAN'S SYNDROME/HYPOPITUITARISM.   Sheehan's syndrome is due to postpartum hemorrhage of such severe degree that it leads to pituitary thrombotic infarction and necrosis. It occurs in 0.01% to 0.02% of postpartum women. Secretion of pituitary hormones including prolactin is usually deficient, and thus the patient may fail to lactate postpartum; this is considered to be a key clinical sign of the syndrome. There have been reports of women with Sheehan's syndrome who do lactate, but the diagnosis had to be established by other means. This is believed to be due to the pituitary lactotropes, which have compensatory activity of hypothalamoadenohypophyseal function.[67] Usually cases manifest hyposecretion of all pituitary hormones, with decreased thyroid and adrenal function. They may experience oligomenorrhea or amenorrhea and utero-ovarian atrophy. Often the obstetric crisis that caused the hemorrhage has also required hysterectomy, however, and these findings are obscured.

Maternal diabetes

Pregnancy has become a more common event in the well-controlled diabetic, and fertility rates compare with those of nondiabetics. Much has been said about labor and delivery in the diabetic and almost nothing about lactation in these mothers. Textbooks on diabetes often do not mention lactation except those written prior to 1960, perhaps reflecting the national trends away from breastfeeding. A mother, although diabetic, should be offered the same opportunity to breastfeed that is offered to all patients unless her disease has so incapacitated her that any stress is out of the question.

Brudenell and Beard[5] indicate that when the diabetic infant's progress is uneventful and he can be treated normally, there is no contraindication to breastfeeding. They believe that lactation is more difficult in diabetic mothers, perhaps as a result of operative delivery or the need to keep the infant in a special care unit for the first few days of life.

During the last stages of pregnancy in normal women, there is a more or less constant excretion of lactose in the urine, with the height reached on the day of delivery. Following delivery, the lactose excretion immediately drops to a low level where it remains for from 2 to 5 days, followed by a sudden large excretion of lactose in the normal woman. Lactosuria in the diabetic may lead to diagnostic confusion. It occurs normally late in pregnancy and in the postpartum period before the infant takes much milk, if the mother does not nurse, or if the supply of milk exceeds the requirement of the infant. Lactose reabsorbed from the breasts is excreted in the urine.

In the diabetic lactating woman, the concentration of lactose in the breast milk remained remarkably constant despite very marked elevations or depressions of the blood glucose concentration, according to Joselin and associates.[23] During lactation, lactosuria occurs physiologically and must be distinguished from glucosuria. Lactation is recorded by Wilder[72] as decreasing the blood sugar level. The sparing effect of lactation on the insulin requirement has been observed by many, including Joselin et al.[23] The depression of the level of the blood sugar in normal nursing diabetic women may lead to hypoglycemic symptoms. The simultaneous lactosuria may be misdiagnosed as glucosuria and excessive insulin be taken. The improved tolerance has been explained by the transference of sugar from the blood to the breast for conversion to galactose and lactose. Joselin and colleagues[23] report that the majority of patients at the Joselin Clinic, as well as those at Johns Hopkins Hospital, breastfeed in whole or in part. They recommend the increased administration of the B vitamins for the diabetic during lactation, based on work by Tarr and McNeile.[63]

DIET FOR THE LACTATING DIABETIC. Although it is clearly demonstrated that all lactating mothers have an increased energy requirement, it is critical to the diabetic to identify this need and provide for it in dietary adjustments. The 300 kcal required by the infant initially means at least 500 to 800 additional kcal in the mother's diet. Since the milk is synthesized from maternal stores and substrates, the plasma glucose levels in the lactating diabetic will be lower. The daily maternal insulin requirement is usually much less. The balance is a significant one between the needs of the infant and the energy and nutrition production in the mother. Most postpartum women, including the diabetic, have fat stores developed during pregnancy in preparation by the body for lactation. The diabetic, when balancing diet and insulin, needs to consider that the course of lactation mobilizes these fat stores as substrate for the mammary gland. It has been recommended by Tyson[64] that the diet include no less than 100 g of carbohydrate and 20 g of protein. This will permit the continued mobilization of fat stores to produce the glucose needed for mother and milk. When a diabetic increases fat metabolism, there is always the risk of ketonemia and ketonuria. This indicates a need for increased kilocalories in both the diabetic and the nondiabetic. With some careful observations of blood and urine sugar levels and anticipatory guidance, lactation can be managed without hypoglycemia or hyperglycemia.

ADJUSTMENTS TO LACTATION FOR THE DIABETIC.   The literature is singularly devoid of any specific discussion of the management of lactation for the diabetic with the notable exception of a personal experience recorded by Miller.[37] Miller points out that management depends on the classification of the diabetes.

The mild, or class A, diabetic whose condition can be controlled by diet alone will have to modify her diet to include the increased caloric needs, taking adequate protein, in particular. It has been stated by O'Brien[45] and Vorherr[67] that little or no tolbutamide or other antidiabetic agents appear in breast milk. It should be noted, however, that most diabetic specialists believe there is no place for these oral medications in females in the childbearing years. The mother with insulin-dependent diabetes will usually be able to increase her diet and maintain her insulin level, although some may find insulin requirements will be reduced also. Monitoring blood sugars and acetone will be necessary at first to achieve the correct balance.

Although hypoglycemia does not cause a reduction in lactose in the milk, the phenomenon of hypoglycemia itself will cause increased secretion of epinephrine in insulin shock. The epinephrine will inhibit milk production and the ejection reflex. Miller[37] points out the necessity of using a method of testing the urine that measures only glucose, such as Tes-Tape.* Otherwise the physiologic lacturia may cause inappropriate conclusions as to insulin requirements. Acetone signals a need for increased calories and carbohydrate. In addition, elevated acetone can cause increased acetone in the milk itself, which is a stress to the newborn liver. If one merely increases insulin to clear the acetone, it may predispose the patient to hypoglycemia. Each mother will identify the point below which she cannot reduce her insulin dosage without producing acetonuria.

Usually the insulin requirements are proportional to needs during pregnancy. One who takes large doses may even have to drop the dose by 50% and increase her dietary intake 100%. While the infant is nursing exclusively at the breast, adjustment is usually smooth. Weaning may present some need for day-to-day adjustment, since the amount of milk taken by the infant varies. Many infants take more 1 day and less the next, and it is less predictable. If blood sugars cannot be controlled by diet during this time, then insulin will have to be decreased. If the weaning is gradual and continuous, the adjustment will be similar.

SPECIAL FEATURES OF LACTATION FOR THE DIABETIC.   Some diabetics enjoy a postpartum remission of their diabetes that may be minimal or complete. The remission may last through lactation; it may last several years. This remission has been attributed to the hormone interactions that affect the hypothalamus and pituitary gland during pregnancy, labor, delivery, and lactation. Many diabetics report a feeling of well-being during lactation.

---

*Tes-Tape is manufactured by the Lilly Co.

Diabetics are prone to infection, and therefore mastitis presents a particular problem. With careful anticipatory care, avoidance of fatigue, and antibiotics for at least 10 days when indicated, mastitis should not pose a threat. Monilial infections are more common because of the glucose-rich vaginal secretions, and most diabetic women are alert to the early signs of a fungal vaginitis. Infection of the nipples can also occur due to *C. albicans,* even though the infant does not have obvious thrush. Early specific treatment with nystatin ointment to the breast and nystatin suspension for the infant whenever sore nipples do not respond to the usual nonspecific treatment is recommended. Treatment of both mother and infant simultaneously is necessary or they will reseed each other.

The advantages of breastfeeding to the diabetic beyond the experience of nurturing and nourishing include the advantages of transient amenorrhea. The decrease or absence of menstrual bleeding preserved iron stores. In addition, it keeps chances of pregnancy minimal as the postpartum infertility of the lactating diabetic is thought to be more consistent and predictable than in the nondiabetic. Miller concludes, "The diabetic mother who chooses to nurse her baby presents a situation about which little is known. In addition to the usual advantages that nursing affords the baby, it is highly beneficial to the mother because lactation is an antidiabetogenic factor. The metabolic process of milk production and lactose supply added to the hormone balance during lactation serves to improve the health of the diabetic mother on both the clinical and physical levels. The chief problem to overcome is adjusting the diet and insulin to correspond with the mother's requirements during this remission."[37]

Infants of diabetics present a special problem in breastfeeding, as noted by Lubchenco,[33] because they are often premature, frequently have respiratory distress syndrome and hyperbilirubinemia, and may be poor feeders at first. Hypoglycemia is the immediate problem and its management may initially preclude dependency on breast milk as the sole source of nourishment. Since less than half do develop problems, many need not be separated from their mothers. For those requiring special or intensive care, lactation may have to be postponed briefly, depending on the infant's status.

The hypoglycemia of the infant of a diabetic occurs early and is proportional to the level of hyperglycemia in the mother at the time of delivery. Cord blood sugar and Dextrostix at ½ and 1 hour of age will give the curve of glucose disappearance and potential for hypoglycemia. If lactation can be established, the glucose can be managed by breastfeeding but it must be closely monitored so that intervention can be initiated when necessary. There is also a high incidence of hypocalcemia in infants of diabetic mothers; however, phosphorus and calcitonin levels are normal, which is believed to be due to functional hypoparathyroidism.[43] The role of magnesium in this balance has not been clearly defined.

Thyroid disease

The thyroid gland is intimately involved with hormone activity of pregnancy. The metabolic and hormonal demands of pregnancy alter the thyroid gland. Conversely, the outcome of pregnancy may be altered by changes in the thyroid gland. The thyroxine-binding globulin increases secondary to the increased estrogens. The normal pregnant woman may be euthyroid, yet there are changes in the basal metabolic rate, radioactive iodine uptake, and thyroid size.

Thyroid disease is four times more common in women than men and thyroid abnormality is common in pregnancy. The diagnosis is more difficult to make during pregnancy because of problems with the interpretation of thyroid function tests. Treatment must take into account the presence of the fetus once the management decision is made.

MATERNAL HYPOTHYROIDISM.   It has long been held that hypothyroidism is associated with infertility. There is a low incidence of hypothyroidism during pregnancy. Because of the difficulty in maintaining pregnancy in hypothyroid individuals, the number of women who are truly hypothyroid at delivery is also low. There are women who are maintained on thyroid treatment for one reason or another who do have children. If hypothyroidism is diagnosed, it should be treated with full replacement therapy equivalent to 3 grains of desiccated thyroid daily. The medication should be continued after delivery. The mother should be permitted to breastfeed without question. Previous reports have indicated that thyroid does not appear in human milk. Data from Bode et al.[4] indicate there is measurable thyroid in the milk of normal women. In any event, breastfeeding is not contraindicated. If the mother is truly hypothyroid, particular care should be used to rule out hypothyroidism in the infant, using neonatal screening with thyroxine (T_4) and thyroid-stimulating hormone (TSH) if necessary. Diagnosis can be performed by evaluating blood values and is not a hazard to the nursling.[65]

HYPERTHYROIDISM.   The diagnostic procedures and therapeutic management of the mother with possible hyperthyroidism presents some hazards to the breastfed infant. The diagnosis can be made without radioactive material. The combination of an elevated serum T_4 and a normal resin triiodothyronine (T_3) uptake is helpful. These two determinations can be combined to obtain a free T_4 index, which reflects these determinations in a single value. Whether the patient is operated on eventually or not, her thyrotoxicosis must first be medically stabilized.

The treatment includes antithyroid medication with thiourea compounds, which inhibit the synthesis of thyroid hormone by blocking iodination of the tyrosine molecule. Propylthiouracil (PTU) and methimazole (Tapazole) are the treatments of choice for the mother. The major difficulty in their use in pregnancy is that PTU may cause fetal goiter and possibly hypothyroidism. The goiter is thought to be the result of inhibition of fetal thyroid hormone production by PTU with resulting increase in fetal TSH and thyroid gland enlargement. In 41 pregnancies in 30 patients receiving antithyroid medication, five infants developed goiters. Goiter development was not dose related. It has been recommended that the maternal therapy also include desiccated thyroid on the basis that the various components of thyroid metabolism cross the placenta at different rates.[6]

The lactating mother presents a somewhat similar problem. Vorherr[68] reported 4.5% to 6% of PTU appears in breast milk, which could become an undesirable cumulative dose when the infant is nursed six to eight times per day. Reevaluation of the levels of PTU in milk were reported by Kampmann et al.,[26] who calculated that minimal amounts reach the milk. They found no evidence of effect in the infants with careful follow-up with T_4 and TSH measurements. It has been suggested that the infant can be breastfed and monitored biochemically. Now that microtechniques are available for determining T_3, T_4, and TSH levels, monitoring should not be a technical problem.[65] Physical examination would reveal bradycardia or other signs of hypothyroidism and goiter. It has also been suggested that the infant may be given 0.125 to 0.25 grain of thyroid daily. Certainly this situation should be under close medical surveillance and continually monitored by microanalysis. The clinical judgment rests with the physician as to whether sufficient medication is reaching the infant. The older infant (over 6 months of age) who is getting other diet such as solids would be at less risk than the newborn, who depends solely on breast milk.

Cystic fibrosis

Patients with cystic fibrosis are living longer and enjoying more stable lives as diagnostic and therapeutic advances in the disease continue. Reports have appeared indicating that a number of women with cystic fibrosis have become pregnant and have delivered normal infants. A case was reported of such a mother who had high sodium levels (132 and 280 mEq/L) in her milk. It happens that this mother had not been breastfeeding and expressed her milk for the studies only. As pointed out by Alpert and Cormier,[1] milk from involuting breasts is different and sodium may be closer to serum levels. Since that time, Welch et al.[70] reported one case and Alpert and Cormier[1] reported two cases of successful breastfeeding with maternal cystic fibrosis. Sodium and chloride levels in the milks were normal. These studies demonstrate that mothers with pulmonary and pancreatic disease of cystic fibrosis can breastfeed and their infants do well. It is appropriate, however, to test milk samples occasionally for sodium and chloride.

Malignancy and other situations requiring radioactive exposure

The treatment of a lactating woman with malignancy may well necessitate the use of radioactive compounds for diagnosis and treatment or the use of antimetabolites. Since the breast is a minor route of excretion for most of these compounds, it is probably inappropriate to continue nursing during such exposure. Although the dose of the material in a single aliquot of milk may be small, the effects are cumulative (Appendix F). There are no long-range studies to indicate the outcome of offspring exposed in utero. In addition, a mother with malignancy should be encouraged to spare all her resources to overcome the disease. Lactation is as draining in such a situation as pregnancy.

Diagnostic or therapeutic measures using radioactive materials are contraindicated in pregnancy and lactation, since they tend to accumulate in the fetoneonatal thyroid and the maternal breast. If radioactive testing is deemed essential before treatment can be carried out, a test dose of ^{131}I can be given and breastfeeding discontinued for 48 hours. The validity of the test during lactation has been questioned because the mammary gland may divert a disproportionate amount of ^{131}I to the milk. The milk should be expressed during the 48-hour period and discarded.[69]

An additional question about the young cancer patient is what additional risk lactation adds to long-range prognosis of the mother. The automatic response tends to be not to become pregnant and, in any event, not to breastfeed. This question was examined by Hornstein et al.,[19] who indicate that "the current data suggest that pregnant women with early breast carcinoma may be treated in the same way as nonpregnant women without affecting the pregnancy." The disease that is detected toward the end of pregnancy may be treated with surgery immediately and then the patient may receive adjuvant therapy if indicated after delivery. Advanced disease should be treated aggressively and the infant delivered and not breastfed. During lactation, the diagnosis of breast carcinoma requires the immediate suppression of lactation by medications other than estrogens. The carcinoma is then treated by standard methods. When a woman has already had a radical mastectomy for breast cancer, she can have subsequent pregnancies but they should be delayed until the period of greatest risk is over (i.e., at least 3 to 5 years). She may also breastfeed.

The authors report that 7% of fertile women have one or more pregnancies after mastectomy.[25] Seventy percent of these pregnancies have occurred within 5 years after treatment. Women who have pregnancies after potentially curative mastectomy have survival rates of 5 to 10 years—as good or better than those who do not become pregnant. The patients with the best prognosis, however, may be a function of selection because they are healthier and thus able to become pregnant. Uneventful pregnancy does not guarantee cure, although the highest rate of recurrence is in the first 3 years and gradually declines. It is never zero. Metastases to the axilla increase the risk. Recurrence in the chest wall during pregnancy can be treated with local shielded radiation, but anything more extensive requires aggressive intervention. The importance of careful monitoring during pregnancy is obvious. One of the major contributors to a more grave prognosis of the original disease that appears during pregnancy and lactation is not the underlying disease, but the difficulty detecting the lesion during pregnancy and lactation and the reluctance of patient and doctor to make a diagnosis and initiate treatment. The greatest risk of neoplastic growth occurs in the first 20 weeks of pregnancy, when the immune system is suppressed and growth of the mammary tissues is at its peak under the stimulus from estrogen, progesterone, and prolactin levels.[32] The authors give no data on the influence of postmastectomy lactation on long-range survival. There are women who have wished to nurse on the remaining breast. The decision would necessitate consideration of the individual situation. It represents a different risk/benefit ratio than pregnancy itself. Extensive epidemiologic studies of large populations of women do not show any evidence that breastfeeding has any relationship to the overall risk of breast cancer. Epidemiologic data about breastfeeding on the remaining breast are not available.[32] The incidence of cancer in the remaining breast has fueled the question of prophylactic contralateral mastectomy. The women who are at greatest risk for cancer in the second breast are those who have a family history of breast cancer in their mother or sister, who have had onset in childbearing years, or whose original cancer involved multiple lesions in the primary breast. In their discussion of the other breast, Leis and Urban[32] state that if a postmastectomy patient were to become pregnant and deliver, "it would be rare indeed that the patient would allow or the attending physician would condone the use of the remaining breast for nursing." Although some women cherish the remaining breast, most in the experience of Leis Urban are ashamed of it and keep it hidden.

Renal transplantation

Pregnancy following renal transplant is relatively safe when renal function is adequate before conception and when maintenance immunosuppressive therapy is instituted. Most patients receive azathioprine and prednisone or methylprednisolone. Breastfeeding has been discouraged because of the effect of these medications on the infant especially from the major metabolite of azathioprine, 6-mercaptopurine. The actual levels of these compounds were studied in two patients, one of whom breastfed her infant.[10] Measurements of IgA were also done because of the concept that immunosuppressed women might produce immunoincompetent milk.

The levels of 6-mercaptopurine averaged 3.4 ng/ml in one patient and 18 ng/ml in the other. The therapeutic level is 50 ng/ml with the use of the normal daily dose. The levels of methylprednisolone in the milk (daily dose 6 mg) were at or below the levels measured in normal drug-free controls. The IgA determination in the milk was similar in both transplant and control mothers. The breastfed infant whose mother had a transplant had normal blood cell counts, no increase in infections, and an above-average growth rate.

Smoking

Mothers who smoke choose bottle feeding more frequently than women who do not smoke. Of those smokers who are breastfeeding on discharge from the hospital, more have discontinued breastfeeding by 6 weeks than those who do not smoke.[34]

The pharmacologic effects of nicotine have been studied in the fetuses of experimental animals. The active components of cigarette smoke, nicotine and carbon monoxide, have been implicated in the birth-weight reduction seen in infants of mothers who are heavy smokers. Nicotine has acetylcholine-like actions on the CNS, skeletal muscle, and upper sympathetic and parasympathetic ganglia. Nicotine initially stimulates and then depresses. Nicotine has been shown to interfere with the let-down reflex, but it does not appear to disrupt lactation once it has been initiated. Smoking has been associated with a poor milk supply. It has been reported that women who smoke 10 to 20 cigarettes a day have 0.4 to 0.5 mg of nicotine/L in their milk. Calculations indicate this is equivalent to a dose of 6 to 7.5 mg of nicotine in an adult. In an adult, 4 mg of nicotine has produced symptoms, and the lethal dosage is in the range of 40 to 60 mg for adults. On the basis of gradual intake over a day's time the neonate would metabolize it in the liver and excrete the chemical through the kidney. Low-grade responses to nicotine would be subtle in the neonate and require specific monitoring to detect.

When a group of lactating women who smoked more than 15 cigarettes a day were compared with lactating women who did not smoke at all, the basal prolactin levels were significantly lower in smokers, but suckling induced acute increments in serum prolactin and oxytocin-linked neurophysin were not influenced.[2] These experiments showed no influence on oxytocin when two cigarettes were smoked before a feeding. Serum nicotine and plasma epinephrine but not dopamine or norepinephrine were significantly increased in the mothers during smoking. The smokers weaned their babies more quickly than nonsmokers.[34] The heavy smokers had the lowest prolactin levels and weaned earliest.

In counseling the nursing mother who smokes, consideration should be given to the data. The data suggest that mothers should not smoke while nursing, or at least until they have initiated let-down, that they should not blow smoke in the infant's face, and that they should be cautious about the hot ashes. If it is not possible to stop, they should cut down and also consider low-nicotine cigarettes.

If the mother smokes marijuana, an entirely different risk is created. Animal studies have shown that structural changes occur in the brain cells of newborn animals nursed by mothers whose milk contained cannabis. Nahas et al.[38,39] describe impairment of DNA and RNA formation and of proteins essential for proper growth and development. Results seen in some humans suggest that serious and long-lasting effects can occur. Impairment of judgment and behavioral changes may actually interfere with an individual's ability to care for the infant or adequately breastfeed. If the mother smokes while nursing, there is not only the drug in her milk but the effect of the smoke that the infant inhales from the environment. Since brain cell development is still taking place in the first months of life, any remote chance that DNA and RNA metabolism is altered should be viewed with concern.

The mother who requires hospitalization

EMERGENCY ADMISSION. The mother who suddenly develops an emergency condition that requires hospitalization presents a unique problem in management. It is patently obvious that the emergency condition must be dealt with appropriately medically, surgically, or psychiatrically. It is equally important in all three situations to deal with her as a lactating mother, since failure to do so may have an impact on the successful outcome of the primary condition.

Medical admission. Medical problems such as acute infection or metabolic disturbances should be analyzed in relationship to lactation and to the infant and, in addition, to any other children at home. Is it contagious? In the case of lactation, will the drugs pass into the breast milk? If so, are there alternative treatments? What is the prognosis for recovery? Is the recovery phase less than 2 weeks and is maintaining lactation justified? This decision should not be made in the abstract without an understanding of the mother's commitment to further breastfeeding. If the prognosis is poor for recovery or the drugs involved are contraindicated for the infant but necessary for the mother, provision should be made for the mother's adjusting. It should be kept in mind that abrupt cessation of lactation can cause a flulike syndrome, which will confuse the management picture. It may be advisable to include the mother's obstetrician or pediatrician in the discussion to provide the mother with the necessary support to accept alternatives (Chapter 11).

Surgical admission.   Surgical emergencies such as trauma, appendicitis, or chylocystitis will require immediate attention, including anesthesia and surgery. If it is a self-limited disease with a short postoperative course, as in appendicitis, the mother can go back to breastfeeding on her return home. If the hospitalization will be more prolonged, as in trauma with immobilizing fractures, different considerations are important. It is possible to have the infant brought to the hospital several times a day for nursing. Unless the mother is mobile enough to provide some of the infant's bedside care, rooming-in is too taxing to the recovering patient. It is also stressful to other patients and staff who are not equipped for neonates. The mother would require a single room. If she has provision for her own nursing care or if the nursing staff is agreeable, an arrangement could be worked out. The only contraindication would be whether it would interfere with recovery. When bone healing is important, attention should be given to the dietary demands of bone healing and lactation, especially in calcium, phosphorus, and vitamin intakes. If the mother is to be cared for but immobilized at home, nursing is easier but provision for ample assistance would be mandatory. The needs for assistance would not differ for the breastfed or bottle fed infant of the same age.

Psychiatric admission.   The onset of a psychiatric crisis in a lactating mother is rarely a problem unless the mother has already been identified as having a psychiatric problem. Childbirth has an established etiologic role in postpartum psychosis. There is a report in the literature, however, of a case of mania precipitated in a mother each time she weaned her children from the breast but at no other time. We had treated a patient with a known psychiatric disorder who decompensated during pregnancy, did well during lactation, and had difficulty after weaning. With her fourth child, she weaned abruptly at 3 months and committed suicide 2 weeks later.

As the number of women who breastfeed increases, there will be increased understanding of the relationship of these physiologic events to psychiatric disease. The role of the mother in lactation will be a part of her psychiatric care, and the decision to breastfeed or not should be worked out with her psychiatrist. Most psychiatric wards can accommodate young infants whether they are breastfed or bottle fed, so it is less of a novelty than on the medical and surgical wards. The management of postpartum psychosis includes the concerns of the mother caring for the infant as part of recovery. The drugs used when the mother is nursing should be appropriate for both mother and nursing infant.

ELECTIVE MATERNAL ADMISSION TO THE HOSPITAL.   There are occasions when a lactating mother may have to plan for hospitalization. The urgency will be determined by the underlying disease. If the admission date can be made for over a month away, there is time for gradual weaning of the infant if this is necessary. If weaning is appropriate and/or necessary, the impact will largely be determined by the age of the infant. A very young infant who would profit greatly by continued breastfeeding is one type of problem. If the child is a year old, it may be less traumatic for him to be weaned when the separation time is going to be greater than 48 to 72 hours. A child who is also receiving solids and some other liquids from a cup can sustain himself during the separation without much more than sadness. If the caretaker and the surroundings are familiar, the support of this infant is easier. For the mother of the older child the impact of forced separation during hospitalization is also easier and less likely to produce "milk fever."

The young infant can be sustained by bottle feedings or "cross-nursing" by another lactating mother until he can be breastfed by his own mother again. The mother in the first few months of lactation will have more problems with engorgement, discomfort, and even malaise. Provision should be made to express or pump milk to maintain the supply if the mother will be nursing again or pumping minimally for comfort if lactation is to be discontinued. Milk can be collected in sterile bottles and sent home for the infant. When the admission is elective, plans can be made in advance to have a pump available, renting one if the hospital is not equipped. Methods for collecting, refrigerating, and getting milk home to the infant can be planned along with her other needs, such as a baby-sitter.

During an elective admission for a self-limited disease, rooming-in for the infant may be possible if the circumstances of the illness permit. It should be pointed out that the prime purpose of the hospitalization is to treat an illness. If surgery is involved, rooming-in should not be a stress to the mother when she is in the operating room, in the recovery room, or heavily medicated.

The purpose of this section is to point out that it is possible to maintain lactation when hospitalization is necessary for the mother. It is possible to have the infant accompany the mother or vice versa in a rooming-in arrangement. The theoretic threat of infection in the hospital setting is outweighed by the advantages of human milk in most cases. On the other hand, the decision rests with the physician in charge of the case, who will have the responsibility of looking at the total picture including the medical problem in question, the necessary treatment, and the short-range prognosis for resuming normal breastfeeding. Here again the expertise of the mother's obstetrician and the infant's pediatrician may be invaluable.

The evaluation of nipple discharge

Most nipple discharges are due to benign lesions and many do not require surgical intervention. They could, however, represent a malignant condition and deserve careful investigation. Nipple discharges associated with lactation have a different etiologic incidence profile, but they are no less significant. In general, discharge is more common in older women. Most texts discussing discharge from the nipple are written by surgeons and the distinction regarding the relationship to breastfeeding is not made.[14]

MILKY DISCHARGE. Persistent bilateral lactation is the presentation following breast-feeding and, as noted, may represent pituitary disease. If there is no surgical disease such as an adenoma, medical treatment to suppress prolactin such as estrogens is usually employed. In the nonlactating woman this finding is called galactorrhea and is a spontaneous, milky, multiduct, bilateral discharge.[47]

MULTICOLORED AND STICKY DISCHARGE. Duct ectasia, so called "comedomastitis," is the most common cause of multicolored sticky discharge.[47] It begins as a dilation of the terminal ducts and may occur during pregnancy, although is most common between the ages of 35 and 40. It is rare in virgins and most common in women who have lactated. An irritating lipid forms in the ducts producing an inflammatory reaction and nipple discharge. Cytology shows debris and epithelial cells. Duct ectasia may be associated with burning pain, itching, and swelling of the nipple and aerola. Palpation reveals a wormlike tubular feeling once called varicocele tumor of the breast. As the disease progresses, a mass may develop that mimics cancer and chronic inflammation leads to fibrosis. Surgery is not indicated unless the discharge becomes bloody. The disease is usually treated with thorough cleansing with pHisoHex or povidone-iodine (Betadine) daily and avoidance of nipple manipulation. Lactation would aggravate preexisting diseases but would not be an absolute contraindication.

PURULENT DISCHARGE. Purulent discharge is due to acute puerperal mastitis, chronic lactation mastitis, central breast abscess, or plasma cell mastitis. It is usually unilateral, involving one or two ducts. Once it is diagnosed, the treatment is with antibodies. When an abscess does not clear after cessation of lactation and adequate treatment, a biopsy should be done to rule out secondary necrosis and infection of an underlying lesion.

WATERY, SEROUS, SEROSANGUINEOUS, AND BLOODY DISCHARGES. Nipple discharges are primarily of surgical significance. They are the second most common indication for breast surgery. Watery or colorless, serous or yellow, serosanguineous or pink and sanguineous discharges are more common over the age of 50 but younger women do not escape them.[47] Bloody discharge in pregnancy and lactation is most commonly due to vascular engorgement or trauma of the breast. The next most common causes in pregnancy and lactation are intraductal papilloma (50%) and fibrocystic disease (31%). Because the type of discharge does not identify the malignant or nonmalignant nature of the problem, all patients with unusual discharge should be seen by an appropriate surgeon for diagnosis.

In intraductal papilloma, the discharge is usually spontaneous, unilateral, and from a single duct. It is occasionally associated with a nontender lump in the subareolar area. Symptoms may include bleeding, which is usually painless during pregnancy. It is possible to excise the involved duct and wedge of tissue, leaving the rest intact in order to preserve mammary function, when surgery is required for intraductal papilloma. Painless bleeding during pregnancy may be bilateral or unilateral and may cease after delivery. After serious disease has been ruled out, lactation is possible.

To be significant a discharge should be true, persistent, spontaneous, and nonlactational. Single-duct unilateral discharges are more apt to be surgically significant. A true discharge comes from a duct to the surface of the nipple. Pseudodischarges occur on the surface and may be associated with inverted nipples, eczematoid lesions, trauma, herpes simplex, infections of the Montgomery glands, and mammary duct fistulas. Discharges are more common in women taking oral contraceptives, tranquilizers, or rauwolfia and in those who are postmenopausal and menopausal. Cytologic examination should be part of any examination for an abnormal discharge from the breast, although there is a high percentage of false negatives and there are some false positives. Absence of a mass is reassuring but should not dissuade one from further diagnostic studies.

Lumps in the breast

The lactating breast is lumpy to palpation, and the lumps shift day by day. The most common cause of a persistent lump is a plugged duct (see Chapter 8); the second most common cause is a mass associated with mastitis. Lumps that persist beyond a few days and do not respond to palliative treatment deserve review.

Fibrocystic disease

Fibrocystic disease is a diffuse parenchymal process in the breasts that has many synonyms, none of which is satisfactory. The process involves hormonally produced benign proliferations of the alveolar system of varying degrees that occur in response to the normal menstrual cycle. In a full-blown case there are pain, tenderness, palpable thickenings, and nodules of varying sizes that are most symptomatic with menses. The disease is prominent in the childbearing years and regresses during pregnancy. It is not a contraindication to breastfeeding. Some women have achieved relief by totally eliminating caffeine and related products from their diet.

Breast cysts

Benign cysts of the breast are being identified in younger and younger women, probably because of the more careful self-examination of the breast now recommended. They should be removed and biopsied but do not interfere with lactation. Fibroadenomas that are due to disturbance in the normal menstrual cycle usually proliferate and regress before the age of 30. Pregnancy and lactation stimulate their growth. They are firm, smooth, lobulated masses and are freely movable without fixation. They can be diagnosed radiologically and do not interfere with lactation. They can be removed under local anesthesia if necessary without stopping breastfeeding.

Lipomas

Lipomas are very common in the breast, which has considerable fat in its stroma. They are usually solitary, asymptomatic, slowly growing, freely movable, soft, and well delineated. They can be easily identified radiologically in the lactating breast, which has less fat present.

Fat necrosis

Fat necrosis is usually associated with trauma and is caused by local destruction of fat cells with release of free lipid and variable hemorrhage. Organization with fibrosis may lead to fixation. Fat necrosis can be identified radiologically and looks like a fat density or oil cyst with a capsule.

Hematomas

Hematomas of the lactating breast may occur from trauma or in women on anticoagulant therapy. They generally regress without treatment.

Plastic surgery of the breast

AUGMENTATION MAMMOPLASTY.   Augmentation mammoplasty has become a more acceptable procedure and techniques have improved tremendously.[61] The implantation of inert material is the approach. Young women may request it and then wish to lactate. There should be no destruction of breast tissue or interruption of ducts, nerve supply, or blood supply to the gland or nipple, so that breastfeeding is possible and successful (Fig. 15-1). Injections of silicone are no longer used. The silicone did cause fibrosis and duct destruction.

Postlactation involution of a severe degree occasionally occurs. Some women note

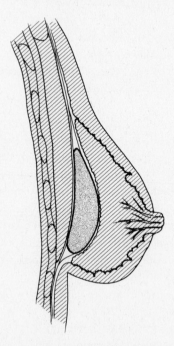

Fig. 15-1. Placement of implant in augmentation mammoplasty. There is no interruption of vital ducts, nerve supply, or blood supply.

considerable regression and seeming atrophy after weaning, which alarms them. The fat deposition has not recurred when the ducts regress. In most of these women the breasts return to their normal contour in about 3 years if there has been no further pregnancy or lactation. Loss of tissue turgor and fat padding occurs without pregnancy or lactation as well (Fig. 15-2). Certainly augmentation is possible if desired once the childbearing is completed.

REDUCTION MAMMOPLASTY.   There are women with breasts so large they cause shoulder and back pain, deep grooves in the shoulders from brassiere straps, and negative self-image. These women sometimes wish surgical correction. Reduction mammoplasty

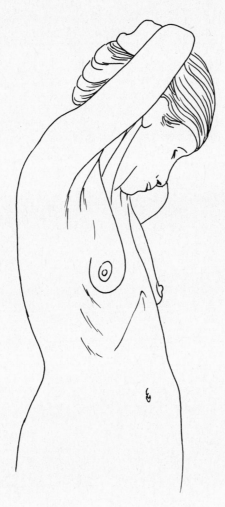

Fig. 15-2. Extreme postlactation involution.

is more destructive than augmentation because of the necessity of replacing the nipple symmetrically, which requires interrupting the ducts.[62] Although plastic surgeons report that these women do not wish to breastfeed, it is our experience that many of them do wish to breastfeed later when they bear a child and are suddenly aware of their maternal role. At the time of surgery they are consumed with their perceived affliction. The surgeon should clearly discuss the options with the patient or provide a procedure that leaves the ducts intact. If the ducts are intact, breastfeeding can be successful postoperatively.

In general, surgery of the breast for nonmalignant lesions does not preclude breastfeeding unless the ductal structure has been interrupted. Surgeons need to consider mammary function in counseling young women about breast surgery.

REFERENCES

1. Alpert, S.E. and Cormier, A.D.: Normal electrolyte and protein content in milk from mothers with cystic fibrosis: an explanation for the initial report of elevated milk sodium concentration, J. Pediatr. **102:**77, 1983.
2. Andersen, A.N., et al.: Suppressed prolactin but normal neurophysin levels in cigarette smoking breast-feeding women, Clin. Endocrinol. **17:**363, 1982.
3. Andersen, A.N. and Tabor, A.: PRL, TSH and LH responses to metoclopramide and breast feeding in normal and hyperprolactinaemic women, Acta Endocrinol. **100:**177, 1982.
4. Bode, H.H., Vonjonack, K., and Crawford, J.T.: Mitigation of cretinism by breast feeding, Pediatr. Res. **11:**423, 1977.
5. Brudenell, M., and Beard, R.: Diabetes in pregnancy, Clin. Endocrinol. Metabol. **1:**691, 1973.
6. Burrow, G.N., and Ferris, T.F.: Medical complications during pregnancy, Philadelphia, 1975, W.B. Saunders Co.
7. Committee on Fetus and Newborn/Committee on Infectious Disease, Academy of Pediatrics: Perinatal herpes simplex virus infections, Pediatrics **66:**147, 1980.
8. Committee on Infectious Disease: Report of the Committee, Red Book, ed. 19, Evanston, Ill., 1982, Academy of Pediatrics.
9. Corey, L., et al.: Genital herpes simplex virus infections: clinical manifestations, course, and complications, Ann. Intern. Med. **98:**958, 1983.
10. Coulam, C.B., et al.: Breastfeeding after renal transplantation, Transplant Proc. **14:**605, 1982.
11. Crumpacker, C.S.: Hepatitis. In Remington, J.S., and Klein, J.O., editors: Infectious disease of fetus and newborn infant, ed. 2, Philadelphia, 1976, W.B. Saunders Co.
12. Dunkle, L., Schmidt, R.R. and O'Connor, D.M.: Neonatal herpes simplex infection possibly acquired via maternal breast milk, Pediatrics **63:**250, 1979.
13. Dworsky, M., et al.: Cytomegalovirus infection of breast milk and transmission in infancy, Pediatrics **72:**295, 1983.
14. Gallager, H.S., et al.: The breast, St. Louis, 1978, The C.V. Mosby Co.
15. Gillin, F.D.: Unpublished data, 1983.
16. Glass, R.K., et al.: Protection against cholera in breast-fed children by antibodies in breast milk, N. Engl. J. Med. **308:**1389, 1983.
17. Hanshaw, J.B.: Cytomegalovirus. In Remington, J.S., and Klein, J.O., editors: Infectious disease of fetus and newborn infant, ed. 2, Philadelphia, 1976, W.B. Saunders Co.
18. Hayes, K., et al.: Cytomegalovirus in human milk, N. Engl. J. Med. **287:**177, 1972.
19. Hornstein, E., Skornick, Y., and Rozin, R.: The management of breast carcinoma in pregnancy and lactation, J. Surg. Oncol. **21:**179, 1982.
20. Huber, G.L.: Tuberculosis. In Remington, J.S., and Klein, J.O., editors: Infectious disease of fetus and newborn infant, ed. 2, Philadelphia, 1976, W.B. Saunders Co.
21. Ingall, D., and Norins, L.: Syphilis. In Remington, J.S., and Klein, J.O., editors: Infectious disease of fetus and newborn infant, ed. 2, Philadelphia, 1976, W.B. Saunders Co.
22. Jelliffe, D.B., and Jelliffe, E.F.P.: Human milk in the modern world, Oxford, 1978, Oxford University Press.

23. Joselin, E.P., et al.: The treatment of diabetes mellitus, Philadelphia, 1959, Lea & Febiger.
24. Kakkar, V.V., et al.: Low doses of heparin in prevention of deep vein thrombosis, Lancet 2:669, 1971.
25. Kalache, A., Vessey, M.P., and McPherson, K.: Lactation and breast cancer, Br. Med. J. 1:223, 1980.
26. Kampmann, J., et al.: Propylthiouracil in human milk, Lancet 1:736, 1980.
27. Kenny, J.F.: Recurrent group B streptococcal disease in an infant associated with the ingestion of infected mother's milk, J. Pediatr. 91:158, 1977.
28. Kilham, L.: Mumps virus in human milk and in milk of infected monkey, JAMA 146:1231, 1951.
29. Kohn, J.L.: Measles in newborn infants (maternal infection), J. Pediatr. 3:176, 1933.
30. Kulski, J.K., Smith, M., and Hartmann, P.E.: Normal and caesarean section delivery and the initiation of lactation in women, Aust. J. Exp. Biol. Med. Sci. 59:405, 1981.
31. Langer, H.: Repeated congenital infection with Toxoplasma gondii, Obstet. Gynecol. 21:318, 1963.
32. Leis, H.P., and Urban, J.A.: The other breast. In Gallager, H.S., et al., editors: The breast, St. Louis, 1978, The C.V. Mosby Co.
33. Lubchenco, C.O.: Infants of diabetic mothers, an editorial, Keeping Abreast J. 1:107, 1976.
34. Lyon, A.J.: Effects of smoking on breast feeding, Arch. Dis. Child. 58:378, 1983.
35. Magno, R., et al.: Anesthesia for caesarian section. IV. Placental transfer and neonatal elimination of bupivacaine following epidural anlages for elective cesarean section, Acta Anaesthesiol. Scand. 20:141, 1976.
36. Merson, M.H. et al.: Maternal cholera immunization and secretory IgA in breast milk, Lancet 1:931, 1980.
37. Miller, D.L.: The diabetic nursing mother, Keeping Abreast J. 1:102, 1976.
38. Nahas, G.G.: Marijuana, JAMA 233:79, 1975.
39. Nahas, G.G., et al.: Inhibition of cellular mediated immunity in marijuana smokers, Science 183:419, 1974.
40. Nahmias, A.J., and Visintine, A.M.: Herpes simplex. In Remington, J.S., and Klein, J.O., editors: Infectious disease of fetus and newborn infant, ed. 2, Philadelphia, 1976, W.B. Saunders Co.
41. Nahmias, A.J., Alford, C., and Korones, S.: Infection of the newborn with Herpesvirus hominis. In Schulman, I., editor: Advances in pediatrics, Chicago, 1970, Year Book Medical Publishers, Inc.
42. Neifert, M.R., McDonough, S.L., and Neville, M.C.: Failure of lactogenesis associated with placental retention, Am. J. Obstet. Gynecol. 140:477, 1981.
43. Noguchi, A., Eren, M., and Tsang, R.C.: Parathyroid hormone in hypocalcemic and normocalcemic infants of diabetic mothers, J. Pediatr. 97:112, 1980.
44. Numazaki, Y., et al.: Primary infection with human cytomegalovirus: virus isolation from healthy infants and pregnant women, Am. J. Epidemiol. 91:410, 1970.
45. O'Brien, T.E.: Excretion of drugs in human milk, Am. J. Hosp. Pharm. 31:844, 1974.
46. Paulus, D.D.: Benign diseases of the breast, Radiol. Clin. North Am. 21:27, 1983.
47. Pilnik, S., and Leis, H.P.: Nipple discharge. In Gallager, H.S., et al., editors: The breast, St. Louis, 1978, The C.V. Mosby Co.
48. Quinn, P.T., and Lofbera, J.V.: Maternal herpetic breast infection: another hazard of neonatal herpes simplex, Med. J. Aust. 2:411, 1978.
49. Remington, J.S., and Desmonts, G.: Toxoplasmosis. In Remington, J.S., and Klein, J.O., editors: Infectious disease of fetus and newborn infant, ed. 2, Philadelphia, 1976, W.B. Saunders Co.
50. Riordan, J.: A practical guide to breastfeeding, St. Louis, 1983, The C.V. Mosby Co.
51. Scalon, J.W., et al.: Neurobehavioral responses and drug concentrations in newborns after maternal epidural anesthesia with bupivacaine, Anesthesiology 45:400, 1976.
52. Schiff, G.M., Sutherland, J., and Light, L.: Congenital rubella. In Thalhammer, O., editor: Prenatal infections. International Symposium of Vienna, Sept. 2-3, 1970, Stuttgart, 1971, George Thieme Verlag.
53. Schreiner, R.L., et al.: Possible breast milk transmission of group B streptococcal infection, J. Pediatr. 91:159, 1977.
54. Schweitzer, I.L., et al.: Factors influencing neonatal infection by hepatitis B virus, Gastroenterology 65:227, 1973.
55. Schweitzer, I.L., et al.: Viral hepatitis B in neonates and infants, Am. J. Med. 55:762, 1973.
56. Shinefeld, H.R.: Staphylococcal infections. In Remington, J.S., and Klein, J.O., editors: Infec-

tious disease of fetus and newborn infant, ed. 2, Philadelphia, 1976, W.B. Saunders Co.

57. Sinata, F.R., et al.: Perinatal transmitted acute icteric hepatitis B in infants born to hepatitis B surface antigen-positive and anti-hepatitis B$_e$-positive carrier mothers, Pediatrics **70:**557, 1982.

58. Skaug, K., et al.: Chlamydial secretory IgA antibodies in human milk, Acta Pathol. Microbiol. Immunol. Scand. **90:**21, 1982.

59. Stagno, S., et al.: Breast milk and the risk of cytomegalovirus infection, N. Engl. J. Med. **302:**1073, 1980.

60. Sullivan-Bolyai, J.Z., et al.: Disseminated neonatal herpes simplex virus type I from a maternal breast lesion, Pediatrics **71:**455, 1983.

61. Synderman, R.K.: Augmentation mammoplasty. In Gallager, H.S., et al., editor: The breast, St. Louis, 1978, The C.V. Mosby Co.

62. Synderman, R.K.: Reduction mammoplasty. In Gallager, H.S., et al., editors: The breast, St. Louis, 1978, The C.V. Mosby Co.

63. Tarr, E.M., and McNeile, O.: Relation of vitamin B deficiency to metabolic disturbances during pregnancy and lactation, Am. J. Obstet. Gynecol. **29:**811, 1935.

64. Tyson, J.E.: The diabetic nursing mother, (editorial), Keeping Abreast J. **1:**106, 1976.

65. Varma, S.K., et al.: Thyroxine, tri-iodothyro-nine, and reverse tri-iodothyronine concentrations in human milk, J. Pediatr. **93:**803, 1978.

66. Vergeront, J.M., et al.: Recovery of staphylococcal enterotoxin F from the breast milk of a woman with toxic-shock syndrome, J. Infect. Dis. **146:**456, 1982.

67. Vorherr, H.: The breast, morphology, physiology, and lactation, New York, 1974, The Academic Press, Inc.

68. Vorherr, H.: Drug excretion in breast milk, Postgrad. Med. **56:**97, 1974.

69. Weaver, J.C., Kamm, M.L., and Dobson, R.L.: Excretion of radioiodine in human milk, JAMA, **172:**872, 1960.

70. Welch, M.J., Phelps, D.L. and Osher, A.B.: Breast-feeding by a mother with cystic fibrosis, Pediatrics **67:**664, 1981.

71. Whitley, R.J., et al.: The natural history of herpes simplex virus infection of mother and newborn, Pediatrics **66:**489, 1980.

72. Wilder, R.M.: Clinical diabetes mellitus and hyperinsulinism, Philadelphia, 1940, W.B. Saunders Co.

73. Young, N.A.: Chickenpox, measles, and mumps. In Remington, J.S., and Klein, J.O., editors: Infectious disease of fetus and newborn infant, ed. 2, Philadelphia, 1976, W.B. Saunders Co.

16

Human milk as a prophylaxis in allergy

THE NATURAL HISTORY OF ATOPIC DISEASE

The association of allergy with cow's milk has been documented in the literature for decades.[6,28] The incidence of this allergy in the general population has been noted to increase progressively since the original comments on the subject by Rowe[38] in 1931. The incidence has been said to have increased 10 times in 20 years and has been attributed to increased recognition, increased incidence of exposure to known allergens, and a gradual decrease in infection as a source of morbidity due to the use of antibiotics and immunization revealing an underlying allergic component to chronic symptoms. Glaser[8] attributed this rapid increase in the development of allergic diseases to the abandonment of breastfeeding when safe pasteurized milk became available. It was noted that 20% of all children were allergic by 20 years of age. Studies of office pediatrics[43] have shown that one third of the visits are due to allergy. One third of all chronic conditions under age 17 are due to allergy, and one third of the days lost from school are due to asthma. In the evaluation of 2000 consecutive unselected newborns in pediatric practice, it was found that 50% had allergic family histories. Grulee et al.[12] observed as early as 1934 that eczema was seven times more common in infants fed cow's milk than in those who were breastfed. McCombs et al.[36] reported in 1979 that asthma caused more than 2000 deaths and the loss of 94 million days of activity and initiated 183,000 hospital admissions and more than one million hospital days in 1 year in the United States alone. The disease costs the American public over a billion dollars annually.

The question of heredity

There is no question that heredity plays a part in the development of allergic disease, an observation first recorded by Maimonides in his *Treatise on Asthma* in the twelfth century. Most studies in the past 60 years have concurred with the concept of a recessive mode of inheritance.[19]

Kern[27] has noted that the outstanding etiologic factor in human hypersensitivity is heredity. He states that there are few diseases in which heredity is so clearly identified and so common.

Hamburger[7] reported that children with both parents atopic had 47% chance of developing atopic disease. When only one parent was atopic, there was a 29% chance of developing atopy; when neither parent was allergic, there was only a 13% risk of the disease. Falliers et al.,[4] in a study of asthmatic monozygotic twins, observed similar serum IgE, blood eosinophil counts, and positive skin tests to allergens in both twins, but dissimilar responses to infection and methacholine. This finding suggests there is also an acquired component to bronchial hyperactivity. There are apparently several mechanisms involved in antigen processing. To identify infants at high risk for developing atopy, several approaches have been suggested. Cord serum total IgE levels of greater than 100 U/ml are associated with five to ten times greater risk than lower levels. Eosinophilia and lymphocytes may prove to be markers, but at present only the family allergic history and the cord blood IgE have been significantly reliable predictors according to Bousquet et al.[1]

Glaser speculated in the 1930s that if a child was at high risk for developing allergy, prophylaxis should be able to change the outcome. The original work on prophylaxis was done by Glaser and Johnstone[11] and reported in 1953. Only 15% of a group of children whose mothers controlled their own diet in pregnancy and controlled the infant's diet and environment at birth did develop eczema, whereas 65% of the sibling controls and 52% of nonrelated controls receiving cow's milk developed similar allergic illnesses. Although as a retrospective study it was open to some criticism, it did begin to look at a very significant issue, that is, reducing the incidence of allergic manifestations in high-risk individuals by a new type of preventive measure.

A second study was designed in 1953 and carried out prospectively by Johnstone and Dutton[20] to investigate dietary prophylaxis of allergic disease. They observed a difference over 10 years in the incidence of asthma and perennial allergic rhinitis in those fed soybean milk (18%) and those fed evaporated milk (50%). No infant in this study of 283 children was breastfed, however. Halpern[14] reported the study of 1753 children fed breast milk, soy milk, and cow's milk from birth to 6 months of age who were followed until they were 7 years or older. The children included those with high-risk, low-risk, and no-risk family histories for allergy. They reported in 1973 no difference in outcome related to early diet. There was a relationship to the family history, however.

In a prospective study to identify the development of reaginic allergy, infants of allergic parents were placed in a study or control group. The study group followed an allergen-avoidance regimen, including breastfeeding. At 6 months and 1 year there was less eczema than the controls had had at 6 months. Lower serum total IgE levels were also reported.[33]

PROPHYLAXIS OF ATOPIC DISEASE

Efforts to alter the incidence of atopic illness have continued to challenge investigators who now have access to increased methodologic sophistication. Prevention of IgE-mediated disorders could be directed at interfering with any of the major forces responsible for the phenotypic expression of atopy. Practically, however, it is not yet possible to mask IgE genes, or manipulate cellular components of the response organ. Clinicians are limited to manipulating the effect of the environment by reducing the allergenic load.

Review of the plethora of studies directed at measuring the impact of dietary manipulations on the incidence of atopic disease demonstrates that retrospective studies show little or no difference in the incidence of asthma and eczema, whereas prospective studies tended to demonstrate a significant reduction in atopic disease in the treated group. These are summarized in Table 16-1. In looking at these data, it is important to recognize that in some studies the risk of the population developing atopic disease on a hereditary basis was not considered. In other studies, breastfeeding may have been carried out for only a few weeks or months. The evidence is clear that 6 months or longer

Table 16-1.   Prevention of atopy: prospective studies

Authors	Year	Number years followed	Number subjects*	Type feeding	Impact on atopy†
Johnstone & Dutton[20]	1953	10 yr	235	Soy-cow's milk	↓ asthma and rhinitis
Mathew et al[33]	1977	1 yr	53 (26)	Breast and soy milk	↓ eczema
Chandra[3]	1979	>24 mo	134	Breast milk	↓ eczema and asthma
Saarinen et al[39]	1979	3 yr	(256)	Breast milk	↓ eczema, food allergy, and asthma
Hamburger[17]	1981	1 yr	(300)	Breast milk	↓ eczema and asthma
Kaufman et al[25,26]	1981	2 yr	(94)	Breast milk	↓ asthma
Hide & Guyer[18]	1981	1 yr	843 (266)	Breast <6 mo, soy milk, cow's milk (maternal diet not controlled)	↓ eczema slight and rhinitis
Gruskay[13]	1982	15 yr	908 (328)	Breast milk 4 mo, soy milk, cow's milk	breast ↓ symptoms; soy no effect
May et al[34]	1982	6 mo	67 normal	Soy/cow's/modern formula	↑ antibodies no disease symptoms
Businco et al[2]	1983	2 yr	(101)	Breast milk <6 mo, soy/cow's milk	↓ asthma and eczema
Kajosaari & Saarinen[24]	1983	1 yr	(135)	All breast milk <6 mo, ½ solid foods early	↑ eczema and food intolerance in those fed solids

Modified from Busino, L., et al.: Ann. Allergy 51:206, 1983.
*Number in study; parentheses indicate number at risk for atopy.
†Arrows indicate decrease or increase compared with the control group.

of exclusive breastfeeding makes a difference. In addition, some studies did not control the breastfeeding mother's diet.

Hamburger et al.[17] carried out prospective prophylactic studies to include measuring IgE and skin radioallergosorbent test (RAST) on mother, father, and infant. They found a significant correlation between maternal IgE and infant IgE and potential allergy in the infant (Tables 16-2 and 16-3). This study had been done by controlling the environment and the diet. The process had been initiated in pregnancy to protect the fetus and continued at birth. Considerable attention, therefore, has been directed toward breastfeeding in this and other studies.

The effect of breastfeeding on allergic sensitization is both direct through the elimination of nonhuman milk protein as an exposure to antigen and indirect by affecting the absorption of antigen through the intestinal tract.[28] Maternal antibody is transferred to the breastfed infant as a part of what has been called the enteromammary immune system[29] (Fig. 16-1). The secretory IgA antibody present in the milk is the result of enteric immune response of the mother to antigens in her gut. This IgA in her milk provides protection against bacterial, viral, and toxic exposures. Prospective studies in infants have shown that infants at high risk for atopic illness from a hereditary standpoint had significantly less disease when breastfed and also reared in a protected environment with delayed use of solid foods, compared with children of similar risk fed cow's milk and regular solid foods. Serum IgE concentrations were also markedly reduced under 6 months and 12 months of age in the breastfed group. Infants with a low incidence of T-lymphocytes were at greater risk to develop allergies if fed cow's milk

Table 16-2. Relationship of maternal total serum IgE level to cord and 4 month serum IgE level in prophylaxis group infants

Maternal IgE U/ml	Cord IgE <0.5 Number (%)	(U/ml) ≥0.5 Number (%)	4 Month IgE <5.0 Number (%)	(U/ml) ≥5.0 Number (%)
≥100	35 (71)	14 (29)	41 (87)	6 (13)
>100	14 (42)	19 (58)	24 (73)	9 (27)
TOTAL	49	33	65	15

From Hamburger, R.N., et al.: Ann. Allergy 51:281, 1983.
P<0.01 by chi square for maternal IgE <100 vs >100 for cord IgE with a trend (p<0.08) at 4 month IgE.

Table 16-3. Relationship of paternal total serum IgE level to cord and 4 month serum IgE level in prophylaxis group infants

Paternal IgE U/ml	Cord IgE <0.5 Number (%)	(U/ml) ≥0.5 Number (%)	4 Month IgE <5.0 Number (%)	(U/ml) ≥5.0 Number (%)
≥100	29 (63)	17 (37)	40 (83)	8 (17)
>100	10 (56)	8 (44)	14 (82)	3 (18)
TOTAL	39	25	54	11

From Hamburger, R.N., et al.: Ann. Allergy 51:281, 1983.

rather than breast milk, according to work of Juto.[21,22] Infants with reduced T cells fed cow's milk also demonstrated higher serum IgE levels and peripheral eosinophil counts.[21,23] Juto also reported that with careful prophylaxis, greater than 50% of infants in whom both parents have serum IgE levels above 100 μ/ml evidenced both elevated cord and 4-month IgE levels. More than 80% of those infants whose parents had IgE levels below 100 μ/ml, however, had both low cord blood and low 4-month IgE levels. Such data confirm the genetic effect of both maternal and paternal genes.

IMMUNOLOGIC ASPECTS OF ALLERGY

Interest in identifying the immunologic aspects of clinical allergy led to a number of additional studies.[15,16] Kletter et al.[30] reported that hemagglutinating antibodies to cow's milk were present in the sera of some newborns but usually at levels lower than those of the mother. The earliest rise in titer was detected at 1 month and a peak was seen at 3 months in infants given cow's milk from birth. Antibodies belonged mainly to the IgG group with their rise and fall paralleling hemagglutinating antibodies. IgA antibodies were in low titer and IgM rarely detected. The delayed exposure to cow's milk in breastfed infants resulted in lower mean values of milk antibodies, and peak values were attained more slowly. An inverse relationship exists between duration of breastfeeding and levels of titers of humoral antibodies.

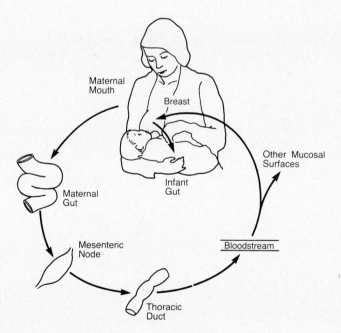

Fig. 16-1. Maternal serum antibodies affect the passage of foreign antigens into the milk, affecting the processing of antigen in the infant's intestine. (Redrawn from Kleinman, R.J.: Ann. Allergy **51:**222, 1983.)

Antibody-facilitated digestion and its implications for infant nutrition have been presented by Freed and Green.[5] They suggest a model of digestion in which oligopeptides in the small bowel are bound to secretory antibodies, which hold them in contact with proteases. This facilitates the breakdown and utilization of the oligopeptides. They consider immunity and digestion to be closely related. Breastfeeding, they point out, with colostrum and then mature human milk provides the immature gut of the infant with both immunity and "digestivity."

Eighteen patients with documented malabsorption of cow's milk, which improved by feeding them human milk, were studied by Savilahti[40] after challenge with powdered milk. Eight patients had clinical reactions; the number of IgA- and IgM-containing cells increased by almost two and a half times in the intestinal mucosa. When breast milk resumed, the findings returned to normal. There was a rise in serum antibodies of both hemagglutination and IgA. There was no change in IgE antibodies or serum complement. Multiple other findings, including villous atrophy and round cell infiltration, were noted. After the age of 2, all the infants became tolerant of milk, which the researchers suggest indicates immunologic immaturity is part of the pathogenesis. Walker presented similar arguments and conclusions in a symposium discussion.[46]

The role of heredity in allergy was studied by Kaufman and Frick.[25] They described unilateral family history as allergy in one parent, bilateral as involving both parents. They followed 94 infants from birth for 24 months. Significantly more infants developed allergy if they were from a bilaterally allergic family. In the first 3 months there was less atopic dermatitis in the breastfed infants with unilateral history than with bilateral history. Businco et al.[2] present similar relationships to family history in a study of breastfed infants.

These data are augmented by findings by Murray[35] examining nasal-secretion eosinophilia in relationship to respiratory allergy, associated with a screening procedure for hearing loss. In a group of children with a history of allergy in the immediate family, an association between early introduction of solid food and the presence of a nasal-secretion eosinophilia was significantly positive.

Although modern processing of cow's milk has diminished the problem, it has not eliminated it, and it would appear that given high-risk factors or strong family history of allergy, an effort to avoid unnecessary exposure to known allergens is an easy way to avoid some medical problems (Table 16-4).

Recommendations for management

Intrauterine sensitization and allergy in the newborn breastfed infant were described by Matsumura[32] and his colleagues in Japan. Glaser[9] also identified the fact that under certain conditions an infant with a predisposition for allergy may become actively sensitized in utero because of the mother's overindulgence in certain foods in pregnancy. Shannon[42] demonstrated the presence of egg antigen in human breast milk, for instance, in 1922. The infant will then respond to reexposure with allergic symptoms on first contact with that same food.[7,31] Infant colic associated with maternal ingestion of cow's

Table 16-4. Some diseases possibly preventable by protecting relatively immunodeficient infants from adverse antigen experience

Disease	Status
Eczema	Established
Asthma	Probable
Hay fever	Probable
Infantile gut and respiratory infection	Probable
Intestinal allergy	Probable
Septicemia and renal *E. coli* infection	Probable
Sudden death	Probable
Ulcerative colitis	Possible

From Soothill, J.T.: Proc. R. Soc. Med. **69:**439, 1976.

milk is discussed in Chapter 14. Kuroume et al.[31] showed in intrauterine sensitization that hemagglutinating antibody titers against lactalbumin and soybean in the amniotic fluid were high. They suggest this measurement of amniotic fluid as an instrument to predict future allergy.

It has been suggested that for the first 6 weeks or so of life, the intestinal tract is immature anatomically and immunologically. The early absorption of protein macromolecules in young animals is well recognized.[41] The subepithelial plasma cells of the lamina propria mucosae and lymph nodes do not make IgA initially. Gradually the levels increase until they reach adult values at 2 years of age. Children with a strong family history of allergy have a more prolonged deficiency of IgA, lasting 3 months or longer. The early introduction of foods other than human milk has been associated with a rise in antibodies in the blood and eosinophilia, as noted earlier. Providing the infant with breast milk to which he will not become sensitized is the most direct way of dealing with the problem.[10]

The total approach to the potentially allergic individual should include diet in pregnancy to exclude known common food allergens plus any known to cause problems in the members of that family[44] (Table 16-5). From birth until 6 months the infant should receive no cow's milk formula. In addition, the diet of the mother should be restricted as in pregnancy and the environment made as allergen free as possible. If the infant is not breastfed, he should receive cow's milk–free formula. Even though this regimen will not totally prevent all the potentials for allergy, it will help to minimize the insults by foreign protein (Appendix M).

Walker[46] summarizes by saying that it has been shown that antigens cross the intestinal barrier in physiologic and pathologic states. He states it is most important to prevent excessive penetration of antigens in patients that are susceptible to the disease via the following steps:

1. Identify the population at risk
2. Encourage breastfeeding in infancy
3. Decrease antigen load with elemental formulas
4. Continue to conduct direct research at identification and prevention

Table 16-5.   Idealized strategy and mechanisms for the prevention of allergic diseases in man

Strategy	Mechanisms
Identify at-risk families	Document IgE reactivity in parents with history of allergic disorders or with existing atopic child
Prevent intrauterine sensitization	Reduce maternal dietary allergenic load during last trimester
Prevent postnatal sensitization to	
1. Food allergens	
a. Transmitted through breast milk	Continue maternal avoidance diet during lactation
b. Ingested by infant	Withhold *all* nonbreast foods except Nutramigen for at least 6 months
2. Environmental allergens	Encourage, instruct, and document avoidance of animals, mite, dust and molds as well as unnecessary medications
Maximize immunologic competence	Encourage, instruct, and support breast feeding for at least 6 months
Minimize nonspecific enhancing factors	Discourage parental smoking; avoid viral illnesses (?), delay pertussis immunization (?)

From Hamburger, R.N., et al.: Ann. Allergy **51**:281, 1983.

REFERENCES

1. Bousquet, J., et al.: Predictive value of cord serum IgE determination in the development of "early-onset" atopy, Ann. Allergy **51**:291, 1983.
2. Businco, L., et al.: Prevention of atopic disease in "at-risk newborns" by prolonged breastfeeding, Ann. Allergy **51**:296, 1983.
3. Chandra, R.K.: Prospective studies on the effect of breast feeding on incidence of infection and allergy, Acta Paediatr. Scand. **68**:691, 1979.
4. Falliers, C., et al.: Discordant allergic manifestations in monozygotic twins: genetic identity vs. clinical, physiologic, and biochemical differences, J. Allergy **47**:207, 1971.
5. Freed, D.L.J., and Green, F.H.Y.: Hypothesis antibody-facilitated digestion and its implications for infant nutrition, Early Hum. Dev. **1**:107, 1977.
6. Gerrard, J.W.: Allergy in infancy, Pediatr. Ann. **3**:9, Oct, 1974.
7. Gerrard, J.W., and Shenassa, M.: Sensitization to substances in breast milk: recognition, management and significance, Ann. Allergy **51**:300, 1983.
8. Glaser, J.: Prophylaxis of allergic disease in infancy and childhood. In Speer, F. and Dockhorn, R.J., editors: Allergy and immunology in children, Springfield, Ill., 1973, Charles C Thomas, Publisher.
9. Glaser, J.: Intrauterine sensitization and allergy in the newborn breast fed infant (editorial), Ann. Allergy **35**:256, 1975.
10. Glaser, J., Daeyfuss, E.M., and Logan, J.: Dietary prophylaxis of atopic disease. In Kelley, V.C., editor: Brennemann's practice of pediatrics, vol II, Hagerstown, Md, 1976, Harper & Row, Publishers, Inc.
11. Glaser, J., and Johnstone, D.E.: Prophylaxis of allergic disease in newborn, JAMA **153**:620, 1953.
12. Grulee, G.G., Sanford, H.N., and Herron, P.H.: Breast and artificial feeding, JAMA **103**:735, 1934.
13. Gruskay, F.L.: Comparison of breast, cow, and soy feedings in the prevention of onset of allergic disease, Clin. Pediatr. **21**:486, 1982.
14. Halpern, S.R., et al.: Development of childhood allergy in infants fed breast, soy, or cow milk, J. Allergy Clin. Immunol. **51**:139, 1973.

15. Hamburger, R.N.: Allergy and the immune system, Am. Sci. **64:**157, 1976.
16. Hamburger, R.N.: Development of atopic allergy in children. In Johansson, S.G.O., editor: International symposium on diagnosis and treatment of IgE-mediated diseases, Amsterdam, 1981, Excerpta Medica.
17. Hamburger, R.N., et al.: Current status of the clinical and immunologic consequences of a phototype allergic disease prevention program, Ann. Allergy **51:**281, 1983.
18. Hide, D.W., and Guyer, B.M.: Clinical manifestations of allergy related to breast and cows' milk feeding, Arch. Dis. Child. **56:**172, 1981.
19. Johnstone, D.E.: The natural history of allergic disease in children. Advances in Pediatric Allergy workshop proceedings, Rome, 1982.
20. Johnstone, D.E., and Dutton, A.M.: Dietary prophylaxis of allergic disease in children, N. Engl. J. Med. **274:**715, 1966.
21. Juto, P.: Elevated serum immunoglobulin E in T-cell-deficient infants fed cow's milk, J. Allergy Clin. Immunol. **66:**402, 1980.
22. Juto, P., and Bjorksten, B.: Serum IgE in infants and influence of type of feeding, Clin. Allergy **10:**593, 1980.
23. Juto, P., and Strannegard, O.: T lymphocytes and blood eosinophils in early infancy in relation to heredity for allergy and type of feeding, J. Allergy Clin. Immunol. **64:**38, 1979.
24. Kajosaari, M., and Saarinen, V.M.: Prophylaxis of atopic disease by six months' total solid food elimination, Acta Paediatr. Scand. **72:**411, 1983.
25. Kaufman, H.S., and Frick, O.L.: The development of allergy in infants of allergic parents: a prospective study concerning the role of heredity, Ann. Allergy **37:**410, 1976.
26. Kaufman, H.S., and Frick, O.L.: Prevention of asthma, Clin. Allerg. **11:**549, 1981.
27. Kern, R.A.: Prophylaxis in allergy, Ann. Intern. Med. **12:**1175, 1939.
28. Kleinman, R.E.: The role of developmental immune mechanisms in intestinal allergy, Ann. Allergy **51:**222, 1983.
29. Kleinman, R.E., and Walker, W.A.: The enteromammary immune system: an important new concept in breast milk host defense, Dig. Dis. Sci. **24:**876, 1979.
30. Kletter, B., et al.: Immune response of normal infants to cow milk. I. Antibody type and kinetics of production, Int. Arch. Allergy **40:**656, 1971.
31. Kuroume, T., et al.: Milk sensitivity and soybean sensitivity in the production of eczematous manifestations in breast-fed infants with particular reference to intrauterine sensitization, Ann. Allergy **37:**41, 1976.
32. Matsumura, T., et al.: Congenital sensitization to food in humans, Jpn. J. Allergy **16:**858, 1967.
33. Matthew, D.J., et al.: Prevention of eczema, Lancet **1:**321, 1977.
34. May, C.D., Fomon, S.J., and Remigio, L.: Immunologic consequences of feeding infants with cow milk and soy products, Acta Paediatr. Scand. **71:**43, 1982.
35. Murray, A.B.: Infant feeding and respiratory allergy, Lancet **1:**497, 1971.
36. McCombs, R., Lowell, F., and Ohman, J.: Myths, morbidity, and mortality in asthma, JAMA **242:**1521, 1979.
37. Ratner, B.: A possible causal factor of food allergy in certain infants, Am. J. Dis. Child. **36:**277, 1928.
38. Rowe, A.H.: Food allergy, Philadelphia, 1931, Lea & Febiger.
39. Saarinen, V.M., et al.: Prolonged breast-feeding as prophylaxis for atopic disease, Lancet **2:**163, 1979.
40. Savilahti, E.: Intestinal immunoglobulins in children with coeliac disease, Gut **13:**958, 1972.
41. Shannon, W.R.: Demonstration of food proteins in human breast milk by anaphylactic experiments in guinea pigs, Am. J. Dis. Child. **22:**223, 1921.
42. Shannon, W.R.: Eczema in breast-fed infants as a result of sensitization to foods in the mother's diet, Am. J. Dis. Child. **23:**392, 1922.
43. Soothill, J.T.: Some intrinsic and extrinsic factors predisposing to allergy, Proc. R. Soc. Med. **69:**439, 1976.
44. Soothill, J.F.: Prevention of atopic allergic disease, Ann. Allergy **51:**229, 1983.
45. Stevenson, D.D., et al.: Development of IgE in newborn human infants, J. Allergy Clin. Immunol. **48:**61, 1971.
46. Walker, W.A.: Antigen absorption from the small intestine and gastrointestinal disease, symposium on gastrointestinal and liver disease, Pediatr. Clin. North Am. **22:**731, 1975.

17

Induced lactation and relactation (including nursing the adopted baby)

Induced lactation is the process by which a nonpuerperal woman is stimulated to lactate, in other words, breastfeeding without pregnancy. Relactation is the process by which a woman who has given birth but did not initially breastfeed is stimulated to lactate. This may also apply to the situation in which a mother may have initially breastfed her infant, weaned him, and then wishes to reinstitute lactation. Induced lactation and relactation are not new concepts but rather are well known to history and to other cultures. The motivation historically has been to provide nourishment for an infant whose mother has died in childbirth or is unable to nurse him for some reason. A friend or relative would take on the care of the child and with it the responsibility to nourish the infant at the breast, since there were no other alternatives. Relactation has been used in times of disaster or disease to provide safe nutrition to weaned or motherless infants. Numerous accounts of induced lactation are recorded in medical literature and reviewed in the writings of Foss and Short[12] as well as Brown.[5] Mead[21] recorded the phenomenon in her writings about New Guinea in 1935. Other anthropologists have made similar observations in other preindustrialized societies of women who have not borne children who, after a few weeks of placing the suckling infant to the breast, produce milk adequate to nourish the infant. Until recently, Western world literature reported the phenomenon as an anecdotal report as part of the discussion of aberrant lactation. Cohen[9] reported in 1971 a patient who had been nursing an adopted child very successfully for weeks when first seen in his pediatric office.

Today the interest in induced lactation in the industrialized world stems from a desire on the part of some adopting mothers to nurture the adopted child at the breast even if she was unable to carry the infant in utero. The interest in relactation comes from mothers of sick or premature infants who wish to breastfeed their infants after the days and weeks of neonatal intensive care are over. These mothers, although postpartum, have not been lactating.

The process of induced lactation is separate from galactorrhea, or inappropriate lactation, which has been described in the medical literature for over 100 years.[28] Abnormal lactation has been observed in a number of circumstances in nulliparous and parous women and even in males.[12] There are many eponyms for these conditions, usually based on the name of the physician who first described the syndrome, such as Chiari-Frommel and Ahumada-del Castillo-Argonz. Normally in the absence of suckling, lactation ceases 14 to 21 days after delivery. Milk flow that continues beyond 3 to 6 months after abortion or any termination of pregnancy is termed abnormal or inappropriate lactation, or galactorrhea. Also included in this group of galactorrhea is lactation in a woman 3 months after weaning or the secretion of milk in a nulliparous woman in association with hyperprolactinemia and amenorrhea. Although these cases are pathologic in nature and therefore different from the groups under discussion, it is noteworthy that some knowledge of the initiation and maintenance of lactation has been gained from the study of these syndromes.

Lactation has been induced for scientific and commercial purposes in nonpregnant and nonparturient animals by the continual systematic application to the mammary gland of the suckling animal or mechanical milking apparatus.[19] The response is effected through the release of mammotrophic hormone from the anterior pituitary gland. This effect is abolished if the pituitary stalk is transected. Ruminants respond to the addition of estrogen or estrogen-progesterone combinations, which facilitate mammary growth. Experiments in goats first involved applying ointment containing estradiol benzoate to the udders of virgins, which resulted in development of the udder and milk yield almost comparable to normal postpartum animals.[10] It was subsequently shown that a combination of estrogen-progesterone not only had a better milk yield but histologically the lobuloalveolar growth was normal, whereas with estrogen alone growth was cystic and irregular. It was also demonstrated that ovariectomized goats could be stimulated to lactation with these two hormones, with normal histology of the udder and good milk production. Initiation of regular milkings had a significant impact on production of milk. The fact that lactation can be stimulated when the ovaries have been removed but not when the pituitary stalk has been severed has significance for understanding of some of the postpartum lactation failures in women. Again in ruminants, growth hormone and thyroid hormone have been shown to increase milk yield, although prolactin does not. This suggests that prolactin is not deficient in ruminants. Selye and McKeown[24] showed in 1934 that suckling stimulus inhibits sexual cyclicity in rats. They further showed that when the main milk ducts to all the nipples are cut and the escape of milk has been rendered impossible, the mechanical stimulation of the nipples by nursing would also inhibit the sexual cyclicity of the normal estric, nonlactating adult rat. These studies demonstrate the significance of suckling in triggering the lactation cycle.

Because the motivation, goals, and physiologic problems may be slightly different, induced lactation and relactation shall be considered separately.

INDUCED LACTATION

When a mother wishes to nurse her adopted infant, the goal is usually to achieve a mother-infant relationship that may also have the benefit of some nutrition. Put in that perspective then, success can be evaluated on the basis of whether or not the infant will suckle the breast and achieve some comfort and security from this opportunity and close relationship with his new mother. As has been well described by Avery,[3] this is nurturing with the emphasis on nursing, not on "breast-feeding" or nutrition. She further notes that "breast-feed" is not an actual word whereas nurse is defined as nourish or nurture. A mother who is interested in inducing lactation to nurse an adopted infant may need to understand that she may never be able to completely sustain the infant by her milk alone without supplementation. Neither the physician nor the mother should be disappointed. The nurturing goal is still achieved.

Preparation for induced lactation

Normally the breast is prepared through pregnancy for the time when lactation will begin by the proliferation of the ductal and alveolar system.[21] Thus it is not inappropriate to assume that a period of similar preparation should take place in induced lactation. It has been suggested that the woman should begin systematically to express the breasts manually and stimulate the nipples for up to 2 months prior to the arrival of the infant, if time permits. A hand pump or other pumping devices can be used, but manual expression may work as well or better. Sometimes some secretion can be produced in this manner if it is carried out systemically on a uniform schedule throughout the day. The schedule should be practical, that is, include times when a mother could take a moment for this activity, such as morning and night plus any times she uses the bathroom.

In other cultures in which lactation is induced as a survival tactic for the infant, no period of preparation is available. The infant is put to the adoptive mother's breast and allowed to suckle. Stress has been placed on herbal teas and good nourishment for the mother, while the infant is also given prechewed food, gruel, or animal milk. Mead attributes much of the success of induced lactation in New Guinea to the ingestion of ample supplies of coconut milk by the new mother.

Adoption is not an easy process, and in fact, it can be quite stressful to become an instant parent. In assisting such a mother, consideration should be given to the infant's age, previous feeding experience, and any medical problems that may exist. Provision for additional nourishment during the process of establishing some milk secretion is most important. Onset of lactation varies from 1 to 6 weeks, averaging about 4 weeks after initiation of stimulation with the appearance of the first drops of milk. When the infant is actually nursing at the breast and being nourished by supplements, milk may appear as early as 1 to 2 weeks.

Some infants are easily confused by switching back and forth between breast and bottle because the sucking technique is slightly different. Other nourishment can be offered by dropper or as solid foods. There is, however, a unique system for providing nourishment for the infant while suckling at the breast. It is called Lact-Aid Nursing Trainer System and is described on p. 425 and Appendix H.

Drugs to induce lactation

As described in Chapter 2, estrogen and progesterone stimulate the proliferation of the alveolar and ductal systems. These hormones work in association with an increase in prolactin production. Although the prolactin level is high during pregnancy, milk secretion is inhibited by the presence of the estrogen and progesterone. After delivery has occurred and the placenta is removed, there is a marked fall in estrogen and progesterone, and prolactin initiates milk production.[26] Efforts to simulate this hormonal stimulation have had variable success and are not recommended in this situation because of the possible effect on the infant via the milk. Women taking birth control pills have been noted in some cases to have breast enlargement. In addition, although estrogen and progesterone may enhance proliferation, they may inhibit lactation per se. The dosage recommended by Waletzky and Herman[30] of conjugated estrogens is 2.5 mg twice a day for 14 days beginning on the fourth day of a regular menstrual cycle. Giving 0.35 mg norethindrone once daily with the morning dose of estrogen prevents breakthrough bleeding. Medication is given for 2 weeks and is comparable in dosage to 2 weeks of birth control pills. This may be accompanied by some side effects. This regimen has been followed in concert with other efforts to stimulate lactation.

Oxytocin, on the other hand, is a critical component in the milk ejection reflex and may be helpful in the early initiation of ejection. Physiologically stimulation of the nipple in the lactating woman results in the release of oxytocin by the hypothalamus, which then triggers the release of milk by stimulating the contraction of the myoepithelial cells and the ejection of milk (see Chapter 8). The effect of intranasal administration of oxytocin on the let-down reflex in lactating women was well described by Newton and Egli.[22] (Oral administration by tablet has not been as effective, since oxytocin is destroyed in the stomach.) Since that time, oxytocin nasal spray has been utilized in nonpuerperal lactation with some success in enhancing let-down but not necessarily altering the volume produced. Continued use of oxytocin over weeks has been associated with diminished effect or even suppression of lactation. The chief benefit of oxytocin is often to break the cycle of failure and instill a feeling of confidence once it has been demonstrated that some secretion can be produced.

Chlorpromazine has been observed to act as a galactagogue as well as a tranquilizer when given to patients in large doses (up to 1000 mg or more). The effect has been observed in both male and female patients in mental institutions. The drug has been reported to increase pituitary prolactin secretion severalfold. It acts via the hypothalamus, probably by reducing prolactin inhibitory factor levels. Using this information, women well motivated to lactate who have attempted induced lactation by suckling a normal infant have had the process enhanced by small doses of chlorpromazine, according to Brown.[7] In a program to induce lactation in refugee camps in India and in Vietnam, nonlactating women were given 25 to 100 mg of chlorpromazine three times a day for a week to 10 days while infants were initially put to breast. Brown reports apparent enhancement of lactation with this treatment.[6] Chlorpromazine has the added pharmacological effect of acting as a tranquilizer. The program of management in these women was supportive in other ways and also included the usual herbal medicines associated with lactation in these Eastern cultures. There was no control group. It is possible that the drug contributed to both the physiologic and psychologic well-being of the women wishing to lactate. It has been suggested that the wish to lactate is a strong component of success, since women whose breasts are frequently stimulated sexually do not begin to lactate. Theophylline can also increase pituitary prolactin secretions, according to Vorherr[23]; therefore both tea and coffee should enhance prolactin secretion and thus lactation. However, excessive amounts may inhibit let-down.

Since the role of prolactin is the initiation and maintenance of lactation, whereas oxytocin regulates the glandular emptying via the milk-ejection reflex, it is reasonable to speculate that enhancing prolactin release would be productive in inducing lactation. The exact activating mechanism of the neuronal reflex arc from breast to brain has not been deciphered. Secretion of prolactin appears to be influenced, if not controlled, by changes in hypothalamic dopamine turnover. Correspondingly, suckling has been observed to deplete dopamine stores.

Investigation of other drugs that are known to stimulate prolactin release has identified some possible therapeutic materials. McNeilly et al.[20] have reported metoclopramide induces prolactin release regardless of the route of administration. Prolactin levels are increased three to eight times normal levels within 5 minutes when a 10 mg dose is given either intravenously or intramuscularly. The effect is achieved within an hour when metoclopramide is given orally. The effect persists for 8 hours. No reports are available for its use in nonpuerperal women at this time, although metoclopramide has been used to enhance lactation and for relactation (p. 420) (see Table 17-5).

The regulation of prolactin secretion in humans has been studied to further the understanding of abnormal lactation as well as provide information on the regulation of pituitary function of the brain. It has been shown experimentally that the hypothalamus secretes PIF, which acts on the mammotropin-releasing cells of the pituitary to inhibit release of the hormone prolactin. The hypothalamus can also regulate prolactin secretion by a stimulatory mechanism, the secretion of thyrotropin-releasing hormone (TRH). When human volunteers (nonpregnant, nonlactating) are given infusions of TRH, increases in thyrotropin and prolactin are observed within minutes of injection with values peaking in 20 minutes. The level of thyroid hormone in the volunteers initially influences the results. Hypothyroid patients have been observed in secrete excessive amounts of prolactin, whereas hyperthyroid patients are relatively insensitive to TRH. This may explain some of the variable results obtained with prolactin-stimulating drugs used in the practical application to stimulate lactation. Studies of relactation have been done using TRH but not of de novo induced lactation.

Table 17-1 summarizes the influence of drugs on prolactin secretion.

Jelliffe[15] points out that the most important factor for continued production of milk is not drugs or hormones but "mulging." He explains that *mulging* (stimulation) is a word created in 1975 by N.W. Pirie to mitigate the confusion between the words *sucking* and *suckling*. The word comes from the Latin *mulgere*, to milk.

Composition of milk in induced lactation

Concern has been expressed that the composition of the milk produced by stimulation of suckling rather than as a result of pregnancy might indeed differ from "normal human milk." Such induced milk is not different in other species that have been studied extensively, including bovine and rat. In developing countries the fact that the infants showed normal growth and weight gain was taken as evidence that the milk is adequate. Vorherr[28,29] reported the analysis of the galactorrheal secretion produced by the breast following hyperstimulation. The comparative analysis is shown in Table 17-2. The induced lactational milk did not differ from puerperal milk. Brown[5] reported higher values of fat, protein, and lactose in galactorrheal milk, but the volume of secretion was small in these subjects.

The composition of the breast secretion produced by two women who induced lactation artificially by breast hyperstimulation was close to the composition obtained for women with normal lactation, according to Kulski et al.[18] (Table 17-2). These investi-

Table 17-1.   Influence of drugs on prolactin secretion

Pharmacologic agents	Plasma prolactin concentration	Mechanism of drug action
L-Dopa	Decrease	Increase in hypothalamic dopamine-catecholamine levels, leading to enhanced activity of prolactin-inhibiting factor (PIF)
Ergot alkaloids (ergocornine, ergocryptine)	Decrease	Direct inhibition of adenohypophyseal prolactin secretion; possible increase of hypothalamic PIF activity (continued PIF function)
Thyrotropin-releasing hormone (TRH; pyroglutamyl-histidyl-prolinamide)	Increase	Direct stimulation of adenohypophyseal lactotrophs for increased prolactin secretion
Theophylline Phenothiazines (chlorpromazine) Amphetamine α-Methyldopa	Increase	Decrease in hypothalamic dopamine-catecholamine levels, leading to diminution of PIF activity
Metoclopramide	Increase	Inhibition of hypothalamic PIF secretion through dopamine antagonism
Sulpiride	Increase	Increase in hypothalamic prolactin-releasing hormone

From Vorherr, H.: Human lactation and breast feeding. In Larson, B.L., editor: Lactation, New York, 1978, Academic Press, Inc., p. 182.

gators also examined the milk of a woman in whom lactation had occurred when medicated with a psychotropic drug (haloperidol). She had had a pregnancy 4 years previously. Her galactorrhea lasted 38 months. Her milk had composition like that of
colostrum for a week but resembled mature milk at 1 month. A woman with hypothyroidism and elevated prolactin and TSH had colostrum-like milk for 53 days of sampling. Two women with galactorrhea and amenorrhea associated with pituitary tumor
and hyperprolactinemia had transient colostrum-like secretion, which changed to mature
milk. Protein values of milk samples from five mothers without biologic pregnancies
were measured by Kleinman et al.[17] Two of the mothers had nursed previous babies
and three had never been pregnant and had never breastfed. These authors did not
distinguish between them. The mean total protein concentration of milk samples from
the "nonbiologic" mothers differs from the "biologic" mothers (Figs. 17-1 and 17-2).
If the goal of induced lactation is nurturing, these differences are clinically unimportant;
however, such data may help to unravel the mysteries of lactation physiology. The
clinician may also wish to keep these values in mind when counseling a mother-infant
dyad about induced lactation nutrition, especially if the infant was premature or small
for gestational age. It is probably of little value to try to analyze a given mother's
secretions, since there is no evidence to question the composition. In tandem nursing,
when a mother continues to nurse an older child and puts an adopted newborn on the
breast simultaneously, the composition of the milk might be in question.

Management of the mother and infant when lactation is induced

The collected experience of counseling women in the Western world who wish to
induce lactation has been reported by Hormann[14] and Avery[3]; the latter author has now
had contact with several thousand such women. Others have had experience with

Table 17-2. Composition of normal breast milk and "galactorrhea milk"

Milk components and properties	Normal breast milk	"Galactorrhea milk"	Induced lactation
Components			
Fat (g/100 ml)	3.7	3-8	
Lactose (g/100 ml)	7.0	3-5	5.4
Total protein (g/100 ml)	1.2	2-7	1.6
Sodium (mg/100 ml)	15	70	22.0
Potassium (mg/100 ml)	50	5	19.8
Calcium (mg/100 ml)	35	38	
Chlorine (mg/100 ml)	45	50	18.4
Phosphorus (mg/100 ml)	15	2	
Ash (mg/100 ml)	20	40-70	
Properties			
Specific gravity	1030-1033	1031	
Milk pH	6.8-7.3	7.3	
Daily volume	400-800 ml	1-120 ml	

From Vorherr, H.: The breast: morphology, physiology and lactation, New York, 1974, Academic Press, Inc.; and Kulski, J.K., et al.: Obstet. Gynecol. **139**:597, 1981. Reprinted with permission from the American College of Obstetricians and Gynecologists.

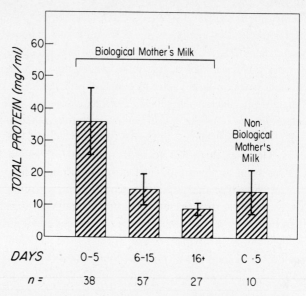

Fig. 17-1. Total protein changes with time: biologic versus nonbiologic mother's milk, protein value ± SD. (From Kleinman, R., Jacobson, L., Hormann, E., and Walker, W.A.: J. Pediatr. **97:**613, 1980.)

smaller series. The request for information and advice is increasing and becoming widespread throughout the United States and other Western countries.

Because there are simple means of supplementing the nutritional needs of the infant, the counseling should center on the relationship and the nurturing aspects. When the process is undertaken in preindustrialized nations, the antiinfective properties become important even though total nourishment may not be possible. Success is measured by having the infant content to nurse at the breast.

The woman should be encouraged to come to the physician's office for a counseling visit prior to the arrival of the adoptive infant to discuss the process of induced lactation. Actually, parents who are planning to adopt an infant should have a preliminary visit with their pediatrician so that some understanding of parenting can be discussed, just as any couple should do prior to the birth of their first child. At this visit to discuss lactation with the couple, it is helpful to explore their motives and general concepts of what is involved. It has been pointed out by all authors on the subject that the husband's interest in and support of lactation is critical to success. His participation in the preparation of the breasts may be a means by which the father can share intimately and constructively in the process. Instruction of the mother in preparation of the breast for suckling is also critical in induced lactation, whereas with puerperal lactation it may not be necessary at all. Exercises to stimulate the nipple should be undertaken several times a day and will be most successful if they are scheduled for times when and situations in which it is easy, feasible, and readily remembered. A few minutes multiple times a

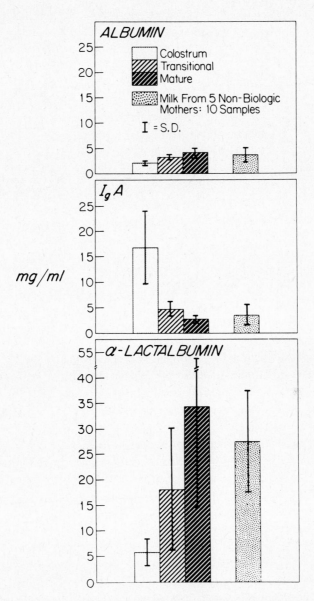

Fig. 17-2. Protein changes with time: biologic versus nonbiologic mother's milk. (From Kleinman, R., et al.: J. Pediatr. **97:**614, 1980.)

day is more successful and less likely to *overemphasize* milk versus mothering than rigid excessive exercises once or twice a day. Manual manipulation with gentle traction or horizontal and vertical stretching can be suggested. Avery[3] suggests that the father be encouraged to assist in breast massage and other techniques. She notes that ''many adoptive parents felt that this technique (fondling and suckling of the breasts by the husband) added to the mutual sharing in preparation for adoptive nursing similar to the closeness many couples experience in preparing for natural childbirth.'' Raphael[23] reports that among 40 adoptive nursing mothers there were dozens of variations on the theme of preparation. A positive attitude seemed to be the only consistent factor.

The need for dietary counseling is obvious. Lip service in behalf of well-balanced nutritious meals is not enough. Discussion should center around the absolute needs in kilocalories, fluids, and nutrients to produce milk (Chapter 9).

The physician should point out that stimulation of the nipples may well cause amenorrhea. Although the variation in menses is not uniform, it should be explained that decreased flow, irregular cycles, or total cessation of menstrual flow is possible. On the other hand, the menstrual cycle may be maintained and the flow of milk may seem to vary during menses. Changes in breast size, heaviness, and feeling of fullness may accompany the induced lactation. There may be an associated weight gain of 10 to 12 pounds, on the average, according to Avery,[3] attributed to the response of the body to developing stores for lactation, just as in pregnancy (i.e., increased fluid retention and appetite increase). The weight gain may be a simple phenomenon of excessive intake. However, there is no need to gain excessive weight during this experience. Mothers (who may be nutritionally depleted) in non-Western countries who induce lactation are given added diet, nourishment, and herbal teas but do not usually gain weight. Failure to experience change in breast size, menstrual regularity, or weight should not be construed as a failed response.

Auerbach and Avery[2] reported a retrospective questionnaire study of 240 women, 83 of whom had never been pregnant or lactated before, 55 of whom had been pregnant but never lactated, and 102 of whom had breastfed one or more biologic children prior to the adoptive nursing (lactation). Most respondents used more than one technique to stimulate their nipples. The most effective method of nipple stimulation, these mothers felt, was nipple exercises combined with infant suckling. Hand-operated pumps caused soreness and irritation. The nipple exercises included nipple stroking, massaging the breast, and rolling the nipple between thumb and finger. In this study, the infant's willingness to suckle improved over time and was related to the age at which he was first put to breast. Infants who were under 8 weeks of age had over a 75% success rate; those over 8 weeks of age had only 50% success. No infants failed to thrive, but nearly all needed some type of supplementation. Mothers who had nursed a biologic baby before were able to wean from supplementation partially or completely. This group was also more disappointed if they had to supplement.

These few simple guidelines, developed as a result of experiences reported by several authors and many mothers, may be helpful to the physician in counseling the mother to induce lactation:

1. Before arrival of baby, initiate frequent brief manual stimulation of nipples. Mechanical pumps cause more nipple soreness than hand stroking, massaging, and exercises.
2. Breastfeed before any other nourishment is provided when putting infant to breast.
3. Avoid stressing baby with hunger.
4. When supplementing, use donor human milk or prepared formula, not cow's milk with its long stomach-emptying time.
5. Avoid rubber nipples and pacifiers to encourage appropriate suckling at breast.
6. Provide supplements by dropper, spoon, or Lact-Aid.
7. Create positive atmosphere—mother the mother.

Rigid conformity to a system of feeding may be a symptom of a more serious problem. Women who are rigid and compulsive may have trouble lactating because of the inability to have a good ejection reflex, which can be inhibited by stress and emotional conflict. Mothers who demonstrate an inordinate attention to volume of production of milk over and above the value of the relationship may feel as if they have failed.

NUTRITIONAL SUPPLEMENTATION. The need to supplement the infant's intake while the milk supply is being developed should be discussed. The older infant who has already been receiving solid foods can be continued on solids by spoon with careful attention to nutritional content so that the diet includes a balance of protein and other nutrients. Supplements with milk or formula should be appropriate to the age of the infant. The infant under 6 months should receive infant formula rather than whole milk if donor breast milk is not available. The milk supplements should be full strength, 20 kcal/oz and provided during the feeding by dropper or Lact-Aid or after the nursing by dropper, spoon, or cup in preference to a rubber nipple, which may confuse the infant in his adaption to nursing at the breast.

The process of induced lactation requires considerable commitment and determination. It is far more arduous a task than initiating postpartum lactation, but it is possible and worth the effort, according to the many mothers who have attempted it. The situation is better managed if a doula is available. It is appropriate for the physician to suggest that in addition to medical support the mother seek counseling from a lactation counselor experienced in induced lactation. Day-by-day contact for verbal support may be helpful, and these needs may be beyond the scope of a busy office practice. The nurse practitioner may be invaluable in this situation, particularly if home visits are made.

Appendix J includes instructions on manual expression of milk.

RELACTATION

The need to relactate exists in a number of circumstances, including the following:

1. A sick or premature infant cannot be fed initially or even until he is several weeks or months old (Fig. 17-3).
2. An infant is weaned prematurely because of illness in the infant or in the mother.
3. An infant who was not previously breastfed develops an allergy or food intolerance.
4. A mother who has lactated weeks, months, or years before is nursing an adopted infant.
5. A mother who is nursing a biologic child begins nursing an adopted child (without benefit of pregnancy).

Historical reviews provide many examples of infants suckled in times of crisis by women who have not lactated for years. The process of reestablishing lactation under these circumstances is generally easier than that of nonpuerperal lactation. Investigations have shown that a breast that has been previously primed by pregnancy to respond to prolactin will produce milk more readily.

Although the general process of nipple stimulation, having the infant suckle the breast, and setting the stage for lactation is similar, the woman who has experienced successful lactation previously may have not only the physiologic but also the psychologic edge.

A prospective study of mothers whose infants were in the neonatal intensive care unit in Durham, North Carolina was reported by Bose et al.[4] The profile of the mothers is listed in Table 17-3. Mother and baby were admitted to the Clinical Research Unit, where they were assisted with relactating including help using the Lact-Aid. The infant's nutritional intake was recorded. Mother and infant were discharged when the mother was comfortable with the Lact-Aid and feeding was established (about 3 days). Follow-up occurred every week or two. All but one infant were initially reluctant to suckle, but all received their entire nutritional intake at the breast, with or without Lact-Aid, within the first week of the study. Most of the mothers had trouble initiating suckling, with the most significant factor being the length of separation from their infant and not degree of prematurity, postnatal age, weight, or feeding regimen. Nipple tenderness occurred in all mothers transiently. All the mothers (except number seven, who was an adoptive mother) produced milk in 1 week, with maximum milk production occurring from 8 to 58 days, proportional to the time since delivery. Although it was done with a small population, this study established some important information. Given appropriate techniques and support, many women appear to be able to relactate and premature infants can learn to breastfeed after initial bottle feeding.

A retrospective study of relactation was reported by Auerbach and Avery[1] in which 366 women responded with a completed questionnaire out of over 500 contacted from a list of names obtained from manufacturer's lists, magazine ads, and requests to breastfeeding support groups. The bias was in favor of well-educated affluent women who

Table 17-3. Historical and clinical data

Case number	Gestational age	Time from delivery to entry into study (days)	Time from last lactation to entry into study (days)	Postpartum breast involution*	Time to first breast milk (days)	Time to half breast milk supply† (days)	Time to complete relactation (days)
1	Term	10	10	None	1	4	8
2	Term	120	120	Incomplete	4	20	28
3‡	Twins, 31 wk	49	49	Complete	7	28	Never
4	32 wk	70	42	Complete	7	39	Never
5	28 wk	150	135	Complete	9	Never	Never
6	32 wk	30	16	None	4	17	58
7	Term (adopted)	5 yr	5 yr	Complete	21	Never	Never

From Bose, C.L., et al.: Pediatrics **67:**565, 1981. Copyright American Academy of Pediatrics 1980.
*Mothers were asked if their brassiere size was different from that before this pregnancy.
†Estimated on the basis of a decrease in formula intake.
‡Ceased to suckle her infant after 28 days in the study in order to return to full-time employment.

had probably obtained their lactation goals. The population included those who had untimely weaning ($N = 174$) following delivery of low–birth weight infants ($N = 117$) and following hospitalization of mother or baby or both ($N = 75$).

Willingness to nurse on the part of the infant was related to his previous suckling experience, but responses in the first week of effort were not directly correlated with ultimate successful suckling. Fifty percent of mothers were able to discontinue supplementing in 1 month and 24% were never able to eliminate supplements completely. Once established, the nursing patterns were similar to those of ordinary breastfeeding. The authors point out that keeping the baby hungry in the mistaken notion that he will nurse more often and for longer periods does not help and may negatively influence outcome. For the professional it is of interest that fewer than 10% of respondents received helpful advice from health-care professionals.

Tandem nursing

Tandem nursing an adoptive child is a phenomenon in which the adoptive mother is still nursing a biologic child and puts an adopted infant to the breast and intends to nourish the newcomer totally. Usually the older child is a toddler and feeding only a few times a day or for comfort and receiving the major nourishment from other food and drink. In biologic tandem nursing, the milk returns to colostrum-like constituency with the birth of the new baby; however, in the absence of a pregnancy the milk volume may increase with increased nipple stimulus while the constituents do not change. Data of milk constituents beyond a year postpartum or in the case of relactation have been noted (see p. 414). In most cases reported anecdotally the adopted infant is several weeks or months old, so the absence of colostrum is less of a problem. On the other hand, the active state of lactation in terms of immediate availability of milk is actually an advantage. An additional concern, as in any situation of tandem nursing, is the development of the older child. The physician will need to be alert to these issues in counseling the family and assuring adequate total nutrition for the adopted child. Eighteen respondents to the survey on adoptive nursing by Auerbach and Avery[2] reported tandem-nursing experiences. Eleven of these mothers were able to discontinue supplements totally (two within the first month). Most of the infants were started on solids by 4½ months, which may be the most effective method of supplementing if nutritional value is maintained. For the physician it is important to be knowledgeable about tandem adoptive nursing and to support the family accordingly.

Drugs to induce relactation

Some medications that have been tried in relactation seem only to work when the breast has been primed by mammogenesis, that is, by pregnancy.

Thyrotropin-releasing hormone (TRH, pyroglutamyl-histidyl-prolinamide) (Thyroliberin), has been used by Tyson and others to induce lactation. Each woman in their study was primed with estrogens beforehand. TRH stimulates the pituitary to release

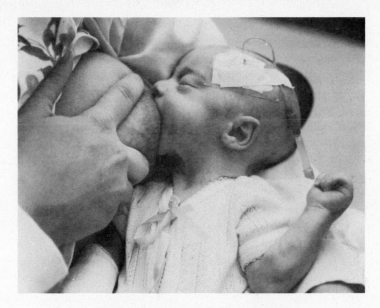

Fig. 17-3. Premature infant (1300 g) at breast.

both TSH and prolactin. Drugs that produce a decrease in hypothalamic catecholamines, such as phenothiazines, reserpine, meprobamate, amphetamines, and α-methyldopa, cause an increase in prolactin secretion by blocking hypothalamic PIF.

The feasibility of pharmacologically manipulating puerperal lactation was demonstrated by Canales et al.[8] using bromocriptine and TRH sequentially. They suppressed lactation using bromocriptine orally for 8 days in four mothers whose infants were premature and/or ill and could not be nursed. These mothers did not lactate during this time. On the eighth day they were given TRH intravenously and then daily orally for 4 days (eighth to twelfth postpartum day). On the fourteenth day they initiated breastfeeding by putting the infant to the breast. Prolactin levels were measured from the day of birth. Levels were depressed by bromocriptine and noted to rise when the TRH was given. The mothers subsequently nursed successfully.

Bose et al.[4] also studied TRH and the basal and stimulated serum prolactin concentrations. Prolactin concentrations were measured followed by levels at 15 and 30 minutes after intravenous infusion of 200 μg of thyrotropin-releasing hormone (TRH). Prolactin levels were also measured before and after suckling at weekly intervals. Serum prolactin levels rose 15 minutes after infusion of TRH (Table 17-4). The absolute rise in prolactin concentrations did not appear to be related to establishment of milk production. The change over time in the basal prolactin levels was not predictably related to lactation progress.

Lactation can be reestablished with metoclopramide, according to Sousa et al.[25]

Table 17-4.   Basal and stimulated serum prolactin concentrations (ng/ml)

Case number	TRH stimulation		Suckling stimulation: presuckling/postsuckling						
	Basal	15 min/30 min	1st wk*	2nd wk	3rd wk	4th-5th wk	6th-7th wk	8th-9th wk
1	179.2	611.1/423.5	136.9/155.4	72.3/123.8	· · · ·	· · · ·	· · · ·	· · · ·
2	38.7	80.9/70.3	17.2/119.3	38.6/214.3	16.6/180.6	186.2/244.5	· · · ·	· · · ·
3	19.9	89.6/77.3	17.9/23.5	· · · ·	· · · ·	· · · ·	· · · ·	· · · ·
4	9.5	89.9/63.4	12.5/12.7	· · · ·	7.0/437.6	5.5/47.3	· · · ·	· · · ·
5	13.9	40.6/36.3	21.1/58.2	37.8/82.0	38.3/57.7	77.2/98.5	24.6/54.2	· · · ·
6	31.7	335.6/274.7	9.5/11.4	· · · ·	16.5/18.4	11.8/16.3	7.8/13.3	· · · ·
7	43.6†	78.8/69.9	8.8/59.6	17.0/77.7	· · · ·	· · · ·	34.4/147.1	19.2/60.5

From Bose, C.L., et al.: Pediatrics 67:565, 1981. Copyright American Academy of Pediatrics 1980.
*Suckling test performed on day 1 or 2 of study.
†In this mother, suckling test was done first, followed one hour later by thyrotropin-releasing hormone (TRH) infusion; thus, 8.8 is the true basal concentration.

Table 17-5.   Data regarding mothers taking metoclopramide

Num- ber	Age of mother (yr)	Age of infant (mo)	Daily dose (mg)	Length of treatment (days)	Side effects	Result	Education level of mother
1	27	2	30	6	None	Increase in milk volume; infant not weaned	University
2	25	10	30	10	None	Same as above	University
3	29	1	20	7	None	Same as above	High school
4	35	3	30	7	None	Same as above	University
5	20	2	20	7	None	Same as above	High school

From Sousa, P.L.R., et al.: J. Trop. Pediatr. 21:214, 1975.

Metoclopramide is a derivative of procainamide, as is sulpiride. Studies done by McNeilly et al.[20] showed that metoclopramide and sulpiride are potent stimulators of prolactin release. These authors demonstrated marked increase in prolactin when metoclopramide is given, as noted earlier in this chapter. Sousa et al.[25] used metoclopramide to reestablish lactation in women who had experienced diminished milk supply. All five mothers experienced increased production of milk when 10 mg was given orally every 8 hours for 7 to 10 days. No side effects were noted, although this drug is known to cause cardiac arrhythmias and extrapyramidal signs in some adults. No side effects were noted in the infants either, but the level of drug was not measured in the milk. The results were encouraging, but further study is needed to determine the minimum dosage necessary to produce the effect and the amount passed into the milk. The summation of the data on patients treated by Sousa et al.[25] is recorded in Table 17-5.

LACT-AID NURSING TRAINER AND OTHER DEVICES

Although many mechanical devices have been developed since Roman times to augment lactation and give other feeding opportunities, the Lact-Aid Nursing Trainer provides a unique ability to nourish an infant adequately while he suckles at the inadequately lactating breast (Fig. 16-4). The suckling stimulates the mother's own supply. On the other hand, the infant continues to suckle the breast because there is milk available. The device has been carefully engineered to provide a source of milk that is obtained by suckling, not by gravity. The capillary tube through which the milk flows can be placed along the human nipple without interfering with suckling. The plastic bags that serve as reservoirs for the supplemental milk are sterile and disposable. The milk is naturally warmed by hanging the bag beside the mother's breast, as shown in Fig. 17-4. See Appendix H for a full description.

Gradual weaning from the Lact-Aid can be provided by putting less and less in the bag each day so that the infant can obtain milk from the breast in increasing amounts as the nipple stimulation effects milk production.

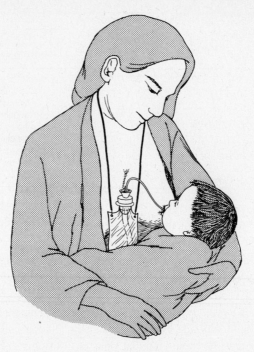

Fig. 17-4. Lact-Aid Nursing Trainer System in use with full-term infant.

Experience in Rochester was initially obtained using Lact-Aid for adoptive induced lactation when the infant was 2 months old or older and needed instant supplementation. An increasing number of mothers wish to nurse their sick premature infants, however. It is often not possible to put the infant to breast for weeks. Meanwhile the mother may pump but only obtains minimal volume. When the infant is finally ready for discharge from the hospital, it is mandatory that he continue to receive reliable nourishment every day. Starving the infant into submission is inappropriate and dangerous. Lact-Aid is an excellent alternative.

For years mothers of premature and sick infants have been assisted in breastfeeding their infants in preparation for discharge from the hospital and during early weeks at home by using dropper feeding, complementary feeds by bottle after each breast-feeding, or solids. The success rate was low and the aggravation for the mother often insurmountable.

Experience has been gained in Rochester with many infants who have thrived with the assistance of supplements from Lact-Aid in these circumstances. Weaning from the Lact-Aid was not a problem for most of the infants. It was a problem, however, for an occasional mother who could not nurse without the Lact-Aid even though it contained less than an ounce of formula per feeding and the breast was supplying the rest. Mother may use the Lact-Aid as a "crutch." Careful anticipatory counseling should avoid this.

Lact-Aid should be started with a full understanding of its role in nourishment of the infant as well as with a plan for weaning from it that begins the first day. Weaning should be appropriate to the age of the infant and his nutritional needs. The nourishment provided should be donor human milk or regular-strength formula, 20 kcal/oz and not just water, sugar water, or diluted formula. Starvation, even for a day or so, in a premature infant compromises the growth, especially of the brain. An infant who has been in the intensive care nursery is in special jeopardy (Fig. 14-13). Several alternative devices have been suggested by professionals interested in the transient supplementation of lactation while a mother increased her milk supply for her full-term baby. Usually these are situations where lactation failure has been the result of inadequate initial advice. The devices use readily available feeding tubes and syringes but lack the special engineering and safety features of the Lact-Aid. Special precautions are advised when employing such hand-made equipment to avoid milk aspiration by the infant, which is the chief hazard. Other devices, such as hand pumps, the Egnell electric pump, and the Whittlestone physiologic breast milker, which are useful in initiating relactation or induced lactation as well as puerperal nursing, are illustrated in Appendix G.

SUMMARY

Careful medical management of the adopted infant who is breastfed is important. Many times the prenatal care of this infant as a fetus in utero has not been optimal. Any failure in growth should be identified quickly so that appropriate supplementation can be provided. In cases of relactation to provide for sick or premature infants, close follow-up is mandatory. A child who does not have a powerful suck may well appear to be very content yet be underfed. This situation was clearly described by Gilmore and Rowland[13] who reported three cases of malnutrition while breastfeeding, attributed to the failure of the mother to recognize signs of growth failure and dehydration.

Relactation and induced lactation are special events requiring the positive support of medical personnel. The physician can serve as a well-informed stable resource in a process that will require considerable effort and commitment by the participants.

Mother-initiated preparation for induced lactation or relactation

1. Nipple stimulation: hand massage and nipple exercises, hand pump, electric "milkers"
2. Diet supplementation: fluids and calories, especially protein
3. Reading, learning, and communication with others with similar experience

Physician-initiated preparation for induced lactation or relactation

1. Knowledgeable, sympathetic support
2. Preparatory hormones and lactagogues to promote mammogenesis
3. Induction of let-down: oxytocin nasal spray to initiate or enhance let-down

4. Counseling about breast preparation and diet supplementation in the context of total care of the mother and the infant
5. Use of nursing supplementing devices

REFERENCES

1. Auerbach, K.G., and Avery, J.L.: Relactation: a study of 366 cases, Pediatrics **65:**236, 1980.
2. Auerbach, K.G., and Avery, J.L.: Induced lactation: a study of adoptive nursing by 240 women, Am. J. Dis. Child. **135:**340, 1981.
3. Avery, J.L.: Induced lactation: a guide for counseling and management, Denver, 1979, Resources in Human Nurturing, International.
4. Bose, C.L., et al., Relactation by mothers of sick and premature infants, Pediatrics **67:**565, 1981.
5. Brown, R.E.: Some nutritional considerations in times of major catastrophe, Clin. Pediatr. **11:**334, 1972.
6. Brown, R.E.: Breast-feeding in modern times, Am. J. Clin. Nutr. **26:**556, 1973.
7. Brown, R.E.: Relactation: an overview, Pediatrics **60:**116, 1977.
8. Canales, E.S., et al.: Feasibility of suppressing and reinitiating lactation in women with premature infants, Am. J. Obstet. Gynecol. **128:**695, 1977.
9. Cohen, R.: Breast-feeding without pregnancy: letter to the editor, Pediatrics **48:**996, 1971.
10. Cowie, A.T., Forsyth, I.A., and Hart, I.C.: Hormonal control of lactation, Monographs on Endocrinology, vol. 15, New York, 1980, Springer-Verlag.
11. Evans, T.J., and Davies, D.P.: Failure to thrive at the breast: an old problem revisited, Arch. Dis. Child. **52:**974, 1977.
12. Foss, G.L., and Short, D.: Abnormal lactation, J. Obstet. Gynecol. Br. Emp. **58:**35, 1951.
13. Gilmore, H.E., and Rowland, T.W.: Critical malnutrition in breast fed infants, Am. J. Dis. Child. **132:**885, 1978.
14. Hormann, E.: A study of induced lactation, La Leche League International bulletin, Franklin Park, Ill., 1976, La Leche League International.
15. Jelliffe, D.B.: Hormonal control of lactation. In Schams, D., editor: Ciba Foundation Symposium no. 45, breast feeding and the mother, Amsterdam, 1976, Elsevier Scientific Publ. Co.
16. Jelliffe, D.B., and Jelliffe, E.F.P.: Human milk in modern world, London, 1976, Oxford University Press.
17. Kleinman, R., et al.: Protein values of milk samples from mothers without biologic pregnancies J. Pediatr. **97:**612, 1980.
18. Kulski, J.K., et al.: Changes in the milk composition of nonpuerperal women, Obstet. Gynecol. **139:**597, 1981.
19. Larson, B.L.: Lactation: a comprehensive treatise. IV. The mammary/gland human/lactation milk synthesis, New York, 1978, Academic Press, Inc.
20. McNeilly, A.S., et al.: Metoclopramide and prolactin, Br. Med. J. **2:**729, 1974.
21. Mead, M.: Sex and temperament in three primitive societies, New York, 1963, Dell Publishing Co., Inc., p. 186.
22. Newton, M., and Egli, G.E.: The effect of intranasal administration of oxytocin on the let-down of milk in lactating women, Am. J. Obstet. Gynecol. **76:**103, 1958.
23. Raphael, D.: Breast feeding the adopted baby. In Raphael, D.: The tender gift: breast feeding, New York, 1976, Schocken Books.
24. Selye, H., and McKeon, T.: The effect of mechanical stimulation of the nipples on the ovary and the sexual cycle, Surg. Gynecol. Obstet. **59:**886, 1934.
25. Sousa, P.L.R., et al.: Re-establishment of lactation with metoclopramide, J. Trop. Pediatr. **21:**214, 1975.
26. Turkington, R.W.: Human prolactin, Am. J. Med. **53:**389, 1972.
27. Tyson, J.E.: Mechanisms of puerperal lactation. In Tyson, J.E., editor: Symposium on pregnancy, Med. Clin. North Am. **61:**153, 1977.
28. Vorherr, H.: The breast: morphology, physiology and lactation, New York, 1974, Academic Press, Inc.
29. Vorherr, H.: Human lactation and breast feeding. In Larson, B.L., editor: Lactation, New York, 1978, Academic Press, Inc., p. 182.
30. Waletzky, L.R., and Herman, E.C.: Relactation, Am. Fam. Pract. **14:**69, 1976.

18

Reproductive function during lactation

FERTILITY

Gonadotropic and ovarian function during lactation have been only minimally investigated. The major body of knowledge has been collected about the postpartum return of the menstrual cycle and ovulation in the woman who is lactating as compared to the nonlactating woman.

The amenorrhea of lactation has been attributed to an imperfect balance of hypothalamoanteropituitary function and gonadotropin secretion. Secretion of follicle-stimulating hormone (FSH) and luteinizing hormone (LH) is generally diminished whenever prolactin is released from the acidophilic cells of the hypothalamoanteropituitary axis. Although the inhibition of FSH and LH has been reported by some, other investigators found no difference between lactating and nonlactating postpartum women. It has been suggested[5] that the ovaries are refractory to gonadotropic stimulation during the early postpartum period and lactation. This has been attributed to the conditions in pregnancy in which high sex steroid plasma levels and large amounts of human chorionic gonadotropin (HCG) led to ovarian inactivity. The ovarian quiescence has been observed in the early postpartum period as well. The antigonadotropic activity of prolaction present during the early months of nursing augments this effect on the ovary. The levels of gonadotropin in all postpartum women for the first weeks of the postpartum period are decreased, which substantiates the theory that there is postpartum ovarian refractoriness. In the first 2 weeks postpartum low levels of FSH are found in urine and plasma. Beling et al.[1] report estrogen excretion to be low with a linear increase during the first 5 to 8 weeks. When lactating postpartum women are given intramuscular gonadotropins, there is no increase in urinary steroids, according to studies by Zarate et al.[32] The prolactin cell predominance may be responsible for the decreased activity of the pituitaryovarian axis postpartum. Myometrial and endometrial involution are also considered to reduce fertility. Animal studies have shown that the release of FSH and LH is inhibited by intense suckling. In addition, animals in which the nipple is stimulated while the milk ducts have been tied off still show a suppression of estrous and menstrual cycles. Selye and McKeown[28] concluded that interruption of sexual cyclicity during lactation is a result of the nursing and not due to the secretory activity of the mammary gland.

Clinically, the perceptible measurement of the return of fertility is the onset of menstruation. Return of reproductive function varies, depending on the length and degree of lactation. Most studies do not, in fact, report the completeness of lactation, that is, whether the infant is totally breastfed or is also receiving solid foods or supplemental bottles.[14] By the end of the third month only 33% of lactating women have had a menstrual period, whereas 91% of nonlactating women have had their period. At 9 months, 65% of those women who are still lactating have had the return of menstruation. Vorherr[31] further reports that 30% become pregnant within 1 year after delivery; 40% of those who became pregnant at 1 year were still lactating. Of the lactating women not using contraception, more than half will become pregnant during the first 9 months of lactation. Another view of the statistics, however, indicates that lactation does exert an inhibitory effect on reproductive function. A mother who nurses at least 20 weeks will postpone menstruation 12 weeks and ovulation 18 weeks.

The period of lactational amenorrhea does offer a measure of conception protection for 3 months. The nonlactating woman has a return of her period at 25 days at the earliest, of ovulation at 25 to 35 days, and a 5% chance of regaining fertility prior to 6 weeks postpartum.

Perez et al.[23] diagnosed the first postpartum ovulation by endometrial biopsy, basal body temperature, vaginal cytology, and cervical mucus in a group of 200 women in a prospective study. The dates of first ovulation, first menses, and nursing status were analyzed. No woman ovulated before the thirty-sixth day, whether lactating or not. The intensity and length of nursing affected the date when ovulation occurred, according to the researchers. About 78% of the women ovulated prior to the first menses. Twelve pregnancies occurred with first ovulation. Of the 170 women who breastfed, 24 ovulated while completely nursing, 49 while partially nursing, and 97 after weaning (Table 18-1).

Following is a general summation of available data on return of ovulation and menstruation[31]:

I. Nursing mothers

   Earliest possible menstruation: 4 to 6 weeks postpartum (pp)

   Most women menstruating: fourth month pp

   Return of menstruation: 6 weeks pp—15%

                          12 weeks pp—45%

                          24 weeks pp—85%

   Earliest possible ovulation: 6 weeks pp

   Return of ovulation: 6 weeks pp—5%

                   12 weeks pp—25%

                   24 weeks pp—65%

Table 18-1. Percentage of ovulatory first cycles by duration from birth and nursing status at time of first bleeding day postpartum*

Ovulatory first cycles	Day of first bleeding			
	0-29	30-59	60 or more	Total
Fully nursing				
No. of patients	—	8	19	27
Ovulatory (%)	—	0	58	41
Partial nursing				
No. of patients	—	7	38	45
Ovulatory (%)	—	29	79	75
Nursing suspended				
No. of patients	—	18	80	98
Ovulatory (%)	—	83	93	91

From Perez, A., et al.: Am. J. Obstet. Gynecol. 114:1041, 1967.
*In the 12 patients who became pregnant during amenorrhea, first bleeding day is defined as ovulation day plus 9.

First ovular cycle: preceded in about 80% by one or more anovular cycles

Early pp: mainly anovular cycles

Later pp: more often ovular cycles

Ovular cycles: in about 50% of regularly menstruating mothers

II. Amenorrheic nursing mothers

Endometrium: state of undifferentiation or hypoproliferation

Return of ovulation: 6 weeks pp—2%

16 weeks pp—10%

After first menstruation—14%

III. Nonnursing mothers

Earliest possible menstruation: 4 weeks pp

Most women menstruating: third month pp

Return of menstruation: 6 weeks pp—40%

12 weeks pp—65%

24 weeks pp—90%

Earliest possible ovulation: 3½-5 weeks pp

Ovular cycles: in about 50% with first menstrual period pp

Early pp ovulation: possible occurrence late in the menstrual cycle—shortening of secretory phase and greater tendency toward irregular menses

Return of ovulation: 6 weeks pp—15%

12 weeks pp—40%

24 weeks pp—75%

IV. Amenorrheic nonnursing mothers

Return of ovulation: 12 weeks pp—20%

16 weeks pp—40%

Data collected in preindustrialized societies show more prolonged lactational amenorrhea, which is probably due to more prolonged total breastfeeding and, to a degree, the relative malnutrition of the mother. Peters et al.[25] indicate that the mean duration of breastfeeding in their study of women in India is 16½ months and of amenorrhea 12 months.

The difference between postpartum and nutritional amenorrhea should be pointed out because true nutritional amenorrhea is predictable on the basis of the height/weight ratio, whereas lactational amenorrhea is hormonal and nutrition has only a trivial effect on postpartum amenorrhea.[11]

Among !Kung hunter-gatherers there are long intervals between births, which has puzzled investigators because the tribes are well nourished, have low fetal wastage, and do not employ contraceptives or prolonged abstinence. Konner and Worthman[17] report that the !Kung have unusual temporal patterns of nursing characterized by highly frequent nursing bouts with short space between nursings. The !Kung nurse several times an hour with only 15 minutes at most between. Serum estradiol and progesterone levels are correspondingly low. Infants are always in the immediate proximity of their mothers until they are weaned, at about 3½ years, during a new sibling's gestation. In Nigeria the effect of duration and frequency of breastfeeding on postpartum amenorrhea is comparable in that Nigerians breastfeed for 16.5 months with a frequency of 4.5 times a day. The mean length of amenorrhea is 12.5 months. Amenorrheic mothers who were lactating had lower levels of serum estradiol and lactic dehydrogenase. There was a significant association of hyperprolactinemia with amenorrhea. The incidence of amenorrhea declined parallel to that of the hyperprolactinemia.[9]

When fertility postpartum during lactation was studied in Edinburgh, suckling was the most important factor inhibiting the return to ovulation.[21] Those mothers who ovulated while breastfeeding had all introduced two or more supplementary feeds per day, and had reduced suckling to under six times a day, with 60 minutes or less suckling time per day. The basal prolactin levels were below 600 μ/L. The mothers who did not ovulate until after 40 weeks postpartum breastfed longest, suckled most intensely, maintained night feeds longest, and introduced supplementary feeds most slowly.[14] The prolactin levels remained substantially above 600 μ/L.

Another review of the effects of hormonal contraceptives on lactation by Hull[15] concludes that there is a significant number of reports of decrease in milk yield. The description of severe growth failure[11] in the nursling, even leading to "contraceptive marasmus," in Egypt and Tunisia is cause for concern.

A significant distinction should be made between token breastfeeding with early solids and more rigid feeding schedules and the ad lib breastfeeding around the clock with no solids until the infant is 6 months old. The amount and frequency of sucking are closely related to the continued amenorrhea in most women. When a totally breastfed infant sleeps through the night at an early age, requiring no suckling for 6 hours or so at night, the suppressive effect on menses diminishes. It has also been shown that if the infant uses a pacifier rather than receives his nonnutritive sucking at the breast, the suppression of ovulation is diminished (Tables 18-2 and 18-3).

Table 18-2. Distribution of natural mothering* sample by months of breastfeeding†

Months of breastfeeding	Number of experiences	Percent of total experiences
12	1	3.5
13-16	5	17.2
17-20	7	24.2
21-24	4	13.7
25-28	6	20.7
29-32	3	10.3
33-36	2	6.9
37	1	3.5

From Kippley, S.: Breast feeding and natural child spacing, New York, 1974, Harper & Row, Publishers, copyright © 1974 by Sheila K. Kippley, reprinted by permission of Harper & Row, Publishers.
*Natural mothering includes, among other things, no pacifiers used, no bottles used, no solids or liquids for 5 months, no feeding schedules other than infant's, presence of night feedings, and presence of lying-down nursing (naps, night feedings).
†N = 29 experiences (22 mothers). Mean months of breastfeeding = 22.8; median months of breastfeeding = 23.0.

Table 18-3. Distribution of natural mothering* sample by months of amenorrhea†

Months of amenorrhea	Number of experiences	Percent of total experiences
1-4	2	6.9
5-8	2	6.9
9-12	7	24.1
13-16	9	31.0
17-20	5	17.2
21-24	2	6.9
25-28	1	3.5
29-30	1	3.5

From Kippley, S.: Breast feeding and natural child spacing, New York, 1974, Harper & Row, Publishers, copyright © 1974 by Sheila K. Kippley, reprinted by permission of Harper & Row, Publishers.
*Natural mothering includes, among other things, no pacifiers used, no bottles used, no solids or liquids for 5 months, no feeding schedules other than infant's, presence of night feedings, and presence of lying-down nursing (naps, night feedings).
†N = 29 experiences (22 mothers). Mean months of amenorrhea = 14.6; median months of amenorrhea = 14.0.

CONTRACEPTION DURING LACTATION
Natural child spacing

Although lactation provides some degree of protection early in the postpartum period, a woman who is seriously concerned about avoiding conception should be informed of her options. If she does not wish to use contraceptives, medications, or devices, she should be instructed in the external signs of ovulation. In most studies of lactation, the initial menses occur prior to the onset of ovulation. The risk of pregnancy during lactational amenorrhea, however, is about 5% unless some effort is made to identify ovulation by basal temperature or cervical secretions.[16]

The sympto-thermal method of fertility awareness during lactation was studied in Canada.[22] A special postpartum chart was designed to record morning temperature, cervical mucus, and other signs of fertility/infertility in relation to dates and postpartum days. The intensity of the breastfeeding was also recorded. There were 54 breastfeeding experiences in 47 women whose ages ranged from 20 to 39. Parity ranged from 1 to 7 with an average of 3.3. The duration of full breastfeeding averaged 3.6 months (range of 3 weeks to 8 months). The duration of breastfeeding ranged from 2 to 28 months with an average of 8.8 months. These mothers found that in general they could predict their fertile times with accuracy while breastfeeding. During times of weaning or change in suckling pattern, special caution was suggested in which the mothers watched for signs of first ovulation.

The effectiveness of periodic abstinence was reviewed for lactating women for *Population Reports*.[24] Long periods of lactational infertility can be identified by either lack of mucus or continuous unchanging mucous flow. As ovulation resumes, irregular mucus patterns occur that are difficult to interpret and therefore require prolonged abstinence. A pregnancy rate with this method was 9.1 per 100 women-years. Because two thirds of the 82 women studied were totally breastfeeding, many of the ensuing postpartum cycles may have been anovulatory or had an inadequate luteal phase, thus helping to keep the pregnancy rate low.

Studies of cervical secretions alone (mucus patterns) during lactation have indicated that the same signs in mucus are reliable during lactation. Charting is carried out in the usual manner and feedings are also recorded. A woman who is following her pattern postpartum should be seen every 2 weeks for guidance until her pattern is well documented. The couple should make careful observations when (1) the infant sleeps through the night, (2) the mother reduces the number of breastfeedings, (3) the infant begins solid foods, (4) the infant begins other liquids or a bottle, or (5) there is illness in either mother or baby. Abstinence is advised until the situation is clear. If there has been no prior ovulation or menstruation when weaning begins, ovulation may occur quite quickly.[6]

Oral contraceptives and lactation

The significant issues related to lactation and the use of oral contraceptives are the potentially adverse effects of oral·contraceptives on milk production, uterine involution, and growth and development of the breastfed infant. A case is reported by Curtis[8] of breast enlargement in a breastfed male infant whose mother began taking norethynodrel with ethynylestradiol 3-methyl ether (Enovid) on the third day postpartum. Breast enlargement began on the third week of life. The mother had noted her milk was not as ''rich'' and started supplements the second week. Nursing was discontinued at about 4 weeks of age and the breasts of the infant returned to normal in 2 to 3 weeks. The additional risks to the mother of thromboembolism, hypertension, and cancer have also been discussed extensively in the literature.

The data available have been well reviewed by Vorherr.[30,31] He summarizes the information by noting that preparations containing 2.5 mg or less of a 19-norprogestogen and 50 μg or less of etinylestradiol or 100 μg or less of mestranol present no hazard to mother or infant. He further points out that milk yield can be decreased with larger doses of combination oral contraceptives containing estrogen and 5 to 10 mg of progestogen/dose. Only two studies of many suggest any variation in the content of the milk (protein, fat, and calcium) (Table 18-4) due to oral contraceptives.

Toddywalla et al.[29] reported the effect of injectable contraceptives as well as oral combinations on milk production. They found an increase in the protein content of the milk and slight increase in quantity from the group given injection of 150 mg of medroxyprogesterone (Depo-Provera) every 3 months. The group receiving 300 mg of medroxyprogesterone every 6 months showed significant increase in quantity but a de-

Table 18-4. Effect of contraceptive steroids on lactation

Agents	Milk yield	Comments
Estrogens		
Ethinylestradiol (50 μg)	No change	Placebo controls
Mestranol (80 μg)	No change	Placebo controls
Progestins		
Depo-Provera*	No change	No placebo controls
(150-250 mg medroxyprogesterone acetate)	No change	No placebo controls
Ethinylestrenol (0.5 mg)	No change	Placebo controls; no adverse effects on infants' weight gain
Lynestrenol (0.5 mg)	No change	No change in infant's growth curve
Norethindrone (10 mg)	No change	No placebo controls
Norethisterone (200 mg)	No change	No placebo controls
Estrogen-progestin combinations		
Anovlar (4 mg norethindrone + 50 μg ethinylestradiol)	Decrease by 40%	No placebo controls
C-Quens*	No change	No placebo controls
(2 mg chlormadinone acetate + 80 μg mestranol, sequential)	Decrease by 32%	No placebo controls; infants' weight gain 10% less than controls
Deladroxate (150 mg dihydroxyprogesterone + 10 mg estradiol enanthate)	Slight decrease	No change in infants' weight
Enovid* (2.5, 5, 10, 20 mg norethynodrel + 100 μg mestranol)		
Enovid 2.5	No change	No placebo controls
	No change	No placebo controls; "patient's acceptance was excellent"
Enovid 5	No change	No placebo controls
Enovid 5, 10, 20	Decrease by 40% to 80%	Textbook information, no details regarding data evaluation
Ovulen* (1 mg ethynodiol diacetate + 100 μg mestranol)	No change	No placebo controls
	"Nursing function occasionally impaired"	No placebo controls
	Decrease by 30%	No placebo controls
	Decrease by 32% to 55%	No placebo controls; infants' weight gain 27% less than controls

From Vorherr, H.: Human lactation and breast feeding. In Larson, B.L., editor: Lactation: a comprehensive treatise, New York, 1978, Academic Press, Inc.
*Consideration of results of various publications.

crease in protein, fat, and calcium as compared with controls (who used mechanical means of contraception). The secretion of hormones in human milk is poorly documented, with only a few infants studied in each hormone combination. In all cases a small but measurable amount was found in the milk. Unfortunately, measurements in the infant's serum are not reported.

The impact of the distribution of oral contraceptives on breastfeeding and pregnancy status in rural Haiti indicated that it did not alter breastfeeding patterns.[3] Women began the pills at 8 to 9 months postpartum. Pregnancy prevalence also decreased as a result.

It is the concern of many that use of any hormone combination to suppress ovulation during lactation is contraindicated because of the potential risk to the infant, not only immediately but also in the long-range view. As discussed earlier, there have been reports of enlargement of the breasts in male and female infants when nursed by mothers taking oral contraceptives with higher dosages of estrogen and/or progesterone than are presently used.

No adverse effects on the infant during the ensuing years in bone maturation, genital development, or impaired fertility have been substantiated. Vorherr responds to the reports of such effects in animal studies by pointing out that (1) only small amounts of progesterone reach the infant and the androgenic capabilities are a fraction of those of testosterone, (2) long-range follow-up from the middle 1950s of nursing mothers given up to 20 mg of progestogen/day showed no bone maturation acceleration in infancy nor impairment of ovarian function and fertility in the infants' reproductive years, and (3) the dosages given the animals in the studies reporting abnormalities were excessive on a comparable weight basis (1 mg in a 6 g newborn rat). It is too early in the history of oral contraceptives to be entirely sure that there is no long-range increase in risk of cancer in the infants so nursed.

Intrauterine devices and other contraceptive methods

Various alternatives to oral contraceptives do exist and have been observed to have different degrees of reliability. The intrauterine devices (IUDs) (95% to 98% effective), cervical caps and diaphragms (85% to 88% effective), condoms (80% to 85% effective), and vaginal suppositories, jellies, or creams (80% effective) have no known contraindication during breastfeeding, since no chemicals are absorbed. The only contraceptive that is 100% effective is abstinence.

A study of 2271 postpartum women who had IUDs inserted between 1976 and 1981 and were followed for 6 to 12 months was reported with careful attention to details of lactation.[7] Data were analyzed separately for IUDs inserted immediately after birth (within 10 minutes of placental expulsion). The results of this analysis indicate that IUD insertion for breastfeeding women would be appropriate either immediately after delivery or later (≥42 days postpartum). When inserted immediately postpartum, the Delta Loop and Delta T were modified by adding projections of chromic sutures, which helps the device remain in the uterus. The sutures biodegrade in 6 weeks, leaving a standard device in place. These authors report that breastfeeding is not a contraindication to IUD insertion. There is not an increased expulsion rate. Conversely the presence of an IUD has no adverse effect on lactation. The appropriate time for insertion should be selected to predate anticipated ovulation but guarantee patient compliance.

A group of 32 women hospitalized for uterine perforation necessitating transperitoneal IUD removal and a matched control group of 497 women who had worn IUDs uneventfully were compared.[13] Of the women in the study, 97% were postpartum compared with 68% of the controls. Of the parous study group, 42% were lactating and of the parous controls, 7% were lactating when the IUD was inserted. The risk of perforation was 10 times greater in the lactating than in the nonlactating women, unrelated to time of the insertion postpartum. In another group hospitalized for difficult transcervical IUD removal, the risk was 2.3 times greater for lactating women. The authors recommend caution, not abandonment of the procedure during lactation, because they feel the IUD is the best form of artificial contraception during lactation. Many cultures and societies place taboos on sexual intercourse for the nursing mother as an effective means of spacing children. Usually there are no medical contraindications to sexual relationships during lactation.

SEX AND THE NURSING MOTHER
Sexual arousal associated with suckling

If one examines the normal adult female in regard to the menstrual cycle, sexual intercourse, pregnancy, childbirth, and lactation, one observes that these events are all influenced by the interaction of the same hormones. Not only the presence of estrogen, progesterone, testosterone, FSH, and LH but oxytocin and prolactin as well. The breast is known to respond during all these phases, enlarging before menstruation, during pregnancy, before orgasm, and during lactation.[10] The nipples also respond during these phases. Furthermore, it is noted that the uterus contracts during childbirth, orgasm, and lactation. Body temperature rises during ovulation, childbirth, orgasm, and lactation. As pointed out in Chapter 3, oxytocin is a critical element in the let-down reflex during lactation. Oxytocin levels also rise during orgasms and labor, and oxytocin causes the uterus to contract and the nipples to become erect. Newton and Newton[20] report other similarities in women during these events, including sensory perception and emotional reactions. Following are the psychophysiologic similarities between lactation and coitus:[20]

1. The uterus contracts.
2. The nipples become erect.
3. Breast stroking and nipple stimulation occur.
4. The emotions experienced involve skin changes (vascular dilation and raised temperature).
5. Milk let-down (or ejection) reflex can be triggered.

6. The emotions experienced may be closely allied.
7. An accepting attitude towards sexuality may be related to an accepting attitude to breastfeeding (and vice versa).

Given the biologic and hormonal similarities of lactation to the other events in the sexual cycle of the adult female, it is not surprising that some women experience some form of sexual gratification during suckling on certain occasions. It has been reported by Masters and Johnson[19] in a study of 111 parturient women, only 24 of whom breastfed, that there was sexual arousal experienced during suckling on some occasions. The exact incidence of this response is unknown, but it is believed to be uncommon. Nursing mothers may have an element of guilt surrounding these experiences and thus it is underreported. It has been suggested that guilt leads to early weaning in some cases. For some women the breasts are highly erogenous. The handling and manipulation of the breast necessary during lactation by both mother and infant can, in the right circumstances and mood, be stimulating. Clearly the majority of women who enjoy breastfeeding have no feelings or responses to the stimulation of the breast that could be construed as sexual arousal, although they enjoy breastfeeding and the intimacy with their infant that it provides. The erotic response to nursing the infant has no significance in terms of being normal or abnormal. The decline of breastfeeding because of feelings of shame, modesty, embarrassment, and distaste has been reported by Bentovim[2] and interpreted as indicating that breastfeeding is viewed as a forbidden sexual activity. For such women any sexual allusions and excitement accompanying breastfeeding are not permissible and cause shame. Such attitudes are more common in lower social groups and need to be considered in counseling mothers about breastfeeding prepartum or when premature weaning takes place. Major changes in the number of women who breastfeed may not be possible until society can accept the breast in its relationship to nurturing the infant and also as an object of less sexual ambivalence.

The sensuousness of breastfeeding has been the topic of discussion in popular women's magazines as more is written about women and their bodies.[25] For the well-educated, well-read woman who breastfeeds her infant because she intellectually arrives at the decision, such discussions are an avenue of increased knowledge.[27] Others may still be uncomfortable about breastfeeding if it is apt to be ''pleasurable.'' The physician may sense this discomfort in his patient prenatally by her responses to bodily change during pregnancy. Cultural attitudes are an important part of this response and are deeply ingrained in an individual by the time she reaches the age of parenting. Professionals need to be sensitive to the patient and cautious about imposing cultural change on a given patient, while being alert to needs for information and openness.

The sexual activity of the nursing mother

A review of the limited data available on lactating women in the Masters and Johnson study[19] does indicate that in their group of 111 postpartum women, the nursing mothers were more eager than nonnursing mothers to resume sexual relations postpartum. The data were independent of the fear of pregnancy. They report that this interest was apparent 2 to 3 weeks postpartum. Individual reports through a questionnaire reported by Ladas[18] indicated that 30% of nursing mothers believed their sexual relationships were improved and 2.5% believed they were worse postpartum. The individual testimonies of nursing mothers reported by Ladas indicated they had a better feeling about themselves as well as their relationships with their husbands and family in general.

More general observations indicate that although some women may have increased interest in sexual relations while nursing, others may experience no interest at all for 6 months or so. Whether this is due to the saturation of the mother's needs for intimate relationship and stimulus through nursing, general fatigue, or fear of pregnancy is debatable. Sexual stimulus may trigger the ejection reflex, and milk ejection may have a negative effect on some men. The total knowledge of nursing and suckling as a biologic phenomenon will help couples to understand such reactions and thus avoid inappropriate response psychologically. The conflict in some adult men over their role in regard to the nursing mother's breasts is usually a result of guilt or upbringing. There is no need to advise against fondling the lactating breast during lovemaking, although physicians have often imposed rigid restrictions on sexual activity in the lactating woman. There is no scientific basis for such restriction and no difference in the incidence of infection and mastitis associated with such activity. Unusually restrictive protocols are often imposed on patients without medical indication. Bradley[4] recommends, in fact, oral and manual manipulation of the breasts by the husband during both pregnancy and lactation to prevent sore nipples.

It is helpful to discuss with the lactating woman that the hormonal effect on the vagina may be excessive dryness with an increase in dyspareunia. The dryness responds to locally applied lubricants and tends to improve over time. A sudden change may actually reflect ovulation. The breast that is being stimulated by feeding frequently may not be as sensitive during lovemaking. Usually this too is only transient. The physician should perhaps remind the mother that some adjustment to attend to the father's needs may be necessary.

NURSING WHILE PREGNANT AND TANDEM NURSING

Pregnancy can and does occur while lactating. When it does occur it produces a number of questions. There is no need to hastily wean the first infant from the breast, which is often ordered by the physician. It is possible to lactate throughout pregnancy and then to have two infants at the breast postpartum. It is now a sufficiently common event to be called tandem nursing. Obviously the amount of nourishment provided the first infant at the breast depends on his age and other supplements. When the infant at the breast is only a few months old when pregnancy occurs, there is some rationale to continued breastfeeding for the benefit of the infant until it is time to wean to solids and other liquids at 6 months of age or so. This child will be about a year old when the new infant arrives and if still at the breast may have demands in excess of the mother's ability to provide. Concern had been expressed that the older infant will take much of the nourishment needed by the new infant. In some societies it is believed that a suckling infant will ''take the spirit'' from the newly conceived fetus; thus weaning is mandated once pregnancy is confirmed. The milk produced immediately postpartum by the mother who never stopped nursing appears to be colostrum. The kangaroo has been observed to have a teat for the older offspring with mature milk and a teat for the new offspring who requires significantly different nourishment. Such a provision does not exist for the human. It has been shown by mothers who wish to maintain both infants at the breast that it can be done without any apparent effect on the nourishment of the new infant. Counseling of such a mother should take into account the mother's resource to get adequate rest, nourishment, and psychologic support to withstand the added demand on her, physically and mentally.

If the first child is older and will be well beyond a year of age when the new infant arrives, the need for physical nourishment is minimal and continuation at the breast is more for the security and psychologic benefits. Abrupt weaning should be avoided, and consideration should be given to the impact of separation when the mother is confined during the birth of the new infant. (Perhaps this is an argument for 12-hour hospitalizations for delivery.) The first few days of colostrum are most vital for the new infant and the supply is not infinite; therefore priorities need to be set as far as the older child is concerned.

Many of the changes in child-rearing practices in recent years have increased the freedom and response to human needs. Carried to extremes, instant gratification becomes a right rather than a privilege. Sometimes a mother may need help in seeing that she need not feel guilty if she decides to wean the older child. If it is only an occasional feeding or suckling experience for added security, especially when security is threatened by the arrival of a new infant, it is tolerable in terms of endurance for the mother and she agrees willingly. When, however, continuing nursing becomes a strain or is painful or stressful, she should feel free to stop. When the mother feels real resentment toward the older child who is nursing, Pryor[26] points out that it is time to gently but firmly wean. If such a situation could be anticipated, it is probably easier for the older child to be weaned prior to delivery of the new infant. As with any such decisions to wean, it is best for the physician to work this decision out in frank discussion with the mother (and father, too, if he is available) so that any misgivings, resentment, or feeling of failure can be dealt with openly. Many patients automatically suspect the physician of being antagonistic to breastfeeding if the physician suggests weaning. Even when the reason is purely but urgently medical, discussion should be open and include options and alternatives and their risks. Pryor[26] expresses it succinctly when she says, ''Weaning is part of the baby's growing up, but it is sometimes part of the mother's growing up, too.''

The dilemma of tandem nursing and weaning the older child has been dealt with in other societies with various manipulations such as painting the breast with pepper or bitter herbs to make it taste terrible. Having the mother leave the child with other caregivers is also done. The provision of love and affection during this difficult adaptation for the child is what makes the difference between a traumatic occasion and a step toward growing up. Equally important is the provision of some opportunity for the mother to express her concerns and doubts during the process to her physician, who should be neither judgmental nor unduly rigid in his medical care plan.

REFERENCES

1. Beling, C.G., Frandsen, V.A., and Josimovich, J.B.: Pituitary and ovarian hormone levels during lactation, Acta Endocrinol. **155**(suppl.):40, 1971.
2. Bentovin, A.: Shame and other anxieties. In Ciba Foundation Symposium no. 45, breast feeding and the mother, Amsterdam, 1976, Elsevier Scientific Publ. Co.
3. Bordes, A., Allman, J., and Verly, A.: The impact on breastfeeding and pregnancy status of household contraceptive distribution in rural Haiti, Am. J. Public Health **72**:835, 1982.
4. Bradley, R.A.: Husband-coached childbirth, New York, 1965, Harper & Row, Publishers, Inc.
5. Brambilla, F., and Sirtori, C.M.: Gonadotropin-inhibiting factor in pregnancy, lactation and menopause, Am. J. Obstet. Gynecol. **109**:599, 1971.
6. Brown, R.E.: Breast-feeding and family planning: a review of relationships between breast-feeding and family planning, Am. J. Clin. Nutr. **35**:162, 1982.
7. Cole, L.P., et al.: Effects of breastfeeding on IUD performance, Am. J. Public Health **73**:384, 1983.
8. Curtis, E.M.: Oral-contraceptive feminization of a normal male infant, Obstet. Gynecol. **23**:295, 1964.
9. Delvoye, P., et al.: Serum prolactin, gonadotropins, and estradiol in menstruating and amenorrheic mothers during two years' lactation, Am. J. Obstet. Gynecol. **130**:635, 1978.
10. Eiger, M.S., and Olds, S.W.: The complete book of breastfeeding, New York, 1972, Bantam Books, Inc.
11. Frisch, R.E., and McArthur, J.W.: Difference between postpartum and nutritional amenorrhea, Science **203**:921, 1979.
12. Gioiosa, R.: Incidence of pregnancy during lactation in 500 cases, Am. J. Obstet. Gynecol. **70**:162, 1955.
13. Hartwell, S. and Latuchi, G.I.: IUD perforation, Obstet. Gynecol. **61**:31, 1983.
14. Howie, P.W., et al.: Fertility after childbirth: infant feeding patterns, basal PRL levels, and post-partum ovulation, Clin. Endocrinol. **17**:315, 1982.
15. Hull, V.J.: The effects of hormonal contraceptives on lactation: current findings, methodological considerations and future priorities, Stud. Fam. Plann. **12**:134, 1981.
16. Kippley, S.: Breast feeding and natural child spacing, New York, 1976, Harper & Row, Publishers, Inc.
17. Konner, M., and Worthman, C.: Nursing frequency, gonadal function, and birth spacing among !Kung hunter-gatherers, Science **207**:788, 1980.
18. Ladas, A.K.: How to help mothers breast feed: deductions from a survey, Clin. Pediatr. **9**:702, 1970.
19. Masters, W.H., and Johnson, V.E.: Human sexual response, Boston, 1966, Little, Brown & Co.
20. Newton, N., and Newton, M.: Psychologic aspects of lactation, N. Engl. J. Med. **277**:1179, 1967.
21. Ojofeitimi, E.O.: Effect of duration and frequency of breastfeeding on postpartum amenorrhea, Pediatrics **69**:164, 1982.
22. Perez, A.: Lactational amenorrhea and natural family planning. In Hafez, E.S.E., editor: Human ovulation: mechanisms, prediction, detection, and induction, Amsterdam, 1979, North-Holland Publishing.
23. Perez, A., et al.: First ovulation after child birth: the effect of breast feeding, Am. J. Obstet. Gynecol. **114**:1041, 1972.

24. Periodic abstinence: how well do new approaches work, Popul. Rep. **[I]:**3, Sept. 1981.
25. Peters, H., Israel, S., and Purshottan, S.: Lactation period in Indian women: duration of amenorrhea and vaginal and cervical cytology, Fertil. Steril. **9:**134, 1958.
26. Pryor, K.: Nursing your baby, New York, 1973, Pocket Books.
27. Riordan, J.: A practical guide to breastfeeding, St. Louis, 1983, The C.V. Mosby Co.
28. Selye, H., and McKeown, T.: The effect of mechanical stimulation of the nipples on the ovary and the sexual cycle. Surg. Gynecol. Obstet. **59:**856, 1934.
29. Toddywalla, V.S., Joshi, L., and Virkar, K.: Effect of contraceptive steroids on human lactation, Am. J. Obstet. Gynecol. **127:**245, 1977.
30. Vorherr, H.: The breast: morphology, physiology and lactation, New York, 1974, Academic Press, Inc.
31. Vorherr. H.: Human lactation and breast feeding. In Larson, B.L., editor: Lactation: a comprehensive treatise, New York, 1978, Academic Press, Inc.
32. Zarate, A., et al.: Ovarian refractoriness during lactation in women: effect of gonadotropin stimulation, Am. J. Obstet. Gynecol. **112:**1130, 1972.

The storage of human milk and cross-nursing

19

STORING HUMAN MILK

Because of the renewed interest in providing human milk for the sick newborn and the premature infant, it is often necessary to store milk for infants, especially in the hospital. The storage of human milk involves two types of milk: mother's milk and donor milk. The distinction becomes important in how the milk is stored and how it is prepared for the infant. It is also important because many states have developed codes for donor milk but fortunately have not regulated mother's milk as yet. Certain guidelines are appropriate for each milk.

Milk banks have been in continuous operation for over 50 years according to Siimes and Hallman,[35] who report the collection of 5000 L/1 million members of the general population annually (24.4 L/donating mother). The indications for use of such milk have been alluded to in other chapters but are briefly summarized as follows:

Mother's milk

1. The mother plans to breastfeed the infant ultimately, but needs to provide pumped milk until he can be put to the breast.
2. The infant requires the special nutritional benefits of human milk (as with those infants who are recovering from intestinal surgery), yet cannot nurse.
3. The infant weighs 1500 g or less and has difficulty digesting and absorbing other milks.

Donor milk

1. The infant is at risk of infection or necrotizing enterocolitis. Although effects are not clearly demonstrated with mature milk, fresh colostrum is held to be especially protective.
2. The physician believes the infant would benefit from the nourishment in human milk

because of prematurity, especially if the infant weighs less than 1500 g.

3. The mother is temporarily unable to nourish a breastfed infant completely. It may be that the mother's supply is inadequate when she first puts the infant to the breast after weeks of pumping or when the mother has been ill or hospitalized. Usually these infants are already at home.

Structure of a milk bank

There has been a resurgence of interest in milk banks in recent years, paralleling the interest in breast milk in general.[30] Banks have been reinstated after years of dormancy. The Mother's Milk Unit in California,[31] for instance, is part of a total transplant program. There are many hospitals, particularly those with intensive care nurseries, that are collecting and storing breast milk for use with hospitalized infants without the fanfare of being labeled a bank. In England and Wales, five large-scale human milk banks provide milk for infants in a large geographic area.

The state of New York passed an amendment to the public health law in 1980 in which it was declared policy that any and all infants requiring human breast milk be assured access to sufficient quantities of wholesome human breast milk donated by concerned lactating mothers on a continued and systematic basis (see Appendix K for entire law). This law resulted in an addition to the rules and regulations of the hospitals' minimum standards, since it was anticipated that the greatest number of infants requiring human milk would be hospitalized in tertiary neonatal units. The administrative rules and regulations were developed with the consultation of experts in milk banking and neonatal care. Because the items cover all of the considerations known to be necessary to provide the safest and most effective human milk for recipients, the regulations are duplicated in Appendix K for reference. Similarly, the Committee on Medical Aspects of Food Policy[6] in the United Kingdom held a Working Party on Human Milk Banks from 1979 to 1980, publishing a formal report in 1981 as an operational guideline for pediatric departments of hospitals that were setting up milk banks. The consultants included pediatricians, obstetricians, dietitians, nurses, and scientists with special expertise in lactation and human milk. The document is available from Her Majesty's Stationery Office (London Reports on Health and Social Subjects, no. 22). The recommendations for the expansion of the human milk banking system have not gone without challenge from neonatologists who offer sincere concerns for the risk/benefit ratio because alteration during storage and contamination may detract from the value of the original product for the mother's own infant. A series of sobering letters[1,28] appeared in the British medical press following the release of the document cautioning that the cavalier feeding of unsterile unsupplemented breast milk to small premature infants may produce iatrogenic problems. Neonatologists everywhere advise caution in providing human milk for infants under 1500 g until its value is proven.

Whether a major project is launched and funds sought for its maintenance or a hospital merely wishes to provide a service for its patients, there are some ground rules that are helpful to follow. The hospital administration should be informed so that proper permissions for donors and for recipients can be provided. Establishment of the hospital's liability should also be investigated because a well-meaning donor or physician could be placed in jeopardy for his or her generous act if these seemingly stringent details are not identified and dealt with. A sample permission sheet is provided in Fig. 19-1.

Most hospitals find it convenient to receive and disburse the milk through a member of the nursery staff, such as the unit manager. The Louisville Breast Milk Program[14]

THE UNIVERSITY OF ROCHESTER
SCHOOL OF MEDICINE AND DENTISTRY
AND
STRONG MEMORIAL HOSPITAL
601 ELMWOOD AVE.
ROCHESTER, NEW YORK 14642

DEPARTMENT OF PEDIATRICS

AGREEMENT WITH STRONG MEMORIAL HOSPITAL
AND MOTHERS DONATING BREAST MILK

I, _____, agree to contribute my milk, which I carefully collect, taking the prescribed precautions in its collection. I am in good health and not on medications. I agree to discard milk collected if I am temporarily ill or temporarily on medication. I understand that Strong Memorial Hospital will pay a small stipend for my contribution. I understand they will provide me with small sterile bottles to be used in refrigerating or freezing the collected milk.

Signed_____ Date_____

Witnessed_____ Date_____

Fig. 19-1. Release form used at Strong Memorial Hospital for mothers who donate their milk to milk bank. (Courtesy Strong Memorial Hospital, Rochester, N.Y.)

has developed a system that involves the hospital pharmacy and a pharmacist as a part-time coordinator. The Mother's Milk Unit of the Northern California Transplant Bank, affiliated with Stanford University School of Medicine, uses a full-time coordinator and has a medical director.[20] The Georgetown University Hospital operates an active Breast Milk Bank near the Neonatal Intensive Care Unit with full-time staff and a medical director (Fig. 19-2). Many other hospital-based as well as free-standing programs have been developed nationwide.

Operation of a milk bank

Experience with milk bank operation in Rochester spans almost 20 years. In the late 1950s and early 1960s, before intravenous alimentation, milk was provided postoperatively for sick newborns who could not tolerate other formulas yet were gradually starving on intravenous fluids alone. Milk was collected fresh from volunteers, usually mothers on the postpartum floor who were not going to breastfeed their own infants. Multiple donors were often used for a single infant; thus much colostrum was provided, which may, in retrospect, be why the infants did so well and infection was no problem. Mothers washed their hands and their breasts and used a sterile hand pump. Milk was refrigerated immediately in sterile bottles or given immediately to the infant. Mothers who were asked to donate had had a normal pregnancy and delivery, were serologically negative, had received no medications, and had no indications of infection. No infant had any infections while taking the milk.

In 1968 the demand for milk had become so frequent, particularly for small infants, that collections were begun from regular donors. These women were healthy and met all the criteria just mentioned but were also nursing their own infants. They continued to contribute as long as they nursed their own infants. When the infant was 6 months old, collections were discontinued to avoid milk of lower protein content. It was also required that the infant be in good health and not have a history of jaundice in the neonatal period. These mothers pumped or manually expressed milk and placed it in sterile bottles provided by the hospital. The milk was immediately placed in the deep freeze in the mother's home until she had collected daily samples for a week or two. The hospital provided transportation for picking up the milk. The milk was labeled with donor name, date, and time. The need for milk became so great that the hospital began to pay the donors by the ounce for milk and in turn they brought the frozen milk to the hospital and received another supply of sterile bottles. This provided a steady supply of easily digested nourishment for infants whose nutritional state was critical. An infant was always given milk from the same donor, and because there was a corps of regular donors, this did not present a problem. Milk was not pooled from multiple donors. If a donor mother was ill or taking medication, she continued to pump to maintain her volume but did not save the milk. Most donor mothers pumped from one breast while their infants nursed on the other, although some mothers pumped first and fed the infant afterward. During the 9 years when the system was active, there were no illnesses attributable to this milk in any infant.

At present the infants whose mothers are willing to provide their own milk are permitted to have breast milk. Because of the expressed concern of some immunologists about host graft reaction in immature infants, no infant receives fresh milk from another mother. Frozen banked donor milk that has been thawed is used when milk is not available from an infant's own mother and before he is ready for gastric feedings of formula, as well as in selected cases when the mother wishes her infant to have only

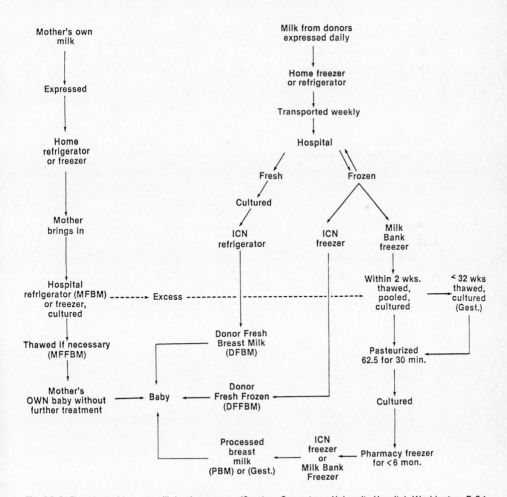

**Georgetown University
Community Human Milk Bank**

HUMAN MILK BANKING
How the Human Milk Bank Program Works

Fig. 19-2. Flowchart of human milk bank program. (Courtesy Georgetown University Hospital, Washington, D.C.)

human milk or when there is a special clinical indication. Mothers also freeze milk for their own infants if the infants are still unable to take it by mouth.

Qualification of donors

A mother who is willing to donate milk should be healthy and fulfill these qualifications:
1. Had normal pregnancy and delivery
2. Is serologically negative for syphilis, hepatitis B surface antigen, and cytomegalovirus
3. Has no infection, acute or chronic
4. Is not taking medications, smoking, or using excessive alcohol
5. Is capable of carrying out sterile technique
6. If donating for other infants, own child is healthy and without jaundice

Pregnancy and delivery should have been relatively uncomplicated. The mother should have a negative VDRL and negative chest x-ray results and be taking no medications, including birth control pills or any nonprescription medications such as aspirin or acetaminophen. Her infant should be well and should not have had neonatal jaundice. Some banks obtain approvals from the mother's obstetrician and pediatrician (Figs. 19-3 and 19-4). If the mother is donating only for her own infant, the state of the infant's health obviously does not prevent her from donating. Anytime the mother becomes ill she should discard milk from the previous 24 hour period and not save milk until the illness is over and any medications stopped (Fig. 19-5).

Discarding milk during maternal illness is the hardest regulation to which a mother must adhere. The wish to contribute may overshadow the mother's understanding of the risk it poses for an infant receiving such milk. On the East coast in 1977 a mother developed diarrhea and continued to contribute for her own infant as well as others. This was the source of a serious outbreak of *Salmonella* in the nursery, resulting in unnecessary death and illness for many infants. This is one factor that has persuaded some banks not to pay donors for fear of developing a problem similar to that of blood banks, in which paid donors have more hepatitis and other problems than volunteers. The one limiting factor in donating milk, however, is that one has to be lactating. Becoming a professional donor of milk today is highly unlikely. The amount of protein has been noted to be lower after 6 months of lactation; thus it is advisable to limit a given mother's contributions to 6 months or, at most, 8 months postpartum.

Technique for collection

It is of prime importance to maintain cleanliness and minimize bacteria in the process of collection. The mother should be instructed in washing her hands and her breasts.

There are two major ways of collecting: letting the milk drip while the infant nurses on the other side and pumping or manually expressing the milk.[17,18,38] In general, the latter is preferable. Dripped milk has been found to have lower caloric value and a higher incidence of contamination. Pumped milk has a higher fat content than dripped or manually expressed milk, and in most individuals the volume is also greater. Any equipment used, such as hand pumps, tubing, and collecting bottles, should be sterile. If an electric pump is used, the parts that come in contact with the milk should be sterile and/or disposable. The Egnell pump has the most advantages (Fig. 19-6). Many hospi-

---

(OBSTETRICIAN)

NORTHERN CALIFORNIA TRANSPLANT BANK
MOTHER'S MILK UNIT

Dear Doctor:

I have volunteered to be a donor to the Mother's Milk Unit of the Northern California Transplant Bank, Institute for Medical Research. If this meets with your approval, please provide them with the information listed below.

Thank you,

_____

_____

TO: Mother's Milk Unit
        Northern California Transplant Bank
        751 S. Bascom Ave.
        San Jose, Calif. 95128

I recommend Mrs. _____ as a donor to the Mother's Milk Unit. To the best of my knowledge she had a normal pregnancy, is free of any condition that will impair the quality of mother's milk. Specifically, I believe her Wasserman and TBN and/or chest x-ray are negative. She has had no evidence of hepatitis, no tumors and is taking no medication. To my knowledge, she has no perinatal viral infection. HAA results:

M.D. _____

_____ M.D.

_____

Fig. 19-3. Communication to donor's obstetrician requesting pertinent medical information and approval of mother's participation in milk banking program of Northern California Transplant Bank. (Courtesy Northern California Transplant Bank, Mother's Milk Unit. San Jose, Calif.)

tals own an Egnell pump or one may be rented from a local rental company or may be available through the local La Leche League. The Louisville bank restricts milk collection to use of the Egnell pump, which they have available on a rental basis. They also suggest preparing the breasts with pHisoHex, which is removed with two gauze squares moistened with sterile water. It would be important to check milk samples for pHisoHex content if this were done daily. A simple soap may be preferable. Providing the mother with a preparatory kit has many advantages.

The bank should provide a program of education for the donors. Samples should be cultured initially to ensure proper technique and the absence of significant contamination. Then samples should be sent for culture on a random basis. Studies have shown that milk collected at home has a higher contamination rate than that collected while the donor is hospitalized or with equipment maintained by the hospital. Collection at the hospital also avoids the transportation problem.

Many hospitals use the 4 oz sterile water-nursing bottles packaged by formula com-

---

(PEDIATRICIAN)

NORTHERN CALIFORNIA TRANSPLANT BANK
MOTHER'S MILK UNIT

Dear Doctor:

I have volunteered to be a donor to the Mother's Milk Unit of the
Northern California Transplant Bank, Institute for Medical Research.
If this meets with your approval, please so indicate below.

Thank you,

_____

_____

- -

TO: Mother's Milk Unit
    Northern California Transplant Bank
    751 S. Bascom Ave.
    San Jose, Calif. 95128

I approve of_____donating milk to
the Mother's Milk Unit.

                                    _____
                                                    M.D.
                                    _____

Fig. 19-4. Communication to donor's pediatrician requesting pertinent medical information and approval of mother's participation in milk banking program of Northern California Transplant Bank. (Courtesy Northern California Transplant Bank, Mother's Milk Unit, San Jose, Calif.)

panies for collections by discarding the water at the time of collection and then filling them with milk. Many programs suggest the use of 50 ml plastic centrifuge tubes,* which are presterilized and have tight-fitting tops. These tubes have the advantage of more appropriate volume and easy measurability and sterility. Whether slightly acid human milk will leach plasticizers from plastic containers when stored in the freezer for weeks or months is unknown.

*No. 25330, manufactured by Corning Glass Works.

NORTHERN CALIFORNIA TRANSPLANT BANK
MOTHER'S MILK UNIT

DONOR INFORMATION

Donor No.:_____

Date:_____

Name:_____ Age:_____ Blood type:_____

Address: _____City: _____

Cross streets:_____Phone No.:_____

Husband's name:_____No. of children:_____

Infant's name:_____ Birth date:_____

Hospital delivered: _____ City:_____

Obstetrician:_____

Address: _____Private:_____ Clinic:_____

Pediatrician: _____

Address: _____Private: _____ Clinic:_____

Home visit:_____By: _____

Permission slip from obstetrician: _____

Permission slip from pediatrician: _____

Skin test (TBN):_____Chest x-ray:_____

Do you smoke?_____ If yes, how many cigarettes a day?_____

Are you taking any medication?_____If yes, what kind and why?_____

Storage facilities: _____Referred by:_____
        Please draw a simple map, on back, of how we find your home.

_____
Donor signature

Fig. 19-5. Intake information sheet obtained on all donors of milk by Northern California Transplant Bank. (Courtesy Northern California Transplant Bank, Mother's Milk Unit, San Jose, Calif.)

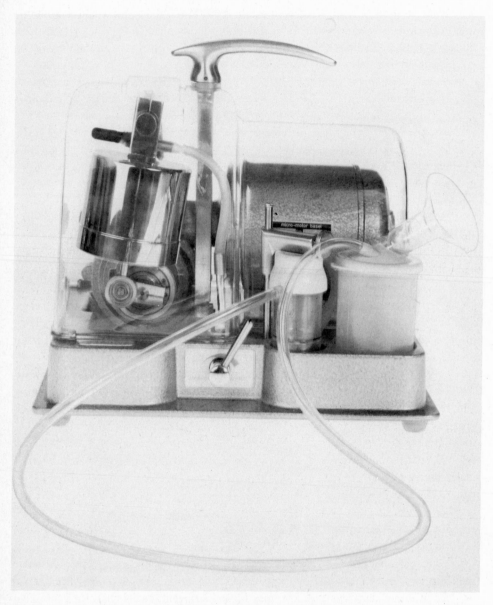

Fig. 19-6. Egnell pump. Egnell pump works with milking action on areola rather than vacuum extraction. Parts of pump that come in contact with milk can either be disposed of or sterilized. (Courtesy Egnell, Inc., Cary, Ill.)

Bank milk collected by manual expression is less likely to be contaminated than that collected by hand pumps, including Lloyd B, even when pumps are boiled or placed in electric dishwasher.[27,40] The rubber bulb of the hand pump that resembles a bicycle horn retains milk and bacteria. Nesty cups have been associated with the highest level of contamination. The contamination has included coliforms, and gentamicin-resistant gram-negative rods were found when donors used pumps at home.

Contaminated breast milk was the source of *Klebsiella* bacteremia in a neonatal intensive care unit according to Donowitz et al.[9] Unpasteurized human milk from a single donor fed via nasogastric and nasoduodenal tubes to sick newborns was found to be contaminated from the safety overflow bottle and tubing of the electric breast pump maintained in the neonatal intensive care unit. This part of the tubing and equipment should be sterilized or disposed of between collections according to the manufacturer's instructions. Strict attention to sterilization of equipment is imperative.

Paxson and Cress[32] have reported a significant difference in the survival of the leukocytes when the milk is collected and stored in plastic containers rather than glass, since the cells apparently stick to the glass. The phagocytosis of these cells, however, is not affected by the container. The researchers further demonstrated that varying the osmolarity or protein concentration does not alter the number or the phagocytosis of the cells. Because they believe the main reason for feeding preterm infants human milk is for the protection against infection, they suggest nasogastric feedings instead of naso-jejunal feeding (to maintain pH in the acid range; in the small bowel, the pH is 6.5 to 8). The milk is collected in sterile plastic containers and maintained in the refrigerator until it is fed to the infant, avoiding heating, freezing, and alkaline solutions.

The effect of the container on the stability of the constituents of milk was investigated by Garza et al.[16] Pyrex and polypropylene containers were found not to interact with water- and fat-soluble nutrients such as vitamin A, zinc, iron, copper, sodium, and protein nitrogen. Polyethylene bags were found to spill easily, to be harder for mothers to fill without contamination, and to be difficult to handle in the nursery. The containers also leaked and punctured easily. Polyethylene also resulted in 60% lower secretory IgA levels because of adherence to the material. It appears that polypropylene plastic containers may have a significant advantage in maintaining the stability of all constituents in human milk collections and may be easier and safer to handle.

Contrary to initial reports, there is no bacteriologic benefit to discarding the first 5 to 10 ml of milk pumped from the breast.[5] Samples had no different bacteriologic counts when this was done. This is particularly important initially when early colostrum and milk are less in total volume but high in value to the infant. At home, later, when production is abundant and technique may be less stringent, discarding 2 to 3 ml might be appropriate.

Rinsing the sterile collecting bottles with a 1% hypochlorite solution so that the solution adhered to the sides of the bottles decreased the bacterial contamination of milk.[23]

Storage and testing of milk samples

Fresh refrigerated unsterilized human milk can be used for 24 hours following collection. Donors are instructed to bring milk to the nursery within 3 hours if it is to be used fresh. If it is to be frozen, this should be done immediately at $0°$ F ($-18°$ C) (standard home freezer) or in top of a refrigerator freezer. The milk stored in the latter should be deep frozen within a week if it is to be stored any length of time. The milk kept at $-18°$ C can be kept for 6 months.

All samples should be labeled with name of donor, date, and time. Milk is stored in the freezer in such a way that the oldest milk is used first, and all milk of a single donor is kept together.

Monitoring for bacterial contamination is done on multiple samples before an individual is accepted as a donor.[11] Studies were done on pooled samples by Siimes and Hallman[35] who believe that pooling provides more stable nutritional content. Testing of milk samples from a given donor should also be done on a regular basis by a bacteriology laboratory approved for testing milk samples.[8] Usually random samples taken every 2 weeks will suffice once a donor has been accepted. When a hospitalized mother is contributing fresh milk to her own infant, it is usually not cultured.

STANDARDS FOR RAW DONOR HUMAN MILK. All raw donor milk should be screened microbiologically before use. There are no generally accepted microbiologic criteria for such milk except that no potential pathogens should be present.[4] Such pathogens include *Staphylococcus aureus,* β-hemolytic streptococci, *Pseudomonas* species, *Proteus* species, and *Streptococcus faecalis.* Some milk that cannot be fed raw can be pasteurized.[44]

Other guidelines include the following:
1. A total aerobic mesophilic colony count of less than 2.5×10^6 colony forming units/ml with a predominance of normal skin flora
2. A count of staphylococci of less than 1×10^5 colony forming units/ml
3. No enterobacteria

STANDARDS FOR PASTEURIZATION OF DONOR HUMAN MILK. Milk suitable for pasteurization should meet minimum standards[44]:
1. A total aerobic count that does not exceed 1×10^6 colony forming units/ml
2. *S. aureus* that does not exceed 1×10^3; there is the risk of feeding heat-treated enterotoxins when *S. aureus* exceeds 1×10^6
3. Presence of organisms defined as being of fecal origin not exceeding 1×10^4
4. Presence of organisms not part of normal flora not exceeding 1×10^7 colony-forming units/L
5. Presence of unusual organisms such as *Pseudomonas aeruginosa,* spore-bearing aerobes, or spore-bearing anaerobes

Testing milk for protein, fat, and carbohydrate is not necessary and is costly and time consuming. A new quick method of analysis has been suggested by Lucas et al.[29] It involves standard hematocrit microtubes and a centrifuge. The percentage of cream or "creamatocrit" is read from the capillary tube. There is a linear relationship to fat and energy content.

$$\text{Fat(g/L)} = \frac{(\text{Creamatocrit [\%]} - 0.59)}{0.146}$$

$$\text{kcal/L} = 290 + (66.8 \times \text{Creamatocrit [\%]})$$

Accuracy is within 10%.

This methodology was validated with further analysis by Lemons et al.,[25] who repeated the studies and confirmed actual measurements of total fat and caloric content. As the protein and lactose content remains relatively constant over time, the variation in fat content is the primary constituent affecting caloric value of the milk. There was no effect of either freezing for up to 2 months or of pasteurization on the creamatocrit. There was no evidence of fat globule degradation during storage that affected the test.

Special cautions while performing this simple test should include the following:

Use a representative, well-mixed sample.

Complete a sample of pumping from at least one breast; do not take just a spot sample.

A well-mixed 24 hour sample can be used.

Use tube at least three fourths filled; seal one end.

Centrifuge for 15 minutes in standard table-top centrifuge.

Occasional small layer of liquid fat on top (free fatty acids) should not be included.

Keep tube vertical.

Make measurement within 1 hour of centrifugation.

The effect of heating and freezing on the various constituents of human milk has been studied by a number of investigators whose data should be considered before deciding how to store milk for special purposes.

HEAT TREATMENT. When human milk was pasteurized at 73° C for 30 minutes, there was little IgA, IgG, lactoferrin, lysozyme, and C_3 complement left, and when the temperature was kept at 62.5° C for 30 minutes there was a loss of 23.7% of the lysozyme, 56.8% of the lactoferrin, and 34% of the IgG, but no loss of IgA, according to work done by Evans et al.[13] Similar studies of heat treatments of graded severity were carried out by Ford et al.[15] (Tables 19-1 to 19-4). The findings were similar. Pasteurization at

Table 19-1.   Immunoglobulin activity (mg/ml) in unheated and heat-treated human milk

Heat treatment	IgA	IgM	IgG
None	0.50	0.10	None detected
56° C 30 min	0.48	0.10	None detected
62.5° C 30 min	0.39	0	None detected
70° C 15 min	0.24	0	None detected
80° C 15 min	0.10	0	None detected

From Ford, J. E., et al.: J. Pediatr. **90:**29, 1977.

Table 19-2. Total lactoferrin and unsaturated iron-binding capacity in unheated and heat-treated human milk

Heat treatment	Lactoferrin* (mg/ml)		Unsaturated iron-binding capacity† (μg of Fe/ml)		
None	3.4	3.7	3.4	3.1	3.1
56° C 30 min	—		3.0	—	—
Holder pasteurization (62.5° C 30 min)	1.2	1.5	1.3	0.7	0.8
65° C 15 min	1.0	1.0	0.6	0.4	0.4
70° C 15 min	0.2	0.1	0.1	0	0
75° C 15 min	0.2	0.2	0	0	0

From Ford, J.E., et al.: J. Pediatr. **90**:29, 1977.
*Duplicate determinations were made on each test sample.
†Each value represents a different preparation of milk.

Table 19-3. Influence of different heat treatments of human milk on its lysozyme activity

Heat treatment	Lysozyme activity (μg of egg white lysozyme equivalent/ml milk)*	
None	98	99
HTST pasteurization	103	107
62.5° C 30 min	103	105
70° C 15 min	62	68
80° C 15 min	35	37
90° C 15 min	7	7
100° C 15 min	2	3

From Ford, J.E., et al.: J. Pediatr. **90**:29, 1977.
*Each value represents a different preparation of milk.

Table 19-4. Influence of different heat treatments of human milk on its capacity to bind added [³H] cyanocobalamin and [³H] folic acid

Heat treatment	Unsaturated binding capacity (ng/ml)	
	Cyanocobalamin	Folic acid
None	43.4	21.9
HTST pasteurization	26.2	—
62.5° C 30 min	22.6	19.7
65° C 15 min	18.4	16.4
70° C 15 min	14.4	14.2
75° C 15 min	14.0	11.5
80° C 15 min	15.0	10.2
85° C 15 min	18.4	4.2
90° C 15 min	21.6	2.4
95° C 15 min	22.8	1.5
100° C 15 min	18.6	1.5

From Ford, J.E., et al.: J. Pediatr. **90**:29, 1977.

62.5° C for 30 minutes (Holder method) reduced IgA by 20% and destroyed IgM and lactoferrin. Lysozyme was stable at 62.5° C but destroyed at 100° C, as was lactoperoxidase and the ability to bind folic acid against bacterial uptake. Growth of *Escherichia coli* increased in heated milk. B_{12}-binding capacity declined progressively with increasing temperature of the heat treatment. These data raise the question as to whether any heat treatment might not increase the risk of enteric infection in the infant. Some milk banks have advocated heating when the bacterial count is at a certain level, which may be too cumbersome to be practical. Ford et al.[15] suggest that for batch processing, 62.5° C for 30 minutes may be the method of choice.

The alterations of the lymphocyte and antibody content after processing were studied by Liebhaber et al.[26] They, too, found significant changes with heat, including a decrease in total lymphocyte count and in specific antibody titer to *E. coli*.

Welsh and May[42] discuss anti-infective properties of breast milk and provide two tables (Tables 19-5 and 19-6) to demonstrate the stability of the antibacterial and antiviral properties of human milk. Siimes and Hallman[35] have relied on heat treatment of their milk samples, 60° C for 10 minutes. They do save fresh milk collected from donors who have been consistently identified to have no bacteria in their milk separately for immediate feeding to high-risk neonates.

Short-time low-temperature pasteurization of human milk was reported by Wills et al.[45] using the Oxford Human Milk pasteuriser. Heating at 56.0° C for 15 minutes destroyed over 99% of the inoculated organisms, which included *E. coli, S. aureus,* and group B β-hemolytic streptococci. The remaining activity of antimicrobial proteins after different time/temperature treatments is shown in Table 19-7.

LYOPHILIZATION AND FREEZING. The impact of lyophilization was similar to that of heating, showing a decrease in total lymphocyte count and in immunoglobulin concentration and specific antibody titer to *E. coli*.

Table 19-5. Antibacterial factors in breast milk

Factor	Shown in vitro to be active against	Effect of heat
L. bifidus growth factor	*Enterobacteriaceae,* enteric pathogens	Stable to boiling
Secretory IgA	*E. coli; E. coli* enterotoxin; *C. tetani, C. diphtheriae, D. pneumoniae, Salmonella, Shigella*	Stable at 56° C for 30 min; some loss (0% to 30%) at 62.5° C for 30 min; destroyed by boiling
C_1-C_9	Effect not known	Destroyed by heating at 56° C for 30 min
Lactoferrin	*E. coli; C. albicans*	Two thirds destroyed at 62.5° C for 30 min
Lactoperoxidase	*Streptococcus; Pseudomonas, E. coli, S. typhimurium*	Not known; presumably destroyed by boiling
Lysozyme	*E. coli; Salmonella, M. lysodeikticus*	Stable at 62.5° C for 30 min; activity reduced 97% by boiling for 15 min
Lipid (unsat'd fatty acid)	*S. aureus*	Stable to boiling
Milk cells	By phagocytosis: *E. coli, C. albicans* By sensitized lymphocytes: *E. coli*	Destroyed by 62.5° C for 30 min

From Welsh, J.K., and May, J.I.: J. Pediatr. **93**:1, 1979.

Table 19-6. Antiviral factors in breast milk

Factor	Shown in vitro to be active against	Effect of heat
Secretory IgA	Polio types 1, 2, 3, coxsackie types A9, B3, B5; ECHO types 6, 9; Semliki Forest virus, Ross River virus, rotavirus	Stable at 56° C for 30 min; some loss (0% to 30%) at 62.5° for 30 min; destroyed by boiling
Lipid (unsat'd fatty acids and monoglycerides)	Herpes simplex; Semliki Forest virus, influenza, dengue, Ross River virus, Murine leukemia virus, Japanese B encephalitis virus	Stable to boiling for 30 min
Nonimmunoglobulin macromolecules	Herpes simplex; vesicular stomatitis virus	Destroyed at 60° C; stable at 56° C for 30 min; destroyed by boiling for 30 min
	Rotavirus	Unknown
Milk cells	Induced interferon active against Sendai virus; Sensitized lymphocytes? Phagocytosis?	Destroyed at 62.5° C for 30 min

From Welsh, J.K., and May, J.T.: J. Pediatr. **93**:1, 1979.

Table 19-7. Influence of pasteurization temperatures on human milk

	% IgA	% Lactoferrin	% Lysozyme
62.5° C	67	27	67
62.5° C 5 min	77	59	96
56.0° C 15 min	90	91	100

Freezing specimens up to 4 weeks showed no change in IgA or *E. coli* antibody titer, although the lymphocyte count was decreased. The technique involved freezing to −23° C and thawing at 1, 2, 3, and 4 weeks. Although there were cells present after freezing, they showed no viability when tested with the trypan blue stain exclusion method. The storage of human milk at 4° C for 48 hours caused a decrease in the concentration of milk macrophages and neutrophils but not of the lymphocytes, which also maintained their activity, according to work reported by Pittard and Bill.[33] The loss of cells may be desirable if the graft versus host reaction in a premature infant who is possibly immunodeficient is of concern. Evans and associates[13] reported their results with 3-month storage −20 ° C and of freeze-drying and reconstitution (lyophilization). They found no significant change in lactoferrin, lysozyme, IgA, IgG, and C3 after 3-month freezing but a small loss of IgG after lyophilization (Table 19-8). Whether factors that promote the growth of normal flora in the gut survive treatment was also investigated.[2] These researchers propose that "human milk should be collected in as sterile a manner as possible and deep frozen shortly after collection. If a donor mother maintains a low bacterial count in her milk, then its use unheated should be considered. Pasteurization, if used, should be at minimum temperature capable of adequate bacterial killing (about 62° C for 30 min)."[13]

Table 19-8.   Effect of deep freezing (3 mo) at $-20°$ C and lyophilization of human milk proteins (mg/100 ml milk)

	Raw milk (mean ± SE)	Deep frozen milk			Lyophilized milk		
		Mean ± SE	Mean as % raw	P	Mean ± SE	Mean as % raw	P
α_1-Antitrypsin (16 samples)	2.38 ± 0.3	1.98 ± 0.2	83.2	<0.05	2.22 ± 0.3	93.3	>0.1
IgA (8 samples)	9.55 ± 0.84	9.25 ± 0.83	96.9	>0.1	9.33 ± 0.74	97.7	>0.1
IgG (16 samples)	0.42 ± 0.05	0.42 ± 0.04	100	>0.1	0.33 ± 0.04	78.6	<0.05
Lactoferrin (11 samples)	332 ± 71.7	338 ± 57.4	102	>0.1	363 ± 79	109.3	>0.1
Lysozymes (11 samples)	5.1 ± 1.26	4.6 ± 0.67	90.2	>0.1	4.8 ± 1.19	94.1	>0.1
C3 (16 samples)	1.35 ± 0.13	1.26 ± 0.11	93.3	>0.1	1.27 ± 0.13	94.1	>0.1

From Evans, T.J., et al.: Arch. Dis. Child. 53:239, 1978.

NUTRITIONAL CONSEQUENCES OF HEAT TREATMENT.   Initially the focus was on the effect of processing human milk on its unique anti-infective properties,[18,21] but attention has been given to the nutritional consequences as well.[34] Storage for 24 hours did not affect vitamin A, zinc, iron, copper, sodium, or protein nitrogen concentrations at 37° C.[39,43] Ascorbic acid levels fell markedly when stored at 37° C and 4° C at 24 and 48 hours. (They remain stable for 4 hours.) Other investigators have found that ascorbic acid levels drop 40% with heating.[16,39]

Levels of unsaturated fatty acids apparently are also affected by heating and cold storage but the data need clarification. It is anticipated that heating or freezing and thawing are capable of damaging membranes surrounding milk fat globules.[34] The fat globule could then undergo fragmentation and allow greater access of milk lipases to triglycerides.[41] The percentages of polyunsaturated fatty acids, linoleic ($C_{18:2}$) and linolenate ($C_{18:3}$), decreased after both heating and freezing, while monounsaturates and saturated fatty acids were unaffected.[41]

Because the nourishment of low–birth weight infants has been the purpose of many bank milks, the ability of preterm infants to utilize treated bank milk is relative. Pasteurization at 62.5° C for 30 minutes was reported not to influence nitrogen absorption or retention in low–birth weight infants.[34] When raw, pasteurized, and boiled human milks were fed to very low–birth weight (<1.3 kg) preterm infants in 3 separate consecutive weeks, fat absorption was reduced by one third in the heat-treated group. There was a reduction in the amount of nitrogen retained in the heat-treated group as well, although the absorption was unaffected. The absorption and retention of calcium, phosphorus, and sodium were unaffected by heating or freezing. The mean weight gain was greater by one third when the infants were fed raw human milk.[43]

Pasteurization decreased B_{12} by about 50% and folate binding capacity by 10%. Sterilization (100° C for 20 minutes), on the other hand, had similar effects on B_{12} binding and completely inactivated folate binding.[39] Vitamins A, D, E, B_2, B_6, choline, niacin, and pantothenic acid were barely affected by pasteurization, whereas thiamin was reduced up to 25%, biotin up to 10%, and vitamin C up to 20%. Refrigeration at 4° C to 6° C for 72 hours allows little bacterial growth and causes no change in nutrients or infection-protective properties. Freezing does have a little effect on both and the milk can be kept for months, whereas heating has significant effect and the milk still requires freezing for storage. Experience feeding donated raw milk to newborns has shown no ill effects if carefully monitored according to Björksten et al.[3]

VIRUSES IN HUMAN MILK.   The dilemma of cytomegalovirus (CMV) is a significant one, since the virus does pass into the milk. In a study of postpartum women, CMV was recovered from the genital tract in 10%, from the urine in 7%, from the saliva in 2%, and from the breast milk in 30%. CMV does persist after storage at 4° C and $-20°$ C in some specimens.[37] It is destroyed at 62° C after 30 minutes.[10] Donor milk should be accepted only from CMV-negative mothers. Mothers who are seropositive may be permitted to provide for their own infants because they have already provided the protection as well.

Hepatitis virus also passes into milk, and donors should therefore be screened and be seronegative. The question of having seropositive women feed their own infants is discussed in Chapter 14.

SPECIAL CONSIDERATIONS.   Thawing milk should be done in the refrigerator and each bottle should be used completely within 24 hours. Defrosting in the microwave oven may lead to separation of layers. Microwaves do decrease vitamin C content but are not known to destroy other factors. The greatest danger of microwaving is that the milk heats and the container does not, so that an infant could be burned or the milk significantly overheated.

Donor milk is at risk for being contaminated with cow's milk by the donor. The California Mother's Milk Bank checks its contributions with a simple test directed at precipitating the casein. They mix 1 ml of donor milk with 1 ml of 8N sulfuric acid and 8 ml water and let it sit at room temperature for 5 hours. If cow's milk is present, it will precipitate.[31]

Financial aspects

Established milk banks have various financial structures. The Louisville bank has demonstrated that given a small amount of seed money, a viable self-sustaining program can be developed. Their income includes charges for equipment rental and for processing milk. Certainly the hospital should recover costs of collecting and processing. This should be a reimbursable item of hospital costs. Precedent for this has been set in the United States. Since legislation has been passed by some states mandating the availability of human milk for all babies who need it, there must be reimbursement for it and funds available for its proper handling.

The recommendations from the State of New York (see Appendix K) suggest that the monitoring of standards of a hospital-based bank be absorbed into existing hospital surveillance. Free-standing banks would be monitored by the state and local health departments. Economic analysis indicates that the primary costs would be administrative overhead costs. The human milk supply is considered a donated product. Also acknowledged are staff costs, minimal equipment costs, and laboratory costs as well as costs to the state health department to administer the system. Much consideration is being given to limiting banks to hospital settings, where health professionals and equipment are readily available.

Siimes and Hallman[35] report that generally $4/L is paid to the donor, which, added to costs of equipment rental and milk processing, brings the cost of feeding an infant to $13/L.

WET NURSING OR CROSS-NURSING

Although feeding an infant by one who is not his mother is an established means of sustaining life, it is uncommon in Western cultures. There are no medical contraindications provided the nursing woman is in good health and taking no medications. The chief obstacle is psychologic or social. Actually women who are trying to develop a supply of milk when their own infant cannot nurse because of prematurity or illness would be greatly benefited by having a vigorous normal suckling infant nurse at their breasts. In contemporary society, the term *cross-nursing* has replaced "wet nursing" in order to disassociate the phenomenon from the negative historical connotations. In cross-nursing the mother continues to breastfeed her own child in addition to the child she takes for a feeding or two per day. The circumstances described in the report by Krantz and Kupper[24] usually involve baby-sitting arrangements, which may be daily and formal or random and informal. They interviewed three women involved in a mutual agreement for baby-sitting purposes. The mothers were married and well educated. The babies were female and 4 months old. There appeared to be no physical effects on the babies according to the mothers. The behavioral reactions of the babies were "looking puzzled" and being disturbed if the surrogate mother spoke. Some difficulty was noticed in let-down, and all three mothers noted a difference in the way each baby suckled.

Another purpose of cross-nursing is for maternal benefit, wherein an experienced vigorous infant is nursed by a woman whose own baby is unable to give proper stimulus to milk production. This has been done by private arrangement and has not caused any known problems. Usually the normal newborn is younger than 2 months. Cross-nursing has also been used to stimulate lactation in adoptive nursing. In this situation the infants are exchanged to stimulate the adoptive mother's breasts and also to show the adopted infant that milk comes from breasts and how to suckle at the breast.

The hazards to cross-nursing are undocumented but worthy of consideration. The physical problems are the potential for infection, either of mother or of baby, interruption of milk supply for the mother's own baby, and the difference in composition of milk if babies are of different chronologic or conceptual ages. The psychologic hazards could include failure of mother to let-down, refusal of infant to nurse (which does occur when infants are introduced to the phenomenon beyond 4 months of age), and negative impact on siblings and household. The long-range effects are not documented.

Reasonable caution is certainly appropriate, taking care to assure that the cross-nursing mother is healthy and well nourished, without any general or local infection, and not taking any medications or smoking. The infants should probably be close in age and also free of infection, especially thrush. If this were a commercial venture in a public day-care setting, regulations of certification screening for tuberculosis, syphilis, hepatitis, CMV, herpesvirus, and other infectious agents might be in order. Documents of liability might be required.

Perhaps as breastfeeding knowledge and understanding reach a greater number of professionals and women, such opportunities may be more common. At present it is significant to recognize this as a viable option.

Breast pumping equipment

In this chapter, several types of breast pumping devices have been alluded to around questions of the sterility of milk collected. Additional issues need to be considered including efficiency, ease of use, potential for breast trauma, availability, and cost. A good pump should be capable of completely emptying the breast and of stimulating production. It should be clean, contamination free, easy to use, and atraumatic (see Appendix G for details of manufacturer and distributor).

HAND PUMPS.   The bicycle horn pump has been marketed in drugstores for years without instructions for use or cleaning. At the museum at the Corning Glass Works in Corning, New York there is a glass and rubber hand pump made by Davol circa 1830 A.D. on display next to glass baby bottles and pewter nipples. The current model is the same, except the glass has been replaced by plastic. The dangers of this pump are legion but can be summarized by saying the milk is contaminated, a squirt of milk can go directly into the bulb, the pump requires constant emptying, and it can be quite traumatic to the nipple, areola, and breast.

Modifications of this style that have been made insert a removable collecting bottle in place of the well in the bicycle horn pump. The modification permits feeding the infant directly from the collecting vessel by placing a nipple on it. Milk does not wash back over the breast and pumping is not interrupted for emptying. The tube and bulb still may harbor bacteria because they are hard to clean. The limitations of the effect of creating a simple vacuum and applying a simple, rigid, sharp-edged flange against the breast are still present. This pump is satisfactory for temporary use, but it takes time to become proficient in its use, and it may never create enough pressure to be effective. A new model (Nurture) with special flexible silicone funnel overcomes these problems.

The cylindric pumps are two all-plastic cylindric tubes that fit inside one another to create a vacuum. A flange to accommodate the nipple and areola is at top of inner tube,

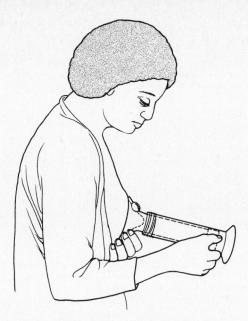

Fig. 19-7. Cylindric pump in use.

which also has gasket for tight fit at other end. The outer tube collects the milk and is adapted for use as feeding unit when a nipple is screwed on top. The mother creates the vacuum by pulling the outer tube and creates rhythm by pushing the outer tube in and out (Fig. 19-7). It is simple, easy to clean, and the milk is usable. This pump is excellent in hands of an experienced, dextrous mother. There are several manufacturers and the product differs slightly. Some have a choice of flanges. The Lloyd-B pump has a trigger handle adapted to a flange mechanism that empties into a collection jar the size of a baby-food jar (not a baby bottle). It does have a vacuum relief switch; however, the entire mechanism requires a certain dexterity and a rather large hand to operate. It is portable and also easily cleaned. There are no parts that harbor bacteria.

There is a pump called Ora'Lac Pump that operates with a mouthpiece through which the mother creates a vacuum (Fig. 19-8). It actually could be created by taking a DeLee trap neonatal suction apparatus and replacing the suction catheter with a flange to apply to the breast. Since one can create only limited negative pressure orally, there is a built-in safety factor. A mother might have trouble maintaining suction for long.

MECHANICAL PUMPS.   Electric pumps are most efficient as the mechanical effort is applied by the motor and the mother can concentrate on applying the cup to her breast, massaging the breast, and relaxing so that adequate let-down can take place. All electric pumps are not equal and some guidance is needed to be sure that the mother understands the principles involved. Nursery staff should be familiar with the equipment. The pumps

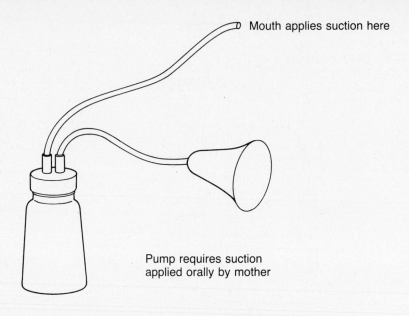

Mouth applies suction here

Pump requires suction
applied orally by mother

Fig. 19-8. Hand pump in which suction is applied orally by the mother.

are no challenge to skilled intensive care nursery nurses who are adept at handling complicated electronic equipment.

A pump that cycles pressure instead of maintaining constant negative pressure will be less likely to cause petechiae or internal trauma. Negative pressures should have a governor mechanism to avoid excessive pressures. Mean sucking pressures of most normal full-term infants range from -50 to -155, with a maximum up to -220 mm Hg/in^2. Manufacturers recommend about 200 mm Hg/in^2 to initiate flow in most women.

A careful study by Johnson[22] of over 1000 patients at the University of Texas using a variety of pumps has confirmed some facts about pumps. The amount of negative pressure possible and the control mechanisms were recorded. The findings are summarized in Tables 19-9 and 19-10.

Although attention is usually given to the pressure mechanisms, equally important is the cup that is applied to the breast. The diameter and the depth of the flare are fixed for the hand pumps and the Gomco electric pump, but a choice is offered for the Egnell, Medela, and Whittlestone pumps. The nipple should have room to be drawn out and the flange should be adequate to transmit pressure or milking action to the collecting ampullae under the areola. The hand pumps are too small; however, bigger is not always better and a mother may find that the smaller model of the two offered may suit her anatomy more physiologically. This feature does not correlate directly with overall size of breast. The ideal range is 68 to 82 mm outer diameter and 35 to 40 mm depth of

Table 19-9.   Electrical pumping devices

Mechanical pump	Advantages	Disadvantages
All mechanical pumps		Expensive Can rent Should be covered by insurance
Egnell/Medela (Fig. 19-6) Rhythmic vacuum Simulates nursing	Helpful in initiating let-down Simulates rhythm of suck- ling Disposable tubing and col- lecting cups	Well serviced by company

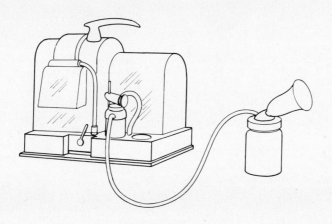

Gomco/Sorenson Adapted from suction apparatus Finger control of T-tube will cycle vacuum	Good visibility Good collection vessel	Poor cup design—painful Continuous negative pressure can run too high Hard to control Not good for long use Noisy

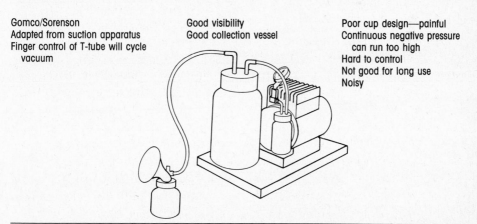

Continued.

Table 19-9. Electrical pumping devices—cont'd

Mechanical pump	Advantages	Disadvantages
Whittlestone Milker (see Appendix G) Physiologic milk with breast cups that milk breast	Excellent milking action Comfortable Initiates and maintains milk supply	Availability Can be rented

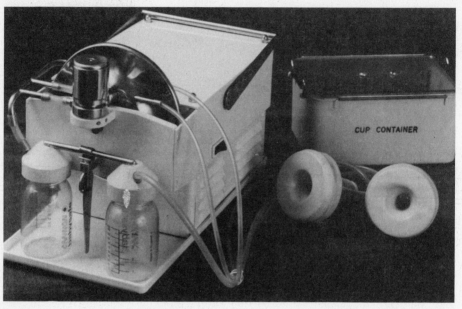

Table 19-10. Hand pumping devices

Hand pump	Advantages	Disadvantages
Bicycle horn pump	Inexpensive Portable Milk washes back over nipple Constantly empties	Difficult to clean Bulb retains bacteria Works as vacuum No instructions Can cause trauma Not appropriate for donor milk

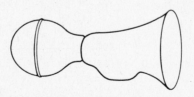

Table 19-10.   Hand pumping devices—cont'd

Hand pump	Advantages	Disadvantages
Evenflo pump	Inexpensive	Difficult to clean, bulb harbors bacteria even when boiled

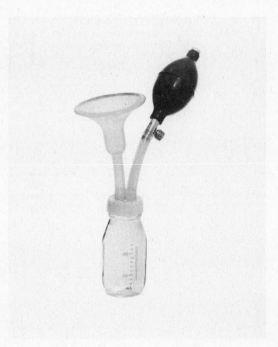

Hand pump	Advantages	Disadvantages
Nurture*	Portable Can feed baby from collecting container	Works well for experienced mother with good let-down

*Nurture model made by Lact-Assist, Inc. is best hand device. This silicone flange can be adopted to any cycling electric pump also.

Table 19-10. Hand pumping devices—cont'd

Hand pump	Advantages	Disadvantages
Cylindric Two all-plastic cylindric tubes that fit inside one another to create vacuum. Inner tube has flange at top and rubber or nylon gasket	Less expensive than electric Portable Can feed baby from collecting container Easily cleaned and sterilized	Requires some dexterity Works as vacuum with some rhythm

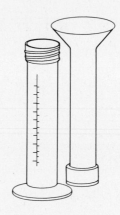

Hand pump	Advantages	Disadvantages
Lloyd B pump Glass flange attached to collecting jar. Trigger handle mechanism creates vacuum; has vacuum relief switch	Less expensive than electric Portable Can be cleaned	Handle difficult to squeeze Hand becomes cramped Awkward Large breast and nipple may hit flange Transfer of milk to feeding unit necessary

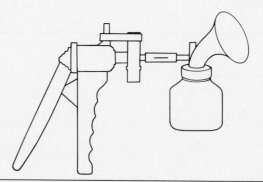

flare[22] (Fig. 19-9). The Nurture silicone funnel adapts well to all sizes and shapes because of its flexibility.

A simple water-powered breast pump was devised by Ellis[12] in Australia, using an ordinary water tap, a simple water aspirator vacuum pump, and an attached breast flange and collecting bottle. It has the advantages of being inexpensive ($20), portable, and dependent on only a water faucet. The pressure is controlled by the mother, who places her finger over the side opening and can cycle the pressure valve. The overall suction pressure can be adjusted by changing the water flow (Fig. 19-10). A similar device, independently reported by Sponsel[36] in England, used a water-driven venturi pump and was proclaimed for its cost-effectiveness and convenience.

The relative efficacy of four methods of human milk expression was measured by Green et al.[19] The electric pump (Egnell) enabled mothers to pump significantly more milk with higher fat content in the 10-minute time allotted for the study than did the Lloyd B, the Evenflo hand pump, or manual expression, all three of which were about equal in efficacy.

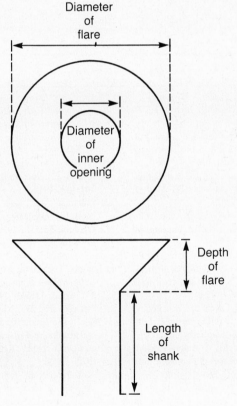

Fig. 19-9. Measurement of nipple cups. (From Johnson, C.A.: Clin. Pediatr. **22:**40, 1983.)

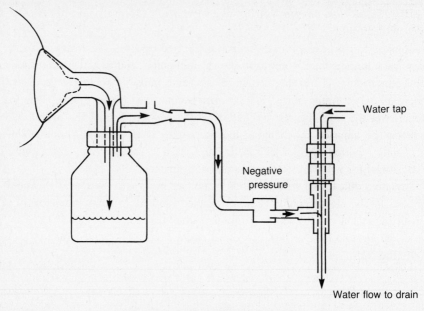

Water tap

Negative
pressure

Water flow to drain

Fig. 19-10. Water-powered breast pump.

REFERENCES

1. Barrie, H.: Human milk bank, Lancet **1:**284, 1982.
2. Beerens, H., Romond, C., Neut, C.: Influence of breastfeeding on the bifid flora of the newborn intestine, Am. J. Clin. Nutr. **33:**2434, 1980.
3. Björksten, B., et al.: Collecting and banking human milk: to heat or not to heat? Br. Med. J. **281:**765, 1980.
4. Carroll, L., et al.: Bacteriological criteria for feeding raw breast-milk to babies on neonatal units, Lancet **2:**732, 1979.
5. Carroll, L., Osman, M., and Davies, D.P.: Does discarding the first few millilitres of breast milk improve the bacteriological quality of bank breast milk, Lancet **2:**898, 1979.
6. Committee on Medical Aspects of Food Policy: The collection and storage of human milk, London, 1981, Her Majesty's Stationery Office.
7. Committee on Mother's Milk, America Academy of Pediatrics: Operation of mother's milk bureaus, J. Pediatr. **23:**112, 1943.
8. Davidson, D.C., Poll, R.A., and Roberts, G.: Bacteriological monitoring of unheated human milk, Arch. Dis. Child. **54:**760, 1979.

9. Donowitz, L.G., et al.: Contaminated breast milk: a source of *Klebsiella* bacteremia in a newborn intensive care unit, Rev. Infect. Dis. **3:**716, 1981.
10. Dworsky, M., et al.: Persistence of cytomegalovirus in human milk after storage, J. Pediatr. **101:**440, 1982.
11. Eidelman, A.I., and Szilagyi, G.: Patterns of bacterial colonization of human milk, Obstet. Gynecol. **53:**550, 1979.
12. Ellis, K.J.: A simple water-powered breast pump, Med. J. Aust. **2:**278, 1978.
13. Evans, T.J., et al.: Effect of storage and heat on antimicrobial proteins in human milk, Arch. Dis. Child. **53:**239, 1978.
14. Fleischaker, J.W., Nowak, M.M., and Quinby, G.E.: The Louisville Breast Milk Program: the organization and operation of an in-hospital human milk bank, Keeping Abreast J. **2:**124, 1977.
15. Ford, J.E., et al.: Influence of heat treatment of human milk on some of its protective constituents, J. Pediatr. **90:**29, 1977.

16. Garza, C., et al.: Effects of methods of collection and storage on nutrients in human milk, Early Hum. Dev. **6:**295, 1982.

17. Gibbs, J.H., et al.: Drip breast milk: its composition, collection and pasteurization, Early Hum. Dev. **1:**227, 1977.

18. Goldblum, R.M., et al.: Human milk banking. II. Relative stability of immunologic factors in stored colostrum, Acta Paediatr. Scand. **71:**143, 1982.

19. Green, D., et al.: The relative efficacy of four methods of human milk expression, Early Hum. Dev. **6:**153, 1982.

20. Harrod, J.R.: Personal communication regarding Mother's Milk Unit, California Transplant Bank, July, 1978.

21. Hernandez, J., et al.: Effect of storage processes on the bacterial growth-inhibiting activity of human breast milk, Pediatrics **63:**597, 1979.

22. Johnson, C.A.: An evaluation of breast pumps currently available on the American market, Clin. Pediatr. **22:**40, 1983.

23. Jones, C.L., Jennison, R.F., and D'Souza, S.W.: Bacterial contamination of expressed breast milk, Br. Med. J. **2:**1320, 1979.

24. Krantz, J.Z., and Kupper, N.S.: Cross-nursing: wet-nursing in a contemporary context, Pediatrics **67:**715, 1981.

25. Lemons, J.A., Schreiner, R.L., and Gresham, E.L.: Simple method for determining the caloric and fat content of human milk, Pediatrics **66:**626, 1980.

26. Liebhaber, M., et al.: Alterations of lymphocytes and of antibody content of human milk after processing, J. Pediatr. **91:**897, 1977.

27. Liebhaber, M., et al.: Comparison of bacterial contamination with two methods of human milk collection, J. Pediatr. **92:**236, 1978.

28. Lucas, A.: Human milk banks, Lancet **1:**103, 1982.

29. Lucas, A., et al.: Creamatocrit: simple clinical technique for estimating fat concentration and energy value of human milk, Br. Med. J. **1:**1018, 1978.

30. McEnery, G., and Chattopadhyay, B.: Human milk bank in a district general hospital, Br. Med. J. **2:**794, 1978.

31. Mother's Milk Unit, California Transplant Bank: A symposium on breast milk banking: procedures and protocols, San Jose, Calif., 1977, The Mothers' Milk Bank: The Institute for Medical Research.

32. Paxson, C.L., and Cress, C.C.: Survival of human milk leukocytes, J. Pediatr. **94:**61, 1979.

33. Pittard, W.B., and Bill, K.: Human milk banking: effect of refrigeration on cellular components, Clin. Pediatr. **20:**31, 1981.

34. Schmidt, E.: Effects of varying degrees of heat treatment on milk protein and its nutritional consequences, Acta Paediatr. Scand. Suppl. **296:**41, 1982.

35. Siimes, M.A., and Hallman, N.: A perspective on human milk banking, J. Pediatr. **94:**173, 1979.

36. Sponsel, W.E.: Simple and effective breast pump for nursing mothers, Br. Med. J. **286:**1180, 1983.

37. Stagno, S., et al.: Breast milk and the risk of cytomegalovirus infection, N. Engl. J. Med. **302:**1073, 1980.

38. Stocks, R.J., et al.: A simple method to improve the energy value of bank human milk, Early Hum. Dev. **8:**175, 1983.

39. Sunshine, P., Asquith, M.T., and Liebhaber, M.: The effects of collection and processing on various components of human milk. In Frier, S., and Eidelman, A.I., editors: Human milk: its biological and social value, Amsterdam, 1980, Excerpta Medica.

40. Tyson, J.E., et al.: Collection methods and contamination of bank milk, Arch. Dis. Child. **57:**396, 1982.

41. Wardell, J.M., Hill, C.M., and D'Souza, S.W.: Effect of pasteurization and of freezing and thawing human milk on its triglyceride content, Acta Paediatr. Scand. **70:**467, 1981.

42. Welsh, J.K., and May, J.T.: Anti-infective properties of breast milk, J. Pediatr. **94:**1, 1979.

43. Williamson, S., et al.: Effect of heat treatment of human milk on absorption of nitrogen, fat, sodium, calcium, and phosphorus by protein infants, Arch. Dis. Child. **53:**555, 1978.

44. Williamson, S., et al.: Organization of bank of raw and pasteurised human milk for neonatal intensive care, Br. Med. J. **1:**393, 1978.

45. Wills, M.E., et al.: Short-time low-temperature pasteurization of human milk, Early Hum. Dev. **7:**71, 1980.

The role of mother support groups and community resources

20

Certain changes in cultural aspects of Western civilization have contributed to the widespread use of artificial feedings for human infants as well as to the changing structure of the family. Urbanization has been associated not only with industrialization but also with the separation of generations from one another. This has produced the nuclear family. Nuclear families are smaller, mobile, isolated families often stranded in a large urban population. The young couple and their new infant are totally without personal human resources. That is, there is no one who cares enough to give individual support to the family. There is no one to turn to, share the experience with, and receive advice, encouragement, and support from.

Rites de passage were described by the French author Van Gennep[23] as the ceremonies and rituals that mark special changes in people's lives. The list includes marriage, motherhood, birth, death, circumcision, graduation, ordination, and retirement. In our present culture there is support for most of these events except birth and motherhood. The most critical *rite de passage* in a woman's life, Raphael[18] points out, is when she becomes a mother. Raphael further distinguishes this period of transition with the term *matrescence,* "to emphasize the mother and to focus on her new life-style." Traditional cultures herald a mother giving birth, whereas our culture announces the birth of an infant. The former highlights the mother, the latter the infant. Matrescence is a time of coddling. In preindustrial societies the mother is coddled for some time after birth, having only the responsibility of the infant's care while the mother's needs are met by doulas. Mothering the mother should be part of the postpartum support for a new mother.

A number of other forces added momentum to the bottle feeding trend that began in the 1920s when manufacturers finally were able to mass-produce an inexpensive container and rubber nipple with which to feed infants cheaply. Pediatrics was a new specialty to guard the health of children. The stress was on measuring and calculating.

473

Physicians seemed more secure when they could prescribe nutrition. The rise in the female labor force has also been credited with having an impact on the method of feeding infants, who were no longer brought everywhere with the mother to be nursed but were instead left behind to be bottle fed. The new technology of the infant food industry was a continuing influence on nutritional thinking of both medical and lay groups.

Breastfeeding was never totally abandoned. There was always a group of women who prepared themselves for childbirth and read and researched feeding and nutrition and chose to breastfeed.[16] In the middle 1940s Dr. Edith Jackson began the Rooming-In Project in New Haven. Families in New Haven who sought "childbirth without fear" and an opportunity to room-in with their infants usually wished to breastfeed. In the rooming-in unit, breastfeeding was often "contagious" because one mother successfully nursing would encourage others to try. Hospital stays averaged 5 to 7 days, during which time the mother-infant couple was cared for as a pair. About 70% of the patients left the hospital breastfeeding. Students and staff who were exposed to the philosophy of this unit went to many parts of the country, taking with them tremendous commitment to prepared childbirth and nurturing through breastfeeding. The classic article on the management of breastfeeding by Barnes et al.[3] was published as a result of counseling hundreds of nursing mothers.

DEVELOPMENT OF MOTHER SUPPORT GROUPS

There still remained the need for nuclear families to have access to support and conversation about healthy infants, mothering, and breastfeeding.[4] The La Leche League was developed to meet these needs in Franklin Park, Illinois, in 1956. The original intent was to provide other nursing mothers with information, encouragement, and moral support. There are now thousands of local chapters and a network of state and regional coordinators who all synchronize their activities with the headquarters in Franklin Park. La Leche League's 4000 groups are in 43 countries, in the United States, Canada, parts of Europe, New Zealand, and Africa, and other parts of the world.[9]

There is an excellent publication, *The Womanly Art of Breastfeeding,*[9] which was prepared by the original group of mothers involved in La Leche League. The publication was revised for the twenty-fifth anniversary of the organization in 1981. La Leche League continues to provide information and updated publications about common questions that arise during lactation. Local groups offer classes to prepare mothers to breastfeed. They help with suggestions about the nitty-gritty details of preparation, nutrition, clothing, and mothering in general. They also provide every mother with a telephone counselor. To be qualified to serve as a consultant to another mother, a member must demonstrate knowledge and expertise in breastfeeding as well as an understanding of how to counsel and render support. "Telephone mothers" do not give medical advice and are instructed to tell a troubled mother to call her own physician for such advice.

Interested local physicians provide medical expertise for the group in situations in which a medical opinion is appropriate. The league provides support for mothers to reduce the time the physician needs to spend counseling on the nonmedical aspects of lactation. Most information needed by the new mother is not medical.

Similar programs have been developed in 15 other countries. A well-established and respected program in Norway is Ammehjelpen, in Australia, the Nursing Mothers' Association of Australia, and in the United Kingdom, The National Childbirth Trust.

The International Childbirth Education Association also provides resources for the new family. Its program makes preparation and training available for couples during pregnancy and afterward as parents. Its scope embraces the entire childbirth concept, of which breastfeeding is part.

Sociologist Alice Ladas[10] studied women who attended La Leche League preparation classes and compared them to a similar group who attempted to breastfeed but did not have this preparation. She was able to demonstrate clearly that the women who attended such programs had more confidence and seemed to profit by receiving accurate, up-to-date and relevant information as well as receiving individual and group support.[11]

Silverman and Murrow[20] studied league activities and concluded that group dynamics are important and feelings of normalcy are reinforced. The information and experience were shown to be important, but the support from the group had the greatest influence on success in breastfeeding.[22] Meara[15] reports similar observations on league activities in a nonsupportive culture.

A follow-up study of breastfeeding in Oxford was carried out by Sloper et al.[21] In this study it was observed that significantly more mothers went home breastfeeding, mothers nursed longer, and solid foods were started later when support was provided. The authors attribute this shift to the change in advice and support given in the hospital and at home visits.

COMMUNITY RESOURCES

Most hospitals provide training in preparation for childbirth. Part of the program is about the new infant and how to plan for his care. These programs often serve as the initial stimulus to consider breastfeeding. Jelliffe and Jelliffe[8] suggest modifications of other health services to promote breastfeeding (Table 20-1).

The YWCA in most communities provides preparation for childbirth. Its classes usually provide programming that appeals to young and unwed women, a group in need of services rarely provided by other sources.

The Visiting Nurses Association and the public health nurses on the staff of the local county health department are special resources particularly skilled at counseling new mothers with their infants. They can provide valuable information to the physician who is working with an infant who fails to thrive at the breast by witnessing the breastfeeding scene at home.

Table 20-1. Possible modifications of the health services designed to promote breastfeeding in a community

Health service	Modifications
Prenatal	Information on breastfeeding (preferably from breastfeeding mothers); breast preparation; maternal diet; emotional preparation for labor
Puerperal	Avoid maternal fatigue/anxiety/pain (e.g., allow mothers to eat in early labor; avoid *unnecessary* episiotomy; relatives and visitors allowed; privacy and relaxed atmosphere; organization of day with breastfeeding in mind); separate mother and newborn as little as possible and stimulate lactation (e.g., no prelacteal feeds; first breastfeeding as soon as possible; avoid *unnecessary* maternal anesthesia; permissive schedule; rooming-in); lactation "consultants" (advisers—preferably women who have breastfed), adequate "lying-in-period"; in hot weather, extra water by dropper or spoon
Premature unit	Use of expressed breast milk (preferably fresh); contact between mother and infant with earliest return to direct breastfeeding
Children's wards	Accommodation in hospital (or nearby) for mothers of breastfed infants
Home visiting	Encourage, motivate, support
Health center	Supplementary food distribution (e.g., formula and weaning foods) according to defined, locally relevant policy
General	Supportive atmosphere from all staff; avoid promotion of unwanted commercial infant foods (e.g., samples, posters, calendars, brochures, etc.); adopt minimal bottle feeding policy and practical health education concerning "biological breastfeeding"

From Jelliffe, D.B., and Jelliffe, E.F.P.: Human milk in the modern world, Oxford, 1978, Oxford University Press, copyright D.B. and E.F.P. Jelliffe 1978.

There are many other organizations, local and national in scope, that have the perinatal period and the family as their focus. Many of these are also interested in promoting breastfeeding as part of their overall goals.

A model program in Rochester was developed as a cooperative effort among The Home Care Program of the Genesee Region, which was already serving the chronically ill and recently hospitalized population, and health-care providers.[1] The pediatricians, obstetricians, and medical society worked with the Home Care staff to devise a program of early discharge from the hospital of mothers and their newborns (less than 24 hours postpartum) followed by daily visits by a specially trained perinatal nurse. A homemaker was also provided to take care of the chores and other children. Laboratory services were provided at home. An important focus of the program has been counseling for successful breastfeeding.[13] The regional Blue Cross pays for the service in its regular contract. The target population is the healthy family that wishes to "normalize" its birth experience.

The government has taken an active interest in the promotion of breastfeeding as well. In the goals for national health prepared by a multidisciplinary task force, it is stated that by 1990 75% of infants leaving the hospital shall be breastfed and at 6 months of age at least 35% will still be breastfeeding.[17] The plan of action to reach these goals has included the development of a Healthy Mothers–Healthy Infants Program. There is also a national committee for the promotion of breastfeeding, which includes representation from major professional organizations of physicians, dietitians, social service workers, nurses, nurse midwives, and hospital administrators. A major thrust of the national effort has been through the Women, Infants, and Children Program (WIC), in which mothers are being encouraged to breastfeed and given nutritional and practical lactation management instruction and support. An instruction manual is available for WIC workers.[5] The Department of Agriculture and the Department of Health and Human Services developed a program that included a national closed circuit television program in April 1983. A videotape of this professional program is now available for purchase or rent from the Department of Maternal and Child Health in the Department of Health and Human Services in Washington, D.C. The Surgeon General conducted a national workshop on breastfeeding and human lactation in Rochester, New York, in June 1984 to develop recommendations for national policy. Publication from the workshop is available from the Government Printing Office in Washington, D.C.

Issues of rural health have begun to include those surrounding birth and the infant's welfare. Programs are being developed to increase breastfeeding among rural people. Although the incidence of breastfeeding has increased among well-educated self-motivated middle Americans, the number of impoverished, less well-educated women who breastfeed remains small. Progress is being made, community by community, by dedicated health-care workers, dietitians, and WIC staff. Health professionals often serve as a catalyst in developing such programs but should always be ready to serve as knowledgeable, supportive consultants to the effort of others.[6]

Lactation centers have been developed in health care centers such as the program developed by Naylor in San Diego or free-standing programs such as the Lactation Institute in Encino, California founded by Marmet and Shell.

The purpose of these programs is to provide consultation services for mothers as well as education and information for health-care workers.[6] Efforts have been made to change hospital policy regarding breastfeeding in order to increase the success rate.[14] A very impressive program was initiated in the Philippines by Relucio-Clavano.[19] She has not only increased the incidence of breastfeeding but improved the morbidity from sepsis, diarrhea, and malnutrition. A logical and effective approach to changing hospital policy has been designed by Hales to promote breastfeeding in hospitals where the complex organizational structure is overwhelming to the busy professional who sees a need but does not know the process.[7,14]

Lactation consultants

For years, many medical and nursing professionals have served as lactation consultants ready to respond to any colleague's request for knowledge and expertise. With the great national movement to embrace breastfeeding, however, a new type of lactation consultant is evolving from the vast pool of women who have served in local mother-to-mother programs to help others breastfeed. While many of these consultants do have the educational credentials one expects from a consultant, many have no such credentials. The health-care professional needs to see that the lactation resources available in the community are truly of professional quality and background. Counseling is a special skill requiring more than personal experience with the situation.

Lactation counselor as a member of the health-care team

Modern medicine has developed a team approach to the management of many patient populations such as the elderly or the handicapped.* There is a team approach to the management of many categories of diseases such as cancer and diabetes. There is also a health-care team that provides medical service for the family during the perinatal period. This team includes an obstetrician and a pediatrician or a family physician; nurse midwives; nurses working in prenatal care, obstetrics, newborn, and public health; social workers; dietitians; and, when a problem develops, perinatologists, neonatologists, and the skilled team from the perinatal center. These team members are well-educated and extensively trained professionals. Together they have improved the morbidity and mortality rates of childbirth. The long-range prognosis for the intact survival of infants has been significantly improved. Thus medical progress has occurred concomitantly with the isolation of the nuclear family. The result is a medically successful birth to a family that is emotionally and socially ill prepared to cope. The family is ill prepared to take over when the mother and baby are discharged from the hospital and instantly placed on their own without a transitional period of adjustment with close support and supervision.

The counselor becomes a very important addition to the health-care team, replacing the traditional family support system. The counselor not only needs to know the role as counselor interacting with the family but also must understand how she interfaces with other members of the health-care team. The professional team members are beginning to understand the importance of the volunteer counselor and how to work most effectively with her. The counselor can fill the gap between the professional and the parents. Some practitioners provide a nurse practitioner whose role is to fill that gap. The counselor will quickly earn the respect of the health-care team if she communicates openly with them, supports the mother in a positive manner, and encourages a relationship of mutual trust and respect between mother and the team.

The peer counselor will complement the work of the health professionals but should never replace the role of the health-care provider.

WHO SHALL COUNSEL.   When one is working closely with people in critical life situations, there are people who make good counselors and there are equally good people who are not appropriate as counselors and should have other jobs in the organization.

Counseling is a profession, and professional counselors are carefully screened, ed-

---

*From Lawrence, R.A.: Introduction. In Lauwers, J., and Woessner, C., editors: Counseling the nursing mother: a reference handbook for health care providers and lay counselors, Wayne, N.J., 1983, Avery Publishing Group, Inc.

ucated, and trained. Therefore, individuals who volunteer to help mothers should be screened, educated, and trained also. They should have some special qualities:

The ability to truly listen

The ability to avoid judgment

The ability to understand other life-styles

The ability to admit it when they do not know

The ability to seek appropriate help from professionals

The ability to recognize incompatibility in a given relationship

In the past few decades, peer counseling has become widespread and has been successful, not only with breastfeeding and childbirth but also with chronic disease such as cystic fibrosis and with devastating illnesses such as cancer. The first thing all these groups have had to acknowledge is that just because one has experienced a life event she is not automatically qualified to counsel others experiencing similar situations.

The candidate must first put her own experiences into perspective and understand what has motivated her to seek this counseling role. Counseling is an opportunity to help by listening, and being a sympathetic listener is the most important quality. This is not a time to talk about the counselor's pregnancies. The counselor cannot have her own agenda and press her personal views or life-style on the mother she counsels, nor should it be used as a personal platform to promote organizational biases.

The counselor must understand that assuming a place on the health-care team is demanding of time and effort. One must be available at the convenience and need of the client, even when this is inconvenient to the counselor.

The most difficult time for any counselor is when she must recognize that the problem is beyond her expertise. This takes sufficient knowledge of the subject matter to recognize the danger signs of a problem that requires other intervention. More difficult is that it takes the inner strength and courage to admit that one is indeed beyond one's own resources and skills before a little problem becomes a serious medical or psychologic crisis. A timeworn adage of the health-care professional is *First, do no harm.*

LEARNING TO HELP MOTHERS. The suggestions put forth to guide a counselor in training must be general overall guidelines about attitude and posture. The emphasis is on listening, encouraging a mother to talk, and ultimately helping her to solve her own problem by understanding it. Professional counselors are trained using didactic sessions, role play, and supervisory sessions until skills are developed. Continued reinforcement of philosophy and techniques forms the basis of growth and improvement. The lay counselor should attend counselor training sessions provided by her parent organization and work closely with her supervisor. Sharing counseling situations with others with more experience will give further insight. Returning to the reference materials again and again will bring to light new thoughts that have been read before but not truly assimilated initially because of lack of experience.

There is no substitute for correct information. Much research is underway in this country and worldwide in the field of human lactation. Working in the arena of breast-feeding counseling mandates continual updating of information. For the past decades this country has experienced a renaissance in the art of breastfeeding. It is only recently that there has been a renaissance in the science of human lactation. The basic reference information about human lactation is available in resource texts. Readers should seek out the original references for a fuller understanding. It is often difficult to sort out the old wives' tales from scientific fact in some of the myriad of lay publications available, so reference material should be selected cautiously. When there is a question of management that requires additional resource material, it is probably a question that should be referred to the mothers' physician.

The lay counselor does not provide medical advice. The counselor can encourage the mother to contact her doctor. When the infant is doing poorly or is sick, the pediatrician should be consulted promptly. The rare condition of failure to thrive while breastfeeding is increasing in frequency, paralleling the increased incidence of breastfeeding. It has serious implications for the infant and for the continuation of breastfeeding unless treatment is initiated promptly by the physician. The physician is powerless to help if he is not consulted. When the infant's problem is identified and it is prudent to continue breastfeeding, the counselor can be an invaluable asset in supporting and reassuring the mother.

Maternal problems such as mastitis should respond well if treated early, but recurrent mastitis may develop when home remedies are substituted for proper treatment. The role of the lay counselor in such situations is significant. Encouraging the mother to seek medical care promptly is most important. Reinforcing medical advice will further enhance its effectiveness. For example, if rest is prescribed, the counselor can help the mother to understand how critical rest is to recovery and then help her figure out how she is going to cope at home with family responsibilities and a newborn and still rest.

The question of maternal drugs during lactation is a complex issue that cannot be resolved without a knowledge of pharmacology, maternal and infant metabolism, and the influences of dose, time, age of infant, and pharmacokinetics. Checking a list of drugs that appear in milk is not sufficient. The physician should be consulted. If more data are needed, the regional Poison Control Center can be consulted by the physician. No counselor should assume this responsibility. On the other hand, when a decision has been reached on the safety of the use of the medication, the counselor can help the mother work through the issues related to her breastfeeding. Perhaps adjustment in dosing and feeding schedule is necessary, and perhaps pumping and discarding the milk is necessary for 24 hours; in any case, managing these lactation modifications can be facilitated by supportive counseling.

The role of the lay counselor is support of the mother. The counselor should work in concert with the medical health-care team, as a team player, not as a competitor or as an adversary, but as a facilitator. The mission of the team is successful lactation, a satisfying mothering experience, and healthy infant. The health-care team will continue to be responsible for the family long after lactation has been discontinued. The confidence and trust developed between the health team and family will be critical to lasting success. The lay counselor should be remembered as a gentle facilitator and a kindly, caring support person who was there through the *rite de passage* of matrescence.

RECOMMENDATIONS OF THE ACADEMY OF PEDIATRICS.   The Academy of Pediatrics[2] has made a statement in support of human milk in 1978.* They have summarized a lengthy presentation with the following:

1. Full-term newborn infants should be breastfed, except if there are specific contraindications or when breastfeeding is unsuccessful.
2. Education about breastfeeding should be provided in schools for all children, and better education about breastfeeding and infant nutrition should be provided in the curriculum of physicians and nurses. Information about breastfeeding should also be presented in public communications media.
3. Prenatal instruction should include both theoretical and practical information about breastfeeding.
4. Attitudes and practices in prenatal clinics and in maternity wards should encourage a climate that favors breastfeeding. The staff should include nurses and other personnel who are not only favorably disposed toward breastfeeding but also knowledgeable and skilled in the art.
5. Consultation between maternity services and agencies committed to breastfeeding should be strengthened.
6. Studies should be conducted on the feasibility of breastfeeding infants at day nurseries adjacent to places of work subsequent to an appropriate leave of absence following the birth of an infant.

---

*Initiated by the Nutrition Committee of the Canadian Paediatric Society, this statement was prepared by both the Committee on Nutrition of the American Academy of Pediatrics and the Nutrition Committee of the Canadian Paediatric Society. Copyright American Academy of Pediatrics, 1978.

REFERENCES

1. Amado, A., Lawrence, R.A., and Roghman, K.: Perinatal Home Care: report on a Blue Cross and Home Care effort, Caring **2:**27, 1983.
2. American Academy of Pediatrics Committee on Nutrition: Pediatrics **62:**591, 1978.
3. Barnes, G.B., et al.: Management of breast feeding, JAMA **151:**192, 1953.
4. Ciba Foundation Symposium no. 45, breast feeding and the mother, Amsterdam, 1976, Elsevier Scientific Publ. Co.
5. Food and Nutrition Service, U.S. Dept. of Agriculture: Promoting breastfeeding: a guide for health professionals working in the WIC and CSF programs, Washington, D.C., 1983, U.S. Dept. of Agriculture.
6. Gussler, J., and Bryant, C.: Helping mothers breast-feed: program strategies for minority communities. Health Action Papers, vol. I, Lexington, Kentucky, 1984, Lexington Fayette County Health Department, University of Kentucky Medical Behavioral Sciences Department.
7. Hales, D.J.: Promoting breastfeeding: strategies for changing hospital policy, Studies in Family Planning **12:**167, 1981.

8. Jelliffe, D.B., and Jelliffe, E.F.P.: Human milk in the modern world, Oxford, 1976, Oxford University Press.

9. La Leche League: The womanly art of breast-feeding, ed. 3, Franklin Park, Ill., 1976, La Leche League International.

10. Ladas, A.K.: How to help mothers breast feed, Clin. Pediatr. **9:**702, 1970.

11. Ladas, A.K.: The less viable option: breast feeding, J. Trop. Pediatr. **18:**318, 1972.

12. Lawrence, R.A.: Introduction. In Lauwers, J., and Woessner, C., editors: Counseling the nursing mother: a reference handbook for health care providers and lay counselors, Wayne, N.J., 1983, Avery Publishing Group, Inc.

13. Lawrence, R.A., Amado, A., and Roghman, K.: Home health care program in the management of breastfeeding, In press.

14. Lewis, L.: Successful breast-feeding programs for low-income, minority mothers, Public Health Currents **22**(1):1, 1982.

15. Meara, H.: A key to successful breast feeding in a nonsupportive culture, J. Nurse Midwife. **21:**20, 1976.

16. Pryor, K.: Nursing your baby, New York, 1973, Harper & Row, Publishers, Inc.

17. Public Health Service: Implementation plans for attaining the objectives for the nation, Public Health Rep. **98**(suppl.): 145, 1983.

18. Raphael, D.: The tender gift: breast feeding, New York, 1976, Schocken Books.

19. Relucio-Clavano, N.: The results of a change in hospital practices, Assignment Child. **55/56:**139, 1981.

20. Silverman, P.R., and Murrow, H.G.: Caregiver during critical role in the normal life cycle, unpublished report, Harvard Medical School.

21. Sloper, K.S., Elsden, E., and Baum, J.D.: Increasing breast feeding in a community, Arch. Dis. Child, **52:**700, 1977.

22. Thompson, M.: The effectiveness of mother to mother help, research on the La Leche League International program, Birth Fam. J. **3:**1, Winter, 1976-1977.

23. Van Gennep, A.: Rites of passage, Vizedom, M.B., and Caffee, G.L., translators, London, 1960, Rutledge & Kegan Paul, Publishers.

Appendix A
Growth and development

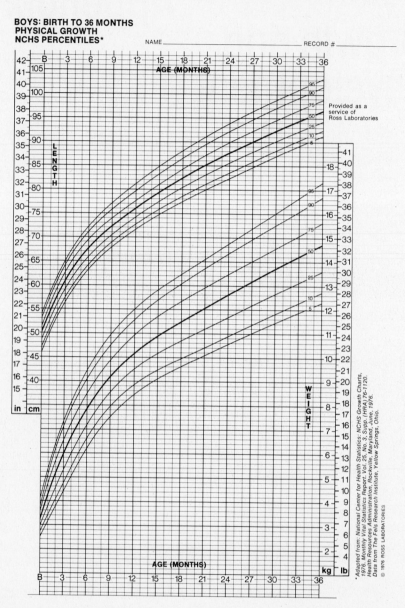

Fig. A-1. Normal males, birth to 36 months. Length and weight. (Courtesy Ross Laboratories, Columbus, Ohio.)

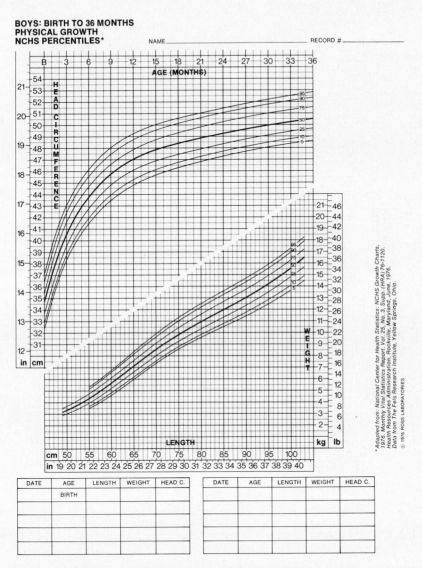

Fig. A-2. Normal males, birth to 36 months. Head circumference and weight/length. (Courtesy Ross Laboratories, Columbus, Ohio.)

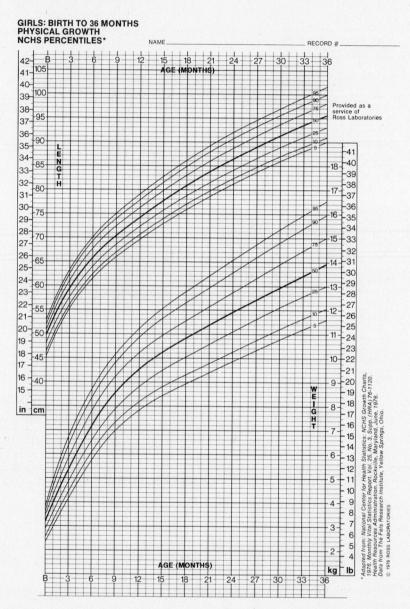

GIRLS: BIRTH TO 36 MONTHS
PHYSICAL GROWTH
NCHS PERCENTILES*

NAME_____ RECORD #_____

Fig. A-3. Normal females, birth to 36 months. Length and weight. (Courtesy Ross Laboratories, Columbus, Ohio.)

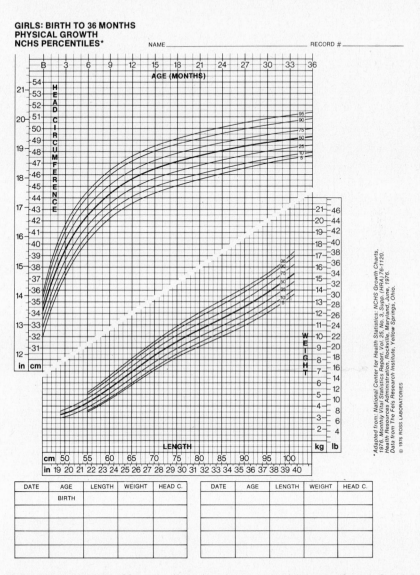

Fig. A-4. Normal females, birth to 36 months. Head circumference and weight/length. (Courtesy Ross Laboratories, Columbus, Ohio.)

Table A-1. Changes in weight and length by low-birth weight and full-size infants during the first 3 years of life

Age interval (mo)	Size appropriate for gestational age (GA)									Size small for GA		
	GA 28-32 wk			GA 33-36 wk			GA 37-42 wk			GA 37-42 wk		
	N	Mean	SD	N	Mean	SD	N	Mean	SD	N	Mean	SD
Males—change in weight (kg)												
0-3	17	2.9	0.6	28	2.9	0.6	123	2.8	0.6	22	2.9	0.5
3-6	17	2.3	0.6	25	2.2	0.5	104	1.9	0.5	19	2.1	0.7
6-9	17	1.4	0.5	26	1.5	0.5	106	1.4	0.4	17	1.3	0.4
9-12	17	1.1	0.4	28	1.0	0.4	121	1.1	0.6	17	0.8	0.3
12-24	16	2.2	0.5	34	2.1	0.6	—	—	—	23	2.1	0.9
24-36	13	2.0	0.5	32	1.8	0.6	114	2.0	0.7	21	2.0	1.2
Males—change in length (cm)												
0-3	17	12.4	1.7	28	12.2	1.6	123	10.6	1.1	22	11.0	1.3
3-6	17	9.7	1.5	25	8.6	1.3	104	6.6	1.6	19	7.5	2.3
6-9	17	6.4	0.9	26	5.6	1.4	106	4.5	1.3	17	5.7	1.3
9-12	17	4.1	1.4	28	4.5	1.1	121	4.0	1.0	17	4.0	1.0
Females—change in weight (kg)												
0-3	22	2.4	0.5	34	2.7	0.5	136	2.4	0.5	32	2.5	0.6
3-6	18	2.1	0.4	34	2.1	0.6	78	1.9	0.5	28	1.8	0.4
6-9	16	1.4	0.3	32	1.4	0.3	78	1.4	0.5	26	1.2	0.4
9-12	18	1.2	0.4	28	0.9	0.4	86	1.0	0.4	27	1.0	0.4
12-24	21	2.6	0.6	34	2.4	0.7	—	—	—	35	2.1	0.6
24-36	21	2.2	0.9	29	2.0	0.7	79	2.2	0.7	35	1.9	0.9
Females—change in length (cm)												
0-3	22	11.7	1.8	34	11.0	1.1	136	10.0	1.1	32	10.9	1.4
3-6	18	9.1	1.5	34	7.9	1.4	78	6.5	1.4	28	6.9	1.3
6-9	16	5.9	1.5	32	4.9	1.0	78	4.8	1.2	26	4.9	0.5
9-12	18	4.6	1.0	28	4.8	1.4	86	4.1	1.0	27	3.8	1.0
12-24	21	12.8	2.1	34	12.3	1.7	—	—	—	35	11.8	1.7
24-36	21	8.8	1.9	29	8.5	1.6	79	8.5	1.2	35	7.9	1.5

From Fomon, S. J.: Infant nutrition, ed. 2, Philadelphia, 1974, W. B. Saunders Co.

Table A-2. Skinfold measurements

Age (mo)	Sex	Number	Biceps (mm)		Triceps (mm)		Subscapular (mm)		Suprailiac (mm)	
			Mean	SD	Mean	SD	Mean	SD	Mean	SD
1	G	81	3.7	0.59	5.8	1.18	6.3	1.11	4.4	1.01
	B	112	3.6	0.74	5.4	1.25	5.7	1.29	4.1	1.08
3	G	81	5.4	1.15	8.3	1.64	7.8	1.58	7.2	1.85
	B	119	5.2	1.14	7.9	1.62	6.9	1.52	6.4	1.97
6	G	86	6.6	1.34	10.3	1.71	8.2	2.01	7.0	1.95
	B	119	6.3	1.55	9.8	1.80	7.3	1.70	6.5	2.13
9	G	86	6.3	1.10	10.1	1.69	7.9	1.66	5.8	1.38
	B	119	6.0	1.30	10.0	1.94	7.3	1.71	5.5	1.76
12	G	86	6.1	1.12	9.9	1.70	7.6	1.52	5.3	1.18
	B	118	5.9	1.28	9.9	1.82	7.3	1.72	5.1	1.42
18	G	86	6.0	1.12	10.0	1.62	7.1	1.46	5.0	1.11
	B	119	5.7	1.06	10.0	1.78	7.0	1.54	4.7	1.22
24	G	85	6.0	1.19	10.3	1.79	6.7	1.33	5.0	1.15
	B	118	5.8	1.12	10.0	1.93	6.5	1.61	4.6	1.27
36	G	85	6.1	1.07	10.4	1.56	6.4	1.52	4.9	0.99
	B	118	5.6	1.04	9.9	1.61	5.8	1.27	4.5	0.99

From Karlberg, P., et al.: Acta Paediatr. Scand. (suppl. 258):1, 1976.

Appendix B
Infant activity

Table B-1. Infant scheduling record*†

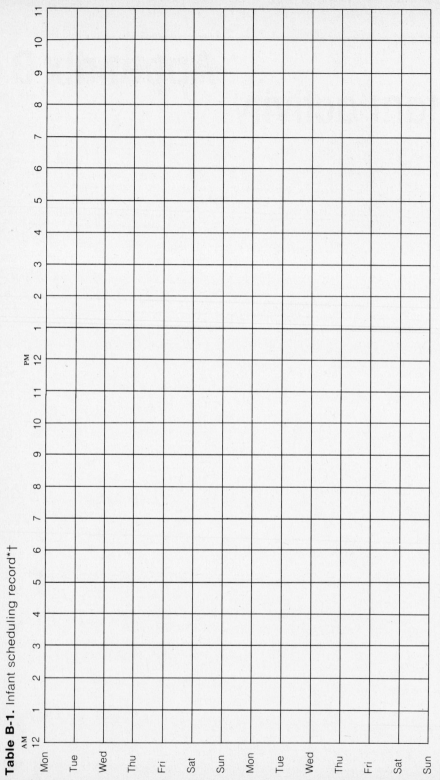

*Chart kept by mother to record infant activity when problems arise around nursing, sleeping, or fussing.
†Record with a line (—) time spent sleeping (—S—), feeding (—F—), and awake but not feeding (—A—), and crying or fussing (—cry—).

Appendix C
Dietary guidance during lactation

Table C-1. Tool A—Food record: diet history

Name _____
Medical record no. _____
Date _____

Meals and snacks		Total food intake				Comments
Time	Place	Food	Description of food items		With whom eaten?	Any related factors?—associated activity, place, persons, money, feelings, hunger, etc.
			Amount	Type or preparation		

From Williams, S.: Handbook of maternal and infant nutrition, Berkeley, Calif., 1976, SRW Productions, Inc.

Table C-2.   Tool B—Nutrition interview: diet history

Name _____ Date _____
Age _____ Height _____ Prepregnant weight _____
Gravida _____ EDC _____ Present weight _____

Activity-associated general day's food intake pattern

LIVING SITUATION

Housing _____
Members of household _____
Culture _____
Occupation: Husband _____
        Self _____
Recreation, physical activity _____

PRESENT FOOD HABITS	**Place**	**Time**
Morning		
Noon		
Evening		
Snacks		
Comments		

Checklist

Protein foods	Breads, cereals, legumes	Vegetables
Milk	Breads (whole-grain	Dark yellow
Cheese	enriched)	Deep green
Meat	Cereals	Potato
Fish	Pastas	Others
Poultry	Dried beans, peas,	Desserts, sweets
Eggs	lentils	Soft drinks, candy
Fruits	Fats and oils	Alcohol
Citrus	Butter	Vitamin, mineral
Others	Margarine	supplements
	Others	Medication, drugs

From Williams, S.: Handbook of maternal and infant nutrition, Berkeley, Calif., 1976, SRW Productions, Inc.

Table C-3. Tool C—Nutritional analysis sheet

Food groups	Major nutrient contributions	Recommended daily intake (number of servings)	Patient intake	Analysis of food needs
Protein-rich foods				
Milk and cheese	Protein (complete, high biological value); Ca, P, Mg; vitamin D; riboflavin	1 qt milk 2 oz cheese or ½ cup cottage cheese		
Eggs and meat	Protein (complete, high biological value); B complex vitamins; folic acid (liver); vitamin A (liver); iron (liver especially)	2 eggs 2 servings meat (3-4 oz each) Liver once a week at least		
Vitamin- and mineral-rich foods				
Grains, whole or enriched, breads or cereals, legumes	Protein (incomplete, supplementary); B complex vitamins; iron, Ca, P, Mg; energy (protein sparing)	4 or more servings		
Green and yellow vegetables	Vitamin A; folic acid	1-2 servings		
Citrus fruits and other vitamin C–rich fruits and vegetables	Vitamin C	2 servings		
Potatoes and other vegetables and fruits	Energy (protein sparing); added vitamins and minerals	1 serving or as needed for calories		
Fats—margarine, butter, and oils	Vitamin A (butter, fortified margarine); vitamin E (vegetable oils); energy (protein sparing)	1-2 tbsp as needed for calories		
Iodized salt	Iodine	Use with food to taste		

From Williams, S.: Handbook of maternal and infant nutrition, Berkeley, Calif., 1976, SRW Productions, Inc.

Table C-4.   Vegetarian food guide

GENERAL GUIDELINES
1. Follow nutrition guide for regular food plan during pregnancy.
2. Eat a wide variety of foods, including milk and milk products and eggs.
3. If no milk is allowed, use a supplement of 4 μg of vitamin B_{12} daily. If goat and soy milk are used, partial supplementation may be needed.
4. If no milk is taken, also use supplements of 12 mg of calcium and 400 IU of vitamin D daily. Partial supplementation will be necessary if less than four servings of milk and milk products are consumed.
5. Select a variety of plant foods (especially grains, legumes, nuts, and seeds) to obtain "complete" proteins by complementary combinations, as indicated in the list below.
6. Use iodized salt.

	Complementary plant protein combinations	
Food	Amino acids deficient	Complementary protein food combinations
Grains	Isoleucine Lysine	Rice + legumes Corn + legumes Wheat + legumes Wheat + peanuts + milk Wheat + sesame + soybeans Rice + brewer's yeast
Legumes	Tryptophan Methionine	Legumes + rice Beans + wheat Beans + corn Soybeans + rice + wheat Soybeans + corn + milk Soybeans + wheat + sesame Soybeans + peanuts + sesame Soybeans + peanuts + wheat + rice Soybeans + sesame + wheat
Nuts and seeds	Isoleucine Lysine	Peanuts + sesame + soybeans Sesame + beans Sesame + soybeans + wheat Peanuts + sunflower seeds
Vegetables	Isoleucine Methionine	Lima beans Green beans Brussels sprouts } + Sesame seeds or Brazil nuts or mushrooms Cauliflower Broccoli Greens = millet or rice

Modified from Lappé, F.M.: Diet for a small planet, New York, 1971, Friends of the Earth/Ballantine; from Worthington, B.S., Vermeersch, J., and Williams, S.R.: Nutrition in pregnancy and lactation, St. Louis, 1977, The C.V. Mosby Co.

Table C-5. Characteristic food choices of ethnic groups

Black	Mexican-American	Japanese	Chinese	Filipino
Protein foods				
Meat	Meat	Meat	Meat	Meat
Beef	Beef	Beef	Pork	Pork
Pork, ham	Pork	Pork	Beef	Beef
Sausage	Lamb	Poultry	Organ meats	Goat
Pig's feet,	Tripe	Chicken	Poultry	Deer
ears, etc.	Sausage	Turkey	Chicken	Rabbit
Bacon	(chorizo)	Fish	Duck	Variety meats
Luncheon	Bologna	Tuna	Fish	Poultry
meats	Bacon	Mackerel	White fish	Chicken
Organ meats	Poultry	Sardines	Shrimp	Fish
Poultry	Chicken	(dried form:	Lobster	Sole
Chicken	Eggs	mezashi)	Oyster	Bonito
Turkey	Legumes	Sea bass	Sardines	Herring
Fish	Pinto beans	Shrimp	Eggs	Tuna
Catfish	Pink beans	Abalone	Legumes	Mackerel
Perch	Garbanzo	Squid	Soybeans	Crab
Red snapper	beans	Octopus	Soybean	Mussels
Tuna	Lentils	Eggs	curd	Shrimp
Salmon	Nuts	Legumes	(tofu)	Squid
Sardines	Peanuts	Soybean curd	Black beans	Eggs
Shrimp	Peanut butter	(tofu)	Nuts	Legumes
		Soybean paste	Peanuts	Black beans
Eggs		(miso)	Almonds	Chick peas
Legumes		Soybeans	Cashews	Black-eyed peas
Kidney beans		Red beans		Lentils
Red beans		(azuki)		Mung beans
Pinto beans		Lima beans		Lima beans
Black-eyed				White kidney
peas		Nuts		beans
Nuts		Chestnuts		Nuts
Peanuts		(kuri)		Cashews
Peanut butter				Peanuts
				Pili nuts
Milk and milk products				
Milk	Milk	Milk	Milk	Milk
Fluid	Cheese	Fluid	Flavored	Flavored
Evaporated	Ice cream	Flavored	Whole milk	Evaporated
in coffee		Evaporated	(used in	Cheese
Buttermilk		Condensed	cooking)	Gouda
Cheese		Cheese	Ice cream	Cheddar
Cheddar		American		
Cottage		Monterey Jack		
Ice cream		Hoop		
		Ice cream		

Modified from Nutrition during pregnancy and lactation, Sacramento, Calif., 1975, California Department of Health; from Worthington, B.S., Vermeersch, J., and Williams, S.R.: Nutrition in pregnancy and lactation, St. Louis, 1977, The C.V. Mosby Co.

Table C-5. Characteristic food choices of ethnic groups—cont'd

Black	Mexican-American	Japanese	Chinese	Filipino
Grain products				
Rice	Rice	Rice	Rice	Rice
Cornbread	Tortillas	Rice crackers	Noodles	Cooked cereals
Hominy grits	Corn	Noodles	White bread	Farina
Biscuits	Flour	(whole wheat:	Millet	Oatmeal
Muffins	Oatmeal	soba)		Dry cereals
White bread	Dry cereals	Spaghetti		Pastas
Dry cereal	Cornflakes	White bread		Rice noodles
Cooked cereal	Sugared	Oatmeal		Wheat noodles
Macaroni	Noodles	Dry cereal		Macaroni
Spaghetti	Spaghetti			Spaghetti
Crackers	White bread			
	Sweet bread			
	(pan dulce)			
Vegetables				
Broccoli	Avocado	Bamboo shoots	Bamboo	Bamboo shoots
Cabbage	Cabbage	Bok choy	shoots	Beets
Carrots	Carrots	Broccoli	Beans	Cabbage
Corn	Chilies	Burdock root	Green	Carrots
Green beans	Corn	Cabbage	Yellow	Cauliflower
Greens	Green beans	Carrots	Bean sprouts	Celery
Mustard	Lettuce	Cauliflower	Bok choy	Chinese celery
Collard	Onion	Celery	Broccoli	Eggplant
Kale	Peas	Cucumbers	Cabbage	Endive
Spinach	Potato	Eggplant	Carrots	Green beans
Turnip	Prickly pear	Green beans	Celery	Leeks
Lima beans	cactus leaf	Gourd (kampyo)	Chinese cab-	Lettuce
Okra	(nopales)	Mushrooms	bage	Mushrooms
Peas	Spinach	Mustard greens	Corn	Okra
Potato	Sweet potato	Napa cabbage	Cucumbers	Onion
Pumpkin	Tomato	Peas	Eggplant	Peppers
Sweet potato	Zucchini	Peppers	Greens	Potato
Tomato		Radishes	Collard	Pumpkin
Yam		(white radish:	Chinese	Radishes
		daikon;	broccoli	Snow peas
		pickled white:	Mustard	Spinach
		takawan)	Kale	Squash
		Snow peas	Spinach	Sweet potato
		Spinach	Leeks	Tomato
		Squash	Lettuce	Water chestnuts
		Sweet potato	Mushrooms	Watercress
		Taro (Japanese	Peppers	Yam
		sweet potato)	Potato	
		Tomato	Scallions	
		Turnips	Snow peas	
		Water	Sweet potato	
		chestnuts	Taro	
		Yam	Tomato	
			Water	
			chestnuts	
			White radish	
			White turnip	
			Winter melon	

Continued.

Table C-5.   Characteristic food choices of ethnic groups—cont'd

Black	Mexican-American	Japanese	Chinese	Filipino
Fruits				
Apple	Apple	Apple	Apple	Apple
Banana	Apricots	Apricots	Banana	Banana
Grapefruit	Banana	Banana	Figs	Grapes
Grapes	Guava	Cherries	Grapes	Guava
Nectarine	Lemon	Grapefruit	Kumquats	Lemon
Orange	Mango	Grapes	Loquats	Lime
Plums	Melons	Lemon	Mango	Mango
Tangerine	Orange	Lime	Melons	Melons
Watermelon	Peach	Melons	Orange	Orange
	Pear	Orange	Peach	Papaya
	Prickly pear	Peach	Pear	Pear
	cactus fruit	Pear	Persimmon	Pineapple
	(tuna)	Persimmon	Pineapple	Plums
	Zapote (sa-	Pineapple	Plums	Pomegranate
	pote)	Pomegranate	Tangerine	Rhubarb
		Plums		Strawberries
		(dried, pickled		Tangerine
		plums called		
		umeboshi)		
		Strawberries		
		Tangerine		
Other				
Salt pork (fat	Salsa	Soy sauce	Soy sauce	Soy sauce
back)	(tomato-pep-	Nori paste	Sweet and sour	Coffee
Carbonated	per-onion	(seasoned	sauce	Tea
beverages	relish)	rice)	Mustard sauce	
Fruit drinks	Chili sauce	Bean thread	Ginger	
Gravies	Guacamole	(konyaku)	Plum sauce	
Coffee	Lard	Ginger (shoga;	Red bean	
Iced tea	(manteca)	dried form	paste	
	Pork cracklings	called denish-	Black bean	
	Fruit drinks	oga)	sauce	
	Kool-aid	Tea	Oyster sauce	
	Carbonated	Coffee	Tea	
	beverages		Coffee	
	Beer			
	Coffee			

Appendix D
History form for evaluation of infant with failure to thrive

No. _____
Date _____

Slow gaining special history

MOTHER

Name _____

A. **Diet**
1. Do you eat regular meals? _____ How do you rate the kind of food you eat? excellent ☐ good ☐ poor ☐
2. Do you take vitamins? _____ If so, what? _____
_____
3. Do you take brewer's yeast? _____
4. Are you worried about your weight? _____
B. **Health**
1. Are you in good health? _____ If not, describe problems _____
_____
2. Are you taking any medications? _____ Birth control pills? _____
Prescriptions? _____ Nonprescription medicines? _____
3. Have you had any thyroid problems at any time in your life? _____ Are thyroid medications being taken now? _____ What kind? _____
_____

Dosage _____ Last time you had your blood tested for thyroid
_____
4. Do you have any blood pressure problems? _____
C. **Habits**
1. Do you smoke? _____ Which brand? _____
How many per day? _____
2. Do you drink coffee? _____ How many cups per day? _____
Do you drink caffeinated sodas? _____ How many caffeinated sodas per day? _____
3. Do you drink alcohol? _____ How much per day? _____
week? _____ month? _____
D. **Nursing**
1. When the infant nurses, do you feel tingling ☐ burning ☐ filling feeling ☐
leaking on other side ☐ nothing ☐
other _____
2. Do you have a quiet environment for nursing? _____ If not, why (describe)? (Example, loud music, freeway noise, dogs barking) _____
3. Do you own a rocking chair? _____
E. **Social environment**
1. Do you have a busy life-style? _____ If so, why (name activities)? _____
_____
2. Marriage relationship is good ☐ average ☐ poor ☐.
3. Do you have other children? _____ Ages _____ Breastfed?
_____ How long? _____
4. Do you have any source of anxiety or tension? _____ If so, describe _____
_____

Modified from form developed by Fleiss, P.M., and Frantz, K.B.

Slow gaining special history—cont'd

INFANT

Name _____ Date of birth _____

1. How often is infant fed? _____
2. Breast milk only? _____ Other? _____
   Does he feed at each breast at each feeding? _____ How long on each breast?
   _____
3. How long does infant take to finish a feeding? _____ Does infant pause often during feeding?
   _____
4. Who initiates end of feeding? you ☐ infant ☐
5. How do you rate his sucking? poor ☐ weak ☐ average ☐ strong ☐
6. Is he burping easily? _____ What technique is used? _____
   When is he burped? _____
7. Is a pacifier used? _____ What kind? _____ How much usage? _____
8. Number of wet diapers per day _____ Are paper diapers used? _____
9. Number of stools per day _____ consistency _____ color _____
10. Infant is active ☐ average ☐ placid ☐
11. Night sleep pattern: time put to bed _____ Is this on a regular basis? _____
    List awake times _____
12. Is infant healthy? _____ Any problems since birth? _____ If so, what? _____
    _____
    Jaundice? _____ How high was the bilirubin level? _____
    Had any medications? _____ If so, what? _____
13. Ever had a urinalysis? _____ When? _____
    Any other test (especially those for slow weight gain)? _____
    If so, what? _____
    Where? _____

BIRTH HISTORY

1. Type of delivery: vaginal ☐ CS ☐ If CS, scheduled ☐ or emergency ☐?
2. Labor: yes ☐ no ☐ Length of time _____
3. Were medications given during labor or delivery? _____ If so, what? _____
   _____
4. Was it a difficult birth? _____ If so, describe problem _____
   _____
5. First time infant put to breast was _____ hr after birth. Did infant take to it easily? _____
6. Where was the birth? Home birth ☐ Hospital with rooming-in ☐ Hospital with infant only in the
   nursery ☐ Were you separated from infant for any length of time? _____ If so, why? _____
   _____
7. Any medications taken during pregnancy? _____ If so, what? _____
8. Any medications taken after birth? _____ If so, what? _____

FAMILY HISTORY

1. Have previous infants or relatives with failure to thrive? yes ☐ no ☐
2. Have history of metabolic or malabsorption disease? yes ☐ no ☐
3. Infant has cystic fibrosis? yes ☐ no ☐
4. Infant has milk allergy? yes ☐ no ☐
5. Other _____

Appendix E
Normal serum values for breastfed infants

Table E-1. Serum chemical values of normal breastfed infants*

Concentration/100 ml of serum	Age 28 days			Age 56 days			Age 84 days			Age 112 days		
	N	Mean	SD	N	Mean	SD	N	Mean	SD	N	Mean	SD
Males												
Total protein (g)	22	5.87	0.50	36	5.96	0.42	29	6.16	0.57	51	6.29	0.51
Albumin (g)	22	4.02	0.35	36	4.14	0.34	29	4.27	0.39	51	4.38	0.40
Globulins (g)												
alpha₁	22	0.14	0.03	36	0.17	0.03	29	0.18	0.03	51	0.17	0.04
alpha₂	22	0.53	0.10	36	0.60	0.11	29	0.74	0.14	51	0.81	0.19
beta	22	0.61	0.11	36	0.67	0.13	29	0.69	0.20	51	0.67	0.11
gamma	22	0.57	0.14	36	0.38	0.09	29	0.28	0.08	51	0.26	0.10
Cholesterol (mg)	21	139	31	32	153	34	25	133	32	47	145	26
Triglycerides (mg)	18	122	36	32	106	57	25	170	76	46	148	57
Urea nitrogen (mg)	43	8.5	3.2	49	6.6	2.1	47	7.0	2.7	51	7.3	4.2
Calcium (mg)	41	10.2	0.8	47	10.3	1.0	42	10.4	0.8	48	10.3	0.8
Phosphorus (mg)	43	6.6	0.7	49	6.4	0.7	47	6.2	0.5	49	6.2	0.7
Alkaline phosphatase†	31	22	6	40	21	7	35	21	8	44	18	7
Magnesium (mg)	40	2.0	0.2	47	2.1	0.2	45		0.2	50	2.2	0.2
Females												
Total protein (g)	18	6.04	0.40	27	5.86	0.44	21	6.21	0.57	42	6.31	0.62
Albumin (g)	18	4.07	0.27	27	4.03	0.35	21	4.29	0.37	42	4.36	0.42
Globulins (g)												
alpha₁	18	0.15	0.02	27	0.17	0.04	21	0.17	0.03	42	0.19	0.04
alpha₂	18	0.55	0.07	27	0.65	0.12	21	0.74	0.18	42	0.78	0.17
beta	18	0.70	0.18	27	0.63	0.11	21	0.71	0.13	42	0.67	0.16
gamma	18	0.57	0.10	27	0.38	0.10	21	0.30	0.06	42	0.31	0.10
Cholesterol (mg)	13	180	35	25	157	37	20	155	29	40	165	36
Triglycerides (mg)	9	157	43	24	112	53	18	195	56	38	170	52
Urea nitrogen (mg)	37	8.3	2.3	33	6.4	2.2	40	6.4	2.2	42	6.6	3.5
Calcium (mg)	37	10.3	0.8	33	10.3	0.8	40	10.3	0.8	42	10.7	0.7
Phosphorus (mg)	39	6.9	0.8	33	6.4	0.8	40	6.1	0.7	42	6.1	0.7
Alkaline phosphatase	31	19	5	28	17	5	32	17	5	36	17	5
Magnesium (mg)	39	2.0	0.4	32	2.0	0.2	40	2.1	0.2	41	2.1	0.3

From Fomon, S.J., et al.: Acta Paediatr. Scand. suppl. 202:1, 1970.
*Bold figures indicate that value is greater than the corresponding value for infants of the opposite sex and that the difference is statistically significant at the 95% level of confidence.
†King-Armstrong units.

Appendix F
Drugs in breast milk and the effect on the infant

The following list of drugs is provided to assist the clinician in making judgments about management for specific drugs in an individual mother and her infant. The clinician is referred to Chapter 11 for the discussion of interpretation of risks and benefits. It is also important to point out that the significance of a given blood level would vary with the pH and the binding capacity of the maternal plasma protein, which may differ for various ethnic and racial groups. Furthermore, it is not merely a matter of understanding the pharmacokinetics of a specific drug, but also of understanding the physiology of milk production and finally, most critically, understanding the absorption and excretion of the drug by the newborn, which changes with conceptual and chronologic age.

The drugs have been grouped by their major use to provide an opportunity to compare therapeutic choices and select the medication that is best for both mother and infant. The drugs have also been labeled I, II, III, or IV if they were rated by the Committee on Drugs of the Academy of Pediatrics who has published a list of drugs that transfer into human milk. When there is no number, the compound is not included in that list. The committee labeling indicates:

I. Drugs that are contraindicated during breastfeeding
II. Drugs that require temporary cessation of breastfeeding
III. Maternal medication usually compatible with breastfeeding
IV. Food and environmental agents: effect on breastfeeding

The classifications of the drugs listed are as follows:

Analgesics and anti-inflammatory drugs (nonnarcotic)
Anticoagulants
Anticonvulsants and sedatives
Antihistaminics
Anti-infective agents
Autonomic drugs
Cardiovascular drugs

Diagnostic materials and procedures
Diuretics
Environmental agents
Gastrointestinal cathartics
Heavy metals
Hormones and contraceptives
Narcotics
Psychotropic and mood-changing drugs
Recreational drugs
Stimulants
Thyroid and antithyroid medications
Miscellaneous

Table F-1. Relationship of drugs to breast milk and effect on infant (The Roman numerals preceding drugs refer to a list from the American Academy of Pediatrics)

Drug	Excreted in milk	Amount in milk after therapeutic dose	Effect on infant	Reference
Analgesics and anti-inflammatory drugs (nonnarcotic)				
III Acetaminophen (Datril, Tylenol)	Yes		Detoxified in liver. Avoid in immediate postpartum period, otherwise no problems with therapeutic dose.	Bleyer and Breckenridge, 1970; Anderson, 1977
III Aspirin	Yes	1-3 mg/100 ml* Metabolic acidosis in 16-day-old infant when mother took 10 grains for arthritis; caution in early infancy	Long history of experience shows complications rare. When mother requires high, continuing level of medication for arthritis, aspirin is drug of choice. Mother should increase vitamin C intake.	Clark and Wilson, 1980
Donnatal (phenobarbital, hyoscyamine sulfate, atropine sulfate, hyoscine hydrobromide)	Yes		Consider for its component parts. Can be given to children but can accumulate in neonate.	PDR, 1984, personal observations
III Flufenamic acid (Arlef)	Yes	0.50 μg/ml (mean)†	No apparent effect on infant when maternal dosage was 200 mg, three times a day. Infant able to excrete via urine.	Buchanan et al., 1969
III Indomethacin (Indocin)	Yes		Convulsions in breastfed neonate (case report). Used to close patent ductus arteriosus. Insufficient data as to effect on other vessels. May be nephrotoxic.	Eeg-Olofsson et al., 1978
III Mefenamid acid (Ponstel)	Yes	Trace amounts‡	No apparent effect on infant at therapeutic doses; infant able to excrete via urine.	Buchanan et al., 1968
III Naproxen (Naprosyn, synaxsyn, naprosine, naxen, proxen)	Yes	1% of maternal plasma; binds to plasma protein	Less toxic in adults than some other organic derivatives.	PDR, 1984; Roth, 1976
III Oxyphenbutazone (Tandearil)	Yes	In milk of 2 of 55 mothers, 10%-80% of maternal plasma level	No known effect	O'Brien, 1974; Knowles, 1974
Paracetamol (Alvedon)		500 mg dose; M/P 0.76; half-life 2.7 hr less than 0.1% dose	At most 3 μmol/100 ml of milk; no problem	Bitzen et al. 1981
Pentazocine (Talwin)	No		Withdrawal in neonatal period from ingestion during pregnancy.	Kopelman, 1975; O'Brien, 1974

*Plasma level was 1-5 mg/100 ml.
†Shown when mean maternal plasma level was 6.41 μg/ml. Mean level in infant's plasma was 0.12 μg/ml; in infant's urine, 0.08 μg/ml. (Maternal plasma level was fifty times that of infant.)
‡0.91 μg/ml mean maternal plasma level showed 0.21 μg/ml mean milk level. Mean infant plasma level was 0.08 μg/ml and mean urine level, 9.8 μg/ml.

Table F-1. Relationship of drugs to breast milk and effect on infant—cont'd

Drug	Excreted in milk	Amount in milk after therapeutic dose	Effect on infant	Reference
Percodan (oxycodone [derived from opiate thebaine] aspirin, phenacetin, caffeine)	Yes		Consider for its component parts. In neonatal period sleepiness and failure to feed, which increase maternal engorgement and neonatal weight loss, have been observed, probably due to oxycodone.	PDR, 1984; personal observations
III Phenylbutazone (Butazolidin)	Yes	0.63 mg/ml 90 min after 750 mg given IM	Very potent drug; risk to infant not well defined but considerable. Not given directly to children; may accumulate in infant.	Gaginella, 1978; Shore, 1970
III Propoxyphene (Darvon)	Yes	0.4% of maternal* dose	Only symptoms detectable would be failure to feed and drowsiness. On daily, around-the-clock dosage infant could consume 1 mg/day.	O'Brien, 1974; Arena, 1970; Ananth, 1978
Anticoagulants				
III Coumarin derivatives Dicumarol (bishydroxycoumarin) Warfarin sodium (Coumadin)	No	None measurable	Drug of choice if mother is to continue nursing; If surgery or trauma occurs, monitor prothrombin time; give vitamin K to infant.	Brambel and Hunter, 1950; Baty et al., 1976; deSweet and Lewis, 1977; L'Earme, 1977; McKenna, 1983
Ethyl biscoumacetate (Tromexan)	Yes	0–0.17 mg/100 ml†	Hemorrhage around umbilical stump and cephalhematoma reported. Prothrombin normal in infants with hemorrhage. Vitamin K has no effect. Contraindicated while nursing.	Illingworth, 1953; Knowles, 1974
Heparin	No		Heparin is not effective orally.	Goodman and Gilman, 1980
I Phenindione (Hedulin) (Dindevan)	Yes		Breast milk a major route of excretion. Reports of serious hemorrhage in infant. Prothrombin times prolonged in infant. Contraindicated while nursing.	Eckstein and Jack, 1970; Knowles, 1974
Anticonvulsants and sedatives‡				
Barbital (Veronal)	Yes	8–10 mg/L after 500 mg dose	May produce sedation in infant. In general, barbiturates pass into milk but do not sedate infant. Watch for symptoms.	O'Brien, 1974

Drug	In milk	Milk levels	Effect/Comments	Reference
III Carbamazepine (Tegretol)			...unkempt appearance. Infant serum levels 0.4 µg/L-1.8 µg/ml.	Sillanpää, 1975; Nau et al., 1982; Lacey, 1974
Chloral hydrate (Notec, Somnos)	Yes	Up to 1.5 mg/100 ml	No significant symptoms, can be given to infants directly.	
Phenytoin (Dilantin)	Yes	1.5-2.6 µg/ml after 300 mg/day dose	One case of hemolytic reaction reported. Other infants appear to tolerate the small doses. Therapeutic plasma level 10-20 µg/ml. Well eliminated. Infant levels 0-0.7 µmol/L. Less than 5% of dose.	Mirkin, 1971; Steen et al., 1982; Nau et al., 1982
Glutethimide (Doriden)	Yes	Mean concentration low after 250 and 500 mg doses; plasma and milk levels similar		Curry et al., 1971
III Magnesium sulfate (MgSO$_4$)	Yes	For 24 hr after infusion stopped; M/P is 2	Infant receives approximately 6.4 mg/100 ml; calcium levels remain the same; Similac Special Care formula has 8.3 mg/100 ml	Cruikshank, 1982
Mephenytoin (Mesantoin) (hydantoin homologue of mephobarbital)	Unknown		Detoxified in liver. No information.	
Pentobarbital (Nembutal)	Yes		Depends on liver for detoxification so may accumulate in first week of life until infant able to detoxify. No problem for older infant in usual doses.	
Phenobarbital (Luminal)	Yes	0.1-0.5 mg when plasma level 0.6-1.8 mg	Sleepiness and decreased sucking possible. On usual analeptic doses infants alert and feed well. On hypnotic doses infant depressed and hard to rouse. No specific data.	Tyson et al., II, 1938
III Phensuximide (Milontin)			No specific data.	
III Primidone (Mysoline)	Yes	M/P 0.72-0.86 half-life 113 hr	Causes drowsiness and decreased feeds. May cause bleeding due to hypoprothrombinemia. Need vitamin K. Avoid drug during lactation.	O'Brien, 1974, Nau, 1982
Sodium bromide (Bromo-Seltzer and across-the-counter sleeping aids)	Yes	Up to 6.6 mg/100 ml	Drowsy, decreased crying, rash, decreased feeding.	Tyson et al., III, 1938
Trimethadione (Tridione)			No specific data.	
III Valproic acid	Yes	Milk levels 3% of serum levels	Levels at birth may be higher than mother's. Low levels in milk and good clearance in neonate. Probably safe if maternal serum levels midrange. Poorly absorbed orally by neonate.	Nau et al., 1981

*Shown by animal experiments. Plasma/milk ratio (P/M) = ½.
†Shown when mean maternal plasma level was 6.41 µg/ml. Mean level in infant's plasma was 0.12 µg/ml; in infant's urine, 0.08 µg/ml. (Maternal plasma level was fifty times that of infant.)
‡Peaks in 6 hr.

Continued.

Table F-1. Relationship of drugs to breast milk and effect on infant—cont'd

Drug	Excreted in milk	Amount in milk after therapeutic dose	Effect on infant	Reference
Antihistaminics				
III Brompheniramine (Dimetane) III Diphenhydramine (Benadryl) Methdilazine (Tacaryl) III Tripelennamine (Pyribenzamine)	Yes	No specific data available All pass into milk	Drug is used in neonates. May cause sedation, decreased feeding, or may produce stimulation and tachycardia. Should avoid long-acting preparations, which may accumulate in infant. When combined with decongestants, may cause decrease in milk.	Arena, 1970; Rivera-Calimlim, 1977; Oseid, 1975
I Clemastine (Tavist)	Yes	M/P 2:1	Drowsiness, irritability.	Kok et al., 1982
Anti-infective agents				
III Amantadine (Symmetrel)	Yes	Not defined	Vomiting, urinary retention, rash. Contraindicated.	O'Brien, 1974
Amoxicillin	Yes	One gram dose up to 1.3 μg/ml; peak at 4+ hr	Passes into milk supply slowly; acidic and low fat solubility probably not a problem.	Kafetzis et al., 1981
Ampicillin (Polycillin, Amcill, Omnipen, Penbritin)	Yes	0.07 μg/ml	Sensitivity due to repeated exposure; diarrhea or secondary candidiasis.	O'Brien, 1974; Savage, 1977; Gaginella, 1978
Carbenicillin (Pyopen, Geopen)	Yes	0.265 μg/ml 1 hr after 1 g given	Levels not significant. Drug is given to neonate.	O'Brien, 1974
Cefadroxil (Duricef, Ultracef)	Yes	Higher levels than other cephalosporins; slow elimination; fat soluble	Would receive less than 2.4 mg/day when mother takes 1 g/day; levels are bactericidal for sensitive organisms.	Kafetzis et al., 1981
III Cefazolin (Ancef, Kefzol)	Yes	1.5 μg/ml or 0.075% dose given	Probably not significant	Yoshioka et al., 1979
Ceftazidime	Yes	2 g every 8 hr × 5 days; peak 1 hr 5.2 μg/ml through 3.8 μg/ml 7½ hr	Levels higher than most cephalosporins; 80% of dose excreted by newborn in 8 hr.	Blanco et al., 1983
Ceftriazone (Claforan)	Yes	Minimal; level 3%-4% of maternal serum; half-life 12-17 hr	Infant clears drug well from birth.	Kafetzis et al., 1983
Cephalexin (Keflex) Cephalothin (Keflin)	Yes Yes	0.2-0.5 μg/ml/1 g dose	μ/P ratio ≤ 50. Peak levels at 2-3 hr.	Kafetzis et al., 1981
III Chloramphenicol (Chloromycetin)	Yes	Half blood level: 2.5 mg/100 ml 14 mg after single 500 mg dose	Grey syndrome. Infant does not excrete drug well and small amounts may accumulate. Contraindicated. May be tolerated in older infant with mature gly-...	Vorherr, 1974, 1976; Gaginella, 1978; Havelka et al., 1968; Plomb et al., 1983

III Chloroquine (Aralen)	Yes	2.7 mg in 2 days*	Can be used to *treat* child under 6 mo of age who is wholly breastfed.	Clyde and Shute, 1956
Clindamycin (Cleocin)	Yes	Wide differences in milk level among individuals; one tenth to three times plasma levels	Caution expressed	Steen and Rane, 1982
Colistin (Colymycin)	Yes	0.05-0.09 mg/100 ml	Not absorbed orally.	Vorherr, 1974
Demeclocycline (Declomycin)	Yes	0.2-0.3 mg/500 ml	Not significant in therapeutic doses. Can be given to infants.	O'Brien, 1974
Erythromycin (Ilosone, E-Mycin, Erythrocin)	Yes	0.05-0.1 mg/100 ml; 3.6-6.2 µg/ml	Higher concentrations have been reported in milk than in plasma. Should not be given under 1 mo of age because of risk of jaundice. Dose in milk higher when given IV to mother.	Gaginella, 1978; O'Brien, 1974
Gentamicin	Unknown		Not absorbed from gastrointestinal tract, may change gut flora. Drug is given to newborns directly.	Remington and Klein, 1976
III Isoniazid (Nydrazid)	Yes	0.6-1.2 mg/100 ml	Infant at risk for toxicity, but need for breast milk may outweigh risk.	Knowles, 1965; Jelliffe, 1978
Kanamycin (Kantrex)	Yes	18.4 µg/ml after 1 g given IM	Infant absorbs little from gastrointestinal tract. Infants can be given drug.	Anderson, 1977
Lincomycin (Lincocin)	Yes	0.5-2.4 mg/100 ml	Not significant in therapeutic doses to affect child.	O'Brien, 1974;
Mandelic acid	Yes	0.3 g/24 hr after dose of 12 g/day	Not significant in therapeutic doses to affect child.	O'Brien, 1974
Methacycline (Rondomycin)	Yes	½ plasma level; 50-260 µg/100 ml	Same precautions as with tetracycline.	O'Brien, 1974; Voherr
Methenamine (Hexamine)	Yes		Not significant in therapeutic doses to affect child.	O'Brien, 1974
II Metronidazole (Flagyl)	Yes	Level comparable to serum†	Caution should be exercised due to its high milk concentrations. Contraindicated when infant under 6 mo, may cause neurologic disorders and blood dyscrasia.	Gray, 1961; Gaginella, 1978; Hervada, 1978
		Single 2 g dose levels peak at 4 hr; clear in 12-24 hr	Withhold breastfeeding 12-24 hr and resume	Erickson et al., 1981; Heisterberg and Branebjerg, 1983
III Nalidixic acid (Neggram)	Yes	0.4 mg/100 ml	Not significant in therapeutic doses beyond neonatal period. Hemolytic anemia in an infant attributed to nalidixic acid in G6PD deficiency or when mother has renal failure.	Catz and Giacoia, 1972; Vorherr, 1976

*When plasma 13.0 µmol/L in milk.
†Shown when mean maternal plasma level was 6.41 µg/ml. Mean level in infant's plasma was 0.12 µg/ml; in infant's urine, 0.08 µg/ml. (Maternal plasma level was fifty times that of infant.)

Continued.

Table F-1.   Relationship of drugs to breast milk and effect on infant—cont'd

Drug	Excreted in milk	Amount in milk after therapeutic dose	Effect on infant	Reference
III Nitrofurantoin (Furadantin)	Yes	Undetectable to 0.5 μg/ml	Not significant in therapeutic doses to affect child except in G6PD deficiency.	Varsano et al., 1973
Novobiocin (Albamycin, cathomycin)	Yes	0.36-0.54 mg/100 ml	Infant can be given drug directly.	Texeira and Scott, 1958
Nystatin (Mycostatin)	No	Not absorbed orally	Can be given to infant directly.	Knowles, 1974
Oxacillin (Prostaphlin)	No			O'Brien, 1974
Para-aminosalicylic acid	No	24-74 μg/100 ml	Animal study suggests it be avoided.	O'Brien, 1974
Penethamate (Leocillin)	No	10-12 units/100 ml	Clinical need should supersede possible	
Penicillin G, benzathine (Bicillin)	Yes		allergic responses.	
Penicillin G, potassium	Yes	Up to 6 units/100 ml; 1.2-3.6 μg/100 ml	Infant can be given penicillin directly. Parents should be told to inform physician that infant has been exposed to penicillin because of potential sensitivity.	Vorherr, 1976; Gaginella, 1978
Piperacillin	Yes	Trace	May alter intestinal flora. Concentrations below any therapeutic or toxic level.	Baier, 1983
Povidone-iodine (Betadine)	Yes	8-25 times higher in milk than serum	Absorbed from vaginal mucosa	Postellow and Aronow (1982)
III Pyrimethamine (antimalarial) (Daraprim, Fansidar)	Yes	0.3 mg/100 ml (3% of dose) Peaks at 6 hr at 3.3 μg/ml; lasts 48 hr after single dose of 25-75 mg	Significant in therapeutic doses when infant under 6 mo and entirely breastfed. Does eliminate parasites in breastfed infant	Clyde and Shute, 1956 Briggs (1983)
III Quinine sulfate	Yes	0-0.1 mg/100 ml after maternal dose of 300-600 mg	In therapeutic doses, no affect to child except rare thrombocytopenia.	Terwilliger and Hatcher, 1939; *Medical Letter,* 1974
III Rifampin (Rimactane)	Yes	1-3 μg/ml	No effects reported when used as antituberculosis drug	Vorherr (1974); Briggs et al. (1983)
Sodium fusidate	Yes	0.02 μg/ml	Not significant in therapeutic doses to affect child.	O'Brien, 1974
Streptomycin	Yes	Present for long periods in slight amounts given as dihydrostreptomycin	Not to be given more than 2 wk. Ototoxic and nephrotoxic with long use. Is given to infants directly.	Knowles, 1965; Takyi, 1970
Sulfanilamide	Yes	9 mg/100 ml after dose of 2-4 g daily	Not significant in therapeutic doses; may cause a rash or hemolytic anemia. Should be avoided for first month postpartum.	Lein et al., 1974; Knowles, 1965; O'Brien, 1974

III Sulfapyridine	Yes	3-13 mg/100 ml after dose of 3 g daily	To be avoided; has caused skin rash.	Lein et al., 1974; Knowles, 1965; O'Brien, 1974
III Sulfathiazole	Yes	0.5 mg/100 ml after dose of 3 g/day	Not significant in therapeutic doses to affect child after 1 mo of age.	Lein et al., 1974; Knowles, 1965; O'Brien, 1974
III Sulfisoxazole (Gantrisin)	Yes	Concentration similar to plasma level < 1% maternal dose	To be avoided during first month postpartum; because of bilirubin deficiency displacement. Contraindicated in G6PD.	Lein et al., 1974; O'Brien, 1974; Kaufman, 1980
III Tetracycline HCl (Achromycin, Panmycin, Sumycin)	Yes	0.5-2.6 µg/ml after dose of 500 mg four times a day	Not enough to treat an infection in an infant. May cause discoloration of the teeth in the infant; the antibiotic, however, may be largely bound to the milk calcium. Do not give over 10 days or repeatedly.	Posner et al., 1955-1956; Shidlovsky et al., 1957-1958
Thiamphenicol	Yes	3.7 µg/ml after 500 mg dose or 17 mg total dose to infant; levels from multiple doses 2.9 µg/ml for 48 hr	Accumulates in newborn; jaundice and grey syndrome.	Plomb et al., 1983
Tobramycin	Yes	Trace to 0.52 µg/ml; maternal dose 80 mg IM; peak 4 hr	Well tolerated by neonate when given 2.5 mg/kg; oral absorption poor.	Briggs et al., 1983
III Trimethoprim (Bactrim, Septra, Trimpex)	Yes	Milk concentration 1.2-2.4 µg/ml; peak 2-3 hr; M/P 1.25	Infants at risk for kernicterus should not be exposed; if child could receive it, therapeutically OK.	PDR, 1984; Briggs et al., 1983;
Autonomic drugs				
Atropine sulfate‖	Yes	0.1 mg/100 ml	Hyperthermia, atropine toxicity, infants especially sensitive; also inhibits lactation. Infant dose 0.01 mg/kg	O'Brien, 1974; Rivera-Calimlim, 1977
III Carisprodol (Soma, Rela)	Yes	Two to four times maternal plasma	Blocks interneuronal activity in descending reticular formation and spinal cord; drowsiness, hypotonia, poor feed.	O'Brien, 1974; PDR, 1984
I Ergot (Cafergot)	Yes	Unknown	90% of infants had symptoms of ergotism. Vomiting and diarrhea to weak pulse and unstable blood pressure. Short-term therapy for migraine should not exceed 6 mg. Cafergot also contains caffeine, 100 mg.	Riviera-Calimlim, 1977; O'Brien, 1974; Knowles, 1965

Continued.

Table F-1. Relationship of drugs to breast milk and effect on infant—cont'd

Drug	Excreted in milk	Amount in milk after therapeutic dose	Effect on infant	Reference
Mepenzolate bromide (Cantil)	No		Postganglionic parasympathetic inhibitor used to diminish gastric acidity and decrease spasm of colon. Oral absorption low.	O'Brien, 1974; *PDR*, 1984
III Methocarbamol (Robaxin)	Yes	Minimal	Too little in milk to produce effect. No known harm to infant.	O'Brien, 1974
Neostigmine	No			McNall and Jafarnia, 1965
Propantheline bromide (Pro-Banthine)	No	Uncontrolled data indicate no measurable levels	Drug rapidly metabolized in maternal system to inactive metabolite. Mother should avoid long-acting preparations, however.	O'Brien, 1974; Takyi, 1970.
Scopolamine (hyoscine)	Yes		Usually given as single dose and of no problem to neonate. No data on repeated doses.	Arena, 1970
Terbutaline	Yes	3.5 ng/ml average concentration in milk	Infant intake up to 0.7% maternal dose; infant receives similar amounts regardless of dosing; not detectable in infant plasma.	Boreus et al., 1982; Lönnerholm and Lindström, 1982
Cardiovascular drugs				
III Atenolol (Tenormin) beta-receptor blocking agent (cardioselective)	Yes	Higher in milk; 1.5-6.5 times higher than maternal serum; 50 mg dose b.i.d.; maximum level, 6.35 μmol/L	Food decreases absorption of atenolol in adult; infant serum is one tenth of mother's serum; no signs of beta-blocker effect in infants.	Liedholm et al., 1981
III Captopril (Capoten)	Yes	100 mg t.i.d dose; 4.7 ng/ml; peak level at 4 hr when serum peaks at 750 ng/ml 1.1 hr	Maximum dose to infant 0.002% of maternal dose; no effects seen; probably safest of group.	Devlin and Fleiss 1981

Diazoxide (Hyperstat)			Arteriolar dilators and antihypertensive, only given IV, not active orally. No data available.	PDR, 1984
Dibenzyline*				
III Digoxin	Yes	0.61-0.96 ng/ml†	Digoxin 20% bound to protein; infant receives <1/100 of dose. If mother at toxic level of 5 ng/ml, milk would have 4.4 ng/ml and infant would receive only 1/20 daily dose. Cord blood level important in neonatal period	Loughnan, 1978; Levy et al., 1977 Finely et al., 1979. Chan et al., 1978.
III Guanethidine (Ismelin)‡	Yes		Not significant in therapeutic doses to affect child.	O'Brien, 1974; Takyi, 1976
Hydralazine (Apresoline)	Yes	>750 mg/L	Jaundice, thrombocytopenia, electrolyte disturbances possible.	Uedholm et al., 1982
III Methyldopa (Aldomet)‡	Yes		Galactorrhea. No specific data except as affects mother's milk production. Maximum dose to infant estimated to be 0.05 mg per feed.	Takyi, 1970; Redmond, 1976
III Metoprolol (Lopressor, Seloken) Beta-receptor blocking agent (cardioselective)	Yes	Higher in milk, 2.6-3.7 times higher 50 mg b.i.d.; peak level 6.35 μmol/L at 6 hr after dose; some subjects had zero		
Mexiletine (antidysrhythmic)	Yes	M/P varied 0.78-2; mean 1.45; peak level 960 ng/ml	Possible dose to infant 1.25 mg/day; therapeutic dose is 8-10 mg/kg.	Lewis et al., 1981; Timmis et al., 1980
III Nadolol (Corgard) Beta-adrenergic receptor blocker	Yes	80 mg daily dose; steady state in 3 days in milk; 360 μg/ml mean level; 4.6 times higher than serum	Infant receives 2%-7% of maternal dose; caution.	Devlin et al., 1981
Propranolol (Inderal)	Yes	40 ng/ml of maternal plasma	Insignificant amount. Infants reported had no symptoms noted. Should watch for hypoglycemia and/or "beta-blocking effects."	Anderson and Salter, 1976
		Peak 2-3 hr after dose; levels 40%-60% less than plasma single of multiple dose	Cord blood level needs to be considered regarding accumulation at 40 mg q.i.d. maximum to infant 21 μg/24 hr or less than 0.1% maternal dose.	Baver et al., 1983; Smith et al., 1983; Lewis et al., 1981; Habib and McCarthy, 1977

*α blocking agent.
†Peak level occurs 4-6 hr after dose given. Maternal plasma level was higher, M/P = 0.9 and 0.8; infant's plasma level was 0.
‡Adrenergic blocking agent.

Continued.

Table F-1. Relationship of drugs to breast milk and effect on infant—cont'd

Drug	Excreted in milk	Amount in milk after therapeutic dose	Effect on infant	Reference
III Quinidine	Yes	6-8 mg/L	Arrhythmia may occur. May accumulate	Oseid, 1975; Hill and Malkasian, 1979
III Reserpine (Serpasil)*	Yes	Similar to serum of mother	May produce galactorrhea, lethargy, diarrhea, or nasal stuffiness.	O'Brien, 1974; *Medical Letter*, 1974
Diagnostic materials and procedures				
Barium	No		Not absorbed.	
III Iopanoic acid (Telepaque)	Yes		Not sufficient to produce problem in infant on single dose. Does contain iodine radical.	O'Brien, 1974
Radioactive compounds				
II Radioactive sodium	Yes	0.5-1.3% of dose/L†	Diminished after 24 hr; discontinue nursing 24-96 hr.	Knowles, 1974
II [⁶⁷Ga] citrate	Yes		Discontinue nursing until ^{67}Ga has cleared, usually 24 hr. May have activity 2 wk.	O'Brien, 1974
II ^{125}I, ^{131}I	Yes	M/P = 0.13 µCi/0.002 µCi‡	^{131}I content in milk proportional to amount of milk. Most excreted in 24 hr. Discontinue nursing for 48 hr or check milk prior to resuming feeding if under 48 hr. Some studies and doses last up to 12 days.	Weaver et al., 1960
^{90}Sr	Yes	M/P = ¹⁄₁₀	Less than in cow's milk. Bottle infant doubles stores in 1 mo.	Widdowson et al., 1960
II ^{99m}Tc	Yes		Reported to clear in 6-22 hr. Discontinue breastfeeding 24 hr. ^{99m}Tc preferentially picked up by breast tissue. Tc macro aggregates found up to 3 days.	O'Connell and Sutton, 1976; Wyburn, 1973; Pulard et al., 1982
Tuberculin test	No		Tuberculin-sensitive mothers can adoptively immunize their infants through breast milk and that immunity may last several years.	Mohr, 1973
X rays	No		No effect.	
Diuretics				
Acetazolamine (Diamox)	Probable	No specific data available but probably similar to sulfonamide	Acts as enzyme inhibitor on carbonic anhydrase nonbacteriostatic sulfonamide. Observe only for dehydration and electrolyte loss by monitoring urine and tumor	Rothermel and Faber, 1975

Drug	In milk	Concentration in milk	Effect	Reference
III Bendroflumazide (Neo-Nuclex)	?		5 mg b.i.d. × 5 days; suppressed lactation in women who did not wish to breastfeed.	Heuly, 1961.
III Chlorthalidone (Hygroton)	Yes	3%-4% of maternal blood levels	Maternal dose 50 mg/day; infant receives 180 ng; long half-life in adults, 60 hr.	Mulley et al., 1978.
III Chlorthiazide	Yes	500 mg single dose less than 1000 ng/ml; less than 0.1 mg/100 ml milk	Less than 1 mg to baby daily; therapeutic dose in neonates 20 mg/kg/day; displaces bilirubin from albumin significantly; requires higher dose in mother.	Wennberg et al., 1977; Werthmann and Krees, 1972
Ethacrynic acid	?	No data	Potent bilirubin-binding replacing; however, safe to give directly to neonate in dose of 1 mg/kg.	Wenneberg et al., 1977
Furosemide (sullamoylanthranilic acid sulfonamide) (Lasix)	?	Probably little	Drug is given to children under medical management. Slow plasma clearance in premature infant; displaces bilirubin from albumin.	Takyi, 1970; O'Brien, 1974 Wennberg et al., 1977; Shankaran and Poland, 1977
Hydrochlorothiazide	Yes	50 mg/day maternal dose; peaked 4 hr after dose of 100 ng/ml; mean level 80 ng/ml	Daily dose to infant 0.05 mg; level in infant undetectable (less than 20 ng/ml).	Miller et al., 1982
Mercurial diuretics (Dicurin, Thiomerin)	Yes		In addition to diuretic effect, there is risk of mercury deposition. However, drug not absorbed orally.	O'Brien, 1974
III Spironolactone (Aldactone)	Yes	Canrenone, a metabolite, appears	Acts as antagonist of aldosterone; causes sodium excretion and potassium retention. The metabolite apparently has some activity.	
III Thiazides (Diuril, Enduron, Esidrix, Hydrodiuril, Oretic, Thiuretic tablets)	Yes	>0.1 mg/100 ml§	Risk of dehydration and electrolyte imbalance, especially sodium loss, which would require monitoring. Watching weight and wet diapers and taking an occasional specific gravity reading of the urine and serum sodium would assure status of infant. Risk, however, is extremely low. May suppress lactation due to dehydration in mother.	Werthmann and Krees, 1972; Catz and Giacoia, 1972

*Adrenergic blocking agents.
†Peak in 2 hr; detectable for 96 hr.
‡27% of dose in 48 hr.
§Linear relationship between plasma and milk. In 1 L of milk at 0.1 mg/100 ml there would be 1 mg/day. Infant dose is 20 mg/kg/day.

Continued.

Table F-1. Relationship of drugs to breast milk and effect on infant—cont'd

Drug	Excreted in milk	Amount in milk after therapeutic dose	Effect on infant	Reference
Environmental agents				
Aldrin	Yes	Varies by location	Not a reason to wean from breast. No need to test milk unless inordinate exposure.	Bakken and Seip, 1976
Chromium	Yes	Approximately 0.4 µg/L	Toxicant 5-15 µg/day.	Wolff, 1983
Cadmium	Yes	3-35 µg/L	Has been found in milk of mothers who smoke.	Wolff, 1983; Buchet et al., 1978
Benzene hexachloride (BHC)	Yes	Varies by location	Not a reason to wean from breast. No need to test milk unless inordinate exposure.	Bakken and Seip, 1976
Carbon disulfide (volatile solvent)	Yes	22-306 µg/L after commercial exposure	Neurovascular and cardiovascular toxin; infant's urine contained 16-71 µg/L; also found on hands and clothing of mothers.	Cai and Bao, 1981
Chlordane	Yes	Metabolizes to oxychlordane		Savage et al., 1981
IV Dichlorodiphenyltrichloroethane (DDT or DDE)	Yes	Varies by location (gen'l public 70-170 µg/L) M/P = 6-7	Not a reason to wean from breast. No need to test milk unless inordinate exposure.	Wurster, 1970; Rogan et al., 1980; Wolff, 1983
IV Dieldrin	Yes	Varies by location (gen'l population 2-7 µg/L) M/P = 6	Also found in permanently mothproofed garments. Avoid these. Not a reason to wean.	Bakken and Seip, 1976; Savage et al., 1981; Wolff, 1983
IV Hexachlorobenzene (HCB)	Yes	Varies by location	Not a reason to wean from breast. No need to test milk unless inordinate exposure.	Bakken and Seip, 1976
IV Heptachlorepoxide	Yes	Varies by location (gen'l pop 2-9 µg/L)	Not a reason to wean from breast. No need to test milk unless inordinate exposure. Found in 63% samples.	Bakken and Seip, 1976; Savage et al., 1981; Wolff, 1983
Malathion	?	Not detected less than 5 ppb in milk of mothers living where sprayed for 3 mo	Allowable level in cow's milk is 500 ppb.	Lönnerdal and Asquith, 1982
Methyl mercury	Yes	500-1000 ng/ml* M/P = 0.9	Infant blood level 600 ng/ml in heavy exposure. Only in excessive exposure is testing and/or weaning necessary.	Amin-Zaki et al., 1976; Wolff, 1983
Mirex	?	Not found in measurable amounts		Savage et al., 1981

Substance	In milk	Amount	Effect	Reference
Nitrate	Yes	0.023 mM after evening meal	Nitrate is concentrated in saliva but not in milk; high levels cause methemoglobin.	Green et al., 1982
Oxychlordane	Yes	Found in 74% of samples of the general population: approximately 3 μg/L	Toxicant 5 μg/L.	Wolff, 1983
IV Polybrominated biphenyl (PBB)	Yes	Varies by location M/P = 3	If mother at high risk from the environment or the diet, milk sample should be measured. If level in milk is high, then breastfeeding should be discontinued. Those at risk are (1) workers who handle PBB/PCB, (2) individuals who eat game fish from contaminated waters. Crash diets mobilize fats and should be avoided especially if PBB or PCB present.	AAP Committee on Environmental Hazards, 1978 Rogan et al., 1980, 1983; Wickizer and Brillant, 1981
IV Polychlorinated biphenyl (PCB)	Yes	Varies by location M/P = 4-10		
^{90}Sr ^{89}Sr (strontium)	Yes	1/10 of that in maternal diet	Cow's milk has six times as much as human milk. Cow's milk-fed infant doubles amount in body in 1 mo.	Staub and Murthy, 1965; Widdowson et al., 1960
Tetrachloroethylene (PCE) (cleaning solvent)	Yes	Depends on exposure; detectable for 2 wk; 1 mg/100 ml when blood was 0.3 mg/100 ml	1 hr after exposure at cleaning plant mother had 10 ppm in milk; infant developed severe jaundice.	Wolff, 1983; Bagnell and Ellenberger, 1977
Gastrointestinal carthartics				
Aloin	Yes	Low	Occasionally gave symptoms, caused colic and diarrhea in infant.	Tyson, I, 1937
Anthraquinone laxatives such as dihydroxyanthraquinone (Dorbane and Dorbantyl)	Yes	High	Caused colic and diarrhea in infant.	Hervada et al., 1978
Calomel	No	None	None	Tyson, I, 1937
Cascara	Yes	Low	Caused colic and diarrhea in infant.	Hervada et al., 1978
Milk of magnesia	No	None	No effect.	Hervada et al., 1978
Mineral oil	No	None	No effect.	Tyson, I, 1937
Phenolphthalein	Unknown	Unknown†	Reported to cause symptoms in some.	Tyson, I, 1937
Rhubarb	Unknown	None	None in syrup form. Fresh rhubarb may give symptoms of colic and diarrhea.	Tyson, I, 1937
Saline cathartics	No	None	No effect.	Hervada et al., 1978
Senna	No	None	None.	Tyson, I, 1937, Baldwin 1963
Stool softeners and bulk-forming laxatives	No	None	No effect.	Hervada et al., 1978
Suppositories (for constipation)	No	None	Not absorbed.	Shore, 1970

*M/P = 8.6% in heavy exposure.
†Reports differ.

Continued.

Table F-1. Relationship of drugs to breast milk and effect on infant—cont'd

Drug	Excreted in milk	Amount in milk after therapeutic dose	Effect on infant	Reference
Heavy metals				
Arsenic	Yes	Can be measured for given patient	Can accumulate. Check infant's blood level if there is reason to suspect exposure.	Arena, 1970
IV Bromide	Yes		Weakness, bromide rash.	Manguren, 1982
Copper	Yes			Arena, 1970
Fluorine	Yes			
I Gold thiomalate (Myocrisin)	Yes	0.022 µg/ml when mother given 50 mg/wk	Monitor for excessive dose. No proteinuria or aminoaciduria observed.	Bell and Dale, 1976
Iron	Yes			Dillon et al., 1974
Lead	Yes	26-29 µg/L; M/P = 1	Nursing contraindicated if maternal serum 40 µg; conflicting reports, breast milk not always cause of lead poisoning in breastfed infant.	Perkins and Oski, 1976; Wolff, 1983
Magnesium	Yes		Not sufficient to be toxic.	Arena, 1970
IV Mercury	Yes		Hazardous to infant.	O'Brien, 1974
Hormones and contraceptives				
Carbimazole (neo-mercazole)	Yes		Antithyroid effect may cause goiter.	O'Brien, 1974
III Chlorotrianisene (Tace)	Yes		Has estrogenic effect although does not change consistency of milk. May have feminizing effect on infant.	
Contraceptives (oral) III Ethinyl estradiol Mestranol 19-Nortestosterone Norethindrone (Norlutin) III Norethynodrel (Enovid)	Yes	1.1% of dose	May diminish milk supply. May decrease vitamins, protein, and fat in milk. Velázquez took norethindrone. Most significant concern is long-range impact of hormone on young infant, which is not certain. Reports of feminization of infant.	Briggs and Briggs, 1974; Barsivala and Virkar, 1973; Ibrahim and El-Tawil, 1968; Kora, 1969; Miller and Hughes, 1970; Velázquez et al., 1976; Ramadan et al., 1972; Nilsson et al., 1977
Corticotropin	Yes		Destroyed in gastrointestinal tract of infant. No effect.	Catz and Giacoia, 1972
Cortisone	Yes		Animal studies show 50% lower weight than controls and retarded sexual development and exophthalmos.	Catz and Giacoia, 1972

Drug	Passes to milk	Amount in milk	Effect on infant	References
Dihydrotachysterol (Hytakerol)	Yes		May cause hypercalcemia; need monitoring of infant serum and urine calcium.	Catz and Giacoia, 1972
Epinephrine (Adrenalin)	Yes		Destroyed in GI tract of infant.	Catz and Giacoia, 1972
III Estrogen	Yes	0.17 µg/100 ml after 1 g	Risks as with oral contraceptives.	Knowles, 1974
Fluoxymesterone (Halotestin, Ora-Testryl, Ultandren)	Yes		Suppresses lactation; masculinizing.	O'Brien, 1974
Insulin	Unknown		Destroyed in gastrointestinal tract.	Catz and Giacoia, 1972
Liothyronine (Cytomel)	No		Synthetic form of natural thyroid.	O'Brien, 1974
III Medroxyprogesterone acetate (Provera)	No			O'Brien, 1974
Phenformin HCl	Yes	Minimal	Not sufficient to cause symptoms in infant. Does not cause hypoglycemia in normal infants. No case reports available.	O'Brien, 1974
III Prednisone	Yes	0.07-0.23% dose/L after 5 mg dose*	Minimal amount not likely to cause effect on infant in short course.	Katz and Duncan, 1975; McKenzie et al., 1975
Pregnanediol	Yes		Unknown risk as with other female hormones over a long period of time.	
Tolbutamide (Orinase)	Yes		Not recommended in the childbearing years.	
Vasopressin (D DAVP)		Very little	Does not parallel serum levels. Less than 1 ng/L.	Burrow et al., 1981
Narcotics				
III Codeine		0 to trace after 32 mg every 4 hr (6 doses)	No effect in therapeutic level and transient usage. Can accumulate. Individual variation. Watch for neonatal depression.	Knowles, 1965; Oseid, 1975; Kwit and Hatcher, 1935
III Meperidine (Demerol)	Yes	Concentration in milk 1.5-2.4 times higher than plasma; at same time peak 1 hr; 60 mg dose >0.1 mg/100 ml†	Trace amounts may accumulate if drug taken around the clock when infant is neonate because infant metabolizes it slowly. Watch for drowsiness and poor feeding.	Talbott, 1969 O'Brien, 1974; Oseid, 1975
III Methadone	Yes	0.03 µg/ml or 0.023-0.028 mg/day‡	When dosage not excessive, infant can be breastfed if monitored for evidence of depression and failure to thrive.	Blinick et al., 1975 and 1976; Kreek et al., 1974

*0.16 µg/ml after 10 mg dose; 2.67 µg/ml after 2 hr.
†Plasma 0.07-0.1 mg/100ml.
‡Mother received 50 mg/day; MP = 0.83. Peak level 4 hr after oral dose. Results obscured if addict also taking the herbal root golden seal.

Continued.

Table F-1. Relationship of drugs to breast milk and effect on infant—cont'd

Drug	Excreted in milk	Amount in milk after therapeutic dose	Effect on infant	Reference
III Morphine	Yes	Trace amount	Single doses have minimal effect. Potential for accumulation. May be addicting to neonate. No longer considered appropriate means of weaning infant of an addict.	Arena, 1970; O'Brien, 1974; Vorherr, 1974, 1976
Psychotropic and mood-changing drugs				
III Amphetamine	Yes		Has caused stimulation in infants with jitteriness, irritability, sleeplessness. Long-acting preparations cumulative.	Arena, 1970; Knowles, 1965, 1974; Vorherr, 1974
Benzodiazepines* Chlordiazepoxide HCl (Librium)	Yes		Not sufficient to affect infant first week when glucuronyl system needed for detoxification. May accumulate. Older infant, no apparent problem.	Catz and Giacoia, 1972; Takyi, 1970; O'Brien, 1974
III Diazepam (Valium)	Yes	90 µg/L†	Detoxified in glucuronyl system. In first weeks of life may contribute to jaundice. Metabolite active. Effect on infant: hypoventilation, drowsiness, lethargy, and weight loss. Single doses over 10 mg contraindicated during nursing. Accumulation in infant possible.	Erkkola and Kanto, 1972; Brandt, 1976; Patrick et al., 1972; Cole and Hailey, 1970; Catz, 1973
III Pineazepam	Yes	5-11.2 ng of metabolite/ml; >1.0 ng of pineazepam/ml‡	No data, probably similar to diazepam.	Pacifici and Placidi, 1977
Haloperidol (Haldol)	Yes	Unknown	A butyrophenone antidepressant; animal studies in nurslings show behavior abnormalities.	Lundberg, 1972
III Lithium carbonate (Eskalith, Lithane, Lithonate)	Yes	⅓-½ maternal plasma levels§	Measurable lithium in infant's serum. Infant kidney can clear lithium; however, lithium inhibits adenosine 3',5'-cyclic monophosphate, significant to brain growth. Also affects amine metabolism. Real effects not measurable immediately. Report of cyanosis and poor muscle tone and ECG changes in nursing infant.	Schou and Amdisen, 1973; Sykes et al., 1976; Tupin and Hopkin, 1978; O'Brien, 1974; Tunnessen and Hertz, 1972

Drug	Inhibits lactation (Yes)	Level in milk	Comments	References
Monoamine oxidase (MAO) inhibitors (Eutonyl, Nardil)			Inhibits lactation.	Dickey and Stone, 1975
III Meprobamate (Miltown, Equanil)	Yes	2-4 times maternal plasma level	If therapy continued, infant should be followed closely.	O'Brien, 1974; Ananth, 1978
Nicotine	Yes	Range less than 20-512 ppb	Reported slow initiation of suck and decreased sucking pressure by infant; decreased prolactin and oxytocin response to suckling; fretful and unsettled (carboxyhemoglobin also found in mother and infant).	Martin et al., 1978; Andersen et al., 1982; Bisdon, 1937; Ferguson et al., 1976; Yaffe and Waletsky, 1976
Penfluridol||	Yes	Unknown	Animal studies show learning abnormalities in sucklings. This is a potent long-acting oral neuroleptic drug.	Janssen et al., 1970; Athlenius et al., 1973
Phenothiazines				
III Chlorpromazine (Thorazine)	Yes	1/3 plasma level¶	Can be safely nursed; minimum in milk. Increases maternal prolactin. No symptoms in infants reported; 5 yr follow-up showed infants normal.	Ananth, 1978; Blacker et al., 1962; Milkovich and Van den Berg, 1976; Vorherr, 1974
III Mesoridazine (Serentil)	Yes	Minimal	Probably no effect.	O'Brien, 1974
III Piperacetazine (Quide)	Yes	Minimal		O'Brien, 1974
III Thioridazine (Mellaril)	Yes	No information	Thioridoxine is less potent in general than other phenothiazines. Probably quite safe.	O'Brien, 1974
Trifluoperazine (Stelazine)	Yes	Minimal	Apparently no accumulation. No infants that have been followed showed symptoms. Watch for depression or failure to feed. Increases maternal prolactin secretion.	O'Brien, 1974
Tricyclic antidepressants				
Amitriptyline HCl (Elavil)	Yes	Minimal amounts		Ananth, 1978; Ayd, 1973; Vorherr, 1974
Desipramine HCl	Yes	Minimal amounts		
(Norpramin, Pertofrane) Imipramine HCl (Tofranil)	Yes	0.1 mg/100 ml**		

*Alcohol enhances effect of this group.
†10 mg or less yields 45 ng of diazepam/ml and 85 ng of metabolite/ml. P/M ratio is variable. Mean P/M ratio of diazepam is 6.14; of metabolite is 3.64. Effect lasts about 4 days.
‡Both drug and active metabolite appear for about 4 days after dose, 5-11.2 ng/ml metabolite, less than 1.0 ng/ml pinezepam.
§0.030 mmol/L in infant's serum, 0.57 mmol/L in infant's urine. Milk level was half of maternal serum level in case report by Sykes et al.
||Neuroleptic drug.
¶If dose <200 mg, milk contains bare trace. Dose of 1200 mg showed trace.
**Plasma level 0.2-1.3 mg/100ml.

Continued.

Table F-1. Relationship of drugs to breast milk and effect on infant—cont'd

Drug	Excreted in milk	Amount in milk after therapeutic dose	Effect on infant	Reference
Recreational drugs				
III Alcohol	Yes	Similar to plasma level	Ordinarily no problem and can be therapeutic in moderation. Infants are more susceptible to effects. Chronic drinking reported to cause obesity in one infant. Ethanol in doses of 1-2 g/kg to the mother causes depression of milk-ejection reflex (dose dependent). No acetaldehyde found in infants, although maternal level rises.	Ananth, 1978; *Medical Letter*, 1974
		Maternal dose of 0.6 g/kg would produce milk level at 1 hr to 16.9 μmol/ml; dose to baby, 180 mg ethanol	On mean intake comparable to 5.9 ounces/day; studies in rats showed infant pup brain growth but normal somatic growth; slow initiation and decreased sucking measured infants of social drinkers; 1-2 g/kg of ethanol to mother caused decreased let-down.	Borges and Lewis, 1982; Martin et al., 1978; Kesäniemi, 1980; Cobo, 1973
III Heroin	Yes		13 of 22 infants had withdrawal; historically breastfeeding had been used to wean addict's infant. This is no longer recommended.	Savage, 1977; Catz and Giacoia, 1972
Marijuana *(Cannabis)*	Yes	105 ng/ml to 340 ng/ml plus metabolites; higher in milk than serum	Shown in laboratory animals to produce structural changes in nursling's brain cells; impairs DNA and RNA formation. Infant at risk of inhaling smoke during feeding when held while smoking. Found in infant's urine and stools.	Nahas, 1974, 1975, 1976; Crumpton and Brill, 1971; Clark et al., 1970; Campbell et al., 1971; Perez-Reyes and Wall, 1982
Phencyclidine (PCP)	Yes	3.90 μg/ml in one case; 9 days after delivery and more than 42 days after exposure; in mice milk level was 10 times that in blood	Infant was not breastfed.	Kaufman et al., 1983; Nicholas, 1982

Stimulants				
III Caffeine	Yes	1% of dose	Accumulates when intake moderate and continual. Causes jitteriness, wakefulness, and irritability. Caffeine present in many hot and cold drinks. Consider if infant very wakeful.	Horning, 1975; Rivera-Calimilim, 1977
Theobromine	Yes	3.7-8.2 mg/L after 240 mg dose*	No adverse symptoms observed in the infants. Chocolate most common cause of exposure.	Resman et al., 1977; Berlin & Daniel, 1981
Theophylline	Yes	10% of maternal dose†	Irritability, fretfulness	Yurchak et al., 1976; Stec et al., 1980
Thyroid and antithyroid medications				
III Carbimazole (neo-mercazole)	Yes	0.47% of dose	May cause goiter. Sufficient in milk to depress thyroid.	Low et al., 1979
I Methimazole (Tapazole)	Yes	M/P > 1 7.0-16.0% of dose	Inhibits synthesis of thyroid hormone but does not inactivate existing thyroid. Can inhibit infant thyroid. ⅛ grain/day of thyroid can be given to infant simultaneously.	Vorherr, 1976; Gaginella, 1978; Kwit and Hatcher, 1935; Tegler and Lindström, 1980
Potassium iodide	Yes	3 mg/100 ml‡	May alter thyroid function of infant; may cause goiter in infant.	Gaginella, 1978; Knowles, 1965, 1974
III Propylthiouracil	Yes	0.077% of dose	Probably safe. Risk of goiter and agranulocytosis minimal. With present microtechniques for T_3, T_4 and TSH, close monitoring of infant is possible.	Low et al., 1979; Kampmann, 1980
Radioactive iodine ^{125}I, ^{131}I (as a treatment)	Yes	M/P > 1	*Treatment* doses are excreted via the breast for 1-3 wk. Milk can be checked by Geiger counter if there is a question. Breastfeeding should be discontinued until milk is clear.	Knowles, 1965, 1974; Weaver et al., 1960
I Thiouracil	Yes	9-12 mg/100 ml§	Contraindicated.	Williams et al., 1944; Vorherr, 1976; O'Brien, 1974
Thyroid and thyroxine	Yes		Does not produce adverse symptoms on long-range follow-up. Noted to improve milk supply of hypothyroid mothers. No contraindication.	

*113 g chocolate bar.
†M/P = 0.7.
‡Dose was 325-650 mg three times a day.
§Maternal plasma level was 3.4 mg/100 ml after a 1.0 g dose; M/P = 3.

Table F-1. Relationship of drugs to breast milk and effect on infant—cont'd

Drug	Excreted in milk	Amount in milk after therapeutic dose	Effect on infant	Reference
Miscellaneous				
Bromocriptine	Yes	?	Suppresses lactation	Kulski et al., 1978
Bupivacaine (epidural anesthesia)	?	None identified; limit of measure is less than 0.02 μg/ml	No symptoms	Naulty et al., 1983
Cimetidine (Tagamet)	Yes	M/P greater than 1	Maximum ingested by infant is 6 mg; has antiadrenergic effects in adults; H_2-receptor antagonist.	Somogyi and Gugler, 1979
I Cyclophosphamide	Yes	Present*	Antineoplastic agent. Any amounts contraindicated.	Wienik and Duncan, 1971
DPT	Yes	Minimal	One case reported; mother breastfed at 3 wk; infant had rapidly decreasing platelets and WBC without affecting mother's levels. Does not interfere with immunization schedule.	*ACOG,* 1971 Durodola, 1979
Halothane	Yes	2 ppm	Nursing mothers who work in environment with halothane should be checked. Exposure in operating room while working as an anesthetist. No symptoms in infant.	Cote et al., 1976
I Methotrexate (Amethopterin)	Yes	Minor route of excretion: M/P = 0.08/1.0	Antimetabolite. Infant would receive 0.26 μg/100 ml, which researchers consider nontoxic for infant.	Johns et al., 1972

Nicotine	Yes	Mean 91 ppb (20-512 ppb)†	Decreases milk production. No apparent effect on infant—perhaps a tolerance is developed in utero. Smoking may interfere with let-down if smoking started prior to onset of a feeding.	Ferguson et al., 1976; Perlman et al., 1942; AAP Committee on Environmental Hazards, 1976; Lancet, editorial, 1974
Poliovirus vaccine	No		Live vaccine taken orally. Not necessary to withhold nursing 30 min before and after dose.	DeForest et al., 1973; Red Book, 1982
Rh antibodies	Yes		Destroyed in gastrointestinal tract; not effective orally.	Knowles, 1965, 1974
Rubella virus vaccine	Yes	Virus may be in milk.	Not contraindicated. Will not confer passive immunity. Mother should not be given vaccine when at risk for pregnancy.	ACOG, 1971
Smallpox vaccine	No		Exposure is by direct contact. Live virus. Contraindicated when mother has infant under 1 yr. No longer given to children routinely.	ACOG, 1971
Sulfasalazine (Azulfidine)	Yes	Splits to sulphapyridine and 5-ASA; 2 g/day gives infant 4 mg/kg. 40% of maternal levels of sulfapyridine; little or no 5-ASA	Risk of recurrent maternal disease outweighs risk to infant unless infant jaundiced, then postpone until jaundice clears.	Järnerot and Into-Malmberg, 1979; Berlin and Yaffe, 1980
Tolbutamide (Orinase)	Yes	2 ppm	Effect on neonate not known; could cause hypoglycemia.	Moiel and Ryan, 1967

*Single 500 mg IV dose in milk at 1, 3, 5, and 6 hr after injection.
†At ½-1½ packs/day. Large variation from single donor.

REFERENCES

Ahlenius, S., Brown, R., and Engel, J.: Learning deficits in a 4 week old offspring of nursing mothers treated with neuroleptic drug, penfluridol, Naunyn Schmeidebergs Arch. Pharmacol. **279:**31, 1973.

Alexander, L., and Moloney, L.: Marijuana, depression and drug dependency, Med. Counterpoint **4:**12, Sept. 1972.

American Academy of Pediatrics Committee on Drugs: The transfer of drugs and other chemicals into human breast milk, Pediatrics **72:**375, 1983.

American Academy of Pediatrics Committee on Environmental Hazards: Effects of cigarette-smoking on the fetus and child, Pediatrics **57:**411, 1976.

American Academy of Pediatrics Committee on Environmental Hazards: PCBs in breast milk, Pediatrics **62:**407, 1978.

American College of Obstetrics and Gynecology: Recommendations regarding rubella vaccination for women, ACOG Newslett., Jan. 1971.

American Medical Association: Queries and minor notes: magnesium sulfate and breast milk, JAMA **146:**298, 1951.

Amin-Zaki, L., et al.: Perinatal methylmercury poisoning in Iraq, Am. J. Dis. Child. **130:**1070, 1976.

Ananth, J.: Side effects in the neonate from psychotropic agents excreted through breast feeding, Am. J. Psychiatry **135:**801, 1978.

Anderson, A.N., et al.: Suppressed prolactin but normal neurophysin levels in cigarette smoking breast-feeding women, Clin. Endocrinol. **17:**363, 1982.

Anderson, P.: Drugs and breast feeding: a review, Drug Intell. Clin. Pharm. **11:**208, 1977.

Anderson, P., and Salter, F.: Propranolol therapy during pregnancy and lactation, Am. J. Cardiol. **37:**325, 1976.

Arena, J.: Contamination of the ideal food, Nutr. Today **5:**2, 1970.

Ayd, F.: Excretion of psychotropic drugs in human breast milk, Int. Drug Ther. Newslett. **8:**33, 1973.

Bagnell, P.C., and Ellenberger, H.A.: Obstructive jaundice due to a chlorinated hydrocarbon in breast milk, Can. Med. J. **117:**1047, 1977.

Baier, R.: Piperacillin in milk, Am. Soc. Microbiol. 1983.

Bakken, A., and Seip, M.: Insecticides in human breast milk, Acta Paediatr. Scand. **65:**535, 1976.

Baldwin, W.: Clinical study of senna administration to nursing mothers: assessment of effects on infant bowel habits, Can. Med. Assoc. J. **89:**566, 1963.

Barsivala, V., and Virkar, K.: The effects of oral contraceptives on concentrations of various components of human milk, Contraception **7:**307, 1973.

Bartig, D., and Cohen, M.: Excretion of drugs in human milk, Hosp. Formul. Manag. **4:**26, 1969.

Baty, J.D., et al.: May mothers taking warfarin breast feed their infants? Br. J. Clin. Pharmacol. **3:**969, 1976.

Bauer, J.H., et al.: Propranolol in human plasma and breast milk, Am. J. Cardiol. **43:**860, 1979.

Bell, R.A.F., and Dale, I.M.: Gold secretion in maternal milk, Arthritis Rheum. **19**(2):1374, 1976.

Bergman, A., and Wiesner, L.: Relation of passive cigarette smoking to sudden infant death syndrome, Pediatrics **58:**665, 1976.

Berke, R.: Radiation dose to breast-feeding child, J. Nucl. Med. **14:**51, 1973.

Berlin, C.M.: Excretion of methylxanthines in human milk, Semin. Perinatol. **5:**389, 1981.

Berlin, C.M., and Daniel, C.H.: Excretion of theobromine in human milk and saliva, Pediatr. Res. **15:**492, 1981.

Bisdom, W.: Alcohol and nicotine poisoning in nurslings, JAMA **109:**178, 1937.

Bitzen, P.O., et al.: Excretion of Paracetamol in human breast milk, Eur. J. Clin. Pharmacol. **20:**123, 1981.

Blacker, K.H., Weinstein, B.J., and Ellman, G.L.: Mother's milk and chlorpromazine, Am. J. Psychiatry **119:**178, 1962.

Blanco, J.D., et al.: Ceftazidime levels in human breast milk, Antimicrob. Agents Chemother. **23:**479, 1983.

Bland, E., et al.: Radioactive iodine uptake by thyroid of breast-fed infants after maternal blood-volume measurements, Lancet **2:**1039, 1969.

Bleyer, W.A., and Breckenridge, R.T.: Studies on the detection of adverse drug reactions in the newborn. II. The effect of prenatal aspirin on newborn hemostasis, JAMA **213:**2049, 1970.

Blinick, G., Jerez, E., and Wallach, R.C.: Drug addiction in pregnancy and the neonate, Am. J. Obstet. Gynecol. **125:**135, 1976.

Blinick, G., et al.: Methadone assays in pregnant women and progeny, Am. J. Obstet. Gynecol. **121:**617, 1975.

Boreus, L.O., et al.: Terbutaline in breast milk, Br. J. Clin. Pharmacol. **13:**731, 1982.

Borges, S., and Lewis, P.A.: A study of alcohol effects on the brain during gestation and lactation, Teratology **25:**283, 1982.

Borglin, N.E., and Sandholm, L.E.: Effect of oral contraceptives on lactation, Fertil. Steril. **22:**39, 1971.

Bounameaux, Y., and Durenne, J.: Un cas de leucèmie chez une Femme allaitante: effects du traitment par le busulfan sur la nourrisson, J. Ann. Soc. Belg. Med. Trop. **44:**381, 1964.

Brambel, C., and Hunter, R.: Effect of dicumarol on the nursing infant, Am. J. Obstet. Gynecol. **59:**1153, 1950.

Brandt, R.: Passage of diazepam and desmethyldiazepam into breast milk, Arzneim Forsch **26:**454, 1976.

Briggs, M., and Briggs, M.: Oral contraceptives and vitamin nutrition, Lancet **1:**1436, 1974.

Buchanan, R., et al.: The breast milk excretion of mefenamic acid, Curr. Ther. Res. **10:**592, 1968.

Buchanan, R.A., et al.: The breast milk excretion of flufenamic acid, Curr. Ther. Res. **11:**533, 1969.

Burrow, G.N., et al.: DDAVP treatment of diabetes insipidus during pregnancy and post-partum period, Acta Endocrinol. **97:**23, 1981.

Cai, S.X., and Bao, Y.S.: Placenta transfer, secretion into mother's milk of carbon disulphide and the effects on maternal function of female viscose rayon workers, Ind. Health **19:**15, 1981.

Campbell, A.M.G., et al.: Cerebral atrophy in young *Cannabis* smokers, Lancet **2:**1219, 1971.

Catz, C.S.: Diazepam in breast milk, Drug Ther. Jan., 1973.

Catz, C.S., and Giacoia, G.: Drugs and breast milk, Pediatr. Clin. North Am. **19:**151, 1972.

Chan, V., Tse, T.F., and Wong V.: Transfer of digoxin across the placenta and into breast milk, Br. J. Obstet. Gynaecol. **85:**605, 1978.

Clark, J.H., and Wilson, W.G.: A 16-day-old breast-fed infant with metabolic acidosis caused by salicylate, Clin. Pediatr. **20:**54, 1980.

Clark, L., Hughes, R., and Nakashima, E.: Behavioral effects of marijuana: experimental studies, Arch. Gen. Psychiatry **23:**193, 1970.

Clyde, D., and Shute, G.: Transfer of pyrimethamine in human milk, J. Trop. Med. Hyg. **59:**277, 1956.

Cobo, E.: Effect of different doses of ethanol on the milk-ejecting reflex in lactating women, Am. J. Obstet. Gynecol. **115:**819, 1973.

Cobrink, R.W., Hood, T., and Chusid, E.: The effect of maternal narcotic addiction on the newborn infant, Pediatrics **24:**288, 1956.

Cole, A.P., and Hailey, D.M.: Diazepam and active metabolite in breast milk and their transfer to the neonate, Arch. Dis. Child. **50:**741, 1975.

Colley, J., Holland, W.W., and Corkhill, R.T.: Influence of passive smoking and parental phlegm on pneumonia and bronchitis in early childhood, Lancet **2:**1031, 1974.

Cote, C.J., et al.: Trace concentrations of halothane in human breast milk, Br. J. Anaesthesiol. **48:**541, 1976.

Cruikshank, D.P., Varner, M.W., and Pitkin, R.M.: Breast milk magnesium and calcium concentrations following magnesium sulfate treatment, Am. J. Obstet. Gynecol. **143:**685, 1982.

Crumpton, E., and Brill, N.: Personality factors associated with frequency of marijuana use, Calif. Med. **115:**11, 1971.

Curry, S.H., et al.: Disposition of glutethimide, Clin. Pharmacol. Ther. **12:**849, 1971.

Curtis, E.: Oral-contraceptive feminization of a normal male infant, Obstet. Gynecol. **23:**295, 1964.

Davis, S., and Wedgwood, R.: Antibiotic prophylaxis in acute viral respiratory diseases, Am. J. Dis. Child. **109:**544, 1965.

Deforest, A., et al.: The effect of breast-feeding on the antibody response of infants to trivalent oral poliovirus vaccine, J. Pediatr. **83:**93, 1973.

deSweet, M., and Lewis, P.J.: Excretion of anticoagulants in human milk, N. Engl. J. Med. **297:**1471, 1977.

Devun, R.G., Duchin, K.L., and Fleiss, P.M.: Nadolol in human serum and breast milk, Br. J. Clin. Pharmacol. **12:**393, 1981.

Devlin, R.G., and Fleiss, P.M.: Captopril in human blood and breast milk, J. Clin. Pharmacol. **21:**110, 1981.

Dickey, R.P., and Stone, S.C.: Drugs that affect the breast and lactation, Clin. Obstet. Gynecol. **18:**95, 1975.

Dillon, H., Wilson, D., and Schaffner, W.: Lead concentrations in human milk, Am. J. Dis. Child. **4:**91, 1974.

Drugs in breast milk, Med. Lett. Drugs Ther. **16**(6):25, March 15, 1974.

Durodola, J.I.: Administration of cyclophosphamide during late pregnancy and early lactation: a case report, J. Natl. Med. Assoc. **71:**165, 1979.

Eckstein, H.B., and Jack, B.: Breast-feeding and anticoagulant therapy, Lancet **1:**672, 1970.

Eeg-Olofsson, O., et al.: Convulsions in a breast-fed infant after maternal indomethacin, Lancet **2:**215, 1978.

Erickson, S.H., Oppheim, G.L., and Smith, G.H.: Metronidazole in breast milk, Obstet. Gynecol. **57:**48, 1981.

Erkkola, R., and Kanto, J.: Diazepam and breast-feeding, Lancet **1:**1235, 1972.

Fahim, M., and King, T.: Effect of phenobarbital on lactation and the nursing neonate, Am. J. Obstet. Gynecol. **101:**1103, 1968.

Ferguson, B., Wilson, D.J., and Schaffner, W.: Determination of nicotine concentrations in human milk, Am. J. Dis. Child. **130:**837, 1976.

Findlay, J.W.A., et al.: Analgesic drugs in breast milk and plasma, Clin. Pharmacol. Ther. **29:**625, 1981.

Finley, J.P., et al.: Digoxin excretion in human milk, J. Pediatr. **93:**340, 1979.

Gaginella, T.S.: Drugs and the nursing mother—infant, U.S. Pharm. **3:**39, 1978.

Galloway, C.: Follow-up on a patient with myasthenia gravis, Am. J. Obstet. Gynecol. **79:**1031, 1960.

Goodman, L., and Gilman, A., editors: The pharmacological basis of therapeutics, ed. 5, New York, 1975, The Macmillan Co.

Gray, M.S., Kane, P.O., and Squires, S.: Further observations on metronidazole (Flagyl), Br. J. Vener. Dis. **37:**278, 1961.

Green, L.C., Tannenbaum, S.R., and Fox, J.G.: Nitrate in human and canine milk, N. Engl. J. Med. **306:**1367, 1982.

Habib, A., and McCarthy, J.S.: Effects on the neonate of propranolol administered during pregnancy, J. Pediatr. **91:**808, 1977.

Halikas, J., Goodwin, D., and Guse, S.: Marijuana use and psychiatric illness, Arch. Gen. Psychiatry **27:**162, 1972.

Harlap, S., and Davies, A.: Infant admissions to hospital and maternal smoking, Lancet **1:**529, 1974.

Havelka, J., et al.: Excretion of chloramphenicol in human milk, Chemotherapy **13:**204, 1968.

Healy, M.: Suppressing lactation with oral diuretics, Lancet **1:**1354, 1961.

Heisterberg, L., and Branebjerg, P.E.: Blood and milk concentrations of metronidazole in mothers and infants, J. Perinat. Med. **11:**114, 1983.

Hervada, A.R., Feit, E., and Sagraves, R.: Drugs in breast milk, Perinatal Care **2:**19, 1978.

Hill, L.M., and Malkasion, G.D.: The use of quinidine sulfate throughout pregnancy, Obstet. Gynecol. **54:**366, 1979.

Hirsh, J.: Fetal effects of Coumadin administered during pregnancy, Blood **36:**623, 1970.

Horning, M., et al.: Identification and quantification of drugs and drug metabolites in human breast milk using GC-MS-COM methods, Clin. Chem. **21:**1282, 1975.

Hosbach, R., and Foster, R.: Absence of nitrofurantoin from human milk, J.A.M.A. **202:**1057, 1967.

Ibrahim, A., and El-Tawil, N.: The effect of a new low-dosage oral contraceptive pill on lactation, Int. Surg. **49:**561, 1968.

Illingworth, R.S.: Abnormal substances excreted in human milk, Practitioner **171:**533, 1953.

Illingworth, R.S., and Finch, E.: Ethyl biscoumacetate (Tromexan) in human milk, J. Obstet. Gynecol. Br. Empire **66:**487, 1959.

Ingall, D., and Zuckerstatter, M.: Diagnosis and treatment of the passively addicted newborn, Hosp. Pract. **5:**101, 1970.

Jakubovič, A., Hattori, T., and McGeer, P.: Radioactivity in suckled rats after giving ^{14}C-tetrahydrocannibinol to the mother, Eur. J. Pharmacol. **22:**221, 1973.

Jakubovič, A., Tait, R., and McGeer, P.: Excretion of THC and its metabolites in ewe's milk, Toxicol. Appl. Pharm. **28:**38, 1974.

Janssen, P.A.J., Niemegeers, C.J.E., and Schellekens, K.H.L.: The pharmacology of penfluridol (R1634), a new potent and orally long-acting neuroleptic drug, Eur. J. Pharmacol. **11:**139, 1970.

Jarnerot, G., and Intro-Malmberg, M.B.: Sulphasalazine treatment during breast feeding, Scand. J. Gastroenterol. **14:**869, 1979.

Jelliffe, D., and Jelliffe, E.F.P.: Human milk in the modern world, Oxford, 1978, Oxford University Press.

John, T.J., et al.: Effect of breast-feeding on seroresponse of infants to oral poliovirus vaccination, Pediatrics **57:**47, 1976.

Johns, D.G., et al.: Secretion of methotrexate into human milk, Am. J. Obstet. Gynecol. **112:**978, 1972.

Jukes, T.: When friends or patients ask about . . . DDT, JAMA **229:**571, 1974.

Kaern, T.: Effect of oral contraceptives immediately postpartum on initiation of lactation, Br. Med. J. **3:**644, 1967.

Kafetzis, D.A., et al.: Ceftriaxone distribution between maternal blood and fetal blood and tissues at parturition and between blood and milk postpartum, Antimicrob. Agents Chemother. **23:**870, 1983.

Kampmann, J.P., et al.: Propylthiouracil in human milk, Lancet **1:**736, 1980.

Kan, M., and Hopkins, G.: Unilateral breast uptake of ^{67}Ga from breast feeding, Radiology **121:**668, 1976.

Katz, F.H., and Duncan B.R.: Entry of prednisone into human milk, N. Engl. J. Med. **293:**1154, 1975.

Kauffman, R.E., O'Brien, C., and Gilford, P.: Sulfisoxazole secretion into human milk, J. Pediatr. **97:**839, 1980.

Kaufman, K.R., et al.: PCP in amniotic fluid and breast milk: case report, J. Clin. Psychiatry 44:269, 1983.

Kesäniemi, Y.: Ethanol and acetaldehyde in the milk and peripheral blood of lactating women after ethanol adminstration, J. Obstet. Gynaecol. Br. Comm. 81:84, 1974.

Kitto, W.: Breast feeding and tolbutamide, JAMA 199:680, 1967.

Knowles, J.A.: Excretion of drugs in milk: a review, J. Pediatr. 66:1068, 1965.

Knowles, J.A.: What is treatment? J. Pediatr. 69:508, 1966.

Knowles, J.A.: Breast milk: a source of more than nutrition for the neonate, Clin. Toxicol. 7:69, 1974.

Kok, T.H.H.G., et al.: Drowsiness due to clemastine transmitted in breast milk, Lancet 1:915, 1982.

Kolansky, H., and Moore, W.: Effects of marijuana on adolescents and young adults, JAMA 216:486, 1971.

Kopelman, A.E.: Fetal addiction to pentazocine, Pediatrics 55:888, 1975.

Kora, S.: Effect of oral contraceptives on lactation, Fertil. Steril. 20:419, 1969.

Krajnovič, P., and Ferič, V.: Untersuchungen zur Frage der Arzheimittelsicherheit in der Frauenheilkunde, Arzneim Forsch 24:1061, 1974.

Kreek, M.J., et al.: Analysis of methadone and other drugs in maternal and neonatal body fluids, Am. J. Drug Alcohol Abuse 1:409, 1974.

Kreuz, D., and Axelrod, J.: Delta-9-tetrahydrocannabinol localization in body fat, Science 179:391, 1973.

Kris, E.B., and Carmichael, D.M.: Chlorpromazine maintenance therapy during pregnancy and confinement, Psychiatry Quart. 31:690, 1957.

Kwit, N.T., and Hatcher, R.A.: Excretion of drugs in milk, Am. J. Dis. Child. 49:900, 1935.

Lacey, J.: Dichloralphenazone and breast milk, Br. Med. J. 4:684, 1971.

Laumas, R.K., et al.: Radioactivity in the breast milk of lactating women after oral administration of ³H-norethynodrel, Am. J. Obstet. Gynecol. 98:411, 1967.

Lebowitz, M., and Burrows, B.: Respiratory symptoms related to smoking habits of family adults, Chest 69:48, 1976.

Le Orme, M., et al.: May mothers given warfarin breast-feed their infants? Br. Med. J. 1:1564 1977.

Levitan, A., and Manion, J.: Propranolol therapy during pregnancy and lactation, Am. J. Cardiol. 32:247, 1973.

Levy, M., Granit, L., and Laufer, N.: Excretion of drugs in human milk, N. Engl. J. Med. 297:798, 1977.

Lewis, A.M., et al.: Mexiletine in human blood and breast milk, Postgrad. Med. J. 57:546, 1981.

Liedholm, H., et al.: Accumulation of atenolol and metoprolol in human breast milk, Eur. J. Clin. Pharmacol. 20:229, 1981.

Liedholm, H., et al.: Transplacental passage and breast milk concentrations of hydralazine, Eur. J. Clin. Pharmacol. 21:417, 1982.

Lien, E.J., Kuwahara, J., and Koda, R.T.: Diffusion of drugs into prostatic fluid and milk, Drug. Intell. Clin. Pharm. 8:470, 1974.

Lipman, A.: Antimicrobial agents in breast milk, Mod. Med. 45:89, 1977.

Livingston, S.: Treatment of epilepsy with diphenylhydantoin sodium, Postgrad. Med. 20:584, 1956.

Llewellyn-Jones, D.: Inhibition of lactation by oestrogens, Br. Med. J. 4:387, 1968.

Lönnerdal, B., and Asquity, M.T.: Malathion not detected in breast milk of women living in aerial spraying areas, N. Engl. J. Med. 307:439, 1982.

Lönnerholm, G., and Lindström, B.: Terbutaline excretion into breast milk, Br. J. Clin. Pharmacol. 13:729, 1982.

Loughman, P.M.: Digoxin excretion in human breast milk, J. Pediatr. 92:1019, 1978.

Low, L.C.K., Lang, J., and Alexander, W.D.: Excretion of carbimazole and prophylthiouracil in breast milk, Lancet 2:1011, 1979.

Lundberg, P.: Abnormal otogeny in young rabbits after chronic administration of haloperidol to the nursing mothers, Brain Res. 40:395, 1972.

McCracken, G., and Nelson, J.: The current status of gentamicin for the neonate and young infant, Am. J. Dis. Child. 124:13, 1972.

McKenna, R., Cole, E.R., and Vasan, U.: Is warfarin sodium contraindicated in the lactating mother, J. Pediatr. 103:325, 1983.

McKenzie, S.A., Selley, J.A., and Agnew, J.E.: Secretion of prednisolone into breast milk, Arch. Dis. Child. 50:894, 1975.

McNall, P., and Jafarnia, M.: Management of myasthenia gravis in the obstetrical patient, Am. J. Obstet. Gynecol. 92:518, 1965.

Martin, D.C., Martin, J.C., and Streissguth, A.P.: Sucking frequency and amplitude in newborns as a function of maternal drinking and smoking, Current Alcohol 5:359, 1978.

Milkovich, L., and Van Den Berg, B.: An evaluation of the teratogenicity of certain antinauseant drugs, Am. J. Obststet. Gynecol. 125:244, 1976.

Miller, M.E., Cohn R.D., and Burghart, P.H.: Hydrochlorothiazide disposition in a mother and her breastfed infant, J. Pediatr. **101:**789, 1982.

Miller, G.H., and Hughes, L.R.: Lactation and genital involution effects of a new low-dose oral contraceptive on breast feeding mothers and their infants, Obstet. Gynecol. **35:**44, 1970.

Mirkin, B.: Diphenylhydantoin: placental transport, fetal localization, neonatal metabolism, and possible teratogenic effects, J. Pediatr. **78:**329, 1971.

Mohr, J.A.: The possible induction and/or acquisition of cellular hypersensitivity associated with ingestion of colostrum, J. Pediatr. **82:**1062, 1973.

Moiel, R.H., and Ryan, J.R.: Tolbutamide orinase in human breast milk, Clin. Pediatr. **6:**480, 1967.

Mulley, B.A., et al.: Placental transfer of chlorthalidone and its elimination in maternal milk, Eur. J. Clin. Pharmacol. **13:**129, 1978.

Nahas, G.: Inhibition of cellular mediated immunity in marihuana smokers, Science **183:**419, 1974.

Nahas, G.: Marihuana: toxicity, tolerance, and therapeutic efficacy, Drug Ther. p. 33, Jan. 1974.

Nahas, G.: Marihuana, JAMA **233:**79, 1975.

Nahas, G., and Paton, W., editors: Marihuana: chemistry, biochemistry and cellular effects, New York, 1976, Springer-Verlag New York, Inc.

Nau, H., et al.: Anticonvulsants during pregnancy and lactation, Clin. Pharmacokinet. **7:**508, 1982.

Nau, H., et al.: Valproic acid and its metabolites: Placental transfer, neonatal pharmacokinetics, transfer via mother's milk and clinical status in neonates of epileptic mothers, J. Pharmacol. Exp. Ther. **219:**768, 1981.

Naulty, J.S., et al.: Bupivacaine in breast milk following epidural anesthesia for vaginal delivery, Reg. Anaesth. **8:**44, 1983.

Nicholas, J.M., Lipshitz, J., and Schreiber, E.C.: Phencyclidine: its transfer across the placenta as well as into breast milk, Am. J. Obstet. Gynecol. **143:**143, 1982.

Nilsson, S., Nygren, K.G., and Johanson. E.D.B.: d-Norgestrel concentrations in maternal plasma, milk, and child plasma during administration of oral contraceptives to nursing women, Am. J. Obstet. Gynecol. **129:**179, 1977.

Nurnberger, C., and Lipscomb, A.: Transmission of radio-iodine (I^{131}) to infants through human maternal milk, JAMA **150:**1398, 1952.

O'Brien, T.: Excretion of drugs in human milk, Am. J. Hosp. Pharm. **31:**844, 1974.

O'Brien, T.: Excretion of diphenylhydantoin in human milk, Am. J. Hosp. Pharm. **32:**14, 1975.

O'Connell, M.E.A., and Sutton, H.: Excretion of radioactivity in breast milk following $^{m}Tc^{99}$-Sn polyphosphate, Br. J. Radiol. **49:**377, 1976.

Oseid, B.J.: Breast feeding and infant health. Clin. Obstet. Gynecol. **18:**149, 1975.

Overbach, A.: Drugs used with neonates and during pregnancy. Part 3. Drugs that may cause fetal damage or cross into breast milk, RN **37:**39, 1974.

Pacifici, G.M., and Placidi, G.F.: Rapid and sensitive electron-capture gas chromatographic method for determination of pineazepam and its metabolites in human plasma, urine and milk, J. Chromatography **135:**133, 1977.

Patrick, M.J., Tilstone, W.J., and Reavey, P.: Diazepam and breast feeding, Lancet **1**(7740):542, 1972.

Perez-Reyes, M., and Wall, M.E.: Presence of Δ^9 tetrahydrocannabinol in human milk, N. Engl. J. Med. **307:**819, 1982.

Perkins, K., and Oski, F.: Elevated blood lead in a 6-month old breast-fed infant: the role of newsprint logs, Pediatrics **57:**426, 1976.

Perlman, H.H., Dannenberg, A.M., and Sokoloff, N.: The excretion of nicotine in breast milk and urine from cigaret smoking, JAMA **120:**1003, 1942.

Perry, J., and LeBlanc, A.: Transfer of nitrofurantoin across the human placenta, Tex. Rep. Biol. Med. **25:**265, 1967.

Physicians' desk reference, Oradell, N.Y., 1984 Medical Economics Co.

Pittard, W.B., Merkatz, R., and Fletcher, B.D.: Radioactive excretion in human milk following administration of technectium Tc99m macroaggregated albumin, Pediatrics **70:**231, 1982.

Plomb, T.A., Thiery, M., and Maes, R.A.A.: The passage of thiamphenicol and chloramphenicol into human milk after single and repeated oral administration, Vet. Hum. Toxicol **25:**3, 1983.

Posner, C., and Konicoff, N.: Tetracycline in obstetric infections. In Welch, H., and Marti-Ibañez, F., editors: Antibiotic annual, 1955-56, New York, Medical Encyclopedia, Inc., p. 345.

Pynnönen, S., and Sillanpää, M.: Carbamazepine and mother's milk, Lancet **2:**563, 1975.

Ramadan, M.A., et al.: The effect of the oral contraceptive ovosiston on the composition of human milk, J. Reprod. Med. **9:**81, 1972.

Redman, C.: Fetal outcome in trial of antihypertensive treatment in pregnancy, Lancet **2:**753, 1976.

Remmington, J.S., and Klein, J.O.: Infectious diseases of the fetus and newborn infant, Philadelphia, 1976, W.B. Saunders Co.

Resman, B., Blumenthal, H.P., and Jusko, W.J.: Breast milk distribution of theobromine from chocolate, J. Pediatr. **91**:477, 1977.

Rivera-Calimlim, L.: Drugs in breast milk, Drug Ther. **2**(12):20, 1977.

Rose, D.P., et al.: Effect of oral contraceptives and vitamin B_6 deficiency on carbohydrate metabolism, Am. J. Clin. Nutr. **28**:872, 1975.

Roth, S.: Anti-inflammatories: exploring new options, Curr. Prescrib. p. 46, May, 1976.

Rothermel, P., and Faber, M.: Drugs in breast-milk: a consumer's guide, Birth Fam. J. **2**:76, 1975.

Savage, E.P., et al.: National study of chlorinated hydrocarbon insecticide residues in human milk USA, Am. J. Epidemiol. **113**:413, 1981.

Savage, R.: Drugs and breast milk, J. Hum. Nutr. **31**:459, 1977.

Schlesinger, E.: Dietary fluorides and caries prevention, Am. J. Public Health **55**:1123, 1965.

Schou, M., and Amdisen, A.: Lithium and pregnancy. III. Lithium ingestion by children breastfed by women on lithium treatment, Br. Med. J. **2**:138, 1973.

Shambaugh, G., Jr.: Prophylactic antibiotics? Arch. Otolaryngol. **77**:459, 1963.

Shankaran, S., and Poland, R.L.: The displacement of bilirubin from albumin by furosemide, J. Pediatr. **90**:642, 1977.

Shore, M.: Drugs can be dangerous during pregnancy and lactation, Can. Pharm. J. **103**:8, 1970.

Shidlovsky, B.A., Prigot, A., and Maynard, A.: Absorption, diffusion, and excretion studies on the phosphate complex salt of tetracycline. In Welch, H., and Marti-Ibañez, F., editors: Antibiotic annual, 1957-1958, New York, Medical Encyclopedia, Inc., p. 459.

Smith, D.: Marijuana: some notes, queries, and answers, Med. Counterpoint p. 29, 1971.

Smith D., and Mehl, C.: The new social drug: cultural, legal and medical perspectives on marijuana, vol. 3, Englewood Cliffs, N.J., 1970, Prentice-Hall, Inc.

Smith, M.T., et al.: Propranolol, proprandol glucuronide and naphthoxylactic acid in breast milk and plasma, Ther. Drug Monit. **5**:87, 1983.

Somogyl, A., and Gugler, R.: Cimetidine excretion into breast milk, Br. J. Clin. Pharmacol. **7**:627, 1979.

Stec, G.P., et al.: Kinetics of theophylline transfer to breast milk, Clin. Pharmacol. Ther. **28**:404, 1980.

Steen, B., and Rane, A.: Clindamycin passage into human milk, Br. J. Clin. Pharmacol. **13**:661, 1982.

Steen, B., et al.: Phenytoin excretion in human breast milk and plasma levels in nursed infants, Ther. Drug Monit. **4**:331, 1982.

Stone, O., and Willis, C.: The effect of stannous fluoride and stannous chloride on inflammation, Toxicol. Appl. Pharmacol. **13**:332, 1968.

Straub, C., and Murthy, G.: A comparison of Sr^{90} component and cow's milk, Pediatrics **36**:732, 1965.

Sykes, P., Quarrie, J., and Alexander, F.: Lithium carbonate and breast-feeding, Br. Med. J. **2**:1299, 1976.

Takyi, B.E.: Excretion of drugs in human milk, J. Hosp. Pharm. **28**:317, 1970.

Talbott, J.: Marihuana psychosis, JAMA **210**:299, 1969.

Tank, G., and Storvick, C.: Caries experience of children one to six years old in two Oregon communities (Corvallis and Albany). III. Relation of diet to variation of dental caries, J. Am. Dent. Assoc. **70**:394, 1965.

Terwilliger, W.G., and Hatcher, R.A.: Morphine and quinine in human milk, Surg. Gynecol. Obstet. **58**:823, 1939.

Texeira, G.C., and Scott, R.B.: Further clinical and laboratory studies with novobiocin. II, Novobiocin concentration in the blood of newborn infants and in the breast milk of lactating mothers, Antibiot. Med. **5**:577, 1958.

Tobacco smoke and the non-smoker (editorial), Lancet **1**:1201, 1974.

Toddywalla, V.S., Joshi, L., and Virkar, K.: Effect of contraceptive steroids on human lactation, Am. J. Obstet. Gynecol. **127**:245, 1977.

Tunnessen, W., and Hertz, C.: Toxic effects of lithium in newborn infants: a commentary, J. Pediatr. **81**:804, 1972.

Tupin, J.P., and Hopkin, J.T.: Lithium for mood disturbances, Rational Drug Ther. **12**(9):1, 1978.

Tyson, R.M., Shrader, E.A., and Perlman, H.H.: Drugs transmitted through breast milk. I. Laxatives, J. Pediatr. **12**:824, 1937.

Tyson, R.M., Shrader, E.A., and Perlman, H.H.: Drugs transmitted through breast milk. II. Barbiturates, J. Pediatr. **13**:86, 1938.

Tyson, R.M., Shrader, E.A., and Perlman, H.H.: Drugs transmitted through breast milk. III. Bromides, J. Pediatr. **13**:91, 1938.

Vagenakis, A., Abreau, C., and Braverman, L.: Duration of radioactivity in the milk of a nursing mother following ^{99m}Tc administration, J. Nucl. Med. **12**:188, 1971.

Varsano, I., Fischl, J., and Tikvah, P.: The excretion of orally ingested nitrofurant in human milk (letters), J. Pediatr. **82:**886, 1973.

Veláquez, J.G., et al.: Effecto de al administracion oral diaria de 0.350 mg. de noretindrona en la lactancia y en la composicion de la lecl Ginecol. Obstet. Mex. **40:**31, 1976.

Vorherr, H.: Drug excretion in breast milk, Postgrad. Med. **56:**97, 1974.

Vorherr, H.: Drug excretion in breast milk, Senologia **1:**27, 1976.

Wagner, J.: Drug bioavailability studies, Hosp. Pract. p. 119, Jan., 1977.

Weaver, J.C., Kamm M.L., and Dobson, R.L. Excretion of radioiodine in human milk, JAMA **173:**872, 1960.

Wennberg, R.P., Rasmussen, L.F., and Ahlfors, C.E.: Displacement of bilirubin from human albumin by three diuretics, J. Pediatr. **90:**647, 1977.

Werthmann, M.N., and Krees, S.: Excretion of chlorothiazide in breast milk, J. Pediatr. **81:**781, 1972.

Wickizer, T.M., and Brillant, L.B.: Testing for polychlorinated biphenyls in human milk, Pediatrics **68:**411, 1981.

Widdowson, E.M., et al.: Absorption, excretion and retention of strontium by breast-fed and bottle-fed babies, Lancet **2:**941, 1960.

Wiernik, P.H., and Duncan, J.H.: Cyclophosphamide in human milk, Lancet **1:**912, 1971.

Williams, R.H., Kay, G.H., and Jandorf, B.J.: Thiouracil: its absorption, distribution and excretion, J. Clin. Invest. **23:**613, 1944.

Wolff, M.S.: Occupationally derived chemicals in breast milk, Am. J. Ind. Med. **4:**259, 1983.

Wurster, C.F.: DDT in mother's milk, ICEA News, vol. 9, Nov.-Dec., 1970.

Wyburn, J.R.: Human breast milk excretion of radionuclides following administration of radio pharmaceuticals, J. Nucl. Med. **14:**115, 1973.

Yaffe, S.J., and Waletsky, L.R.: Drugs and chemicals in breast milk. In Waletsky, L.R., editor: Symposium on human lactation, DHEW publ. no. 79-5107 Arlington, Va., 1976.

Yoshioka, H., et al.: Transfer of cefazolin into human milk, J. Pediatr. **94:**151, 1979.

Yurchak, A.M., and Jusko, W.J.: Theophylline secretion into breast milk, Pediatrics **57:**518, 1976.

Breast pumps

Table G-1. Manufacturers/distributors

Name	Available	Comments and approximate cost
Hand		
Davol	Drugstores	$2.50
Evenflo	Drugstores	$3.50
Lloyd-B	Lopuco Ltd. 1615 Old Annapolis Road Annapolis, MD 21777	$40.00
Nuture	Lact-Assist, Inc. 2103 Crestmoor Road Nashville, TN 37215 (615)383-7179	Special silicone pump fits all; can be used with electric pumps; $35.00
Cylinder pumps		
Kaneson	Okayama, Japan	$25.00
Comfort plus	Marshall Electronics 5435 W. Fargo Ave. Skokie, IL 60077	$25.00
Craftco Manual	Graham-Field Surgical Co. New Hyde Park, NY	$25.00
Electric (all in range of $900-$1000)		
Egnell	Egnell, Inc. 412 Park Ave. Cary, IL 60013	Widest use effective
Medela	Box 386 Crystal Lake, IL 60014	Has a manual adaptor that can be used separately
Axicare	Neonatal Division Colgate Medical Ltd. 1 Blue Hill Plaza Pearl River, NY 10945	
Whittlestone breast milker	P.O. Box 710 Hamilton, New Zealand (available in USA shortly)	Physiologic milking action
Water pump	Nursing Mothers Association of Australia	$20.00

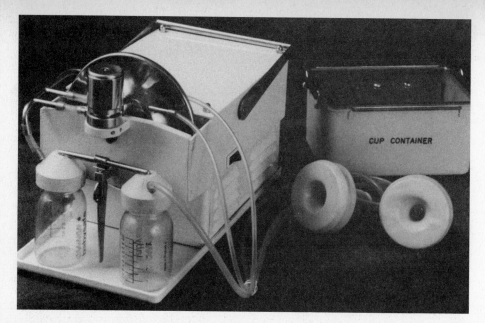

Fig. G-1. Whittlestone physiologic breast milker is intended to simulate the action of sucking infant. This is the only breast milker that applies enough stimulation to increase milk secretion and induce fully effective emptying of breasts. (Courtesy Trigon Industries Ltd., C.P.O. Box 3674, Auckland, New Zealand.)

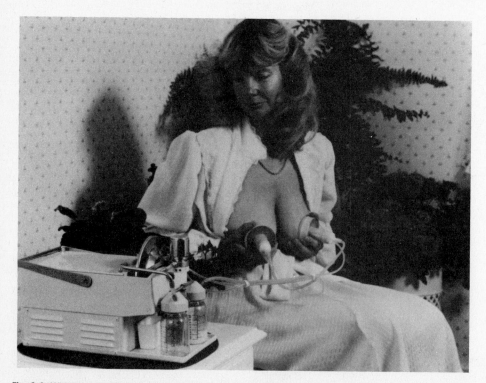

Fig. G-2. Whittlestone physiologic breast milker in use. The breast cups have a foam rubber pad and liner, which contract rhythmically behind the areola, gently stimulating the breast, compressing the milk ducts, and encouraging the ejection of milk into the breast cup. Both breasts are milked simultaneously. Milk is kept sterile and immediately refrigerated in water bath. (Courtesy Trigon Industries Ltd., C.P.O. Box 3674, Auckland, New Zealand.)

THE WHITTLESTONE PHYSIOLOGIC BREAST MILKER _____

The Whittlestone physiologic breast milker has been designed especially for home or hospital, on sound physiologic principles to simulate the action of a sucking baby. It is effective and comfortable.

The breast cups have a soft foam rubber pad and liner that contracts rhythmically behind the nipple area (areola)—gently stimulating the breasts, compressing the milk ducts, and encouraging the ejection of milk into the breast cups. The vacuum can be controlled by the mother to suit her own level of comfort and effectiveness. The vacuum also helps to keep the breast cups in place and removes the milk to the collecting bottles. (Obsolete breast pumps relied on suction alone, which could be damaging to the breast tissue and was often painful and ineffective).

This New Zealand–designed milker is the only one that provides two breast cups. Both breasts are milked simultaneously, taking advantage of the natural let-down reflex and reducing the time involved in expressing breast milk.

The Lact-Aid Nursing Trainer System

Appendix H

Lact-Aid is made up of four parts: (1) the body with permanently attached nursing tube, (2) the clamp ring, (3) the extension tube, and (4) the presterilized Lact-Aid bag with 4 oz capacity.

For convenience in filling and assembling Lact-Aid, a bag hanger and funnel have been specially designed. Six T-shaped end tabs provide easy attachment to the nursing bra.

The filled Lact-Aid is attached to the nursing bra or neck cord between the breasts and is positioned so that the supplement cannot siphon out. The presterilized bag is attached to the body by the clamp ring. The infant suckles the tip of the nursing tube and the nipple of the breast at the same time. As the infant nurses, supplement is drawn from the bottom of the presterilized bag by the extension tube attached to the bottom of the body. This keeps the infant from swallowing any air that might be trapped in the top of the bag. The body has an orifice designed to provide the best rate of flow, slower than milk flows from the breast, but fast enough to keep from overtiring the infant. The nursing tube carries the supplement to the infant's mouth. It is clear, very soft, and flexible and will not cause the infant's mouth or the nipple any discomfort.

When the infant is put to breast, the flow of supplement rewards his nursing efforts. This provides a pleasant incentive for the infant to continue nursing, which in turn provides the breasts with suckling stimulation to build up the milk supply. The Lact-Aid is small enough, even when it contains the full 4 oz capacity of supplement, to enable one to nurse discreetly without it showing.

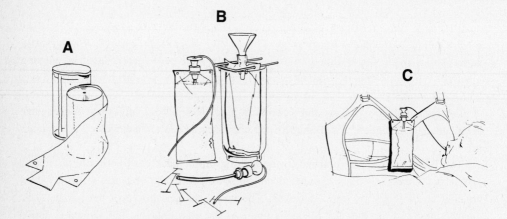

Fig. H-1. A, Presterilized, disposable bags have 4 ounce capacity. **B,** Lact-Aid System includes detailed instruction booklet plus accessories for filling, cleaning, and use. **C,** Filled Nursing Trainer may be attached directly to the nursing bra as shown or suspended by the Neck Cord as depicted in Fig. 17-4. (From Avery, J.L.: Lact-Aid Nursing Trainer Instruction Book, Athens, TN, 1983 Revised Ed., Lact-Aid International, Inc.)

LACT-AID PARTS

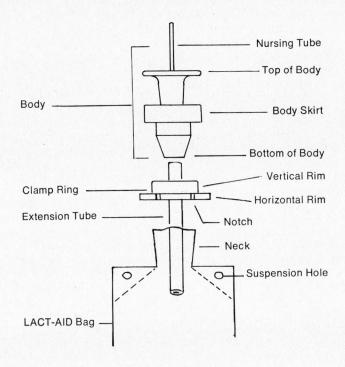

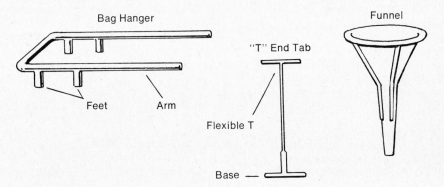

Fig. H-2. Lact-Aid parts. (From Avery, J.J.: Lact-Aid Nursing Training Instruction Book, Athens, TN, 1983 Revised Ed., Lact-Aid International, Inc.)

BIBLIOGRAPHY

Avery, J.L.: A brief discussion of adoptive-nursing: an introduction to the topic, Athens, TN, 1983 Revised Ed. Lact-Aid International, Inc.*

Avery, J.L.: Induced lactation: a guide for counseling and management, Denver, 1973, J.L. Avery.*

---

*Available from Lact-Aid International, Inc., P.O. Box 1066, Athens, TN 80206; hotline-(615)744-9090.

Organizations interested in supporting breastfeeding
Appendix I

Ammehjelpen
Postboks 15
Holmen, Oslo 3, Norway

Arbeitsgruppe and Dritte Welt
Postbach 1007
Bern 300, Switzerland

Association for Improvement of
   Maternity Services
61 Dartmouth Park Road
London NW 5, United Kingdom

Baby Foods Action Group
103 Gower street
London WC1E 6AW, United Kingdom

Center for Science in the Public Interest
1779 Church Street, NW
Washington, D.C. 20036

Health Education Associates
211 S. Easton Road
Glenside, Pa. 19038

International Childbirth Education
   Association
2763 NW 70th Street
Seattle, Wash. 98167

Lact-Aid International, Inc.
P.O. Box 1066
Athens, TN 80206
Hotline-(615)744-9090

LaLeche League International Canadian
   Supply Depot
Box 39
Williamsburg, Ontario, Canada KOC
   2HO

La Leche League International, Inc.
9616 Minneapolis Avenue
Franklin Park, Ill. 60131

National Childbirth Trust
Breast-feeding Promotion Group
9 Queensborough Terrace
London W2 3TB, United Kingdom

Nursing Mothers' Association of
   Australia
99 Burwood Road
Hawthorn, Victoria, Australia 3122

Nursing Mothers Counsel Inc.
P.O. Box 50063
Palo Alto, Calif. 94303

Parents Centres of Australia
148 Hereford Street
Forest Lodge, NSW, Australia 2229

War on Want
467 Caledonian Road
London N.7, United Kingdom

Appendix J

Marmet technique of manual expression of breast milk

EXPRESSING THE MILK

Draining the milk reservoirs

1. **POSITION** the thumb and first two fingers about **1″ to 1½″ behind the nipple.** (C-hold at 12 o'clock and 6 o'clock positions).

–Use this measurement, which is not necessarily the outer edge of the areola, as a guide. The areola varies in size from one woman to another.

–Place the thumb above the nipple and the fingers below as shown.

–Note that the fingers are positioned so that the milk reservoirs lie beneath them.

–Avoid cupping the breast.

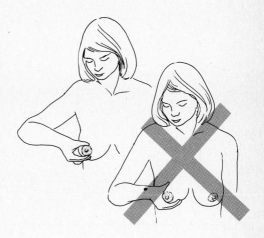

☐ From Chele Marmet Lactation Institute, West Los Angeles, Calif.
For complete instructions and more information about special breastfeeding situations and educational programs, contact The Lactation Institute and Breastfeeding Clinic, 16161 Ventura Blvd., Suite 215, Encino, CA 91436 (213)995-1913.

2. **ROTATE** the thumb and finger position to milk the other reservoirs. Use both hands on each breast. The pictures show hand positions on the right breast.

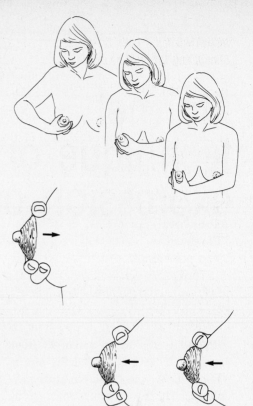

3. **PUSH** straight into the chest wall.
–Avoid spreading the fingers apart.
–For large breasts, first lift and then push into the chest wall.

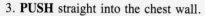

4. **ROLL** thumb and fingers forward as if making thumb and fingerprints at the same time.
–The **rolling motion** of the thumb and fingers compresses and empties the milk reservoirs without hurting sensitive breast tissue.
–Note the moving position of the thumbnail and fingernails in illustration.

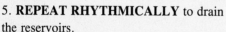

5. **REPEAT RHYTHMICALLY** to drain the reservoirs.
–Position, push, roll; position, push, roll.
Avoid squeezing the breast. This can cause bruising.
Avoid sliding on the breast. This can cause skin burns.
Avoid pulling out the nipple and breast. This can cause tissue damage.

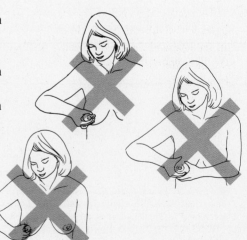

ASSISTING MILK EJECTION
Stimulating the flow of milk

1. **MASSAGE** the milk producing cells and ducts.

–Start at the top of the breast. Press firmly into the chest wall. Move fingers in a circular motion on one spot on the skin.

–After a few seconds move the fingers to the next area on the breast.

–**Spiral** around the breast toward the areola using this massage.

–The motion is similar to that used in a breast examination.

2. **STROKE** the breast area from the top of the breast to the nipple with a light **tickle-like stroke.**

–Continue this stroking motion from the chest wall to the nipple around the whole breast.

–This will help with relaxation and will help stimulate the milk ejection.

3. **SHAKE** the breast while leaning forward so that gravity will help the milk ejection.

Procedure

This procedure should be followed by mothers who are expressing in place of a full feeding and those who need to establish, increase, or maintain their milk supply when the baby cannot nurse.

–Express each breast until the flow of milk slows down.

–Assist the milk ejection (massage, stroke, shake) on both breasts. This can be done simultaneously.

–Repeat the whole process of expressing each breast and assisting the milk ejection once or twice more. The flow of milk usually slows down sooner the second and third time as the reservoirs are drained.

Timing

The ENTIRE PROCEDURE should take approximately 20-30 MINUTES.

- Express each breast 5-7 minutes.
- Massage, stroke, shake.
- Express each breast 3-5 minutes.
- Massage, stroke, shake.
- Express each breast 2-3 minutes.

NOTE: If the milk supply is established, use the times given only as a guide. Watch the flow of milk and change breasts when the flow gets small.

NOTE: If little or no milk is present yet, follow these suggested times closely.

Appendix K

Legislation regarding human milk

STATE OF NEW YORK _____

AN ACT to amend the public health law, in relation to the availability of human breast milk for infant consumption

The People of the State of New York, represented in Senate and Assembly, do enact as follows:

Section 1. Legislative findings. The legislature hereby finds and declares that human breast milk, the preferred food for all infants, provides a superior, well tolerated nutritional source because of its unique components. It contains substances, lacking in other forms of infant nutrition, which help control infection and aid in preventing infant disease. For premature infants or those with a low birth weight or infants who are allergic to cow's milk and infant formulas, human breast milk is essential.

It shall be the declared policy of the state of New York that any and all infants requiring human breast milk be assured access to sufficient quantities of wholesome human breast milk, donated by concerned lactating mothers on a continual and systematic basis. The availability of such a supply of human breast milk should be made known to the public so that health providers and families of infants with particular need for human breast milk will be aware of its accessibility.

§2. The public health law is amended by adding a new section twenty-five hundred five to read as follows:

§2505. Human breast milk; collection, storage, and distribution; general powers of the commissioner. The commissioner is hereby empowered to:

(a) adopt regulations and guidelines including, but not limited to donor standards, methods of collection, and standards for storage, and distribution of human breast milk;

(b) conduct educational activities to inform the public and health care providers of

_____

☐ From Office of Health Systems Management, Bureau of Standards Development, New York State Department of Health, Empire State Plaza, Albany, N.Y., 1984.

the availability of human breast milk for infants determined to require such milk and to inform potential donors of the opportunities for proper donation;

(c) establish rules and regulations to effectuate the provisions of this section.

§3. This act shall take effect immediately.

NEW YORK STATE CODE: Human milk banks
Chapter II
Administrative rules and regulations
Subchapter G
Maternal and child health
Part 68
Human milk banks
(Statutory authority: Public health law § 2505)

Subchapter G of Chapter II is hereby amended to add a new Part 68 to read as follows:

Sec.		Sec.	
68.1	Definitions	68.6	Collection and storage of human milk
68.2	Permit to operate a human milk bank	68.7	Processing of human milk
68.3	Governing responsibility	68.8	Distribution of human milk
68.4	Medical direction	68.9	Records to be maintained
68.5	Qualifications of donors		

68.1 Definitions. As used in this Part:

(a) Human milk bank shall mean an organized service which has been issued a permit to operate by the Commissioner and exists for the selection of donors and for the collection, processing, storage or distribution of human milk for infants other than the donor's own infant.

(b) Donor shall mean a lactating woman who voluntarily contributes milk to a human milk bank for infants other than her own and who does not receive remuneration for human milk.

(c) Single donor milk shall mean the accumulation of milk from one donor.

(d) Multiple donor human milk shall mean the accumulation of human milk from more than one donor.

(e) Collection of human milk shall mean the expression of milk from the breast, placing of the milk into a container and storage of the milk.

(f) Transfer station shall mean the location between the donor site and the milk bank where containers of human milk are held temporarily.

(g) Processing of human milk shall mean the testing of collected human milk for bacterial, and when indicated for viral and/or environmental contamination, and the treatment of milk to reduce or eliminate contaminants.

68.2 Permit to operate a human milk bank.

(a) A valid permit issued by the Commissioner of Health is required for lawful operation of a human milk bank.

(b) A permit will be issued subject to the human milk bank being established, maintained and operated in compliance with this Part.

(c) An applicant for a permit to operate a human milk bank shall submit to the department:

(1) justification for establishment of the service and plan for coordination with other human milk banks;

(2) proposed budget for operation of the milk bank;

(3) the name of the person in charge of the milk bank;

(4) the name of the medical director;

(5) selection criteria for donor participation;

(6) procedures for testing human milk and criteria for determining acceptability of milk for infant consumption; and

(7) the education program for potential donors.

(d)   A human milk bank shall allow admission to a representative of the Commissioner for the purpose of inspecting premises, procedures, equipment, or records to determine compliance with the standards in this section.

68.3   Governing responsibility.   The holder of the permit of the milk bank shall ensure the development and implementation of policies for the operation of the human milk bank, the appointment of a medical director and the designation of the person to be in charge.

68.4   Medical direction.

(a)   Medical direction shall be provided by a physician who is licensed and currently registered with the New York State Education Department and who is eligible for board certification in pediatrics.

(b)   The medical director shall monitor the medical efficacy of the program and shall, as a minimum, develop:

(1) medical criteria for donor participation;

(2) quality standards for milk; and

(3) a policy for priority distribution of human milk when the demand exceeds the supply.

68.5   Qualifications of donor.

(a)   The milk bank shall initially screen and periodically assess the donor for conditions that may adversely affect the quality of milk or impair the donor's health to include but not be limited to:

(1) use of medications, tobacco, alcohol and other substances in quantities likely to be harmful if transmitted through human milk to a recipient;

(2) systemic chronic diseases;

(3) acute and chronic infectious diseases;

(4) emotional and/or behavioral problems;

(5) history of jaundice in own infant after one week of age;

(6) sources of exposures which may be associated with environmental contaminants;

(7) length of postpartum period; and

(8) ability to follow directions.

(b)   There shall be evidence that the donor has been tested for presence of hepatitis B surface antigen (HB_sAg) and has been found negative.

(c)   The milk bank shall obtain informed signed consent from the donor to participate in the milk bank program.

(d)   The milk bank shall provide a program of education for donors which shall include, but not be limited to:

(1) purpose of the milk bank and donor responsibilities;

(2) policies and procedures concerning operation of the milk bank;

(3) procedures for collecting and storing milk;

(4) problems, diseases and medications or other substances contraindicating use of milk;

(5) diet and nutrition; and

(6) breast care and common problems associated with breast feeding.

68.6   Collection and storage of human milk.

(a)   The milk bank shall supply presterilized, leak proof containers and container seals to the human milk donor.

(b)   The human milk bank shall educate and monitor each donor in collection procedures to include but not be limited to:

    (1) cleansing hands and breasts according to currently acceptable techniques;

    (2) use of sterilized containers and container seals and method for sterilization of breast pump or other equipment, if used; and

    (3) procedures for home storage of collected human milk.

(c)   Human milk shall be stored at 45°F (7.2°C) or below for no more than 48 hours after expression; frozen milk shall be stored at 0°F (−18°C) or below for no more than 90 days.

(d)   The container shall be identified by a tag affixed to it which shall show the donor's identification number, the date and the hours the milk was expressed. When frozen human milk is held at a transfer station this tag shall also show the identification of the station, time of receipt and of departure.

(e)   Human milk shall be transported so that it is protected from contamination, thawing and refreezing and maintained at 45°F (7.2°C) or lower if liquid, 0°F (−18°C) or lower if frozen.

(f)   Transfer stations shall not handle liquid milk and when human milk is stored at a transfer station it shall be received in the frozen state, protected from contamination, thawing and refreezing and be stored at 0°F (−18°C) or below.

(g)   The physical facilities of the human milk bank minimize the potential for contamination by:

    (1) locating the human milk bank in a distinct identifiable area and providing a separate refrigerator and freezer for human milk; and

    (2) equipping refrigerators and freezers with a recording thermometer which shall be calibrated against a certified thermometer at least four times a year and which shall be either visually or mechanically monitored for fluctuations in temperature which affect the quality of the milk.

68.7   Processing of human milk.

(a)   Policies, procedures and criteria shall be developed and submitted for review and approval by the Department for:

    (1) routine bacteriological testing of donated human milk;

    (2) virology testing when indicated;

    (3) testing for those environmental contaminants to which the donor is likely to have been exposed because of diet, residence or other factors when a judgment is made to include such a donor in the program;

    (4) random sample testing of donated milk for adulteration; and

    (5) microbiological monitoring to assure the effectiveness of pasteurization.

(b)   The human milk bank shall make arrangements with an approved laboratory to perform the required tests.

68.8   Distribution of human milk.

(a)   The human milk bank shall distribute human milk to infants regardless of whether the infant is hospitalized or is in another setting according to the pre-established priority distribution.

(b)   The human milk bank shall make known the availability of human milk to the public so that health providers and families of infants with particular need for human milk will be aware of its availability.

68.9   Records to be maintained.

(a)   An individual file of each donor shall be maintained and shall include but not be limited to:

(1) findings from the medical history;

(2) results of tests for diseases transmissible through human milk;

(3) a consent form signed by the donor which informs the donor of her obligations and of any risks involved;

(4) documentation of instructions given to the donor for preserving the wholesomeness of donated milk; and

(5) a record of any donor illness reported to the milk bank during participation in the program.

(b)   Records of milk donations filed by donor identification number to include but not be limited to:

(1) information from the identification tag affixed at the time of collection showing date and hour of collection and, if applicable, the identification of the transfer station with recorded times of receipt and departure;

(2) results of all tests performed;

(3) the date of pasteurization, if applicable; and

(4) the date the milk was distributed or used, and if applicable, identifying information regarding milk accumulated from multiple donors.

(c)   Records of information about recipients to include but not be limited to:

(1) infant's age, birth weight and/or weight history and diagnosis which indicated the medical need for human milk;

(2) the dates the service began and terminated;

(3) identification of all milk given to the recipients;

(4) documentation that the risks of consumption by and infant of donated milk have been disclosed to persons legally responsible for the infant.

(a)(10)(i)   The hospital, with the advice of the maternity staff, shall formulate a program of instruction and provide assistance as needed for maternity patients in the fundamentals of [normal] infant care, post pregnancy care and family planning.

(ii) Each maternity patient shall be given the opportunity and the right to breast feed her infant unless there is a medical contradiction which is made known to such patient.

(a) Assistance shall be provided as needed to facilitate breast feeding.

(b) An educational program shall include the nutritional and physiological benefits of human milk, care of breasts, common problems associated with breast feeding, and the sanitary procedures to follow in collecting and storing human milk. The educational program shall also include problems, diseases and medications or other substances contraindicating breast feeding.

(b)(21) Human milk bank shall mean an organized service which has been approved by the commissioner through a construction application to the State Hospital Review and Planning Council and exists for the selection of donors and for the collection, processing, storage or distribution of human milk for infants other than the donor's own infant.

(22) Human milk donor shall mean a lactating woman who voluntarily contributes milk to a human milk bank for infants other than her own and who meets the qualifi-

cations defined in Section 68.5 of Part 68 of Chapter II of this Title, Administrative Rules and Regulations. A human milk donor shall not receive remuneration for human milk.

(c)(3) (vi) *(a)* The preparation, handling and storage of human milk, infant formula ingredients and equipment shall be carried out in accordance with written procedures, copies of which shall be filed with the full-time health officer and kept in the 'formula room'. Such procedures and any changes or amendments thereto shall be subject to the approval of the full-time health officer.

(vii) *(a)* A hospital that is approved to operate a human milk bank shall conform to the provisions of Part 68 of Chapter II of this Title, Administrative Rules and Regulations.

(b) A hospital that does not routinely collect, store or distribute donated human milk and does require donated human milk for a specific infant does not require approval to operate a human milk bank but shall conform to Sections 68.5, 68.6, 68.7 and 68.8 of Part 68 of Chapter II of this Title, Administrative Rules and Regulations.

Appendix L
Vitamin and mineral supplement needs in normal children in the United States

American Academy of Pediatrics— Committee on Nutrition

GUIDELINES FOR SUPPLEMENTATION

Table L-1 summarizes the following guidelines for the use of supplements in healthy infants and children. The indications for vitamin K and fluoride are discussed in the text only.

Newborn infants

Vitamin K administration to all newborn infants is effective as a prophylaxis against hemorrhagic disease of the newborn. This 1961 recommendation was strongly reaffirmed in 1971 to prevent or minimize the postnatal decline of the vitamin K-dependent coagulation factors (II, VII, IX, and X). Vitamin K_1 is considered the vitamin derivative of choice in a single, intramuscular dose of 0.5 to 1 mg or an oral dose of 1.0 to 2.0 mg. In rare instances, the dose may have to be repeated after about four to seven days.

Breast-fed infants

The renewed emphasis on human milk as an ideal food has raised the question whether breast-fed infants require any vitamin or mineral supplements prior to the introduction of solid foods. This subject bears further discussion, particularly with respect to the most widely used supplements: vitamins A, C, D, and E, iron and fluoride.

Table L-1 Guidelines for use of supplements in healthy infants and children*

| Child | Multivitamin-multimineral | Vitamins | | | Minerals |
		D	E	Folate	Iron
Term infants					
Breast-fed	0	±	0	0	±†
Formula-fed	0	0	0	0	0
Preterm infants					
Breast-fed‡	+‡	+	±§	±‡	+
Formula-fed‡	+‡	+	±§	±‡	+†
Older infants (after 6 mo)					
Normal	0	0	0	0	±†
High-risk‖	+	0	0	0	±
Children					
Normal	0	0	0	0	0
High-risk	+	0	0	0	0
Pregnant teenager					
Normal	±	0	0	±	+
High-risk¶	+	0	0	+	+

*Symbols indicate: +, that a supplement is usually indicated; ±, that it is possibly or sometimes indicated; 0, that it is not usually indicated. Vitamin K for newborn infants and fluoride in areas where there is insufficient fluoride in the water supply are not shown.
†Iron-fortified formula and/or infant cereal is a more convenient and reliable source of iron than a supplement.
‡Multivitamin supplement (plus added folate) is needed primarily when calorie intake is below approximately 300 kcal/day or when the infant weighs 2.5 kg; vitamin D should be supplied at least until 6 months of age in breast-fed infants. Iron should be started by 2 months of age (see text).
§Vitamin E should be in a form that is well absorbed by small, premature infants. If this form of vitamin E is approved for use in formulas, it need not be given separately to formula-fed infants. Infants fed breast milk are less susceptible to vitamin E deficiency.
‖Multivitamin-multimineral preparation (including iron) is preferred to use of iron alone.
¶Multivitamin-multimineral preparation (including iron and folate) is preferred to use of iron alone or iron and folate alone.

Rickets is uncommon in the breast-fed term infant, despite the fact that human breast milk appears to contain small amounts of vitamin D (ie, about 22 IU/liter). One possible explanation is that the vitamin D in breast milk is in the form of an easily absorbed sulfate analogue, but this needs to be confirmed. The antirachitic properties of breast milk seem to be adequate for the normal term infant of a well nourished mother. However, if the mother's vitamin D nutrition has been inadequate and if the infant does not benefit from adequate ultraviolet light (due to dark skin color and/or little exposure to light) supplements of 400 IU of vitamin D daily may be indicated.

Vitamin A deficiency rarely occurs in breast-fed infants. Historically, vitamin A supplementation was coupled with vitamin D supplementation because both were provided by cod liver oil. Currently there is little reason to provide vitamin A supplements; thus, there would be no harm in omitting vitamin A from supplements designed to provide vitamin D for infants who are breast-fed. Similarly there is not evidence that supplementation with vitamin E is needed for the normal, breast-fed term infant.

Vitamin B_{12} deficiency has been reported in breast-fed infants of strict vegetarian mothers, but this is relatively rare in North America. The recent report of a 6-month-old infant of a vegan mother with severe megaloblastic anemia and coma is a reminder that the maternal diet strongly influences the concentration of certain water-soluble vitamins in breast milk. Thiamin deficiency can also occur in breast-fed infants of thiamin-deficient mothers, but this situation is virtually restricted to infants in developing countries. In the United States, the rare breast-fed infants of mothers who are themselves malnourished should receive multivitamin supplements.

Iron deficiency rarely develops before 4 to 6 months of age in breast-fed infants because neonatal iron stores can supply the major portion of iron needs during this period. Although breast milk may contain little more than 0.3 mg iron per liter, about half of this iron is absorbed in contrast to the much smaller proportion that is assimilated from other foods. This iron helps to delay the depletion of neonatal iron stores, but other sources of iron are required in midinfancy. In normal, breast-fed term infants, the addition to the diet of iron-fortified cereal after 6 months of age probably is desirable to supply adequate amounts of iron.

The benefit of fluoride supplementation in the breast-fed infant is controversial. This is understandable because of the dearth of evidence that fluoride supplementation in the first six months of life alters the prevalence of dental caries in the secondary dentition. In addition, the low level of fluoride in breast milk, even in areas where water is fluoridated, may provide a teleologic argument for not supplying extra fluoride in early infancy. However, the view that fluoride supplementation is unnecessary during the first six months of life is tempered by the knowledge that unerupted teeth are being mineralized in early infancy; consequently, supplemental fluoride would be expected to have a beneficial effect during this period. In weighing these opposing views, the Committee recently favored initiating fluoride supplements shortly after birth in breast-fed infants, but also recognized that fluoride supplementation could be initiated at 6 months of age.

Fluoride supplements are available alone and in combination with vitamins, with or without iron. Thus, if iron or vitamin D supplements are indicated, it is acceptable to include 0.25 mg fluoride if the water supply contains less than 0.3 ppm of fluoride.

Formula-fed term infants

Infants consuming adequate amounts of commercial cow's milk formulas which are in keeping with the recommendations of the Committee do not need vitamin and mineral supplementation in the first six months of life. They do not require supplements during the latter part of the first year if formula continues to be used in appropriate combination with solid foods. After 4 months of age, iron-fortified formula and/or iron-fortified cereal are convenient sources of iron and are preferable to the use of iron supplements. If powdered or concentrated formula is used, fluoride supplements should be administered only if the community water contains less than 0.3 ppm of fluoride. Ready-to-use formulas are now manufactured with water low in fluoride, and recommendations for fluoride supplementation should be similar to those for breast-fed infants.

Vitamin K deficiency is seen occasionally in infants. It is usually associated with diarrhea and especially with the administration of antibiotics, through a decrease in the synthesis of vitamin K by the intestinal microflora. In the past, the feeding of soy or other non-milk based formulas was associated with vitamin K deficiency, which was related in part to the type of oil used in the formula. In 1976, the Committee recommended that all infant formulas, particularly non-milk-based formulas, be required to contain an appropriate level of vitamin K.

Preterm infants

The needs of preterm infants for certain nutrients are proportionately greater than those of term infants because of the increased demands of a more rapid rate of growth and less complete intestinal absorption.

During the first weeks of life (prior to consumption of about 300 kcal per day or reaching a body weight of 2.5 kg), a multivitamin supplement that provides the equivalent of the RDAs for term infants should be supplied. The components of this supplement should ideally include vitamin E in a form well absorbed by preterm infants, such as d-α-tocopheryl polyethylene glycol 1000 succinate. Folic acid deficiency has been reported in preterm infants, and folic acid should be included in the regimen. Folic acid is not in liquid multivitamin-multimineral mixes because of its lack of stability. However, because the period of administration will generally be in a hospital, folate can be added to a multivitamin preparation in the hospital pharmacy in a concentration to provide 0.1 mg (the US RDA) per daily dose. The shelf life should be limited to one month, and the label should read "shake well" because folate will gradually precipitate. Iron supplementation is best delayed until after the first few weeks of life because extra iron may predispose to anemia when there is insufficient absorption of vitamin E. Neonatal iron stores are still abundant, and iron needs for erythropoiesis are relatively small during the physiologic postnatal decline in hemoglobin concentration.

After several weeks of age, when the infant is consuming more than 300 kcal/day or when the body weight exceeds 2.5 kg, a multivitamin supplement is no longer needed, but it is a convenient method for providing the few specific nutrients that still may be required. These include vitamin D, iron, and possibly folic acid.

There have been sporadic reports of rickets, particularly in breast-fed premature infants. This probably results from the low phosphorus content of breast milk, which has only 150 mg/liter in contrast to about 450 mg/liter in formulas. The condition is also correctable with phosphate supplementation. However, there is also evidence that vitamin D supplementation is helpful. Iron is required at a level of 2 mg/kg/day starting by 2 months of age because neonatal iron stores may become depleted earlier than in term infants—before it is appropriate to supply iron in the form of fortified solid foods. Iron-fortified formula also supplies sufficient iron for the prevention of iron deficiency in preterm infants.

Appendix M
Prenatal dietary prophylaxis of atopic disease

In addition to heredity, the prophylaxis of allergic disease in the potentially allergic child involves four major considerations:

1. The possibility of intrauterine sensitization
2. The nutrition of the newborn infant with particular respect to the fact that human breast milk is the best and only natural food
3. The role of secretory immunoglobulin A (SIgA)
4. The fact that food ingested by the nursing mother may pass through with the breast milk and be immunologically capable of sensitizing a potentially allergic infant or of causing a reaction in a previously sensitized infant

Because specific food allergies occasionally appear to be inherited, the pregnant mother of a potentially allergic child should exclude from her diet not only those foods to which she is allergic but also those foods to which other members of the immediate family are sensitive. Overindulgence in any particular food (pica) is to be avoided, particularly the peanut, which is a rather common offender.

An absolute indication for a strict dietary regimen is the presence in the immediate family of significant asthma or atopic dermatitis. If the prospective mother is sensitive to milk, she should be on a milk-free diet. All of the protein required by the mother may be obtained from beef and other meats and soybean. Adequate vitamins should be supplied, bearing in mind that some of the synthetic coloring, of which tartrazine (FD&C yellow no. 5) is the most common offender, as well as some artificial flavoring materials may cause problems. It is hoped that vitamin products completely free of these materials will eventually be available. Adequate calcium should be supplied and is least expensive when obtained as calcium carbonate powder, reagent quality, one-half tea-

□ From Glaser, J., Dreyfuss, E.M., and Logan, J.: Prenatal dietary prophylaxis of atopic disease. In Kelley, V.C., editor: Practice of pediatrics, vol. 2, Hagerstown, Md., 1976, Harper & Row, Publishers, Inc.

spoon (0.4 g calcium) per day during pregnancy and two-thirds teaspoon (0.5 g calcium) per day during lactation.

If there is no milk allergy in the immediate family a pint of milk (500 ml) daily, boiled 10 minutes, or the same amount of half evaporated milk and half water may be given. In these preparations, bovine γ-globulin, the most heat labile of the milk allergens, followed closely by bovine serum albumin, is rendered immunologically inactive. As a result, milk-allergic individuals sensitive only to these proteins are the only milk-allergic individuals who can tolerate boiled or evaporated milk.

One of the least allergenic substitutes for cow's milk is soybean milk. The preparations designed primarily for infants are rather tasty to adults and may be used as desired. Detailed instructions for their use may be obtained from the manufacturers.

The superheated proprietary milks have been shown to be only somewhat more allergenic than soybean milk. If soybean milk is objectionable, it is reasonable to substitute these milks, not to exceed 1½ pints a day. Bremil, Enfamil, Similac, and SMA are some of the preparations readily obtained at drug stores and supermarkets.

Appendix N

acinus The tube leading to the smallest lobule of a compound gland; it is characterized by a narrow lumen.

adipose tissue *See* panniculus adiposus.

afferent Conducting inward to, or toward, the center of an organ, gland, or other structure or area. Applies to sensory nerves, arteries, and lymph vessels.

alveolus A glandular acinus or terminal portion of the alveolar gland where milk is secreted and stored, 0.12 mm in diameter. From 10 to 100 alveoli, or tubulosaccular secretory units, make up a lobulus.

apocrine A term descriptive of a gland cell that loses part of its protoplasmic substance.

Apt test A test, named after its developer, performed on fresh blood to distinguish between adult and fetal hemoglobin. The blood is suspended in saline, an equal amount of 10% NaOH is added and mixed; adult hemoglobin turns brown, while fetal hemoglobin remains red. A control of known adult blood should also be done.

arborization Development of a branched appearance.

areola mammae Areola. The pigmented area surrounding the papilla mammae, or nipple.

autophagic vacuole Autophagosome. A membrane-bound body within a cell containing degenerating cell organelles.

BALT Bronchus-associated immunocompetent lymphoid tissue, to which the mammary gland may act as an extension. *See* GALT and MALT.

basal lamina The layer of material, 50 to 80 nm thick, that lies adjacent to the plasma membrane of the basal surfaces of epithelial cells. It contains collagen and certain carbohydrates. It is often called the basement membrane.

casein A derivative of caseinogen. The fraction of milk protein that forms the tough curd.

colostrum The first milk. It is a yellow sticky fluid secreted during the first few days postpartum, which provides nutrition and protection against infectious disease. It contains more protein, less sugar, and much less fat than mature breast milk.

columnar secretory cell A type of secretory cell in the shape of a hexagonal prism, which appears rectangular when sectioned across the long axis, the length being considerably greater than the width.

Coopers' ligaments Triangularly shaped ligaments stretching between the mammary gland, the skin, the retinacula cutis, the pectineal ligament, and the chorda obliqua. These underlie the breasts.

corpus mammae The mammary gland; breast mass after freeing breast from deep attachments and removal of skin, subcutaneous connective tissue, and fat.

creamatocrit Measurement for estimating the fat content and, therefore, the caloric content of a milk sample. A microhematocrit tube is filled with milk (usually a mix of foremilk and hind milk) and spun in a microcentrifuge for 15 minutes. The layer of fat is measured as one measures a blood hematocrit.

cross-nursing The breastfeeding by a lactating woman of a baby who is not her own, usually temporarily, in the role of a child-care arrangement.

cuboidal secretory cell A secretory cell whose height and breadth are of similar size.

cytosol Cell fluid.

doula An individual who surrounds, interacts with, and aids the mother at any time within the period that includes pregnancy, birth, and lactation. She may be a relative, friend, or neighbor and is usually but not necessarily female. One who gives psychologic encouragement and physical assistance to a new mother.

efferent Carrying impulses away from a nerve center.

ejection reflex A reflex initiated by the suckling of the infant at the breast, which triggers the pituitary gland to release oxytocin into the bloodstream. The oxytocin causes the myoepithelial cells to contract and eject the milk from the collecting ductules. (Also called let-down reflex or draught.)

engorgement The swelling and distention of the breasts, usually in the early days of initiation of lactation, due to vascular dilation as well as the arrival of the early milk.

eosinophil A granular leukocyte possessing large conspicuous granules in the cytoplasm and containing a bilobed nucleus.

foremilk The first milk obtained at the onset of suckling or expression. Contains less fat than later milk of that feeding (i.e., the hind milk).

galactocele A cystic tumor in the ducts of the breast, which contains a milky fluid.

galactagogue A material or action that stimulates the production of milk.

galactopoiesis The development of milk in the mammary gland. The maintenance of established lactation.

galactorrhea Abnormal or inappropriate lactation.

galactose ($C_6H_{12}O_6$) A simple sugar that is a component of the disaccharide lactose, or milk sugar.

galactosemia A congenital metabolic disorder in which there is an inability to metabolize galactose because of a deficiency of the enzyme galactose-1-phosphate uridyltransferase. It causes failure to thrive, hepatomegaly, and splenomegaly.

GALT Gut-associated lymphoid tissue to which the mammary gland may act as an extension. *See* BALT and MALT.

Golgi apparatus A specialized region of the cytoplasm, often close to the nucleus, that is composed of flattened cisternae, numerous vesicles, and some larger vacuoles. In secretory cells it is concerned with packaging the secretory product. It is also probably concerned with the secretion of polysaccharides in some cells, but its full range of functions has not yet been elucidated.

heterophagic vacuole Heterophagosome. A membrane-bound body within a cell, containing ingested material.

hind milk Milk obtained later during nursing period, that is, the end of the feeding. This milk is usually high in fat and probably controls appetite.

homocystinuria A rare inborn error of amino acid metabolism characterized by mental deficiency, epilepsy, dislocation of the lens, growth disturbance, thromboses, and defective hair growth.

hyperadenia The existence of mammary tissue without nipples.

hypermastia The existence of accessory mammary glands.

hyperthelia The existence of abundant, more or less developed, nipples without accompanying mammary tissue.

immunoglobulin Protein fraction of globulin, which has been demonstrated to have immunologic properties. Immunoglobulins include IgA, IgG, and IgM—factors in breast milk that protect against infection.

induced lactation Process by which a nonpuerperal female (or male) is stimulated to lactate.

lactiferous ducts The main ducts of the mammary gland, which number from 15 to 30 and open onto the nipple. They carry milk to the nipple.

lactiferous sinuses Dilations on the lactiferous ducts at the base of the nipple.

Lactobacillus bifidus Organism of the intestinal tract of breastfed infants.

lactocele Cystic tumor of the breast due to the dilation and obstruction of a milk duct usually filled with milk.

lactoferrin An iron-binding protein of external secretions, including human milk. It inhibits the growth of iron-dependent microorganisms in the gut.

lactogenesis Initiation of milk secretion.

let-down reflex *See* ejection reflex.

lobulus A subunit of the parenchymal structure of the breast made up of 10 to 100 alveoli, or tubulosaccular secretory units. From 20 to 40 lobuli make up a lobus.

lobus A subunit of the parenchymal structure of the breast made up of 20 to 40 lobuli. From 15 to 25 lobi are arranged like the spokes of a wheel with the nipple as the central point.

lymphocyte A mature leukocyte derived through the intermediate stage of lymphoblast from the reticuloendothelium found in lymphatic tissue.

MALT Mucosal-associated lymphoid tissue, which includes gut, lung, mammary gland, salivary and lacrimal glands, and genital tract. There is traffic of cells between secretory sites. Immunization at one site may be an effective means of producing immunity at distant sites. *See* GALT and BALT.

mamilla The nipple; any teatlike structure.

mammogenesis Growth of the mammary gland.

mastitis Inflammation of the breast, including cellulitis, and occasionally abscess formation.

matrescence The state of becoming a mother or motherhood as a new event in an individual's life.

megaloblastic anemia Defective red blood cell formation due to megaloblastic hyperplasia of the marrow; there are often megaloblasts, or primitive nucleated red cells in the peripheral blood.

merocrine Pertaining to the type of secretion in which the active cell remains intact while forming and discharging the secretory product.

mesencephalon The midbrain.

methylmalonic aciduria The condition of the urine being acidic from an accumulation of methylmalonic acid due to an inborn error of metabolism.

milk fever A syndrome of fever and general malaise associated with early engorgement of the breasts or with sudden weaning from the breast.

mitogen A substance capable of stimulating cells to enter mitosis.

Montgomery glands Small prominences, sebaceous glands in the areola of the breast, which become more marked in pregnancy. They number 20 to 24 and secrete a fluid that lubricates the nipple area.

Morgagni's tubercle Small sinuses into which the miniature ducts of the Montgomery glands open in the epidermis of the areola.

myoepithelial cell An epithelial cell, usually lying around a glandular acinus, in which part of the cytoplasm has contractile properties, serving to empty the sinus of its secretion.

nonnutritive sucking The act of suckling the breast with little or no secretion of milk. Infant may suckle when distressed or to be calmed or quieted.

nonpuerperal lactation The production of milk in a woman who has not given birth.

nucleotides Compounds derived from nucleic acid by hydrolysis and consisting of phosphoric acid combined with a sugar and a purine or pyrimidine derivative. The milk nucleotides are secreted from glandular epithelial cells.

opsonic Belonging to or characterized by opsonin, a substance in mammalian blood having the power to render microorganisms and blood cells more easily absorbed by phagocytes.

oxytocin An octapeptide synthesized in the cell bodies of neurons located mainly in the paraventricular nucleus and in smaller amounts in the supraoptic nucleus of the hypothalamus. Oxytocin stmulates the ejection reflex by stimulation of the myoepithelial cells in the mammary gland.

panniculus adiposus Adipose tissue. The superficial fascia, which contains fatty pellicles.

papilla mammae Mamilla. The nipple of the breast.

perinatal Around birth. The time from conception through birth, delivery, lactation, and at least 28 days postpartum.

plasma cell Cell derived from the B cell series, which manufactures and secretes antibodies.

prolactin A hormone present in both male and female and at all ages. During pregnancy it stimulates and prepares the mammary alveolar epithelium for secretory activity. During lactation it stimulates synthesis and secretion of milk. At other ages and in the male it interacts with other steroids.

rachitic Relating to, characterized by, or affected with rickets.

relactation Process by which a woman who has given birth but did not initially breastfeed is stimulated to lactate (also applies to reinstituting lactation after it has been discontinued).

squamous epithelium A sheet of flattened, scalelike epithelium adhering edge to edge.

stroma The connective tissue basis or framework of an organ.

subependymal matrix The layer beneath the ependyma, the layer of ciliated epithelium that lines the central canal of the spinal cord and the ventricles of the brain.

switch nursing Putting the infant to one breast for a short time, usually 5 minutes, moving the infant to the other breast for 5 minutes, and then moving the infant back to the first side in an effort to improve milk production.

tail of Spence The axillary tail of the breast.

transitional milk The milk produced early in the postpartum period as the colostrum diminishes and the mature milk develops.

tubuloalveolar Having both tubular and alveolar qualities.

tubulosaccular Having both tubular and saccular character.

turgescence The swelling up of a part. The unusual turgid feeling resulting from swelling with fluid.

whey protein Protein remaining when the curds of casein have been removed. The mixture of proteins present is complex and includes β-lactoglobulin and α-lactalbumin and enzymes.

witch's milk Product of neonatal galactorrhea due to absorption of placental prolactin.

Index